# Effective Management in Therapeutic Recreation Service

# Effective Management in Therapeutic Recreation Service

Gerald S. O'Morrow

Marcia Jean Carter

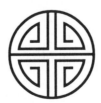

Venture Publishing, Inc.

State College, Pennsylvania

Copyright © 1997

 Venture Publishing, Inc.
1999 Cato Avenue
State College, PA 16801
(814) 234-4561; FAX (814) 234-1651

Production Manager:  Richard Yocum
Design, Layout, and Graphics:  Diane K. Bierly
Manuscript Editing:  Diane K. Bierly, Katherine Young
Additional Editing:  Richard Yocum
Cover Design:  Sikorski Design
Cover Photography:  © Gary Buss 1994/FPG International
Printing and Binding:  Thomson-Shore, Inc.

Library of Congress Catalogue Card Number 96-61938
ISBN 0-910251-87-8

Dedicated to:


Mary, Dianne, Sharon, Patrick, and Stephen O'Morrow who have supported me throughout my professional career in therapeutic recreation.


The memory and love of my family: John and Peg Carter and John, Nancy, Cory, Zachary, and Nathan Carter.

# Contents

## Chapter 3: Functions of Management

# Part 2: Administrative Management

## Chapter 4: Leadership

## Chapter 5: Vision, Mission, Philosophy, and Objectives

## Chapter 6: Organizational Behavior

## Chapter 7: Ethical Perspectives

## Chapter 8: Working with Higher Management

# Part 3: Operational Management

## Chapter 9:  Financial Management and Budgets

## Chapter 10:  Computer and Information Systems

## Chapter 11:  Decision Making, Problem Solving and Conflict Management

## Chapter 12: Marketing

## Chapter 13: Staffing

# Part 4: Human Service Management

## Chapter 14: Effective Communication

## Chapter 15: Motivation

## Chapter 16: Performance Appraisal

# Part 5:  Consumer Management

## Chapter 20:  Service Delivery Management

## Chapter 21:  Risk Management

## Chapter 22:  Quality Service Management

# Appendix A

# Appendix B

# Appendix C

# Appendix D

# Appendix E

# Index

# Preface

No comprehensive therapeutic recreation publications today focus specifically on the therapeutic recreation manager. *Effective Management in Therapeutic Recreation Service* provides theoretical and practical knowledge about the management of therapeutic recreation service in health and human service organizations. The text was written for therapeutic recreation personnel who will eventually be seeking either a management role or are new to a management position. This book also speaks to therapeutic recreation managers who have been in a management position for a period of time and are looking for a practical desk reference and major resource to help improve their performance.

We, the authors, recognize that while therapeutic recreation managers work in a variety of health and human service organizations, this book specifically focuses on the core competencies essential for the therapeutic recreation manager at the first level of managerial responsibility in the organizational chain of command. In other words, we are writing for a therapeutic recreation specialist who has responsibility for managing direct therapeutic recreation service and the assignment and direction of therapeutic recreation staff who deliver the service.

The challenge and excitement of management stems from the opportunity to see what needs to be done in the interest of the consumer. Therapeutic recreation specialists need to be introduced to the concept of management in these terms; it is a challenge. The manager should know how to spark a group of practitioners into getting the job done while understanding the theory underlying the action taken. Effective managers need to have the skills necessary to function in a health and human service delivery system with assurance, knowing they are well-equipped for their role. In addition, they need to be able to speak the language used by other health and human service managers as well as to articulate therapeutic recreation needs to other managers and administrators who have no specific knowledge of therapeutic recreation.

While we admit that all the knowledge that might be useful to a potential manager or practicing manager is not in this one volume, we hope to present the most important portions of management knowledge relevant to therapeutic recreation service in an organized and useful way. In doing so, we emphasize the essentials of management that are pertinent to being an *effective practicing therapeutic recreation manager* in either a clinical setting or a community-based leisure service setting. This means that to achieve the best kind of practice managers must apply and implement management concepts, functions, techniques, and skills to the realities of any situation. As every practicing manager knows, there is no universal "one best way" of doing things in all instances, and the practical application of management theory and science has always recognized the importance of the realities or contingencies in a given situation.

While this text is designed for both upper level undergraduate and graduate students as well as practitioners, it is well to note that some chapters are a brief overview and enhancement of what students undoubtedly considered in their introductory park and recreation administration course.

Where this does occur, the content is associated with the implementation of therapeutic recreation service. Further, the sequence of chapters reflects a management perspective as opposed to a program perspective. Likewise, the chapters are arranged from a practical perspective or functional-process organization. As a result, service matters associated specifically with the consumer are considered in later chapters since consumer service is dependent upon effective accomplishment of earlier managerial functions. Last, because the largest number of therapeutic recreation managers appear to work within some type of a healthcare facility, many of the examples and figures used are from healthcare facilities. At the same time, however, all of the material herein has direct application in other types of settings such as community-based leisure service agencies.

One final note. We recognize that changes are taking place on a daily basis in health and human service organizations which in turn affect therapeutic recreation service and its management. Therapeutic recreation service is expanding rapidly even though reengineering and downsizing is occurring in many health and human service organizations. Tomorrow's health and human service delivery, and quite possibly the delivery of therapeutic recreation service regardless of setting, will look totally different from today's. Hence, we foresee that some statements may not be as appropriate as they were at the time the manuscript was prepared especially as related to the concept of quality management in healthcare facilities.

This book is organized into five parts: After introducing the student to the management discipline and the therapeutic recreation manager's job including transition from practitioner to manager, Part 1 considers the characteristics of management. Chapter 2 is devoted to an overview of the theoretical perspectives in management with particular attention to the human factor of management and contingency theory. Therapeutic recreation managers are able to make clearer sense of complex situations and to formulate the best possible strategies for rational action by using theories. The various functions of managers—planning, organizing, directing, and controlling—are treated in Chapter 3. These functions are generally accepted as the most effective way to describe the management process.

Part 2 examines selective administrative functions that support effective and efficient management. In Chapter 4 consideration is given to leadership. Clearly, one of the keys to being an effective manager is to become an effective leader. Leadership theories, styles, and power are considered in addition to leadership relationships with individuals, groups, and situations. Further attention is given to the supervisor as a leader. Chapter 5 focuses on the development of vision, mission, philosophy, goals, and objective statements of therapeutic recreation divisions or departments within health and human service organizations. Examples of such statements from various organizations

are provided. Chapter 6 provides the therapeutic recreation manager with information on behavior that influences individual and group dynamics in an organization. Chapter 7 considers ethics as an integral part of therapeutic recreation management. Particular attention is given to the values and rights of consumers, major ethical theories, and ethical decision making as a process. The last chapter in Part 2, Chapter 8, discusses how to work effectively with supervisors. Managing the boss is a crucial skill for successful therapeutic recreation managers.

Operational management is the focus of attention in Part 3. The nature and process of financial management and budgets is found in Chapter 9. Attention is given to sources of revenue to support therapeutic recreation services as well as the budget process, types of budgets, budget review, and the role of the first-line manager in the fiscal management process. Chapter 10 provides rudimentary information and knowledge on the recent addition of computers and information systems to assist in therapeutic recreation practice and management.

Chapter 11 concentrates on decision making, problem solving, and conflict management. By considering the components of decision-making and problem-solving processes, the manager will become adept at implementing the most appropriate and effective solution to a given problem. Managing conflict is an important skill to develop because using appropriate solutions to resolve conflict will prevent its potential destructiveness. Marketing of therapeutic recreation services is discussed in Chapter 12. The nature of marketing in health and human services, the marketing process, and the development of a strategic marketing plan for therapeutic recreation are considered in the chapter. Chapter 13 focuses on therapeutic recreation staffing to deliver quality service. Consideration is given to legal and professional regulations and standards, human resource planning, recruiting processes, selection, and practices, and issues affecting staffing.

Part 4 considers elements associated with human service management. The hallmark of an effective manager is effective communication. Chapter 14 reviews the strategies and techniques that foster effective interpersonal communication and the nature of supervisory communication to achieve goals. Consideration is also given to organizational and professional communication respectively. Why do people act as they do? Answers to this question are given in Chapter 15 which covers the subject of motivation. This chapter initially considers individual need fulfillment by examining various motivation theories, and the chapter concludes with a discussion of the therapeutic recreation manager's interaction with the work culture and motivation. Guidelines to follow regarding developing a positive motivational atmosphere are also given. The important managerial function and challenge of performance appraisal is explored in Chapter 16. This function contributes to quality outcomes and ongoing service improvements. Chapter 17 develops for the first-line manager the logic for and composition of staff training and development programs including program implementation and evaluations respectively. Chapter 18 and Chapter 19 focus on two significant topics: volunteers and intern management. Knowledge needed for the successful management, development, implementation, and evaluation of volunteer and internship programs is provided.

Last, Part 5 considers those matters associated with the consumer. Chapter 20 concentrates on a number of factors concerned with therapeutic recreation service delivery management—scheduling of services, therapeutic recreation processes, protocols, documentation, and monitoring and consulting practitioner performance. The management of risk is discussed in Chapter 21. The final chapter, Chapter 22, examines the management of quality service which incorporates a historical overview of quality management in health and human service organizations and the implications of total quality management and quality assurance and continuous quality improvement in therapeutic recreation services.

Each chapter ends with a series of thought-provoking discussion questions which require the student to review and apply the material presented in the chapter. In addition, Appendices to the text are provided. The reader will find in the Appendices an assortment of material which has direct application to therapeutic recreation practice in health and human service organizations.

# Acknowledgments

As might be expected with a text of this kind, the authors are indebted to many people who helped create this publication, some of whom provided manuals, job descriptions, budgeting reports, vision and mission statements, and similar documents from their health and human service organization. We would like to acknowledge the following for their contributions:

Patricia Ardovino, CTRS
Indiana University
Bloomington, Indiana

Missy Armstrong, CTRS
Harborview Medical Center
Seattle, Washington

joan burlingame, CTRS
Idyll Arbor, Inc.
Ravensdale, Washington

Sharon K. Entsminger, CTRS
Chesterfield County Parks and Recreation
    Department
Chester, Virginia

Julie Forker, CLP, CTRS
Maryland National Capital Park and Plan-
    ning Commission
Riverdale, Maryland

Karen M. Indelicato, CTRS
Northern Virginia Mental Health Institute
Falls Church, Virginia

Mead B. Jackson, RTR, CTRS
Los Angeles County/University of South-
    ern California Medical Center
Los Angeles, California

M. Jean Keller, CLP, CTRS
University of North Texas
Denton, Texas

Jerri K. Lerch, CTRS
Lindenview Regional Behavioral Center
Fort Wayne, Indiana

Lynn Mabe, CTRS
Southwestern Virginia Mental Health
    Institute
Marion, Virginia

Carolyn M. Nagle, CLP, CTRS
Fox Valley Special Recreation Association
North Aurora, Illinois

Ann B. Prichard, CTRS
Johnston-Willis Hospital
Richmond, Virginia

Paulette Schuster, RTR, CLP, CTRS
Department of Recreation and Parks
Los Angeles, California

Lisa Silverman, CTRS
Department of Recreation, Parks and Cultural Activities
Alexandria, Virginia

Martha Smith
Mount Vernon Hospital
Alexandria, Virginia

Jean Tague, CTRS
Recreation Resources, Inc.
Austin, Texas

Lisa Turpel, CLP, CTRS
Portland Parks and Recreation Department
Portland, Oregon

Jeffrey Witman, CTRS
Philhaven Behavioral Healthcare Services
Mt. Gretna, Pennsylvania

The authors are also grateful to a number of others for their valuable information concerning and personal experiences in the management of therapeutic recreation service and hospital management. Our thanks go to Angie L. Anderson, CTRS, Director, Recreation Therapy, Iowa Methodist Medical Center, Des Moines, Iowa; Steve LeConey, CTRS, Supervisor of Therapeutic Recreation, Cincinnati Recreation Commission, Cincinnati, Ohio; and Dianne O'Morrow-Snyder, RN, Vice President, Patient Care Services, Cabarrus Memorial Hospital, Concord, North Carolina. In addition, Irene Lamb deserves special recognition for her creative suggestions and editorial assistance throughout the preparation of the drafts and Diane Bierly for her editing and preparation of the manuscript at Venture Publishing, Inc. We also acknowledge Carin Dowdy for her assembly of materials. Likewise, Lynda Kersey and Tari Mole for their typing services associated with various chapter drafts. We would like to extend our thanks for the gratuitous assistance received from the respective library staffs at Radford University and Ashland University. We also thank the publishers who granted permission for their work to be reprinted herein. Last, but certainly not least, is Ann Miller, the senior author's secretary who typed and retyped the manuscript. Her tolerance and sense of humor helped through many corrections and adjustments. Needless to say, she has made the task of putting the manuscript together a lot easier. Thanks Ann.

G.S.O'M.
M.J.C.

# Chapter 1
# Overview

## Introduction

Health and human service organizations consist of those organizations that exist to benefit the consumer. Such organizations include both governmental (federal, state, and local) agencies and private profit and nonprofit organizations which originally grew out of an increased sense of social responsibility.

Since the 1950s there has been an unparalleled growth in the size and scope of health and human service organizations. It was during this same period of time that therapeutic recreation began to emerge as a professional field of service. As the years passed, therapeutic recreation practitioners carried out their responsibility of direct service ably and often imaginatively. In addition, as therapeutic recreation programs and services developed in varied health and human service organizations, therapeutic recreation practitioners moved into positions of management without any formal organized body of practice knowledge and techniques directly applicable to therapeutic recreation management. As noted by Carter, Van Andel, and Robb (1995, p. 157):

> Many fine programs fail, not because they are inadequately planned, implemented, and evaluated, but because the underlying foundations or support systems are weak or inadequately managed.

Given the important role that therapeutic recreation practitioners are likely to play as they assume management positions, it is vital that potential managers have an understanding of the definition of management and management skills and the dimensions of management. This chapter not only addresses these three points, but also explores the role of the therapeutic recreation manager, the dimensions of the therapeutic recreation division or department, and the factors associated with making the transition from practitioner to manager. Initially, however, societal changes that have taken place since the 1950s, the emergence of therapeutic recreation as a profession, the implications of that history for therapeutic recreation service management, and the challenges to therapeutic recreation management today will be examined briefly.

## Decades of Change

Few things in life remain unchanged over time. Individuals, families, communities, and organizations grow and adapt according to events and conditions within their environment. During the past several decades societal, political, economic, technological, and legal forces have influenced the content and context of health and human services and the delivery of these services. In addition, these services and their delivery have been under siege from many individuals and organizations.

In the 1950s legislation was passed for the planning and financing of healthcare. Debate flourished about the notion of healthcare as a basic right, as something more than a privilege for people with economic means. The debate continues today, with the consumer believing strongly that adequate healthcare is a right and at the same time a prerequisite for the good life. In the more generic human services arena, those who worked in and received services from human service agencies began to have a voice in determining the destiny of the agencies and the services being provided. Also during this decade third-party health insurance companies such as Blue Cross and Blue Shield offered an insurance premium plan to pay for healthcare. In addition, systems theory as a management concept emerged at the same time that social scientists recognized that interdependence of individuals, governments, and societies was a basic fact.

The 1960s witnessed federal policy and legislation (e.g., Civil Rights Act of 1964) that increased citizen access to health and human services. Healthcare expenditures in 1960 were 5.3 percent of the gross national product (GNP) (Bush, 1994). Lyndon Johnson's call for a war on poverty led to the passage of a vast array of social welfare programs. While some social agencies expanded to address unmet social needs, others were widely criticized for being unresponsive to changing needs and conditions. Government programs such as Medicare and Medicaid were started. At the same time, a technological explosion occurred based on heavy public investment in medical research. Elaborate technology became available for diagnosis and treatment, and for life support and life extension. During this decade social roles were also changing, and there was much experimentation with new lifestyles.

The 1970s ushered in increased government regulation and mandated community-based planning to limit hospital expansion. The goal was to contain rapidly increasing healthcare costs. Wellness programs designed to promote health and prevent disease gained momentum partly in response to the business community's recognition of rising healthcare costs and insurance premiums. Also, during this period there was a marked increase in legislation that expanded recreation and leisure service opportunities for individuals with disabilities and provided funds for research and demonstration projects.

The 1980s marked the birth of large for-profit hospital chains, the introduction of legislation associated with deregulation and competition, and the inception of marketing to consumers. Also, patients in hospitals came to be redefined as customers. Alternative delivery systems (e.g., substance abuse centers, home health service, outpatient service) proliferated during this period as did new reimbursement arrangements such as prospective payment systems through diagnostic-related groups (DRGs). Preferred provider organizations (PPOs) in their various guises also became common. This movement led to "managed care" as a major feature of the system although the forerunner of managed care began with Kaiser Permanente (Kaiser Foundation Health Plan) in the 1930s (Northern, 1995).[1] At the same time consumers demanded a healthy environment in which to live and work. In fact, the direction of the healthcare industry shifted away from "medical care" and towards "healthcare." This shift incorporated an emphasis on acute illness rather than chronic illness and the importance played by the environment, lifestyle, and social stress in the onset and progression of disease.

Legislation during this time period focused on many aspects of consumer care. Providing access for persons with disabilities so they could participate more fully in society was a major milestone. Congress enacted a hospice option within Medicare benefits in the early 1980s to foster community-based care for the terminally ill. Later in the decade the Omnibus Budget Reconciliation Act (PL 100–203) was passed with reference to Medicaid and Medicare standards and emphasis on the inclusion of therapeutic recreation as part of the rehabilitation process. Last, the U.S. Department of Health, Education, and Welfare was restructured to become the Department of Health and Human Services, while Education became a separate department. Such development during the 1980s permanently changed the nature of health and human services and set the stage for the trends of the 1990s.

The dramatic changes in health and human services in the 1980s did not magically end in 1990. Healthcare expenditures by 1990 had risen to 12.2 percent of the GNP to 14 percent by 1992, and it was estimated that by 1994 it would represent 16 percent of the economy (Bush, 1994). In the early 1990s many health and human service organizations adopted the principles of total quality management (TQM) to improve the quality of their services to consumers. At the same time, the goals and values of health and human services were being rethought.

In the healthcare arena it became apparent that society was no longer willing to pay for escalating healthcare costs but wanted changes in all components of the healthcare delivery system to deal with the emerging healthcare crises. Further, healthcare planners agreed that they needed to know more about the cost-effectiveness, quality, and safety of the methods health practitioners used

---

[1]Managed care is the generic term for a system that attempts to control and influence the way in which healthcare is provided and paid for. The most common form of managed healthcare is that of the health maintenance organization (HMO). An HMO provides basic and supplemental health maintenance and treatment within a defined geographic area to an enrolled group of people for a prepaid capitated amount. The most common of these are independent or individual practice association (IPA), preferred provider organization (PPO), independent practitioner organization (IPO), and exclusive provider organization (EPO). Another system is managed care organizations (MCO). An MCO is an organization that simply manages, administers, or coordinates health services to an enrolled group of people. For more information on HMOs see Boland's *Managed Care Work* (1993).

for the prevention, diagnosis, and treatment of disease. This was the result, in part, of the continued decline in community hospitals since 1977 which provided inpatient acute care services (Hull, 1994). By the mid-1990s many hospitals were being referred to as "health centers" to distinguish them from the older generation of hospitals which focused on inpatient care. New hospitals or health centers were putting greater emphasis on outpatient care and prevention. In addition, the U.S. Department of Labor reported that the healthcare industry was the largest single employer of all the industries monitored by the department, outpacing overall employment in the economy and total population growth (Kronenfeld, 1993). Not only had the numbers of people employed in healthcare increased, but also the types of people had changed and the number of different categories of healthcare workers had increased (i.e., allied health and assistant personnel). Kronenfeld (1993) reported more than 700 different job categories in the health industries.

As one moves into the late 1990s, one can assume that technology will continue to influence health and human services. While health reform is unknown at present, it appears there will be continued attempts to reduce expenditures, and patients will be restricted in their ability to receive some services. By the year 2000, it is anticipated that there will be more demand for pediatric services, older-adult services, geriatric services, preventive care, fitness and wellness programs, rehabilitation services, and outpatient services (Thomas, 1993). In addition, organizations will control healthcare services as opposed to the consumer (Thomas, 1993). According to Petryshen and Petryshen (1993/1994, p. 108), "there is a growing consensus that managed care will shape the future of healthcare delivery, creating new working environments and new ways of providing cost-effective, quality patient care." It would appear that a new healthcare delivery system will emerge through reengineering.

Another perspective of the 1990s reveals that the number of people with disabilities was rising to a higher level of social visibility and responsiveness than in the past. Acknowledgment of their right to equal opportunity and quality of life was noted with the enactment of the Individuals with Disabilities Education Act (PL 101–476, 1990) and the Americans with Disabilities Act (PL 101–336, 1990). The latter was considered to be the most significant piece of legislation of the past decade for disabled persons. This legislation was designed to provide a clear and comprehensive mandate that would end discrimination against individuals with disabilities relative to housing, employment, public transportation, and communication services. Definitions of places of public accommodation include several categories with direct references to recreation facilities and their programs (Stein, 1993). A year later, in 1991, the U.S. Department of Labor (U.S. Department of Labor,

Bureau of Labor Statistics, 1991) reported that recreation therapy was the twelfth fastest growing profession requiring a baccalaureate degree in the United States. In the same year, the importance of active recreation and accessible programs and facilities was documented by the U.S. Department of Health and Human Services in its national health strategy report, *Healthy People 2000: National Health Promotion and Disease Prevention Objectives* and were restated in the 1995 revision (U.S. Department of Health and Human Services, Public Health Service, 1991, 1995).

Concurrent with those factors that influenced health and human services and recreation and leisure services for individuals with disabilities during the last half of this century, therapeutic recreation began to emerge as a specific field of service with a distinctive theory and method of practice between 1950 and 1960. Therapeutic recreation shifted its philosophical basis to include treatment service in addition to participative leisure experiences in both healthcare facilities and community-based leisure service organizations. This practice theory remains a major influence on much of the practice to this day. The emergence of therapeutic recreation was the result of an expansion of healthcare services wherein recreation services became common in settings such as psychiatric institutions and hospitals; residential facilities for the mentally retarded and other specific disabilities; local mental health, mental retardation, and developmental disability centers; skilled and long-term care facilities; rehabilitation units in general medical hospitals, comprehensive freestanding rehabilitation centers, and substance abuse rehabilitation facilities; and other healthcare facilities. At the same time, recreation services for persons with disabilities of all ages were offered more and more through community-based leisure service agencies, primarily parks and recreation departments. Unfortunately, the expansion of therapeutic recreation service with its theory of practice was not accompanied by the development of therapeutic recreation management skills. Managers of therapeutic recreation departments developed their skills on-the-job.

In the three decades since, therapeutic recreation's emergence as a profession gave attention to issues critical to its professionalization including credentialing, accreditation, practice standards, models of service, ethics, advocacy, legislation, definitions, and philosophy of therapeutic recreation. Further, in the healthcare arena therapeutic recreation was included in the standards associated with inpatient and outpatient physical rehabilitation issued by the Joint Commission on Accreditation of Healthcare Organizations (JCAHO). Likewise, therapeutic recreation was included within the medical rehabilitation and behavioral health standards (e.g., alcohol and other drug programs, mental health programs) of the Commission on Accreditation of Rehabilitation Facilities (CARF). The Health Care Financing Administration (HCFA) also included therapeutic recreation services within federal government standards in skilled nursing and long-term care facilities. Last, during the healthcare reform debate in 1994, the American Therapeutic Recreation Society (ATRA) and the National Therapeutic Recreation Society (NTRS) issued a joint statement supporting the commitment of President Bill Clinton and the United States Congress to making healthcare a right of all Americans (ATRA and NTRS, 1994).

Today the scope of therapeutic recreation reveals a wide range of services to individuals with an equally diverse set of problems, disorders, and limitations. Services are provided to individuals in institutional and residential facilities, in community-based health and human service agencies as noted above plus outpatient services, home health agencies, hospices, and various other day treatment and social programs (summer day camp, adult social clubs, inclusion buddy aquatic programs, etc.). According to Connolly and Garbarini (1996), there are 30,000 recreation therapists employed in various settings in the United States as of 1996. Of these, 14,000 are certified by the National Council for Therapeutic Recreation Certification (NCTRC).

A changing, somewhat challenging, environment will probably continue to confront health and human service managers and providers during the remaining years of this decade and into the next century. At no time in the history of the United States have so many powerful forces been exerting their influence. Forces, trends and changes in organizational structures, delivery systems, cost containment, quality management and accountability, consumerism, health problems, and healthcare policy will continue to affect the health and human service professions and the roles, functions, and skill requirements of these professionals. Therapeutic recreation managers and practitioners at all levels of responsibility and in all types of settings will have to respond to ever-changing demands in society and in the field. According to Calloway (1992, p. 11):

> The future success of therapeutic recreation managers will be largely determined by the profession's ability to assess and respond to a changing society that will introduce new challenges and technologies. Therapeutic recreation managers must develop their visionary skills and adopt strategies and new techniques as demanded.

Perhaps the most significant issue that will challenge the therapeutic recreation profession as a result of economic, social, and political changes will be the implementation, delivery, and monitoring of quality therapeutic recreation services regardless of setting. If therapeutic recreation service quality is to improve and meet the demands of the public, the federal government (i.e., HCFA), and of regulatory agencies (i.e., JCAHO and CARF), it must come

through the development of effective procedures that are directed by personnel with management knowledge, understanding, and skills.

# Management Defined

Many definitions of management exist. Perhaps the most widely quoted one, attributed to management theorist Mary Parker Follett, is that "management is the act of getting things done through other people" (Wren, 1979, p. 3). Since management is an authorized activity that is inherent in all formal organizations, it will be defined here as a process of working with others to achieve organizational goals in a changing environment (Kreitner, 1992). This is done by efficient use of resources (i.e., human, financial, physical) in an effective manner (Griffin, 1990). The person responsible for getting the work done in an effective manner is the manager. Numerous barriers will be encountered along the way in getting the job done, but the manager is charged with the responsibility of taking actions that will make it possible for individuals to make their best contribution to organizational goals and objectives.

The manager's job in many respects is analogous to that of an orchestra leader. If the individual musicians played without a common score and without a conductor, what would be the result? Just noise. The purpose of the score and the conductor is to weld the individual instruments into pleasing music. And so it is with the manager.

# Management Skills

In the early 1970s Robert L. Katz (1974) noted that all managers required three basic skills: technical skills, interpersonal or human relation skills, and conceptual skills. In entry-level managerial positions, technical skills tend to be important. On the other hand, the need for conceptual or decision-making skills, although generally less important on the lower rungs of the managerial ladder, tend to increase in importance as one moves up the organizational hierarchy. Interpersonal or human relation skills, however, are equally important for managers at all levels of the organizational hierarchy.

Megginson, Mosley, and Pietri (1992) added administrative skills to the three skills identified by Katz. In addition, they noted that administrative skills are used about the same by all managers. In recent field research as reported by Sandwith (Spring, 1993), five managerial competencies were identified. The new skill added to the previous four is leadership:

1. **Conceptual or creative.** The ability to think in the abstract coupled with the development of new ideas or putting existing ideas into new forms.

2. **Leadership.** The ability to influence others; "... a role model of enthusiasm, competence, diligence, and concern for others' involvement in his or her work efforts" (p. 48).
3. **Interpersonal.** Effective interaction with others and the ability to communicate effectively.
4. **Administrative.** Competency in personnel and financial management. These skills include an administrator's ability to follow policies and procedures, process paperwork, and manage expenditure within the limits set by a budget. This skill, in a sense, is an extension of conceptual skills.
5. **Technical.** Knowledge and skills necessary to accomplish one's specialized activities.

Unfortunately, Sandwith does not clarify leadership's importance relative to managerial levels. Regardless, it appears that in this complex period of time more skills are needed.

# Dimensions of Management

Predicted to characterize health and human service organizational systems where therapeutic recreation managers find themselves are potential problems caused by changing organizational complexity and structure; increasing availability of information; increasing technological use, interdisciplinary teamwork, or collaboration; competition for scarce resources; internal conflict and power struggles; and other problems needing creative solutions. Effective management in such a milieu demands competence in any number of situations. Traditional management processes include goal setting combined with planning, organizing, staffing, cost-effective budgeting, motivating, delegating, directing, and evaluating. Some linking processes associated with management functions include problem solving, idea generation, decision making, increasing job satisfaction, team building, conducting groups and meetings, time management, stress management, conflict management, providing advice and technical instruction, staff development, self-development, and matters representing the discipline of therapeutic recreation and its field of study.

It is important to remember that managers *practice* management. Management is a practice and not a science. Managers do not practice economics or behavioral science; however, these are elements used among them for successful management. While the specifics of the therapeutic recreation manager may be modified and tailored for different circumstances, the principles of management are the same regardless of setting.

# Therapeutic Recreation Manager

While there are various levels of management (i.e., top, middle, and first-line), therapeutic recreation managers in health and human service organizations are considered first-line managers because they are responsible for delivery of therapeutic recreation service, assignment and direction of professional practitioners and volunteers, and interaction with other managers in the same organization or with others in the community who deliver therapeutic recreation services. There may be times however, that the manager may be responsible for providing direct service (e.g., vocation, sick leave, special programs). This management responsibility would be true whether one is managing in a healthcare facility or in a community-based leisure service organization. However, there are exceptions. In some large health and human service organizations (i.e., hospitals, institutions, and public or private freestanding community-based leisure service centers for persons with disabilities) and depending on the organizational structure, therapeutic recreation managers may occupy a middle management position wherein they would be responsible for implementing basic policies and plans developed by top management and for supervising and coordinating the activities of lower level managers. The coordinator or director of an activity therapy department in a state institution responsible for varied disciplines like occupational therapy and music therapy would be an example of middle management.

First-line manager is often the first position held by a practitioner who enters management from the worker or subordinate personnel rank; however, there are some settings in which the first-line manager is also the sole practitioner (e.g., nursing homes and small community-based leisure service organizations). It seems reasonable to assume as has been noted earlier, that most first-line managers have had little or no formal academic preparation in therapeutic recreation management. Their advancement is the result of competency in direct service, program knowledge, and job experience. This is not to say that direct practice experience and program knowledge are not important prerequisites for first-line managers. A recent therapeutic recreation practitioner survey noted that of 854 respondents, nearly one-third indicated they occupy an administrative or supervisor position (O'Morrow, 1995).

Even though the first-line manager holds a bottom-rung managerial position in the organization, it is one of the most critical and valuable roles within the administration of the organization. The manager's responsibility is to turn a management plan into operational reality. Within the context of a program, the first-line manager is primarily involved with developing and facilitating technical and professional processes, as well as identifying areas of knowledge and skill deficiencies, providing opportunities for upgrading them, and evaluating practitioner performance. The first-line manager also serves as a linking agent by advocating and representing the interests of subordinates to the next managerial level and communicating, clarifying, and enforcing the directives of his or her supervisor.

Effective managers have a common affinity for understanding the nature of the larger organization within which they work. In other words, a special effort is made to understand the inner workings of the larger organization of which their department is a part. Realizing that the needed information cannot be uncovered simply from printed documents, managers are relentless in their probing. They observe, inquire, and integrate until they are satisfied that they have a valid conceptual model of the organization.

The majority of objectives for any therapeutic recreation service, regardless of setting, relate to the consumer, and the first-line therapeutic recreation manager is the administrative channel through which these objectives ultimately succeed or fail. This professional person must ensure that quality services for consumers are delivered efficiently in an ever-changing environment of standards and regulations, consumer activism, and budget limitations. Planning for the department, for example, is in vain if the therapeutic recreation manager cannot translate the objectives into concrete action. To perform effectively as a first-line manager requires that one has clear ideas of that role and how it relates to the health and human service organization.

Other characteristics of a successful first-line therapeutic recreation manager would be having the ability to conceptualize ways to resolve problems by using creative solutions. In addition, being able to rebound from the frustrations of today and recognize that tomorrow is another day with its own challenges and rewards is also important. Last, to have a sense of humor is vital; without it the environment can rapidly create management burnout.

Therapeutic recreation managers are also considered functional managers, as opposed to general managers, because they are responsible for a specialized service that is important to the organization. Recently, more and more therapeutic recreation managers in community-based settings are assuming general managerial responsibilities because of their knowledge of the Americans with Disabilities Act (ADA). While manager is the term most frequently used for the role and function examined in this text, other titles may be used such as *administrator, chief, director, head,* or *supervisor.*

In summary, a manager is both an investor in the organization and its goals, and an integrator and interpreter of its functions. The manager has a professional role, an interpersonal role, a business role, and an informational role. A manager's responsibility, as will be explored further is to ensure that functions are carried out and tasks are per-

formed to meet the organizational goals, objectives, and plans. If practiced effectively, the result is quality service to the consumer. These responsibilities are achieved through appropriate behavior and competent use of administrative skills, human resource skills, and technical skills.

# First-Line Manager Responsibilities and Challenges

While some of these responsibilities were mentioned previously and many will be considered in more detail in subsequent chapters, the concern here is highlighting and briefly describing the many and varied responsibilities and challenging aspects of being a first-line manager.

## Setting Objectives

All planning rests on the assumption that the first-line manager has a clear idea of the objectives to be achieved in providing services. These objectives direct activities of the department although they may vary or be supplemented by interim and ad hoc objectives formulated on the basis of the day-to-day situation.

## Planning and Organizing

Reaching objectives entails making a plan concerning what has to be done. This means that the first-line manager analyzes what activities need to be done, sets priorities, and plans the best means to achieve the desired ends. In addition, the plan must assign responsibility, and it must be communicated to staff. The challenge of the first-line manager is to convert planning into action by way of organizing. Planning must deal with the realities of therapeutic recreation service. There is no way the first-line manager can be unrealistic since plans are tied to everyday results, and these results provide loud and clear feedback.

## Communicating and Motivating

It seems absurdly simple to note that the first-line manager tells the staff what is expected of them. It is a step, however, often neglected. The manager may assume that the staff will envision the same objectives as the manager does. This assumption, unfortunately, is often faulty. Even if all staff members are highly motivated to give "good service," there is no reason to assume that all of them mean the same thing by this phrase. Therefore, the manager has a critical obligation to make clear to staff the kind of performance wanted.

As the acknowledged head of the department, the manager lays the groundwork for the exchange of information related to consumer service, organizational matters, and trends. The way information is articulated to staff has a direct bearing on the way it is used and processed.

Effective managers keep communication flowing. Because of the manager's vital role in the organization, the manager's ability to listen to staff is as important as his or her ability to be a good spokesperson. Moreover, managers create an environment conducive to professional behavior when they solicit staff suggestions and act on them.

## *Measuring and Evaluating*

The manager makes expectations explicit and does not assume that staff will always share his or her standards of performance. While staff need to set personal goals that correspond to the department objectives, the manager provides the yardstick against which the individual measures his or her performance. Periodic written evaluations are an essential management tool that should be supplemented by routine feedback on what staff is doing right and what areas need improvement.

The danger in not setting standards is that minimal standards, if any, will prevail. The delivery of quality consumer service depends on each practitioner's striving for excellence. The manager understands that everyone will not perform equally well, but he or she establishes standards to aim for and establishes what is required. Quality assurance (QA) and continuous quality improvement (CQI) form a basis for judging how well a group is performing.

## *Ensuring Consumers' Welfare*

One step the manager can take to ensure quality delivery of service to the consumer is to scrutinize the policies and procedures manual. There are policies and procedures for reporting on and off duty, for transmission of information regarding consumers, for interacting with higher management staff, and for working with interns or fieldwork students and volunteers. All of these practices plus many others have an impact upon consumer service. It is important, therefore, that the manager identify the policies and procedures associated with the department and subject them to scrutiny.

The first-line manager is ultimately responsible for and to the consumer. This means that the manager, depending upon the setting, must have knowledge about the consumer on an ongoing basis including achievements and goals the consumer wants to reach. Likewise, the manager also should know the challenges and problems consumers present to staff. The manager acquires such knowledge through QA and CQI measures primarily.

## *Other Responsibilities and Challenges*

Other first-line managerial responsibilities and challenges that can be organized in terms of personnel, administration, and education are as follows (Whetten and Cameron, 1984):

### Personnel Challenges

1. Organizing and managing time despite so many demands and changes.
2. Managing the frustrations associated with being creative in a bureaucratic agency environment.
3. Managing the guilt feelings regarding the use of supervisory privileges (e.g., conference attendance, travel, larger office).
4. Managing personal job frustrations and insecurities about giving priority to working or to experiencing a lack of knowledge which often requires a commitment to update oneself.

### Administrative Challenges

1. Managing the heavy paperwork demands for accountability.
2. Managing increased work load without increases, or even with reductions, in staff.
3. Translating poorly conceived and untimely administrative directives into a form which staff can understand and implement.
4. Managing interagency conflicts based on jealousy, competition, and poor communication regarding differing service standards.
5. Confronting staff with disciplinary action over inadequate performance after years of inattention by previous supervisors.
6. Managing well-organized unit or staff meetings (e.g., maintaining clear focus and avoiding long, boring meetings).
7. Managing staff's concerns for the quality of work with the manager's concern for the quantity of work.
8. Managing top and middle management who violate the chain of command and subordinates who make "end runs" on the manager to higher authorities.
9. Managing work unit issues, such as staff abuse of privileges (e.g., overuse of compensation time), a dominant worker who undermines morale, jealousies among workers, and translation of agency goals and objectives into viable worker activities.

### Educational Challenges

1. Motivating staff to plan for their own professional growth.
2. Managing to secure the time and money for staff inservice training.

In addition to these responsibilities and challenges, the manager should have knowledge and awareness of other health and human service resources especially those that relate to providing leisure service and ways to make referrals to them. The manager will also possess adequate knowledge and understanding of the therapeutic recreation continuum and therapeutic recreation process and their application regardless of setting. Last, the manager is knowledgeable about the purposes and activities of the national professional membership organizations (e.g., ATRA and NTRS) including state affiliation organizations and the professional certification organization (e.g., NCTRC). The manager is active in these professional organizations, is certified by them and, at the same time, recognizes the importance of certification for his or her staff. The manager is also knowledgeable about other allied health professions and their goals, standards, and services.

In conclusion of this section, Figure 1.1 offers a reflection of the variables that affect the therapeutic recreation manager.

# Therapeutic Recreation Department Dimensions

The therapeutic recreation division or department usually operates within the broader context of the health and human service organization. While the therapeutic recreation department must support the overall mission of any organization as a major dimension, its approach must be grounded in therapeutic recreation's values and beliefs as to what constitutes professional quality. The philosophy and goals of therapeutic recreation, regardless of setting, provide a basis for organization and intradepartmental decision making. They also outline the relationship of therapeutic recreation to the overall organization, define what therapeutic recreation is, and point out its unique contribution to the organization. By using recreation and leisure experience in helping individuals with problems, limitations, and disabilities to achieve their optimal intellectual, physical, emotional, and social well-being, the philosophy and goals of therapeutic recreation are affirmed. The promotion of leisure opportunities and wellness, the prevention of disease, and the treatment of illness have been and will continue to be therapeutic recreation foci.

Within this context, programs are the instruments through which the department accomplishes its goals and objectives. The manager's task is to oversee the therapeutic recreation process which is a model for action that includes establishing outcomes, the nature of the services to be provided, the consumers to be served, and the resources required.

In addition to these major dimensions, therapeutic recreation operating practices need to be in congruence with the organization's overall environment. These practices structure the work of the department and its operations. Department dimensions, while not comprehensive, are shown below:

- mission;
- marketing;
- philosophy;
- programming, scheduling, staffing;
- scope;
- managerial reporting;
- objectives;
- department policies;
- organizational structure;
- personnel policies;
- standards of practice;
- job description;
- budget;
- performance evaluation;
- information processing;
- continuous quality management;
- advocating and networking; and
- negotiating.

# Making the Transition: Practitioner to Manager

It is widely recognized that a sizeable proportion of therapeutic recreation practitioners whose professional training is in direct service move into positions of managerial responsibility at some point in their careers. A major reason for this is that a management position continues to be one of the few options open to practitioners that increases status and salaries. Other reasons for taking a management position might include a desire to achieve; help to change and improve policies and services; reach for power; offer service and give of one's self (French and Raven, 1968). Regardless, a practitioner frequently experiences a high degree of difficulty in making the transition to manager and focusing on getting the job done through other people. To some extent this problem is associated with any new job or practice role. An interesting observation the authors have made is that after a period of three to five years as a manager, "a point of no return" is reached—that is, it would not be feasible to return to the position of individual practitioner. A commitment has been made to a career in professional management.

In what follows, several areas in which problems appear to exist when there is a transition from practitioner to management role are focused on briefly.

The move into a manager's position often affects the nature of relationships with colleagues. While still a practitioner, the new manager is likely to have participated in a

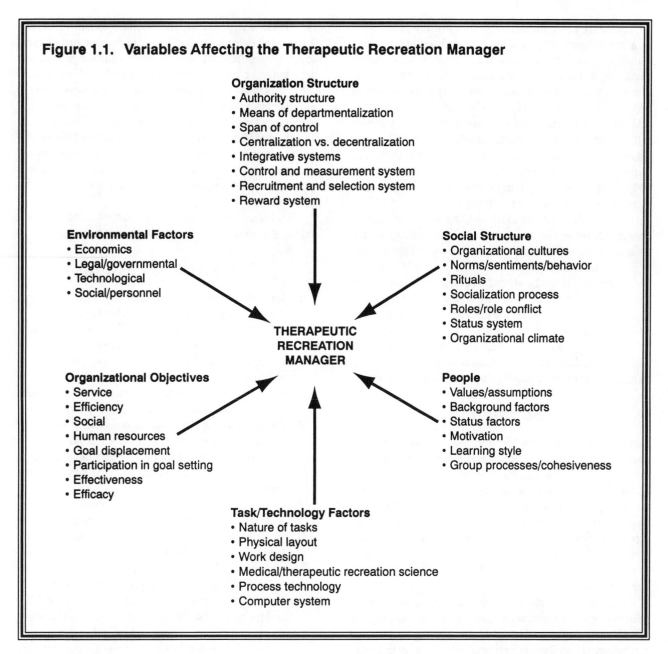

**Figure 1.1. Variables Affecting the Therapeutic Recreation Manager**

**Organization Structure**
• Authority structure
• Means of departmentalization
• Span of control
• Centralization vs. decentralization
• Integrative systems
• Control and measurement system
• Recruitment and selection system
• Reward system

**Environmental Factors**
• Economics
• Legal/governmental
• Technological
• Social/personnel

**Social Structure**
• Organizational cultures
• Norms/sentiments/behavior
• Rituals
• Socialization process
• Roles/role conflict
• Status system
• Organizational climate

**THERAPEUTIC RECREATION MANAGER**

**Organizational Objectives**
• Service
• Efficiency
• Social
• Human resources
• Goal displacement
• Participation in goal setting
• Effectiveness
• Efficacy

**People**
• Values/assumptions
• Background factors
• Status factors
• Motivation
• Learning style
• Group processes/cohesiveness

**Task/Technology Factors**
• Nature of tasks
• Physical layout
• Work design
• Medical/therapeutic recreation science
• Process technology
• Computer system

normative system that valued mutuality and cooperation. He or she probably enjoyed opportunities to ventilate frustration, gain support, and exchange ideas and information. New relationships are likely to be more functionally specific and instrumental. The manager's new status makes it increasingly difficult for him or her to maintain primary group relationships with colleagues who have now become subordinates. The change in structural arrangements usually pushes the manager and practitioners toward an impersonal and neutral level of interaction.

One of the most troublesome areas managers encounter in their first management position is exercising authority over subordinates, especially former colleagues. The problem centers on eliciting support and cooperation in moving toward the goals of the organization, motivating people to change behavior or improve performance, and gaining cooperation with changes proposed by managers. The manager's direct practice knowledge and skill gained as a practitioner usually help in resolving these kinds of problems. However, if various efforts fail, the manager is often faced with the necessity of using the authority of the office to elicit the desired behavior. The manager who consistently shrinks from using the authority of the position when there are problems will eventually lose the ability to coordinate activities toward the organization's objectives.

The new manager needs to have an appreciation of the organization as a functioning system. While the manager will certainly understand the dynamics of the department as a practitioner, he or she now must develop an understanding of the interdependency of the process and events occurring in the organization such as the exchange relationships that must occur between the organization and its task environments; the effects of organization, structure, and climate on such things as communication, practitioner satisfaction, and performance; the importance of ideological and occupational commitments and professional vested interests as determinants of individual and group behavior; and the dynamics underlying various problems like goal displacement, ritualism, and intergroup conflict.

Finally, the manager must understand the differences between direct service and management, and recognize the unique skills and perspectives needed in each of these roles. While the new manager probably has those skills related to direct service, he or she should be particularly aware that management, as has been noted earlier, is itself a professional activity that requires the same level of expertise and dedication required of the practitioner in direct practice.

Attempting to make the transition to management by remaining a *de facto* practitioner, who happens incidentally to manage, is to avoid coming to terms with this reality.

# Summary

Initial consideration was given to those factors that have changed the delivery of health and human services since the 1950s. Coupled with these factors was a brief review of the emerging professionalization of therapeutic recreation. If professionalization is to continue, attention must be given to the implementation and delivery of quality service regardless of setting. However, for this to be accomplished, it must come through the development of effective procedures that are directed by personnel with management skills.

Management was defined as the process of working with others toward goal accomplishment in a changing environment. Skills that effective managers generally use can be sorted into five major types: conceptual or creative, leadership, interpersonal, administrative, and technical. This was followed by consideration of management dimensions. While there are several levels of management, the therapeutic recreation manager in a health and human service organization is considered a first-line manager. In most settings, this manager is usually classified as a functional manager because he or she provides a specialized service.

Therapeutic recreation manager responsibilities and challenges were noted as well as the dimensions of a therapeutic recreation department with special attention given to incorporating the philosophy, values, and beliefs of therapeutic recreation.

Final consideration was given to factors associated with making the transition from practitioner to manager.

# Discussion Questions

1. Identify the different skills of a therapeutic recreation manager. Give an example of each.
2. Does the type of organization affect the type of skills needed by a therapeutic recreation manager within the organization? Indicate which are more desirable relative to the organization.
3. Interview a therapeutic recreation manager about how he or she works. Discuss findings in class.
4. On the basis of your present personality and management experience, what managerial skills appear to be the highest priority for further development? What strategies can you use to assist you in developing these skills?
5. Of the five types of skills—conceptual, leadership, interpersonal, administrative, and technical—which would you think is the easiest for a manager to learn? Which is the most difficult? Considering the broad responsibilities and challenges of a manager, develop a list of the activities and identify thereafter the relative importance you attach to each activity and the amount of time you would give to the activity. Use different settings wherein therapeutic recreation service is provided and you are the manager of the department.

# References

American Therapeutic Recreation Association (ATRA) and National Therapeutic Recreation Society (NTRS). (1994). *Therapeutic recreation: Responding to the challenges of healthcare reform* [Brochure].

Boland, P. (1993). *Managed care work.* Gaithersburg, MD: Aspen Publishers, Inc.

Bush, D. D. (1994, Spring). The insurer's point of view. *Hanover Quarterly,* 10–13.

Calloway, J. (1992). Organizational and management styles in therapeutic recreation. In R. M. Winslow and K. J. Halberg (Eds.), *The management of therapeutic recreation service* (pp. 1–26). Arlington, VA: National Recreation and Park Association.

Carter, M. J., Van Andel, G. E., and Robb, G. M. (1995). *Therapeutic recreation: A practical approach* (2nd ed.). Prospect Heights, IL: Waveland Press, Inc.

Connolly, P., and Garbarini, A. (1996). *Healthcare management and recreation therapy: Cost benefits.* Thiells, NY: National Council for Therapeutic Recreation Certification.

French, J. R. P., Jr., and Raven, B. (1968). The base of social power. In D. Cartwright and A. Zander, (Eds.), *Group dynamics* (3rd ed., pp. 262–268). New York, NY: Harper & Row.

Griffin, R. W. (1990). *Management* (3rd ed.). Boston, MA: Houghton Mifflin Co.

Hull, K. (1994). Hospital trends. In C. Harrington and C. L. Estes (Eds.), *Health policy and nursing* (pp. 150–168). Boston, MA: Jones & Bartlett Publishers.

Katz, R. L. (1994, September–October). Skills of an effective administrator. *Harvard Business Review, 51,* 90–102.

Kreitner, R. (1992). *Management* (5th ed.). Boston, MA: Houghton Mifflin Co.

Kronenfeld, J. J. (1993). *Controversial issues in healthcare policy.* Newbury Park, CA: Sage Publications, Inc.

Megginson, L. C., Mosley, D. C., and Pietri, P. H., Jr. (1992). *Management: Concepts and applications* (4th ed.). New York, NY: HarperCollins Publishers.

Northern, L. (1995, June 7). Stirring alphabet soup? *Rehab Rap,* 1–2.

O'Morrow, G. S. (1995). *Therapeutic recreation practitioner analysis, 1994.* Arlington, VA: National Recreation and Park Association.

Petryshen, P. M., and Petryshen, P. R. (1993/1994). Managed care: Shaping the delivery of healthcare and creating an expanding role for the caregiver. *Annual in Therapeutic Recreation, 4,* 108–114.

Sandwith, P. (1993). A hierarchy of management training requirements: The competency domain model. *Public Personnel Management, 22:1,* 43–62.

Stein, J. O. (1993). The Americans with disabilities act. In *Leisure opportunities for individuals with disabilities: Legal issues* (pp. 1–11). Reston, VA: American Alliance for Health, Physical Education, Recreation and Dance.

Thomas, R. K. (1993). *Healthcare consumers in the 1990s.* Ithaca, NY: American Demographics Books.

U.S. Department of Health and Human Services, Public Health Service. (1995). *Healthy people 2000: Midcourse review and 1995 revisions.* Sudbury, MA: Jones & Bartlett Publishers.

U.S. Department of Health and Human Services, Public Health Service. (1991). *Healthy People 2000: National health promotion and disease prevention objectives.* Washington, DC: Government Printing Office.

U.S. Department of Labor, Bureau of Labor Statistics. (1991). *Occupational handbook.* Washington, DC: Government Printing Office.

Whetten, D. A., and Cameron, K. S. (1984). *Developing management skills.* Glenview, IL: Scott, Foresman and Company.

Wren, D. A. (1979). *The evolution of management thought* (2nd ed.). New York, NY: John Wiley & Sons.

# Part 1

# Characteristics of Management

# Chapter 2
# Theories of Management

## Introduction

Today therapeutic recreation managers, primarily those in the various healthcare facilities, operate in an environment that is in a state of flux. As a result, managers must be thoroughly familiar with a plurality of factors that influence the conditions under which service-giving resources are managed. It is imperative that the most current information be available because information is essential to the understanding of facts. For therapeutic recreation managers facts generally imply problems, and problems require solutions.

What approaches are available to therapeutic recreation managers for securing solutions to problems? Certainly, managers use different approaches in the interpretation, analysis, and solution of management problems, and they vary from setting to setting. Through experience and knowledge, therapeutic recreation managers can scan the problem and secure a preliminary decision that may be appropriate. However, such a decision might not be sufficient for finding a solution in other cases.

Managerial approaches to problem solving may be classified by various categories. For purposes of this discussion, the approaches are categorized as historical, parasitic, and professional.

The historical approach is used by managers who, in addressing problems, follow the same processes and techniques that were handed down from the past. These managers lack innovative ideas. Consequently, they base their solution on the repetition of previous approaches to problems much like some therapeutic recreation practitioners who consistently use a specific activity in association with specific consumer goals. The prevailing hope of the historical manager is that the present problem is sufficiently similar to the past problem and that the old solution will be relevant to the new problem. Historical managers expend much energy in attempting to "force fit" the new problem into the old solution. Of course, this approach does not consider the extent of changes occurring in the new environment, either internal or external. The degree of this changing environment is well-described by Alvin Toffler in *Future Shock* (1971). As a result, this approach is a contradistinction to the prevailing dynamism so evident in the therapeutic recreation manager's working environment.

The parasitic approach consists of observing and learning from the action of other managers. This approach differs from the historical one in that managers attempt to copy the behavior and actions of contemporary colleagues rather than duplicating the methods of a predecessor. Although some improvement in managerial decision making can be learned from this approach, it still presents the problem of fitting the solution to the right problem.

Managers who use the professional approach are characterized by the use of theoretical systems in search of solutions to problems. The pretension of restricting actual therapeutic recreation problems to fixed solutions is not logical and is, at best, erroneous. Such restrictions on therapeutic recreation managers result in ineptness and are evidenced by the Peter Principle in action. To preclude such ineptness, it is important that future managers be aware of the various theories or schools of management.

In preparation for reviewing the various theories of management it is important to outline how theory is of use to managers:

1. **Organization.** A theory provides a framework in which one can organize ideas and experiences. It helps detect similarities, differences, and other patterns in data and provides explanation for these patterns.
2. **Perspective.** A theory also provides a perspective, a certain way of looking at things. Using a particular theory influences how one interprets what one sees.
3. **Explanation.** Theories not only organize information, but they also provide explanations of events. Theories are general statements that help one understand *why* certain things do or do not happen. Why, for example, does therapeutic recreation specialist A work harder than therapeutic recreation specialist B? One management theory will say that it is because A receives a larger salary than B. Another theory will say that it is because B is not interested in working with that group of consumers on that unit. A third will say that both factors are operating: A has interesting, stimulating work and is paid more than B, who is dissatisfied with her work in several ways.
4. **Prediction.** A theory should also help one predict what is likely to happen in a given situation. Developmental theory predicts that certain crises will occur during adolescence, including conflicts between parent and teenagers. Familiarity with this theory enables a specialist to provide leisure guidance to a family with an at-risk youth in a leisure counseling program.
5. **Application.** A theory that predicts what is likely to happen in a given situation can provide some direction regarding what action is to be taken. Management theories serve as guides for selecting the most effective action.

Although this discussion will be brief, more detailed presentations can be found in many good texts on management and organization in the library as well as in the reference publications in this chapter.

# Theories

As one begins the consideration of the various theories of management one should recognize that the actual practice of management has been in existence for thousands of years and can be traced back to the Egyptians. The mere physical presence of the pyramids forces one to accept that there had to exist formal plans, organizations, leadership, and control systems. The study of management from a scientific perspective did not begin until the late nineteenth century.

From a historical perspective, management thought, according to Griffin (1990) has been shaped by three sets of forces: social forces (the norms and values that characterize the people in culture), economic forces (associated with economic systems and general economic conditions and trends), and political forces (governing institutions and general governmental policies and attitudes toward business).

There is no single theory of management to explain all human behavior that is universally accepted. Further, it is not unusual to become frustrated in the study and review of management theories. To help put different theories in perspective, this section shall discuss the five conventional approaches keeping in mind there is overlap or refinement from one theory to the next. These five approaches are:

1. the classical approach,
2. the behavioral approach,
3. the quantitative approach,
4. the systems approach, and
5. the contingency approach.

## Classical Management Theory

Classical theory is built around four elements: division and specialization of labor, chain of command, structure of the organization, and span of control. Classical theory has had a number of labels since the turn of the century including scientific management, management science, and operations management.

While several theorists have contributed to classical management theory, Frederick W. Taylor, who played a dominant role in its early development, is considered "the father of scientific management" (Wren, 1987). His innovations in the workplace resulted in higher quality products and improved employee morale.

In his book, *The Principles of Scientific Management,* published in 1911, Taylor offered four principles of scientific management to maximize individual productivity:

- develop a "science" for every job by studying motion, standardizing the work, and improving working conditions;
- carefully select workers with the correct abilities for the job;
- carefully train these workers to do the job and offer them incentives to produce; and
- support the workers by planning their work and by removing obstacles (Wren, 1987).

Henry Gantt, Frank and Lillian Gilbreth, and Morris Cooke added to scientific management. Gantt humanized Taylor's differential piece-rate system by combining a guaranteed day rate (minimum wage) with an above-standard bonus (Kreitner, 1992). The Gilbreth's devoted their efforts to motion analysis, or "least-waste" method, of labor. Their approach focused not on how long it took to do a piece of work but rather on the best way to do it. The "one best way" was the one that required the fewest motions to accomplish (Wren, 1987). Cooke broadened the ideas of scientific management to include their application in universities and municipal organizations. He recognized that the concepts of efficiency, so valuable to the profit sector, could be equally valuable in nonprofit and service organizations (Robbins, 1980).

Although Taylor, Gantt, the Gilbreths, and Cooke focused on the techniques that management might use in the production of goods through the use of individual employees and improving organization efficiency, none of them addressed management as a function distinct and separate from techniques and individuals.

It was Henri Fayol who attempted to develop a broad and more functional universal approach to management—managing the total organization. In 1916 he published a study concerned with the principles of general management entitled *General and Industrial Management* (Fayol, 1949). Fayol primarily studied the upper echelon of organizations and felt that the need for managerial ability increased in relative importance as an individual advanced in the chain of command (Fayol, 1949). Fayol's work provided definitions regarding the basic functions for management which are planning, organizing, commanding, coordinating, and controlling. If goals are to be accomplished, these functions must be carried out (Fayol, 1949).

Fayol defined management in these words:

> To manage is to forecast and plan, to organize, to command, to coordinate, and to control. To foresee and provide means examining the future and drawing up the plan of action. To organize means building up the dual structure, material and human, of the undertaking. To command means binding together, unifying and harmonizing all activity and effort. To control means seeing that everything occurs in conformity with established rule and expressed demand. (Fayol, 1949, pp. 5–6)

Fayol came to the conclusion that there was a set of management principles that could be used in all types of management situations regardless of organization. Further, these principles should be used to implement the five functions.

Fayol (1949, pp. 19–20) listed the principles of management as follows:

1. division of work,
2. authority,
3. discipline,
4. unit of command,
5. unit of direction,
6. subordination of individual interest to the general interest,
7. remuneration,
8. centralization,
9. scalar chain (line of authority),
10. order,
11. equity,
12. stability or tenure of personnel,
13. initiative, and
14. esprit de corps.

While not specifically associated with classical theory or scientific management, the work of Luther Gulick and Lyndall Urwick expanded on the contribution of Fayol's management functions. Gulick (1947) enlarged on Fayol's contribution, using the acronym POSDCORB to represent the functions of management. The acronym stands for planning, organizing, staffing, directing, coordinating (or communicating), reporting, and budgeting. Variations of this management scheme are still used by many managers today as well as the authors of this book. Urwick (1944) indicated that administrative skill within management functions is a practical art that improves with practice and requires hard study and thinking. From his work Urwick concluded that there are three principles of administration. He described the first principle as that of *investigation* and stated that all scientific procedure is based on investigation of the facts. Investigation takes effect in planning. The second principle is *appropriateness* which underlines forecasting, entering into process with organization and taking effect in coordination. Exercising the third principle the administrator looks ahead and organizes *resources* to meet future needs. Planning enters into the process with command and is effected in control.

Oliver Sheldon departed from earlier writings in scientific study of management by noting the importance of ethics in management and that managers have a social responsibility to their community. Lending itself also to the field of scientific study was the work of Leonard White. He argued that management should be separate from politics and that the mission of management is economy and efficiency (Robbins, 1980).

Although Max Weber is identified more with organizational theory, it is important to note his relationship to scientific management. Weber (1947) is credited with attempting to create the ultimate efficient organization by proposing a rational bureaucracy of integrated activities and positions with inherent activities. Employees occupied roles that were assigned on the basis of technical qualifications that, in turn, were determined by formalized impersonal procedures. Rules and regulations were developed for each position regardless of the person who occupied it. The concept of role became paramount in Weber's system with employees conceived almost as preprogrammed interchangeable robots. Weber's impersonal bureaucracy seemed to outlaw the development of personal relationships in legitimate organizational activities. However, this impersonal bureaucracy contributes to the stability of any organization and the predictability of its performance (Shortell, Kaluzny, and associates, 1988).

The overall approach of Taylor, Gantt, the Gilbreths, Fayol, and others was to provide a rational basis for management and place it on a more objective and scientific foundation. As the classical management theory developed, it examined in more detail the functions of managers. The result was a refinement of the classical theory. According to Hax and Majluf (1984), Weber, Taylor, and Fayol have had a lasting impact on management and organizational design.

## Behavioral School

As more managers began operating under the principles of the classical management thought, it became apparent that results were not totally compatible with expectations. Many managers felt that the classical approach did not take into account human relations in that people desire social relations, respond to group pressures, and search for personal fulfillment. As a result the management field moved gradually from a mechanical approach of following a series of concepts of rules to an attempt to understand the worker. Studies focused on democratic structure, multidirectional communications, and promotion of general satisfaction of the worker. Self-development, individualization, initiative, and creativity were identified as attributes to be promoted and encouraged. Since the therapeutic recreation manager may not have too much to say about the way in which the organization is structured, behavioral theory may have special significance for the manager.

Behavioral management theory was stimulated by a number of writers, but the primary catalyst for this movement was Elton Mayo (1933) and his studies at Western Electric Company's Hawthorne Plant concerned with the physical environment and productivity. Mayo initiated a series of studies that were intended to contribute to the concepts of scientific management but which ultimately demonstrated the impact of small group dynamics upon production. Small groups of women and men were selected for an intensive study focusing on the impact of physical working conditions, the psychological capacity

of the worker on productivity, and how monetary incentives played a role in work behavior. Mayo found that physical comfort and pay had less impact on productivity than the way workers related to each other socially and economically (i.e., being paid for the group's output rather than individual output). After several years of the Hawthorne experiments concerned with increasing productivity, the researchers concluded that "other factors," or human factors and the social processes, accounted for increased productivity.

Mayo (1933) points out in *The Human Problems of Industrial Civilization* that emotional factors are important in productivity. He also urged managers to provide work that stimulated personal satisfaction. He did not argue against the bureaucratic structure approach to management as outlined by Weber, but he proposed that improvements be made by making the structure less formal and by permitting more employee participation in decision making. The implication of Mayo's studies relative to the therapeutic recreation manager is quite clear. Sometimes the only thing required to meet people's needs is to pay attention to them. This applies to consumers, peers, and other health and human service staff.

Mary Parker Follett is another behavioral scientist who suggested to managers that employees are a "complex conviction of emotions, beliefs, attitudes, and habits" (Kreitner, 1992, p. 52). Because she believed that managers had to recognize the individual's motivating desires to get employees to produce more, she suggested that managers motivate performance rather than demand it.

In the development of the behavioral school, Chester Barnard (1938) is recognized as one of the outstanding contributors. Associated with the systems approach to management, Barnard's work was primarily drawn from sociological approaches to management in which he attempted to find answers underlying the process of management. Barnard established a theory for a system of cooperation: willingness to serve, common purpose, and communication are the principle elements in an organization. This theory basically emphasized the need of individuals to solve the limitation of themselves and their environment through cooperation with others. In addition it is necessary that formal authority work with individuals for success (Kreitner, 1992). Barnard's work brought forth the recognition of the organization as a social organism that must interact with environmental pressures and conflict.

Later theorists, such as Kurt Lewin (1951), Abraham Maslow (1954), Douglas McGregor (1960), and others influenced a humanistic approach to management. Maslow is well-known for his theory based on a hierarchy of needs—physiologic, safety, love, belonging, self-esteem and self-actualization. Organizations and management theories, according to Maslow, ignore the human being's intrinsic nature and are detrimental to the psychic and physical health and well-being of employees. Although these needs, especially higher level ones, may be suppressed, ignoring basic human needs would contribute to lower productivity, high absenteeism, high turnover, low morale, and job dissatisfaction. Maslow's theory of hierarchy of needs led to theories on motivation (Maslow, 1968).

McGregor furthered the human relations movement. His theme was that people are basically good, and in order to stimulate their performance, one should humanize work with this philosophy: Let people participate and take an active role in those decisions that affect them, have trust and confidence in people, and reduce external control devices. He developed a set of assumptions called Theory X and Theory Y about human behavior which are reflected in Figure 2.1. In McGregor's view, Theory X focused on the tasks to be done. In contrast, Theory Y was a more appropriate view for managers to take in regard to viewing employees since its focus was on the employees and their job satisfaction (McGregor, 1960). According to Robbins (1995), there is no evidence to confirm that either set of assumptions is valid. In recent years a Theory Z (Ouchi, 1981) has been proposed that suggests a middle ground between Theories X and Y and will be discussed shortly.

In summary, the behavioral school brought together newly developed theories, methods, and techniques of the relevant social sciences on the study of inter- and intrapersonal phenomena, ranging from the personality dynamics of individuals at one end to the relation of cultures at the other end. According to the advocates of the behavioral approach to management today technology, work rules, and standards do not guarantee good job performance. Success depends on motivated and skilled individuals who are committed to organizational objectives.

On the other hand, a common criticism of the human relations approach is that most managers function in a bureaucratic environment in which one organizational structure is adopted and little enthusiasm is given by management for individuality.

## Quantitative Management Theory

Quantitative management theory approach never really claimed to be the overall conceptual base for management theory that advocates have implied it to be. However, the approach does use tools that provide management with a greater power for the analysis of problems. Quantitative management theory incorporates two interrelated branches: management science (not related to scientific management) and operations management. Together they focus on decision making, economic effectiveness, formal mathematical models, and the use of computers to stimulate and solve problems. Of note here is decision making. It concentrates on a rational approach to making a decision whereby it becomes the central focus of all management, implying thorough consideration of alternatives prior to the selection of a course of action (Koontz, 1961).

## General Systems Theory

An organization is a complex sociotechnical system (DeGreen, 1973). In the 1950s von Bertalanffy described a general systems theory that provided a consistent operational model for studying systems at all levels of science from a single cell to complex social systems such as business firms, healthcare facilities, political states, and so on (Kast and Rosenzweig, 1985). According to von

---

### Figure 2.1   Theory X and Theory Y

**Theory X Assumptions:**
1. People do not like work and try to avoid it.
2. People do not like work so managers have to control, direct, coerce, and threaten employees to get them to work toward organizational goals.
3. People prefer to be directed, to avoid responsibility, to want security; they have little ambition.

**Theory Y Assumptions:**
1. People do not naturally dislike work; work is a natural part of their lives.
2. People are internally motivated to reach objectives to which they are committed.
3. People are committed to goals to the degree that they receive personal rewards when they reach their objectives.
4. People will both seek and accept responsibility under favorable conditions.
5. People have the capacity to be innovative in solving organizational problems.
6. People are bright, but under most organizational conditions, their potentials are underutilized.

Source: McGregor, D. (1960). *The human side of enterprise,* (pp. 33–34, 47–48). New York: McGraw-Hill. Reprinted with permission of the McGraw-Hill Companies. Copyright 1960.

Bertalanffy (1972, p. 411), "In order to understand an organized whole we must know both the parts and the relations between them." General systems theory is interdisciplinary in its study approach; it is based on the assumption that everything is part of a larger, independent arrangement.

A system can be defined as a unitary whole composed of two or more elements in interaction and differentiated by an identifiable boundary from its environment. It is characterized by input (i.e., materials, employees, money, consumers), the transformation process (i.e., technology, operating system, management systems), output (i.e., services, well consumers, employees' behaviors), and feedback (i.e., consumer, factors in the environment) to the system. Feedback enables a system to regulate itself. Feedback gives the system the ability to control its input and output. For example, in the community, laws, rules, and regulations regulate the behavior of citizens. In the family system, parents provide feedback to children to regulate behavior (Kast and Rosenzweig, 1985).

The Gunn and Peterson (1978) publication *Therapeutic Recreation Program Design: Principles and Procedures* takes a systems approach to programming. The therapeutic recreation process has some characteristics of an open system: it is open, flexible, and dynamic; it is planned and goal directed; it interacts with the environment; and it emphasizes feedback. Input (data) from the consumer and practitioner is transformed by the process of analyzing, planning, and implementing, all of which occur throughout the therapeutic recreation process. The output (consumer response) is then evaluated.

The Input Process Output (IPO) model of Carter, Van Andel, and Robb (1995) is another example of a systems approach to program design. Moreover, the IPO model is associated with Riley's (1991) outcome evaluation model and quality of care indicators.

There are any number of characteristics associated with systems. For example, systems are either open or closed. Closed systems are usually self-contained. However, there is disagreement on whether or not a truly closed system exists. The assumption is that the most important feature of organizations have to do with their internal structure and processes which are relatively isolated from the external environment. Open systems, on the other hand, interact with the surrounding environment for survival (see Figure 2.2). Environmental factors include political, social, and economic variables which influence system performance. By taking into account its environment the organization's structure, process, and performance are centrally influenced by the nature of the inputs taken in from the environment and the outputs produced. Organizations such as hospitals and departments of parks and recreation are open systems since their survival depends on interaction with the surrounding environments.

Another important assumption made by systems theory is that systems are made up of subsystems—a system within a system. According to Kreitner (1992), there are hierarchies of systems ranging from very specific systems (e.g., communication, decision making) to general ones. While subsystems have some degree of autonomy, they are also dependent on the next subsystem. A therapeutic recreation department within physical medicine and rehabilitation (PM and R) can function somewhat independently, but it is eventually dependent on PM and R which is in turn dependent on the hospital. A therapeutic recreation division within a community-based parks and recreation department is dependent on the community-based department, and the department is dependent on the community. Thus, there is a constant interdependence among various departments.

Sentience, the capacity for thought, abstraction, and feeling, is another characteristic of systems. It brings into play the uniquely human importance of emotions, values, and personal and culture-bound meanings (remember the human relations approach found in the behavioral school). People are not simply aware of the world around them, they are actively involved in trying to make sense of it by attempting to organize or influence their environment (Boulding, 1968).

Although various management theories from the past have been integrated into general systems theory in a positive way, there are critics of the systems theory because it lacks an empirical research base.

## Contingency Theory

Today virtually any health and human service organization must cope with an environment that is more complex, more changeable, and, therefore, more uncertain than the environments healthcare organizations faced in the past. Likewise, departments of parks and recreation will increasingly be forced to cope with changes in service delivery as a result of the Americans with Disabilities Act. To meet the challenge of change, a new approach to theory and practice of management has emerged.

Most books about management today recognize that it is largely contingency-based. Contingency theory suggests that appropriate managerial behavior is contingent on a variety of elements (Kast and Rosenzweig, 1973). These elements may be the environment (consumers, third-party payers), personnel (training, shortage of staff), technology, department or organization size and goals, administrator's power and influence, and clarity and equity of reward systems. According to Shetty (1974, p. 27), "The effectiveness of a given management pattern is contingent upon multitudinous factors and their interrelationship in a particular situation." Taking a universal approach to this theory, Koontz, O'Donnell and Weihrich (1980, p. 17) note:

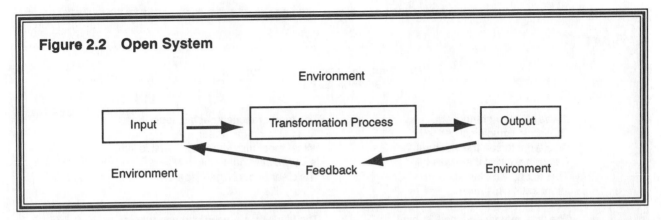

**Figure 2.2  Open System**

Environment

Input → Transformation Process → Output

Environment          Feedback          Environment

that there is no one best way to plan; there is no one best way to lead; there is no one best way to organize a group; and there is no one best way to control the activities of an organization. The best concepts and techniques can be selected only after one is aware of the particular circumstances he is facing. . . .

Consequently, what has worked in the past, such as a concept or technique to solve a problem, may not be appropriate in a different situation or under different circumstances. The approach to the delivery of services in a hospital setting is going to be much different from a community parks and recreation department.

Although still not fully developed, the contingency approach is helpful to management because it emphasizes situational appropriateness. As noted by Kreitner (1992, p. 60), "People, organizations, and problems are too complex to justify rigid adherence to universal principles of organizations."

While other management theories have emerged during the past decade, not all have yet undergone extensive empirical testing. A number of contemporary theories reflect promise. One such perspective of the study of management is from the best seller *In Search of Excellence* (Peters and Waterman, 1982). Researchers identified the common attributes that presumably led to the excellence in business of 62 companies. Two attributes applicable to therapeutic recreation managers are closeness to the customers (i.e., learn from their customers) and spending time observing and talking to practitioners who are performing "hands-on" functions.

The Theory Z model (Ouchi, 1981) attempts to integrate common business practices from the United States and Japan into one middle-ground framework. Theory Z takes a humanistic viewpoint and focuses on developing better ways to motivate people. In fact, many of the management theories discussed in this chapter are directly associated with leadership theories and motivation which will be discussed in a later chapter. In addition, Theory Z em-

phasizes collective or participative decision making, collective responsibility as opposed to personal responsibility, and a recognition of mutual dependence (Ouchi, 1981).

# Theory Application to Therapeutic Recreation

Although the theories just presented and their application to effective therapeutic recreation management will be considered throughout this text, it is well to note that there is no single theory that is universally accepted. Figure 2.3 (page 22) humorously illustrates the dilemma in management theory: where one is and what perspective one takes determines what one sees. Each has its limitations because organizations today are unique, changing, and complex. Consequently, therapeutic recreation managers should use management theory in an elective way.

To assist in this decision-making process, as a therapeutic recreation manager one may want to ask the following questions:

1. **Is the theory internally consistent?** Are the different parts of the theory congruent with each other, or is there some inconsistency in the way human behavior is explained or predicted?
2. **Does the theory provide useful guidelines for practice?** The purpose for considering theories that explain human behavior is to apply them to specific situations. However, some theories are so broad or narrow that it is difficult to apply them to specific situations.
3. **Has empirical testing yielded evidence in support of the theory?** Some theories have a natural appeal that tempts one to accept them without sufficient evaluation.
4. **Is the theory congruent with one's values and one's philosophy of therapeutic recreation as well as with the organization's?** A management theory that supports the growth and development of the individual employee implies a very different set of

**Figure 2.3**

### The Blind Men and the Elephant
### By John G. Saxe

It was six men of Indostan,
To learning much inclined,
Who went to see the elephant
(Though each of them was blind,)
That each by observation
Might satisfy his mind.

The first approached the elephant,
And happening to fall
Against his broad and sturdy side,
At once began to bawl:
"God bless me! but the elephant
Is very much like a wall!"

The second, feeling of the tusk,
Cried: "Ho! what have we here
So round, and smooth, and sharp?
To me 'tis very clear
This wonder of an elephant
Is very like a spear!"

The third approached the animal,
And happening to take
The squirming trunk within his hands,
Thus boldly up he spake:
"I see," quoth he, "the elephant
Is very much like a snake!"

The fourth reached out his eager hand,
And fell upon the knee:
"What most this wondrous beast is like,
Is very plain," quoth he;
"Tis clear enough the elephant
Is very like a tree!"

The fifth who chanced to touch the ear
Said: "E'en the blindest man
Can tell what this resembles most:
Deny the fact who can,
This marvel of an elephant
Is very like a fan!"

The sixth no sooner had begun
About the beast to grope,
Then, seizing on the swinging tail
That fell within his scope,
"I see," quoth he, "the elephant,
Is very like a rope!"

And so these men of Indostan
Disputed loud and long,
Each in his own opinion
Exceeding stiff and strong,
Though each was partly in the right,
And all were in the wrong!

Source: Saxe, J. G. (1936). The blind men and the elephant. In H. Felleman (Ed.), *The best-loved poems of the American people*, pp. 521–522. New York, NY: Doubleday and Company.

values from one that supports immediate termination when the skills of the specialist are no longer needed. In addition, the theory must be in agreement with the health and human service organization.

In the development of classical management theory, the work of Fayol and his basic functions of management stand out. Although these functions have been modified and expanded, they will provide the nucleus for the discussion of what management is and what managers do. In addition, his guidelines or principles of management, and those of Gulick and Urwick, are intertwined throughout the discussion of the management process.

It can also be noted from the review of these theories that goal achievement (i.e., quality service) within any setting is getting things done through people. Further, these people have human needs, perceptions, and aspirations. Material surroundings, wages and hours, or work cannot be considered in isolation from their value in relating a person

to a setting. No therapeutic recreation practitioner should be viewed as motivated strictly by economic or rational considerations. Values, beliefs, and emotions are inextricably involved in each practitioner's behavior. Successful goal achievement depends on good human relations, job satisfaction, and an understanding of what motivates people. A sensitive manager is aware of individual differences. A humanistic management atmosphere, with an emphasis on management theories to improve service, is essential for effective organizational goal achievement.

A last point is the approach to management. Today's environment demands diverse approaches to management to cope with more complexity and more uncertainty. It is naive to think that the form of management best for the delivery of therapeutic recreation service in one setting would be appropriate for all settings. While there are similarities, there are also differences, and these differences represent a wide range of factors. The optimal form of management suggested is contingent upon the factors faced by the therapeutic recreation manager in any setting—providing the highest possible level of consumer care and service while at the same time meeting other conflicting goals such as staying within budget, keeping staff practitioners satisfied, and so on. The contingency theory of management complemented by the systems approach (i.e., open systems, subsystems) offers a viable management approach. Being aware of a variety of theoretical frameworks helps therapeutic recreation managers know that, as they seek to organize and develop their programs and services, they do have choices. These choices are made even more complex, however, by the very nature of health and human service organizations.

# Summary

Therapeutic recreation managers operate in a dynamic environment that places heavy demands on them to cope with a range of factors influencing the delivery of therapeutic recreation service. Managerial approaches to decision making were defined as historical, parasitic, and professional. Professional therapeutic recreation managers were characterized as those who use theoretical systems in search of problems and solutions to problems coupled with work experience.

It was noted that management is influenced by social forces, economic forces, and political forces. The various theories of management were reviewed as follows: the classical theory, the behavioral theory with its human relations approach, the quantitative management theory, the general systems theory, and the contingency theory. Within these theories the contributions of various individuals such as Taylor, Fayol, Mayo, Maslow, and McGregor were highlighted. The systems theory and contingency theory were discussed as potential approaches to management.

Last, consideration was given to the application of these theories to therapeutic recreation management. Initial consideration was given to questions the manager might want to ask regarding what theory is best to use in a particular situation. Thereafter it was indicated that the management functions outlined by Fayol and expanded on throughout the years will be used as a guide in this text. Further, goal achievement cannot be obtained without consideration of individual needs, perceptions, and aspirations. Perhaps the most logical theoretical approach to management discussed was the use of the contingency theory which stresses situational appropriateness in solving complex problems of today.

# Discussion Questions

1. Why should a student in therapeutic recreation who is considering therapeutic recreation management as a career goal know management theory?
2. What weaknesses in scientific management led to the emphasis on human relations?
3. Taylor gave us some scientific principles of management. Contingency proponents now argue that "it all depends." Do you agree or disagree with the contingency proponents? Explain your position.
4. What do you perceive as the main difference between managing a human service division or department such as a therapeutic recreation department and managing a small business? Would the same skills, attitudes, and body of knowledge be appropriate for each?
5. Do you think the contingency approach will succeed? Why or why not?
6. Why review the historical development of management thought? Why not simply review the current state of management knowledge?
7. Of the principle management theories or approaches discussed, which one do you find most appealing to you as a therapeutic recreation manager of a therapeutic recreation department in a general medical hospital and in a community-based parks and recreation department?

# References

Barnard, C. I. (1938). *The functions of the executive.* Cambridge, MA: Harvard University Press.

Boulding, K. E. (1968). General systems theory—The skeleton of science. In W. Buckley, *Modern systems research for the behavioral scientist.* Chicago, IL: Aldine Publishing.

Carter, M. J., Van Andel, G. E., and Robb, G. M. (1995). *Therapeutic recreation: A practical approach* (2nd ed.). Prospect Heights, IL: Waveland Press, Inc.

DeGreen, K. B. (1973). *Sociotechnical systems.* Englewood Cliffs, NJ: Prentice Hall.

Fayol, H. (1949). *General and industrial management* (C. Starrs, Trans.). London, UK: Isacc Pitman and Sons.

Griffin, R. W. (1990). *Management* (3rd ed.). Boston, MA: Houghton Mifflin Co.

Gulick, L. (1947). Notes on the theory of organizations. In L. Gulick and L. F. Urwick (Eds.), *Papers on the science of administration* (pp. 15–30). New York, NY: Columbia Press.

Gunn, S. L., and Peterson, C. A. (1978). *Therapeutic recreation program design: Principles and procedures.* Englewood Cliffs, NJ: Prentice Hall.

Hax, A. C., and Majluf, N. S. (1984). *Strategic management: An integrative perspective.* Englewood Cliffs, NJ: Prentice Hall.

Kast, F. E., and Rosenzweig, J. E. (1985). *Organizations and management: A systems approach* (4th ed.). New York, NY: McGraw-Hill.

Koontz, H., O'Donnell, C., and Weihrich, H. (1980). *Management* (7th ed.). New York, NY: McGraw-Hill.

Koontz, H. (1961, December). The management theory jungle. *Journal of the Academy of Management, 4:3,* 178–188.

Kreitner, R. (1992). *Management* (5th ed.). Boston, MA: Houghton Mifflin Co.

Lewin, K. (1951). *Field theory in social science.* New York, NY: Harper.

McGregor, D. (1960). *The human side of enterprise.* New York, NY: McGraw-Hill.

Maslow, A. (1968). *Toward a psychology of being* (2nd ed.). New York, NY: Van Nostrand.

Maslow, A. (1954). *Motivation and personality.* New York, NY: Harper.

Mayo, E. (1933). *The human problems of an industrial civilization.* New York, NY: Macmillian.

McGregor, D. (1960). *The Human Side of Enterprise.* New York: McGraw-Hill.

Ouchi, W. G. (1981). *Theory Z: How American business can meet the Japanese challenge.* Reading, MA: Addison-Wesley Publishing Co., Inc.

Peters, T. J., and Waterman, R. H., Jr. (1982). *In search of excellence.* New York, NY: Warner Books.

Riley, B. (1991). Quality assessment: The use of outcome indicators. In B. Riley (Ed.), *Quality management: Applications for therapeutic recreation* (pp. 53–67). State College, PA: Venture Publishing, Inc.

Robbins, S. P. (1995). *Supervision today.* Englewood Cliffs, NJ: Prentice Hall.

Robbins, S. P. (1980). *The administrative process.* Englewood, NJ: Prentice Hall.

Saxe, J. G. (1936). The blind men and the elephant. In H. Felleman (Ed.), *The best-loved poems of the American people* (pp. 521–522). New York, NY: Doubleday and Company.

Shetty, Y. K. (1974). Contingency management: Current perspective for managing organizations. *Management International Review, 14:6,* 114–123.

Shortell, S. M., Kaluzny, A. D., and associates. (1988). *Healthcare management: A text in organization theory and behavior* (2nd ed.). New York, NY: John Wiley & Sons.

Toffler, A. (1970). *Future shock.* New York, NY: Bantam Books.

Urwick, L. F. (1944). *The elements of administration.* New York, NY: Harper & Row.

von Bertalanffy, L. (1972, December). The history and status of general systems theory. *Academy of Management Journal, 15,* 447–465.

Weber M. (1947). *The theory of social and economic organizations* (A. Henderson and T. Parsons, Trans.). New York, NY: The Free Press.

Wren, D. (1987). *The evolution of management theory* (3rd ed.). New York, NY: John Wiley & Sons.

# Chapter 3
# Functions of Management

## Introduction

The management process is universal. It is used in one's personal and professional life. It applies to management of oneself, a consumer, a group of consumers, or a group of practitioners.

The management process is composed of four major functions: (1) planning, (2) organizing, (3) directing, and (4) controlling. They represent the breaking down of the managerial job into its principal parts. However, one should recognize that managers' jobs are shaped by the organizations in which they work. As the organization and its environment change, so does the managerial role (Shortell, Kaluzny and associates, 1988).

Planning is an organized managerial function of establishing the basic direction and objectives and of laying out a design for reaching the objectives. It is deciding what to do, how to do it, and who is to do it. Further, it is a disciplined way of implementing the sequence of major tasks to meet goals. Because planning bridges the gap from where one is to where one wants to be, it is the most basic of the four functions. Organizing involves determining the activities necessary to accomplish the plans, grouping them, assigning them to specific positions and individuals, and delegating the requisite authority. Directing is principally the managerial function of leading or supervising subordinates toward the achievement of objectives. Finally, the controlling function compares performance with established objectives and, if necessary, initiates corrective action. Each of these functions and the activities associated with these functions is performed by every professional manager at every management level. The differences are in magnitude and frequency.

While in theory there is a distinct sequence in performance of the management process, in practice, however, things do not work out so neatly. Ideally a therapeutic recreation manager would plan a specific program, organize for its accomplishment, direct the staff who would be involved in the delivery of the program, and ultimately control its progress. Unfortunately, any one of these functions could be short-circuited. A final confounding factor is that few managers have the luxury of working on only one project at a time. The typical manager is involved in several, if not many, undertakings simultaneously.

Are some managerial functions more important than others? No! Clearly, all functions are of equal importance because in the aggregate they comprise the managerial job. Neglecting any one function will lead to ineffective performance. On the other hand, not all managers spend an equal amount of time on each function. Researchers have noted that the amount of time spent on each function is influenced by management level. For instance, top-level managers spend most of their time on strategic adaptation, planning and organizing functions. Middle managers spend most of their time on directing and organizing functions, system support and maintenance, and first-line managers spend most of their time on directing and coordinating the activities of subordinates (Gray and Smeltzer, 1989).

Given this very brief introduction to the management process and its functions, this chapter will now review in somewhat more depth these functions including time management. Each section offers an overview of what is involved in that function from a broad perspective as well as highlighting one or two elements as they relate to therapeutic recreation management.

# Management Functions

## *Planning*

The first element of management defined by Fayol (1949) is planning. He defined it as making a plan of action to provide for the future. In most instances, planning is proactive although it may be reactive. Reactive planning is done in response to a problem (e.g., failure to achieve approval of services by a regulatory agency).

As was noted earlier, planning is the foundation and framework for all of the other management functions. It is a comprehensive process that includes setting goals, developing plans, and incorporating related activities. It is sort of a plan or perish concept. Every manager has a planning function to perform. Planning is not only concentrated among top-level managers. Although it is true that top managers may devote more of their time to planning and work with more vital issues than do managers at the middle or lower levels, the fact remains that every manager has planning to perform within his or her particular area of activities.

If correctly done, planning takes much of the risk out of decision making and problem solving. Moreover, planning improves with yearly experiences, gives sequence in activities, and protects against undesirable organizational changes. Last, it helps to ensure that probable outcomes will be desirable ones in terms of the use of human resources, budget, and service. As an example, Figure 3.1 depicts those management tasks required of a therapeutic recreation manager in association with program planning within a community-based leisure service agency as suggested by Carter, Browne, LeConey, and Nagle (1991). One will note that the therapeutic recreation process format is used in the management plan.

The statement of the vision, mission, purpose, philosophy, goals, objectives, standards, policies, and procedures are all consequences of planning. Conceptual thinking and problem solving are also crucial in planning. Data are gathered and analyzed so that alternatives can be identified and evaluated in the decision-making process. The manager must forecast what is needed for the future, set objectives for the desired results, and develop strategies for how to achieve the goals. Priorities must be set, and strategies need to be sequenced in a time frame to accomplish the goals. Policies and procedures are developed in the planning phase. Policies are standing decisions concerning recurring matters and procedures of standardized methods.

Budgets are used as planning and controlling tools to allocate resources. Planning is the basis for time management which will in turn facilitate the implementation of the plans.

Planning is the essential link between good intentions and action. Without it good ideas rarely become realities. Good planning requires that a manager have a broad knowledge of the organization's operations and goals, detailed knowledge of the division or department, technical knowledge, and intuition. A keen awareness of the changes and current internal and external trends affecting the area of service delivery is also needed.

Planning is the assessment of the therapeutic recreation department's strengths and weaknesses, covering factors that affect performance and facilitate or inhibit the achievement of objectives.

Planning implies writing specific, useful, realistic objectives (the *why*) that will reflect both strategic and operational goals for the department of therapeutic recreation and its personnel. Objectives become the reasons behind an operational therapeutic recreation management plan (the *what*) that will detail activities to be performed, the target dates or time frames for their accomplishment (the *when*), the persons responsible for accomplishing them (the *who*), and strategies for dealing with the technical, economic, social, and political aspects. These operational plans will have control systems for monitoring performance and providing feedback. To recall general systems theory, planning is an open system. The summary of planning describes the work of the department; it gives outsiders a bird's-eye view of its totality.

Many practitioners falsely believe that once a plan has been developed and published it is, in fact, "carved in stone." This is definitely not the case. Flexibility is essential in the planning process. The written plan represents only an interim report. Therefore, planning is not simply an act at a point in time but rather an ongoing process that does not have a final conclusion or finite end point. This dynamic nature of planning is essential to ensure the relevancy of the plan and its resultant decisions to reality. If plans are not revised and reevaluated on an ongoing basis, they soon develop a greater divergency with reality and this divergency increases with the passage of time. Competent managers advocate changing plans at any moment along the way if the change will bring in facilitative resources and alterations. The incompetent manager is one who sticks to the original plan even though it is outdated and changes would be productive.

Planning is an intellectual process based on facts and information, not on emotions or wishes. Planning is a continuous process of assessing and establishing goals and objectives, and implementing and evaluating them (Figure 3.2). The process is subject to change as new facts become known so as to ensure or achieve organization goals for the present and the future.

### Figure 3.1 Management Plan Tasks

**Assessment:**
- Identify assessment techniques and resources
- Prepare assessment instruments
- Organize advisory committee
- Collect data from participants
- Collect data from agency
- Collect data from community
- Analyze collected data

**Planning:**
- Develop philosophy and program structure
- Select program content
- Identify leadership needs
- Prepare management plan
- Prepare participant and staff schedules
- Prepare program resources
- Develop operating policies and procedures
- Develop risk management plan
- Oversee budget functions
- Prepare documentation and recordkeeping procedures
- Develop staff training
- Prepare marketing program
- Develop evaluation plan

**Implementation:**
- Conduct program registration
- Complete individual participant assessments
- Write individual participant plans
- Conduct activities
- Complete formative participant/program evaluations
- Monitor budget functions and staffing
- Conduct staff supervision and development
- Inspect and document health/safety and participant involvement
- Monitor and communicate with market audiences
- Adjust programs and services

**Evaluation:**
- Conduct summative evaluations on participants/programs
- Analyze collected data
- Update participant files
- Update documentation and recordkeeping procedures
- Adjust budget, staff, programs, and services
- Revise risk management, marketing, and staff training programs
- Prepare transition information
- Prepare final program report
- Present report to Advisory Committee

Source: Carter, M. J., Browne, B., LeConey, S. P., and Nagle, C. J. (1991). *Designing therapeutic recreation programs in the community.* Reston, VA: American Alliance for Health, Physical Education, Recreation and Dance. Reproduced with permission from the American Alliance for Health, Physical Education, Recreation and Dance, Reston, VA 22091.

### Figure 3.2 The Continuous Planning Process

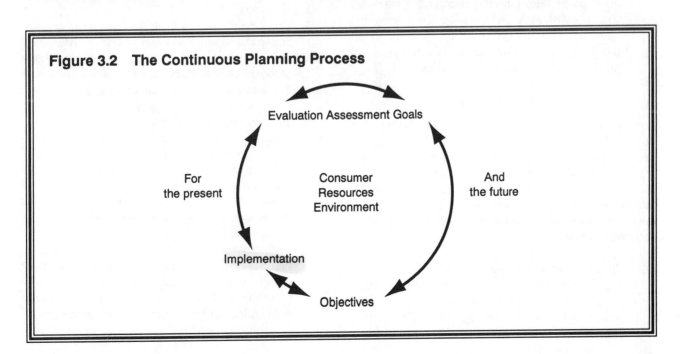

## Resistance to Planning

Unfortunately, many managers resist planning. Absence of formalized planning leads to uncertainty, chaos, and failure. Planning is so basic to management that it must be done whether managers find it easy or not. Understanding factors which contribute to the avoidance of the planning process may help therapeutic recreation managers develop strategies to offset the resistance. According to Kolb (1974), failure of managers to plan may be attributed to one or more of the following factors:

1. Managers may lack knowledge of the philosophy, goals, and working of the organization.
2. Managers may not understand the significance of the planning process, that success or failure of work activities relate directly to the quality of the plan.
3. Time spent on planning often seems wasted in relation to the day-to-day doing of one's job. Planning is only one of many activities competing for the manager's attention.
4. Some managers fearing failure may lack confidence. Planning often involves thinking, paperwork, and "time alone" activities. The manager may feel insecure in his or her ability to formulate plans and does not want anyone else to know the plans were poorly thought out or could not be accomplished.
5. Some managers prefer to act on immediate problems because they generate immediate feedback. Planning deals with the future, and rewards (if any) are deferred.
6. Planning may bring unwanted change. A general fear or reluctance may exist because there are so many possibilities for unexpected and/or unfavorable results or that implementation of plans may require new activities and goals that the manager is unwilling or unable to engage in. The manager may prefer the security of established goals.

## Reasons for Planning

If planning is difficult and most managers would prefer to do other things, why should managers plan? There are good and valid reasons for doing so. The following list is a compilation of reasons given by Douglas Gehrman (1989), manager of the Exxon Company U.S.A. that applies to therapeutic recreation administration, as well. Collectively, the reasons for planning include efficiency, effectiveness, accountability, and morale:

1. **Planning increases chances of success by focusing on results, not activities.** Most studies on planning have been done in the business sector and have shown that although planning does not guarantee success, planners consistently outperform non-planners. Planning helps focus on objectives, and employees can see the result of their labor. Knowing the objectives of the enterprise helps employees relate what they are doing to meaningful outcomes. This principle can be applied to hospitals and other healthcare agencies.
2. **Planning forces analytical thinking and evaluation of alternatives, thus improving decisions.** Through the reasoning process the manager seeks to minimize risk and maximize opportunity.
3. **Planning establishes a framework for decision making consistent with top management's objectives.** The overall planning process in any organization is a top-to-bottom proposition. Top managers set broader objectives with longer term horizons than do lower level managers. In effect, this downward flow of objectives creates a mean-end chain.
4. **Planning orients people to action instead of reaction.** For any given period, the best use is made of available resources, guesswork is eliminated, and the manager can successfully direct his or her activities with foresight, influence, and action.
5. **Planning includes day-to-day managing as well as future-focused managing.** The daily pressures of determining how specific tasks can best be accomplished on time with available resources are important and must be addressed, but the manager must look beyond the immediate focus to the future and plan how to pursue the organization's long-term goals.
6. **Planning helps avoid crisis management and provides decision-making flexibility.** When plans anticipate emergencies, they allow the worker to function more calmly and efficiently when an actual crisis occurs.
7. **Planning provides a basis for measuring organizational and individual performance.** Managers can evaluate the environment, resources, and employees' effectiveness when the expected is known. The entire planning process leads to a continuous inspection of assessment, goal and objective setting, and implementation of plans.
8. **Planning increases employee involvement and improves communications.** Although time-consuming, employee involvement in how things are to be done and by whom creates a feeling of ownership and therefore a strong commitment achievement.
9. **Planning helps one discover the need for change.** Planning can point out opportunities for new or different services. It guides management thinking to future desirable activities, indicates how best to make change, and directs attainment of goals. Change is occurring in all sectors and certainly in the health field which has become one of the biggest industries in the United States.

10. **Planning is cost effective.** Costs of health services are accelerating at a rapid rate. Although many fiscal matters are beyond the manager's control, particularly at the lower levels of management, some costs can be contained through planning for efficient operation.

Efficiency is always desirable. The aim is to achieve goals with a minimum of cost and effort. This occurs only through careful planning which is an anticipatory process. In therapeutic recreation, regardless of setting, practitioners and resources are limited so it is particularly important to provide services as efficiently as possible.

Effectiveness is extremely important. If activities are not planned, the desired results may not be achieved. In therapeutic recreation service, the main goal is, of course, to help people. If practitioner efforts and organization and department resources are diffused, and planning involving unity of purpose and integration of effort does not occur, the level of achievement will be low. Thus the therapeutic recreation manager must do effective planning to create an environment in which therapeutic recreation practitioners will give the service desired and needed by consumers.

Planning is needed for evaluation and accountability. Today public-spirited citizens, legislators, community leaders, and top managers are asking valid questions. What are the results of therapeutic recreation services? Can one afford them? Can one improve them? These and other questions can be answered only as therapeutic recreation managers plan carefully in relation to specific objectives and evaluation procedures for measuring their programs and services. Proper planning makes it possible to carry out an objective evaluation of services.

Careful planning is essential for the morale of the therapeutic recreation department. Practitioners need feelings of achievement and satisfaction in order to perform their best. Such feelings are engendered when the manager and practitioners work together in the planning process making it possible for each practitioner to feel needed and effective. A department that makes it possible for each practitioner to understand exactly what to do and how to do it provides an emotional and administrative climate that is conducive to high morale. How the staff feels will make a difference in the delivery of therapeutic recreation services.

## Strategic, Operational, and Contingency Planning

Strategic planning refers to determining the long-term objectives within the organization and the policies used to achieve these objectives. It means looking at where one is, where one wants to go, and how to reach the desired destination. This type of planning is usually carried out by the chief administrator of the hospital or the superintendent or director of the department of parks and recreation. Although lower level managers (e.g., middle and first-line managers) are not directly involved in strategic planning, they are affected by the strategic plan since it will determine both the objectives they must achieve and the means by which they can do so.

Strategic planning provides a forecast for anywhere from three years to more than ten years. Strategic planning establishes a mission, collects and analyzes data, assesses strengths and weaknesses, sets goals and objectives, uses strategies, operates on a timetable, gives operational and functional guidance to the therapeutic recreation managers, and evaluates. It is important that therapeutic recreation managers have input into strategic planning; however, it is realized that such an opportunity will vary within each organization. Turpel (1992, p. 72) sees the benefits of the strategic planning process as follows:

1. identifies unique strengths and builds strategies for the future on the basis of those strengths;
2. provides a workable mechanism for cooperation among all "players;"
3. separates fact from fiction and tests conventional "wisdom;"
4. places critical issues and problems in the perspective of larger trends;
5. focuses available energy and resources on the top priorities;
6. shapes a vision of the future that provides a touchstone for all involved parties;
7. recruits and develops the leaders of tomorrow; and
8. fosters effective action (gets things done).

Operational planning is performed at the department or service level. Operational planning is usually associated with a specific service within the therapeutic recreation department. For example, a therapeutic recreation manager would assist or have input into developing the overall strategic plan but would only develop departmental goals, objectives, and operational plans related specifically to the department.

Operational plans consist of everyday working management plans. They are developed from both short- and long-range goals and objectives based on the strategic planning process. In development of operational plans new strategic objectives can emerge or old ones can be modified. Strategic plans and objectives are made into operational plans and carried out at all levels of management, not just at the first-line management level.

First-line managers develop strategies, goals, objectives, and time frames in order to accomplish the overall strategic plan. They match each department goal or objective to a strategic goal or objective. Departmental goals and objectives may be more detailed and specific than the overall strategic goals and objectives. There can also be numerous departmental objectives that support one strategic objective.

Goals are critical not only to the organization but also to the department. Goals serve four important purposes as noted by Richards (1986). First, they provide guidance and a unified direction for the practitioners in the department. Goals can help practitioners understand where the department is going and why getting there is important. Second, as an outgrowth of guidance, planning is facilitated. Goals and planning are interrelated. Third, goals can serve as a source of motivation and inspiration for staff. Goals that are specific and moderately difficult can motivate people to work harder, especially if attaining the goal is likely to result in rewards. Last, goals provide an effective mechanism for evaluation and control.

Operational planning at the department level is related to the delivery of direct program services. It involves matching practitioners to responsibilities, developing policies and procedures specific to the delivery of services, identifying training needs, preparing and conducting training programs, supervising personnel, and evaluating. Evaluation takes place on a continuing basis. Depending on the results, modifications are made in the implementation of the plan as deemed appropriate.

Contingency planning refers to identifying and dealing with the many problems that interfere with getting work done. Some examples of potential problems are new, inexperienced staff who do not know the policies and procedures of the organization well and may not be very committed to it; volunteer tardiness or staff absenteeism which leaves the department short of personnel (sick days, holidays, weekends, or vacations); physician request for a special service or program and unavailability of supplies or equipment at that time; and staff quitting without giving notice. Once aware of possible contingencies, the therapeutic recreation manager must be alert to detect their occurrence before they are out of control. Finally, therapeutic recreation managers should ask themselves what activities are necessary to prevent problems from happening and what the plans are for dealing with problems once they have occurred? For example, does the department have plans for dealing with certain kinds of disasters—external disasters, like the floods in the Midwest and the earthquakes in California in 1993 and 1994 that prevented therapeutic recreation practitioners from getting to work, or internal disasters such as loss of power?

The statement of the department vision, mission or purpose, philosophy, goals, objectives, policies, and procedures are all consequences of planning and will be considered in forthcoming chapters.

## Organizing

Organizing is the second managerial function which grows out of the planning phase. It refers to the grouping of activities and resources into organizational units such as departments or sections and staffing these departments. In addition, organizing includes the assignment of such groupings to a manager who has authority for supervising each group and the defined means for coordinating appropriate activities with other departments, horizontally and vertically, to achieve organizational objectives. Last, organizing involves establishing an organizational structure in order to develop and attain the organization's mission including goals and objectives.

The grouping of activities and resources into a department is usually based on function according to similarity of skills or tasks necessary to accomplish a goal. This arrangement by function, according to Gray and Smeltzer (1989), is far and away the most prevalent method of grouping activities. Logical and simple, it minimizes coordination, contributes to economical operation, and reduces the need for interdependence. Moreover, functional structures are usually stable, foster good communication, and managing the coordination of tasks is easily achieved. In addition, recruitment is enhanced because a cadre of professional colleagues can help attract other professionals.

Functional structures also have their disadvantages. Functional structures are rigid and frequently neither prepare practitioners for the future nor train or test them. Functional managers are confronted with situations involving only their narrow field of specialty. In addition, professional skills are emphasized over organizational goals. Its inherent stress on specialization has a tendency to push the decision-making process upward, because only at the top does one find the confluence of all input required for a final decision.

Having organized, a manager now considers personnel to implement the mission of the department with efficiency and effectiveness. Relationships are delineated relative to the department structure and described in position descriptions that define the scope of responsibilities, relationships, and authority. Job analysis, evaluation, and design help define qualifications for practitioners in each position within the structure (see Chapter 13, Staffing). Finally, physical resources that are needed are identified.

Therapeutic recreation specialists practice in many different types of health and human service organizations. The nature of the structure of these organizations can vary extensively based on the type of ownership (e.g., not-for-profit or for-profit), goals, needs, size, environment, and resources of the organization. In healthcare facilities, the range of healthcare services according to West (1995, p. 159), include "diagnosis, treatment, rehabilitation, education, and prevention and health promotion." Furthermore, a significant development in the last ten years in healthcare (e.g., hospitals) has been the growing trend toward multihospital mergers which have taken on varied corporate forms. As a result there is disagreement among organizational theorists as to what kind of structure is best for specific organizations (Hammer and Champy, 1993). Therapeutic recreation in the community is another example of how organization or program structure affects the task of therapeutic recreation management (see Figure 3.3).

A structure can be highly centralized and specialized or systems based depending on decision-making responsibility and participation. It can be departmentalized by joining all the people who perform a specific function, or it can build teams of people with differing but complimentary skills. It can use traditional hierarchical designs or experiment with task forces, committees, or even leaderless groups. More about teams and leaderless groups is found in Chapter 6.

Without effective structural organization, people are working in a situation of uncertainty and, perhaps, even chaos. They do not know who is responsible for what.

They do not know who has authority for decision making. They do not know how the various jobs and departments are linked together. Obviously, such a state of affairs is a serious impediment to individual and group productivity. Efficiency, effectiveness, and morale would go down.

Basically, most healthcare organizations and community-based leisure service agencies are conservative in the way they are structured. The hierarchical structure is still largely predominant because managers believe the hierarchic format offers a model for placing large numbers of people into a structure that can be easily identified and programmed. It also provides for easy performance evaluation, promotion based on seniority and achievement, and more fair distribution of awards.

Recently, teams have begun to surface in some healthcare organizations as well as in the matrix organizational structure. The latter structure combines service and functional structure, is less rigid than the traditional functional structure, and opens horizontal barriers that a strictly functional structure imposes. According to the gurus of reengineering, Hammer and Champy (1993), the matrix

---

## Figure 3.3  Management Continuum: Therapeutic Recreation in the Community

**Autonomy**

| | | | |
|---|---|---|---|
| Therapeutic recreation program as distinct entity | Therapeutic recreation as a distinct unit parallel to other health and social service units | Therapeutic recreation grouped with another professional group, such as social work or occupational therapy | Therapeutic recreation under another professional group |

**Settings**

| | | | |
|---|---|---|---|
| Private camp, special recreation associations | Public leisure service departments, nonprofit agencies | Education and school models, advocacy groups | Youth agencies, private consulting agencies |

**Philosophy**

| | | | |
|---|---|---|---|
| Provide comprehensive service continuum, enhance client functional capacity, maintain health status and community quality of life | Provide comprehensive service continuum, focus on education, health promotion and maintaining functional capacity in the community | Service focus on education, health promotion, and maintaining community quality of life | Service focus on education, health promotion, community leisure experiences |

**Tasks**

| | | | |
|---|---|---|---|
| Complete array of management tasks | Management tasks focus on training, marketing, funding, advocacy, resource utilization, as well as direct service | Management tasks include advocacy, funding, marketing, as well as direct service | Management of direct services, fundraising, marketing |

Source: Carter, M. J., Van Andel, G. E., and Robb, G. M. (1995). *Therapeutic recreation: A practical approach* (2nd ed.). Prospect Heights, IL: Waveland Press, Inc. Reproduced with permission.

structure is the structure to be used because healthcare organizations are so complex today. (Reengineering is defined as "the fundamental rethinking and radical redesign of business processes to achieve dramatic improvement in critical, contemporary measures of performance, such as cost, quality, service, and speed" [Hammer and Champy, 1993, p. 32].)  Blancett and Flarey (1995, p. 83) note the following regarding reengineering healthcare facilities:

> Through reengineering newer organizational structure will evolve.  These newer structures will be focused on simplicity so that organization can respond more quickly to rapid changes in both the internal and external environments.

Regardless of what evolves, the success of any organizational design is largely dependent on the manager's skills.

The following figures depict various organizational structures through organizational charts.  The reader needs to remember that an organizational chart is a drawing that shows how the parts of an organization are linked.  It depicts the formal organizational relationships, areas of responsibility, persons accountable, and channels of communication.  However, an organizational chart is meaningful only to the extent that the system represented on paper is a reality.  The organizational chart, like milk, may be dated but not fresh.  Its precision sometimes masks what is actually taking place in the organization.  In addition, organizational charts alone do not explain functions in great detail but must be joined by written job descriptions that can provide additional information.

Figure 3.4 shows the conventional midsize hospital hierarchical organization chart while Figure 3.5 (page 34) presents a hospital matrix organization design which illustrates the dual reporting relationships wherein the practitioner reports to the department manager as well as the unit manager (e.g., rehabilitation unit).

The organization chart of Sheltering Arms Physical Rehabilitation Hospital, a freestanding rehabilitation hospital in Richmond, Virginia, is shown in Figure 3.6 (page 35).  Therapeutic recreation services are found within the Inpatient Services (i.e., Team I and II) and Outpatient Services and Referral Development (i.e., Day Rehabilitation Program within Neuro Services).  The Day Rehabilitation Program has two community site locations.  In Teams I and II, therapeutic recreation practitioners are integrated into interdisciplinary teams providing individual treatment programs while co-leading and participating in co-treatment groups.  In the Day Rehabilitation Program (i.e., outpatient) at both sites, customers are seen individually in therapeutic recreation in addition to co-treatment groups and community outings as needed.  Recently, Sheltering Arms initiated a Community Recreation Program which is open to any interested disabled individual and is not limited to individuals currently receiving treatment or those who have previously received treatment from Sheltering Arms.  The program includes clinics, tournaments, and special events which are leisure and recreational activity oriented as well as providing individualized activity skill development within the community.

A community-based leisure service agency, the Los Angeles Department of Recreation and Parks' organizational chart is shown in Figure 3.7 (page 36).  Therapeutic recreation is found within the Adaptive Recreation Section which is in the organizational structure of Special Recreation Services (see Figure 3.8, page 37).

A factor that needs to be remembered in the organizational structure of a healthcare facility (e.g., hospital) is the unique relationship between the authority of the healthcare organization and the authority of its medical staff.  Consequently, a healthcare facility frequently has parallel structures rather than one organizational structure.  This arrangement is often called the "shadow organization" (Trent, 1986).  The medical staff usually is separate and autonomous from the organization; it has its own admission requirements, hierarchy, rewards, and sanctions.  In recent years however, physicians have taken on greater management and administrative responsibilities (e.g., medical director or vice president for medical services) within general medical hospitals as the result of hospital mergers, rapidly changing concepts of delivery of healthcare, healthcare costs, and the expertise and judgment of physicians to assist the administrative staff in decision making to name a few reasons.

## Governance Structure

Regardless of setting or type of ownership the function of the governance structure is best understood as an interface between the demands of the external world and the operations of the internal organization.

Traditional government community-based leisure service agencies have a recreation board or commission governance structure which reflect both policy and advisory responsibilities.  The members are either appointed or selected to the governance body as part of the political process.  In addition, the commission is responsible for selecting (and firing) the director of the department.  In summary, the director selects and supervises all other employees of the department, coordinates the design and operation of the organizational structure, and represents the commission internally and externally.  Literally, the director is an agent for the commission and in essence is the servant of the commission.

Private community-based leisure service agencies, nonprofit voluntary organizations, community agencies serving specific disabilities, and various other types of community

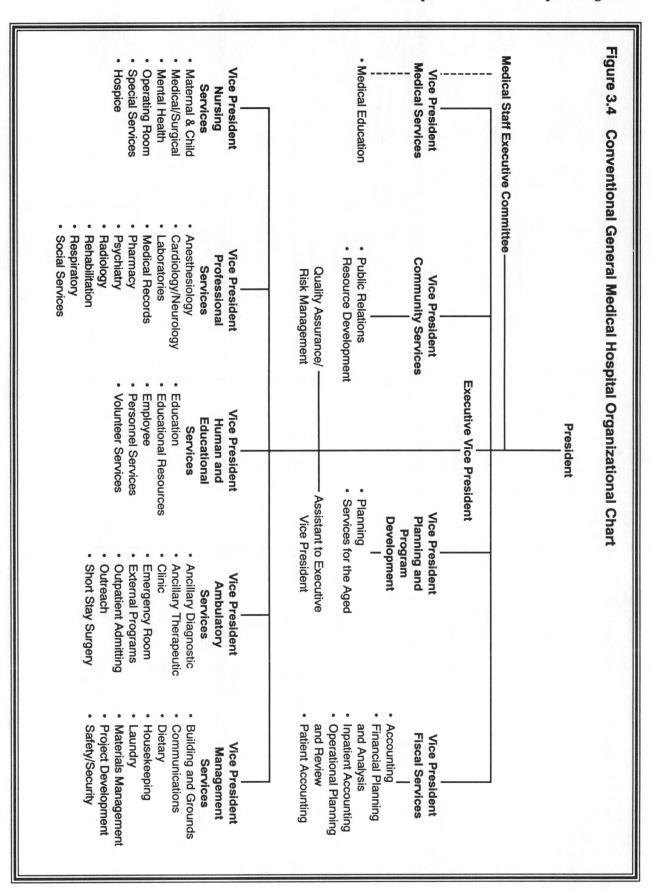

**Figure 3.4 Conventional General Medical Hospital Organizational Chart**

**Figure 3.5   Matrix Organization Design**

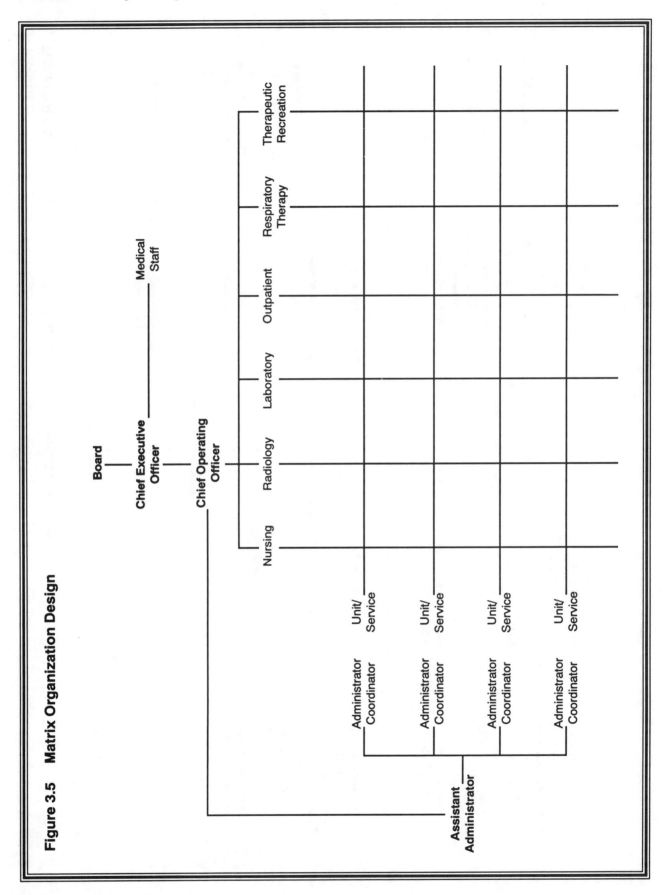

**Figure 3.6   Organizational Chart, Sheltering Arms Physical Rehabilitation Hospital**

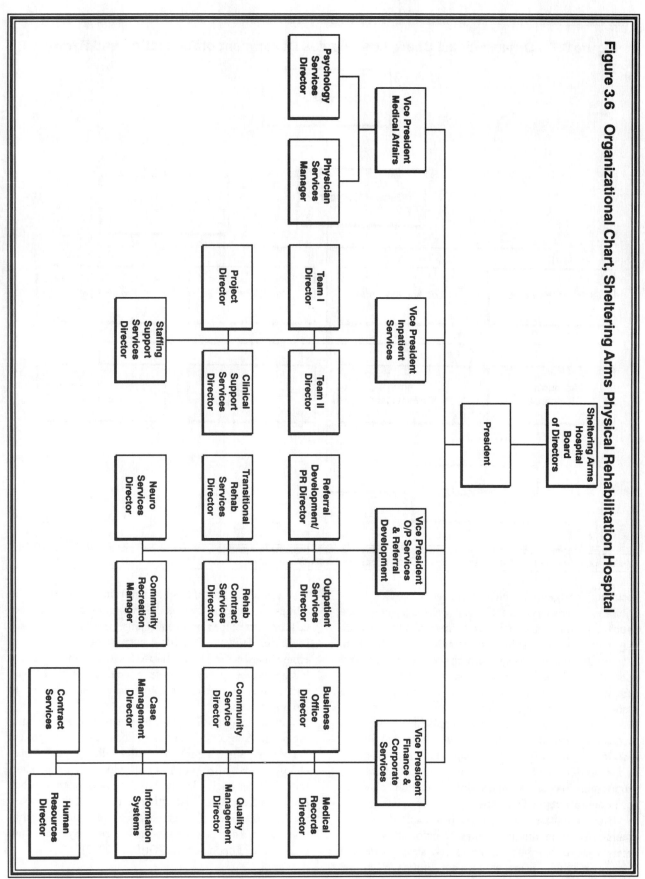

Used by permission of Sheltering Arms Physical Rehabilitation Hospital, Richmond, VA.

**Figure 3.7   Organizational Chart, Los Angeles Department of Recreation and Parks**

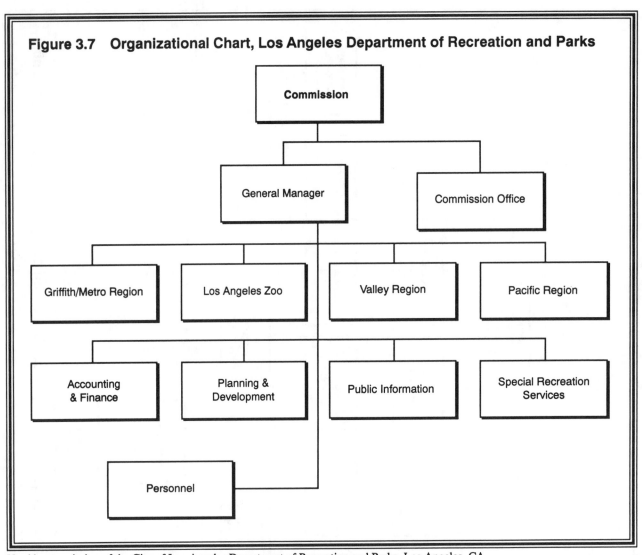

Used by permission of the City of Los Angeles Department of Recreation and Parks, Los Angeles, CA.

social service agencies which coordinate or provide recreation and leisure services and resources have a governance structure similar in nature to the public sector although each may have a unique variation in its organization and function.

Similar in nature to a governing board is the advisory committee. There are many public community-based leisure service agencies which have an advisory committee associated with their therapeutic recreation department. This committee usually has a liaison relationship with the recreation board and commission. Its membership reflects individuals who assist in identifying the recreational needs of the disabled and may also represent special interest groups (e.g., Special Olympics, United Cerebral Palsy, Association for Retarded Citizens).

The committee's major input is associated with the planning function although it may be involved with budgetary matters. Its legal status varies from state to state, and it may or may not operate within a constitution or bylaws.

Administration of hospitals and similar healthcare facilities has become increasingly complex in the past decade because of the significant changes that have taken place in service delivery. The basic purpose of a hospital governing board is similar in nature to that of community-based leisure service agencies—to set policy, review the budget, and represent views of the community or shareholders to the organization.

In the for-profit hospital, the focus is upon maximizing profit. Subject to legal restrictions designed to protect the owners, board members, usually called directors, may choose to maximize profit in either the long or the short run. They may sell all or part of the assets whenever they choose and they may discontinue all parts of the business and liquidate assets if investment is not profitable. In addition, they are compensated for their service by salary and/or investment opportunities (Griffith, 1992).

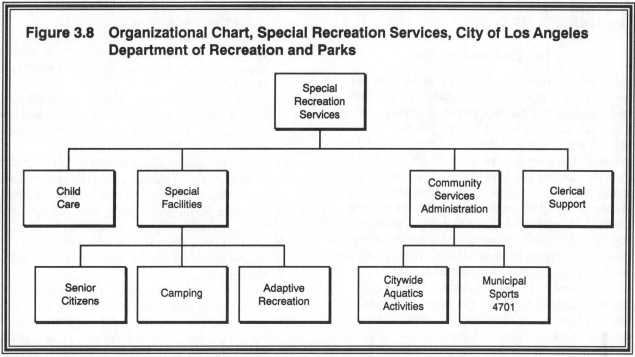

**Figure 3.8 Organizational Chart, Special Recreation Services, City of Los Angeles Department of Recreation and Parks**

Used by permission of the City of Los Angeles Department of Recreation and Parks, Los Angeles, CA.

In not-for-profit hospitals the governing board consists of trustees who are nominated and selected to serve on the board. Their purpose is accepting the assets of the hospital in trust for the community. Profits derived from the operation of the hospital are put back into the hospital and used for the healthcare needs of the community. Trustees may or may not be compensated for service. If compensated, it is usually out-of-pocket expenses associated with board meetings (Griffith, 1992).

Some hospitals owned by large units such as churches, government agencies, and multihospital systems may have no governing board. A director, committee, or group performs the essential functions of a board (Griffith, 1992).

At the corporate level (e.g., Columbia/HCA Healthcare Corporation [for-profit], Carilion Health System [not-for-profit]), the function of the directors or trustees is to elect officers, to establish corporate policies, to supervise the affairs of the corporation, and to carry out the expressed purposes of the bylaws. As related to the hospitals within the corporation, each hospital may only have a director or manager who reports back to the corporation as noted in the previous paragraphs. During the past decade there has been an ever increasing number of healthcare corporations.

While the governing board in either a for-profit or not-for-profit hospital is legally responsible for everything that goes on in the hospital, it delegates this authority and overall responsibility for making decisions for the organization and placing the hospital in a place of effectiveness and efficiency to the chief executive officer (CEO) or president of the hospital. In addition to this specific responsibility,

the board does carry out a number of other essential functions as noted by Griffith (1992, p. 145):

1. establish the vision, mission, and long-range plan;
2. approve the annual budget;
3. appoint members of the medical staff; and
4. monitor performance against plans and budgets.

In most community-based leisure service agencies, the agency director and hospital CEO are empowered to implement the decisions of the commission or board as well as to assist these bodies in making decisions. In order to manage the day-to-day operations, the agency director and CEO rely on an administrative staff with specialized knowledge in financial management, personnel management, public affairs, strategic planning and development, and professional services. In healthcare facilities there is usually a chief operating officer (COO) or senior vice president who is responsible for most of the operating expectations (e.g., resource and revenue expectations, quality of care, quality of work life). In meeting these expectations he or she works through subordinates with titles such as vice president, associate administrator, or assistant administrator depending on the scope of the responsibilities involved. The number of executive or specialized senior administrative staff will depend on the size of the setting and the services provided. In addition, these senior administrators make up an "administrative council" type of structure to promote participative management. They usually meet one or more times a week. All major problems, plans, and budgets are brought by the administrators to these meetings for discussion and resolution (Griffith, 1992).

## Departmentalization

Departmentalization is the allocation of function and responsibilities designed to achieve goals through a formalized arrangement of human and material resources in organizational units. It is the result of the grouping in organizing, as noted earlier, including both advantages and disadvantages. Departmentalization is most appropriate where there is a need for highly specialized expertise to be consolidated. Thus, the therapeutic recreation department in a healthcare facility is considered a functional structure since it provides a specialized service and practitioners perform similar tasks. Special recreation or therapeutic recreation divisions in community-based leisure service organizations would also be considered a functional structure.

The place of the therapeutic recreation department within a healthcare facility and on the organizational chart will vary from facility to facility and influence its scope of service. It may be a separate department reporting to a middle-management administrator, or it may be a unit within a physical medicine and rehabilitation (PM and R) department (see Figures 3.4 and 3.6, pages 33 and 35 respectively). It may even be considered a service wherein therapeutic recreation practitioners are assigned to various treatment teams but have no specific department identification. More and more it appears that therapeutic recreation practitioners are being assigned to interdisciplinary teams but remain identified with a therapeutic recreation department.

A PM and R department is a form of departmentalization since it is considered a functional structure providing specialized services. In this department it is the grouping of activities (e.g., physical therapy, occupational therapy, speech therapy, therapeutic recreation) which might be carried on in other departments or independently but which are brought together in a specialized department for purposes of better service, efficiency, control, or all three.

In community-based leisure service organizations, therapeutic recreation may be an independent division within a department or a special service unit or program section of a department (see Figure 3.8, page 37). Therapeutic recreation services may also be found in a freestanding voluntary agency which focuses specifically on the disabled (i.e., Recreation Center for the Handicapped, San Francisco, California). A study of therapeutic recreation practitioner (N = 833) employment characteristics conducted in 1994 by O'Morrow (1995, p. 8), noted the following location of practitioners within the organizational structure:

8% a unit, section, or division within a municipal park and recreation department;

4% a special recreation district or association;

24% an autonomous unit, section, or department within a general medical hospital or freestanding rehabilitation facility;

16% a unit, section, or department within a rehabilitation unit of a general medical hospital with discipline designations (i.e., occupational therapy, physical therapy, therapeutic recreation);

16% a unit, section, or department within an activity therapy service of a psychiatric institution, residential facility for the mentally retarded, nursing home, etc., with discipline designations (i.e., occupational therapy, physical therapy, therapeutic recreation);

8% a unit, section, or department within an activity service or rehabilitation division with no discipline designations;

5% a unit, section, or department within an occupational therapy or physical therapy department; and

31% other (home healthcare agencies, wellness centers for the disabled, day care centers, camps, group homes, private practice, etc.).

## *Directing*

After the manager has planned and organized, consideration is given to directing personnel and activities to accomplish the goals of the organization. A majority of first-line managers give 50 percent or more of their time to directing (Robbins, 1995; Kraut, 1989). Directing is the connecting link between organizing for work and getting the job done. Directing assures some uniformity of quality and quantity in the work of the staff. Knowledge of one's leadership style, managerial philosophy, sources of power and authority, and political strategies are important. In order to get work done by others, the manager must resolve conflicts, motivate, and discipline staff. All these tasks require good communication skills and assertive behavior.

There are many definitions and concepts of directing. Robin, Fry, and Plovnick (1978), for example, wrote about directing in terms of theories of leadership effectiveness, group dynamics, values and value conflicts, effective interpersonal relationships, working with teams, and managing teams in organizations. Fulmer and Franklin (1982, p. 6) define a manager or supervisor as "someone who is responsible for directing the performance of one or more workers so that organizational goals are accomplished." Rowland and Rowland (1980) note that among the activities of directing are delegation, communication, training, and motivation. On the other hand, Robbins (1995) notes that directing is within the management process of leading. According to Robbins (1995, p. 8): "When managers motivate employees, direct the activities of others, select the most effective communication channel, or resolve conflicts among team members, they are leading."

One may conclude from these definitions and statements that directing is a physical act of therapeutic recreation management—the interpersonal process by which therapeutic recreation personnel accomplish the objectives of the therapeutic recreation department.

To understand fully what directing entails, the therapeutic recreation manager examines the conceptual functions of therapeutic recreation management (i.e., planning and organizing). The therapeutic recreation manager develops management plans of the organization from the statements of vision, mission or purpose, the statement of philosophy or beliefs, and written goals and objectives. Developing such plans involves the process by which methods and techniques are selected and used to accomplish the work of the therapeutic recreation department. Directing or leading is the process of applying the management plans to accomplish therapeutic recreation goals and objectives. It is the process by which therapeutic recreation practitioners are inspired or motivated to accomplish work. Figure 3.9 is an example of a community-based special recreation association vision, mission, and goal statements.

Chapter 6 is entirely devoted to statements of vision, mission, philosophy, and objectives and their development.

The amount of direction needed varies with the knowledge, experience, and initiative of individual practitioners and the staff as a whole. It may take a strict form (e.g., emphasis on clear-cut delegation of responsibility and formal communication), or it may be loose, low-awareness direction (e.g., flexibility, with fluid lines of responsibility and communication). However, everyone needs some direction no matter how small the department. Staff practitioners need to know (1) what is expected of them, and (2) how to do it. A knowledgeable staff practitioner will either know how to do the assigned responsibility or how to obtain information to complete the task. Nevertheless, he or she will still need some direction as to how the responsibilities have been divided among staff. The less experienced, less knowledgeable staff member will also need assistance with the "how to do it" part. This assistance does not necessarily have to come from the therapeutic recreation manager; it may be delegated to an experienced staff practitioner.

The therapeutic recreation manager is responsible for motivating personnel. No matter how fine the plans, nothing usually happens until the people who make up the

---

**Figure 3.9   Vision, Mission, and Goal Statements**

**Vision Statement**
This special recreation association (SRA) is committed to delivery of quality services that enhance the functional capacity, health status, and quality of life of district members with impairments that impact cognitive, psychological, physical, spiritual, social, and leisure well-being. SRA professionals are dedicated to operating with integrity and within the guidelines of professional standards of practice. This SRA intends to augment and enhance member districts' and communities' programs and resources so participants achieve socially appropriate inclusive living and leisure opportunities.

**Mission Statement**
The intent of this SRA is to provide recreational, educational, social, and skill development programs and supportive resources in conjunction with member park districts to individuals with disabilities in order to enhance their social, physical, mental, emotional, spiritual, and leisure well-being, and facilitate their inclusion in the community.

**Goal Statements**
To provide participants the opportunity to participate in year-round social, skill development, educational, and recreational services and programs.
    To provide participants the opportunity to participate in member districts' programs through transitional and integrated programs and services.
    To provide students with opportunities to participate in programs supportive of their educational plans through cooperative programs with the special education district.
    To provide opportunities to community residents that promote awareness of and enhance leisure experiences with individuals with disabilities through information dissemination and public relations.
    To provide opportunities for SRA staff, volunteers, caregivers, and peer professionals to participate in training and education programs.

Source: Carter, M. J., Van Andel, G. E., and Robb, G. M. (1995). *Therapeutic recreation: A practical approach* (2nd ed.). Prospect Heights, IL: Waveland Press, Inc. Reproduced by permission.

department are stimulated to perform. Although money is a motivating power, personnel seek in their work the intrinsic qualities of recognition, achievement, growth, and advancement as was noted in the previous chapter. Frederick Herzberg (1976), called the father of job enrichment, came to the conclusion from his many studies of workers that salaries and salary increases were important factors in fulfilling basic needs but that they were not major motivating factors in work production. Motivation is considered in depth in Chapter 15.

The manager must also be able to communicate effectively, bring about necessary changes, and manage conflict within and between his or her department and other departments. Change, conflict, and communication are three highly interwoven concepts. Some practitioners resist change yet it is necessary if the therapeutic recreation department is to be adaptable. Resistance to change can create conflict; at the same time, conflict can bring about change. Effective communication can facilitate the acceptance of change and help minimize destructive conflict. See Chapter 14 for further discussion of effective communication.

Effective directing increases the contribution of practitioners to the achievement of therapeutic recreation management goals. Effective directing creates harmony between therapeutic recreation management goals and the goals of the therapeutic recreation practitioner. Effective directing operationalizes the principle of unity of command; a practitioner is answerable to one boss as completely as possible. An effective director seeks to understand change, conflict, and communication in order to lead his or her practitioners more effectively.

In addressing responsibilities of the first-line manager, Hellriegel and Slocum (1986) have noted the following criteria:

1. formulates goals and objectives for services that are realistic for the organization, consumer, and therapeutic recreation staff;
2. gives first priority to the needs of the consumer;
3. provides for coordination and efficiency among divisions, departments, and units that provide support service;
4. identifies responsibility for all activities for which the therapeutic recreation staff is responsible;
5. provides for safe, continuous service;
6. considers need for variety in task assignment and for development of personnel;
7. provides for manager's availability to staff for assistance, teaching, counsel, and evaluation;
8. trusts members to follow through with assignments;
9. interprets protocol for responding to incidental requests;
10. explains procedures to be followed in emergencies;
11. gives clear, concise formal and informal directions; and
12. uses a management control process that assesses the quality of service and care given and evaluates the individual performance.

Aspects of directing from a supervisory, leadership, teaching, coaching, decision-making, problem-solving, and conflict management perspective will be considered in more detail in later chapters.

## Controlling

Controlling is the last step in the management process. Fayol (1949, p. 107) defined control as:

> verifying whether everything occurs in conformity with the plan adopted, the instructions issued, and principles established. It has for its object to point out weaknesses and error in order to rectify them and prevent recurrence.

Controlling is closely related to planning for therapeutic recreation managers. The planning function provides the basis upon which the control function is predicated. Feedback from the planning function provides input for the modification and adjustment of the organizational plan. Therefore, one should view planning and control as being closely linked, each influencing the other.

Control includes coordinating numerous activities, making decisions related to planning and organizing activities, and gaining information from directing and evaluating each practitioner's performance. The control function is also concerned with records, reports, organizational progress, and effective use of resources. Finally, control uses standards, regulation, and evaluation to attain organizational goals and objectives.

In healthcare facilities review and regulation of activities are vital because quality of service and care is at stake. Careful monitoring of the cost and use of supplies is a necessity in healthcare facilities and community-based leisure service agencies because of the limited resources available to meet service and care needs.

A systems theory is used in controlling. Feedback and adjustment comprise the control element of therapeutic recreation management. Output is described or defined in terms of the consumer in the program and is measured by quality assurance indicators. When the outcomes or indicators fall short, the information is fed back to the therapeutic recreation practitioner who makes adjustments in the program or treatment plan. Both the consumer and the practitioner are systems input, while the process consists of therapeutic recreation actions related to consumer outcomes and managerial actions related to setting goals for practitioners' behavior. Quality assurance (QA) and continuous quality improvement (CQI) are the processes by which therapeutic recreation is measured and action is taken to correct deficiencies.

Similarly, systems theory can be applied to performance evaluation. For example, input is still the consumer and the practitioner, with process being the managerial actions related to goals of the therapeutic recreation practitioner. A performance evaluation and/or improvement plan between the therapeutic recreation manager and staff practitioner spells out agreed-upon performance goals. The output is corrected actions.

A prime element of the management of therapeutic recreation service is a system for evaluation of the total effort. This includes a system for evaluation of the management process as well as the practice of therapeutic recreation and the delivery of quality service. Evaluation requires standards that can be used as yardsticks for gauging the quality and quantity of services. The key sources for these standards which are available for both management and practice are the American Therapeutic Recreation Association (ATRA) *Standards for the Practice of Therapeutic Recreation and Self-Assessment Guide* (1993) and the National Therapeutic Recreation Society (NTRS) *Standards of Practice for Therapeutic Recreation Service and Annotated Bibliography* (1995), supplemented by the Joint Commission on Accreditation of Healthcare Organizations (JCAHO) and Commission on Accreditation of Rehabilitation Facilities (CARF) standards associated with therapeutic recreation in hospitals and rehabilitation facilities.

Several yardsticks can be developed using these source documents which can be of assistance in developing department objectives. Performance standards can be used for individual performance, and criteria can be developed for evaluation of delivery service. Koontz and Weihrick (1988) have noted that standards are an established criteria of performance based on elements such as planning goals, strategic plans, physical or quantitative measurement of service, cost, programs, and others not specifically related to therapeutic recreation.

A financial control system is implemented by a budget which is defined as a tool for planning, monitoring, and controlling cost, or a systematic plan for meeting expenses (Hellriegel and Slocum, 1986). Budgets form the last link in the management process that began with goals and strategies; they are the most detailed management practice used to ensure that organization and department goals are achieved. Budgets are powerful instruments because they serve as a guide for therapeutic recreation performance and allocation of personnel, supplies, support services, and facilities.

A well-designed therapeutic recreation control system incorporates the following characteristics as suggested by Fulmore and Franklin (1982):

1. controls must reflect the nature of the activity;
2. controls should report errors promptly;
3. controls should be forward-looking;
4. controls should point out exceptions at critical points;
5. controls should be objective;
6. controls should be flexible;
7. controls should reflect the organizational pattern;
8. controls should be economical;
9. controls should be understandable; and
10. controls should indicate corrective action.

In conclusion, control is necessary because internal and external forces affect the intent of departmental goals. Establishing standards is perhaps the first step in the control process. Standards are the gauge against which performance is measured, and different types of standards must be established to measure the various functions within the department.

# Time Management

While one likes to think that the various management functions discussed here can be divided into distinct equal time elements, in reality it is not true. Few managers have the luxury of working on only one project at a time. Time can be a tyrant if one does not learn how to manage it effectively.

The skill of time management enables the first-line manager to separate the important from the unimportant. Time management is a habit pattern characterized by the following points but is not limited to:

1. **Making a written list of "things to do" today.** It is a common sense rule that implies the need to do some advance planning each day in response to upcoming problems and demands and not rely solely on memory.
2. **Prioritize tasks.** Arrange the things to do in order of priority as determined by the expected payoff of each item. Keep in mind that these priorities usually take in both short- and long-term tasks. Don't spend the whole day on one task.
3. **Learn to delegate.** There are many positive reasons for effective delegation. One such reason is that delegation demonstrates a manager's trust and confidence in subordinates which leads to more effective performance and better interpersonal relationships for all.
4. **Control interruptions.** Meeting visitors in the doorway helps managers maintain control of their time by controlling the use of office space. Other factors

associated with this one include having someone else answer calls, having a place to work uninterrupted, and going to practitioners' offices if matters warrant it.

5. **Minimize routine work.** List a few five- or ten-minute tasks. This helps use the small bits of time almost everyone has during his or her day. One can accomplish a lot by doing more than one thing at a time when tasks are routine, trivial, or require little thought.

6. **Know one's own productivity period.** Most individuals know their productivity period. Some are morning people, while others are afternoon people. Managers should handle their most demanding problems during their peak period.

## Summary

This chapter highlighted the traditional four functions of management: planning, organizing, directing, and controlling. It was noted that planning, a principal duty of all managers, is a dynamic, intellectual, future-oriented process directed toward meeting objectives once objectives have been defined. Reasons were given as to why some managers avoid planning. Likewise, reasons were given for planning. Organizing is the grouping of activities into organized units to achieve goals. While there exists various organizational structures, the therapeutic recreation department is a functional structure because it provides a specialized service and practitioners perform similar tasks. Directing initiates and maintains action toward objectives although the amount of direction needed varies with the knowledge, experience, and initiative of the practitioner and the staff as a whole. A list of responsibilities associated with directing and first-line managers was also given. Controlling, the final element of the management process, is the process of seeing that actual expenditures and activities conform to plan. A systems approach is used frequently in controlling. Through this process, standards are established and then applied, followed by feedback that leads to improvement. The process is kept continuous. The last section, time management, considers suggestions for managers in managing their time as related to these management functions.

## Discussion Questions

1. What is the relationship between planning and each of the other management functions?
2. Is any one of the four functions that a manager performs more important than the others? Discuss.
3. In which of the four management functions do you feel your performance would be best? In which, the weakest?
4. Visit a healthcare facility and/or local park and recreation department and note where therapeutic recreation is on the organization chart. Discuss its relationship to middle management and top-level management.
5. Think about a therapeutic recreation division or department, regardless of setting, with which you are familiar. Is it well-managed? How could its effectiveness be improved? Which managerial functions are being performed most effectively?
6. To what extent do you believe that the therapeutic recreation managers you know, regardless of setting, have a clear understanding of their division or department objectives? If, in your opinion, they do not, how would you suggest they go about setting them?

# References

American Therapeutic Recreation Association (ATRA). (1993). Standards for the practice of therapeutic recreation and self-assessment guide. Hattiesburg, MS: Author.

Blancett, S. S., and Flarey, D. L. (1995). *Reengineering nursing and healthcare: The handbook for organizational transformation.* Gaithersburg, MD: Aspen Publishers, Inc.

Carter, M. J., Browne, B., LeConey, S. P., and Nagle, C. J. (1991). *Designing therapeutic recreation programs in the community.* Reston, VA: American Alliance for Health, Physical Education, Recreation and Dance.

Carter, M. J., Van Andel, G. E., and Robb, G. M. (1995). *Therapeutic recreation: A practical approach* (2nd ed.). Prospect Heights, IL: Waveland Press, Inc.

Fayol, H. (1949). *General and industrial management* (C. Starrs, Trans.). London, UK: Isacc Pitman and Sons.

Fulmer, R. M., and Franklin, S. G. (1982). *Supervision: Principles of professional management* (2nd ed.). New York, NY: Macmillan Publishing Co.

Gehrman, D. (1989). Why plan. In R. Kreitner, *Management* (4th ed.). Boston, MA: Houghton Mifflin Co.

Gray, E. R., and Smeltzer, L. R. (1989). *Management: The competitive edge.* New York, NY: Macmillan Publishing Co.

Griffith, J. R. (1992). *The well-managed community hospital* (2nd ed.). Ann Arbor, MI: Health Administration Press.

Hammer, M., and Champy, J. (1993). *Reengineering the corporation: A manifesto for business revolution.* New York, NY: Harper Business.

Hellriegel, D., and Slocum, J. (1986). *Management* (4th ed.). Reading, MA: Addison-Wesley Publishing Co., Inc.

Herzberg, F. (1976). *The managerial choice: To be efficient and to be human.* Homewood, IL: Don Jones-Irwin.

Kolb, D. A. (1974). *Organizational psychology: An experimental approach* (2nd ed.). Englewood Cliffs, NJ: Prentice Hall.

Koontz, H., and Weihrick, H. (1988). *Management.* New York, NY: McGraw-Hill.

Kraut, A. I. (1989). The role of the manager: What's really important in different management jobs. *Academy of Management Executive, 3:4,* 286–293.

National Therapeutic Recreation Society (NTRS). (1995). *Standards of practice for therapeutic recreation service and annotated bibliography.* Arlington, VA: National Recreation and Park Association.

O'Morrow, G. S. (1995). *Therapeutic recreation practitioner analysis, 1994.* Arlington, VA: National Recreation and Park Association.

Richards, M.D. (1986). *Setting strategic goals and objectives* (2nd ed.). St. Paul, MN: West Publishing.

Robbins, S. P. (1995). *Supervision today.* Englewood Cliffs, NJ: Prentice Hall.

Robin, I. M., Fry, R. E., and Plovnick, M. S. (Eds.). (1978). *Managing human resources in healthcare organizations.* Reston, VA: American Alliance for Health, Physical Education, Recreation and Dance.

Rowland, H. S., and Rowland, B. L. (Eds.). (1980). *Nursing administration handbook* (2nd ed.). Rockville, MD: Aspen Systems Corporation.

Shortell, S. M., Kaluzny, A. D., and associates. (1988). *Healthcare management: A text in organization and theory behavior* (2nd ed.). New York, NY: John Wiley & Sons.

Trent, W. C. (1986). Some unique aspects of healthcare management. *Hospitals and Health Services Administration, 31,* 122–132.

Turpel, L. T. (1992). Strategic management. In R. M. Winslow and K. J. Halberg (Eds.), *The management of therapeutic recreation services* (pp. 71–83). Arlington, VA: National Recreation and Park Association.

West, R. (1995). Management of therapeutic recreation in clinical settings. In M. J. Carter, G. E. Van Andel, and G. M. Robb (Eds.), *Therapeutic recreation: A practical approach* (2nd ed., pp. 157–188). Prospect Heights, IL: Waveland Press, Inc.

# Part 2

# Administrative Management

# Chapter 4

# Leadership

## Introduction

What is leadership? It has been widely discussed, many theories have been developed, and examples of leadership abound. Yet if one asked five different people to define leadership there probably would be five different responses. Mintzberg (1989), for example, views leadership as only one of ten roles that managers play. Robbins (1995, p. 322) defines leadership as "the ability to influence a group toward the achievement of goals." Leadership, according to Yukel (1989), may be defined as both a position and an ability. As a *position,* it means that a person is responsible for the control of certain situations and is in a direct or guiding position. A leader may be the top manager of an organization, department, or activity. Leadership *ability* refers to the capacity or skill to influence relationships with others so that they will follow the path taken by the leader. Leadership involves the ability to bring about a desired change or actions from or with others. Leadership implies a kind of movement for others to follow suit in their thinking, feeling, or actions. A leader encourages people to act.

Since this text is concerned with first-line management, the application of these definitions to therapeutic recreation in the workplace might read as follows: the ability of the therapeutic recreation manager to influence department practitioners to work toward the attainment of the organization, department, and consumer objectives. Without effective leadership, the organization and department will be simply a collection of practitioners, consumers, and resources. It is only through leadership that individuals will be drawn together and motivated to accomplish goals and objectives. Leadership, then, is the unifying and motivating force that brings reality to the department from a stage of mere potential. Effective therapeutic recreation managers are those who blend the qualities of leadership and apply the principles of management to practice.

Before proceeding, the authors will clarify the age old concern about leaders and managers. Managers, regardless of level, are usually appointed. They have a legitimate power base and can reward and punish. Their ability to influence is founded upon the formal authority inherent in their positions. The manager as has been noted frequently, is concerned with coordination and integration of resources through planning, organizing, directing, and controlling in order to accomplish specific organization or department goals and objectives. In contrast, leaders may either be appointed or emerge from within a group. Leadership is an interpersonal relationship in which the leader employs specific behaviors and strategies to influence individuals and groups toward goal setting and attainment in specific situations. One must keep in mind, however, the fact that a person can influence others does not indicate whether that person can also plan, organize, or control. One of the few common threads between both management and leadership literature is that effective leaders are important to a successful organization (Robbins, 1980). In other words, effective managers must be effective leaders. Thus, *ideally* all managers should be leaders. But one is cautioned that not all leaders necessarily have capabilities in other management functions.

A body of knowledge and theory germane to therapeutic recreation leadership is in its embryo stage. Although no compendium or consensus exists regarding leadership, it is still important to provide a brief overview of the more well-known leadership theories since the wise and systematic *use of self* influences the achievement of organization and department objectives. The authors have cited a perspective that leadership theory has evolved in response to changes in society and culture. Since man's society and culture are ever-evolving, even the most recent interactionist leadership theories will probably be insufficient to describe, explain, or predict leadership behavior in the twenty-first century. However, these theories do provide a springboard for action to be taken by therapeutic recreation managers.

Following the presentation of leadership theories, other key concepts inherently associated with leadership will be considered—styles and power. Other key concepts related to leadership such as communication, motivation, and organizational behavior will be considered in future chapters.

# Leadership Theories

Two early theories are referred to as the *Great Man Theory* and the *Charismatic Theory*. The former argues that few people are born with the necessary characteristics to be great. Many find this theory unattractive because of its premise that leaders are born and not made which suggests that leadership cannot be developed. The charismatic theory suggests that a person may be a leader because he or she is charismatic, but relatively little is known about this intangible characteristic. What constitutes charisma? Most agree that it is an inspirational quality which some people possess that makes others feel better in their presence. The charismatic leader inspires others by obtaining emotional commitment from followers and by arousing strong loyalty feelings and enthusiasm (Fiedler and Chemers, 1974).

Recently, the charismatic theory is again reviewing attention under a different label (Transformational Leadership) which will be discussed shortly.

## *Trait Theories*

Until the mid-1940s the trait theory was the basis for most leadership research. By 1950 the list had grown to over 100 characteristics identified as essential to successful leadership (Adorno and others, 1950). It postulated that individuals possessing a certain combination of physical, personal, and social traits would be effective leaders. Bass (1981) lists 16 personality traits that have been positively correlated with leadership. Dominance and self-confidence are most frequently related to leadership; emotional control, independence, and creativity are the next most frequent. Social skills, such as sociability and administrative ability, have also been associated with leadership. The fol-

lowing list by Hein and Nicholson (1990) is an example of other common leadership traits associated with this theory:

1. Leaders need to be more intelligent than the group they lead.
2. Leaders mostly possess initiative or the ability to perceive and start courses of action not considered by others.
3. Creativity is an asset.
4. Leaders also possess emotional maturity, integrity, a sense of purpose and direction, persistence, dependability, and objectivity.
5. Communication skills are important.
6. Persuasion often is used by leaders to gain the consent of followers.
7. Leaders need to be perceptive enough to distinguish their allies from their opponents and to place subordinates in suitable positions.
8. Leaders participate in social activities. They can socialize with all kinds of people and adapt to various groups.

While research studies have shown the importance of some traits, they have not consistently identified traits that are common to all leaders. Trait theory does not view personality as an integrated whole, does not deal with subordinates, and avoids environmental influences and situational factors (Stogdill, 1974). On the other hand, Gibb (1969) concludes that the traits associated with leadership are contingent upon the nature of the task, the goal pursued, and the characteristics of group members. This view is supported by McGregor (1966, p. 73) who states, "research findings to date suggest that it is more fruitful to consider leadership as a relationship between the leader and the situation than as a universal pattern of characteristics possessed by certain people." Megginson, Mosley, and Pietri (1991) concluded after a review of the leadership literature associated with the traitist approach that leaders have vision, communicate well, are highly motivated, and motivate their followers. As the traitist approach did not prove completely valid, theorists moved toward examining leadership in relation to the groups being led. It is interesting to note, however, that despite their limitations and contradictions, aspects of trait theory are often used as the basis for management decisions. The most physically imposing or most highly skilled therapeutic recreation practitioner in a group may be chosen as a manager on the basis of this particular leadership trait.

## *Behavioral Theories*

The behavioral theorists, sometimes called functional theorists, concentrated on the leader's action rather than the traits of the leader. Among the most popular and comprehensive of the behavioral research and theories are those of Rensis Likert's (1967) Michigan Studies, the Ohio State University group (Stogdill, 1974), Blake and Mouton's (1964) managerial grid, and Douglas McGregor's (1966) Theory X and Theory Y.

The behaviorists viewed leadership as including not only the qualities of the leader but also the task, expectations, and capabilities of the group. Groups have two major functions. The first function is the performance of a task or achievement of a goal. In therapeutic recreation service the goal is the delivery of quality service. The second function of a group is to strengthen the group itself. In therapeutic recreation service this would include professional development and actions taken to maintain high staff morale.

In relation to these functions, leadership functions have been described primarily by the Ohio State University group (Stogdill, 1974) as "initiating structure" or *task-oriented* and "consideration" or *human-oriented*. Other terms for task-oriented leadership are *job-centered, production-oriented* (Likert, 1967), and *autocratic*. According to Robbins (1980), structure or task refers to the extent to which the leader is likely to define his or her role and those of subordinates in the search for goal attainment. Behaviors that attempt to organize work, work relationships, and goals are also included in this definition. This task oriented behavior reflects McGregor's (1966) Theory X authoritarian (or autocratic) management style (Megginson, Mosley, and Pietri, 1986). Terms for human-oriented leadership are *employee-centered, people-oriented* (Likert, 1967), and *democratic*. Human-oriented is described as the extent to which a person is likely to have job relationships that are characterized by mutual trust, respect for subordinates' ideas, and regard for their feelings. A leader high in human factors could be described as one who helps subordinates with personal problems, is friendly and approachable, and treats all subordinates as equals (Robbins, 1980). Theory Y is employee-centered (McGregor, 1966) and Kurt Lewin's ideas are based on democratic management (Megginson, Mosley, and Pietri, 1986).

Taking the dimensions developed by the Ohio State University and Michigan groups respectively, Blake and Mouton (1964) proposed a managerial grid. The grid was based on the styles of "concern for people" and "concern for production" using a high-low axis. Results showed that administrators perform best where they facilitate task efficiency and high morale by coordinating and integrating work-related activities.

In reality, the behaviorists found very little success in identifying consistent relationships between patterns of leadership behavior and successful performance. The ideal leadership behavior according to the behaviorists is one which combines structure (task) with consideration (human). As an example, the therapeutic recreation manager using the ideal approach would focus on accomplishing the goals, while at the same time maintaining open communication and an environment of mutual trust and respect among staff members.

## Situational Theories

Situation theories became popular during the 1950s and developed from the failure of the other types of theories to address the significance of the environment, organization, goal, or situation on leadership. In addition, reference to these models is sometimes found under the heading of leadership styles. A number of situation or contingency theories exist and are explained below.

### Fiedler's Contingency Model

One of the earliest situational theories was Fiedler's Contingency Model of Leadership Effectiveness (Fiedler, 1967). The focus of attention in this model was on the performance of the group. There must be a group before there can be a leader. He argued that effective group performance depends upon the proper match between the leader's style of interacting with subordinates and the degree to which the situation gives control and influence to the leader. He identified three aspects of a situation that structure the leader's role: (1) leader-member relations, (2) task structure, and (3) leader position power.

Leader-member relations involve the amount of confidence and loyalty the subordinates have in their leader. Task structure refers to the degree to which a task can be defined and measured in terms of progress towards completion. Structure is generally high if easy to define and measure and low if it is difficult to define and measure. Position power relates to the leader's authority in the organization (i.e., hiring, firing, reward, punishment).

Fiedler states that the more positive the leader-member relationship, the more highly structured the task, and the greater the position power, the greater the influence. In addition, of the three situational dimensions, the most important is leader-member followed by task structure. The least important is position power. In summary, Fiedler (1967, p. 32) said that "successful leadership was an interaction of leadership styles and the situation."

### Life-Cycle Model

The life-cycle theory of Hersey and Blanchard (1982) states that the leader's behavior will vary based on the maturity of the subordinates and the situation. Job maturity is defined by the individual's technical knowledge and skill in performing a task. This is combined with the individual's feeling of self-esteem and confidence. An individual can be extremely mature, both personally and in relation to the task, in one particular situation. If the situation changes, the person will experience a decrease in maturity in relation to either the task itself or feelings of self-confidence. For example, an experienced psychiatric therapeutic recreation practitioner understands his or her role, has the knowledge skills necessary to provide quality service to the patient, and is confident in the relationship with both peers and other professionals. The therapeutic recreation manager gives this practitioner a great deal of program freedom and finds ways of intellectually challenging the staff member. If this practitioner transfers to the physical rehabilitation unit within the hospital, the practitioner will have to learn new skills and develop a new set of relationships. Temporarily, the practitioner will experience feelings of insecurity. Both personal and job maturity will decrease and the practitioner will require direction from the manager in this unit. As the practitioner gains knowledge and confidence, the manager allows more freedom and supports the practitioner in making decisions and implementing service. The life-cycle model therefore emphasizes the importance of the maturity level of the staff. Thus the leader needs to adapt leadership styles accordingly.

### Path-Goal Model

According to House and Mitchell (1974), the leader will look at the situation and the characteristics of the individual involved and determine what leadership style (directive, supportive, participative) will increase the subordinate's motivation to perform the task or reach the goal. The leader helps subordinates access needs, explore alternatives, and make the most beneficial decisions. The leader also rewards personnel for task achievement and provides additional opportunities for satisfying goal accomplishment. In brief, the leader shows the way down the "path" to reach the goal and provides rewards for the individual as an incentive. According to Robbins (1995, p. 331), this theory is the "best situational explanation for leader effectiveness. . . ."

## Interactional Theories

Interactional theories can be viewed as the compilation of everything that has been theorized before in an attempt to pull together the three elements of leader, follower, and environment. Schein (1970) proposed a complex man and open systems framework in an attempt to synthesize trait, behavior, motivation, and situation theories. Schreisheim, Mowday, and Stogdill (1979) emphasized the interdependence between the leader and group in any given complex situation as determining the leadership process.

Prentice (1983) stated that a leader's ability to understand and relate to individuals as complex and unique beings was a major factor in the leader's effectiveness. This interpersonal activity resulted in a leader being able to marshal individual collaboration toward goal achievement successfully. The leader is cognizant of his or her own

contribution to the effectiveness of the organization, but in the interpersonal relationship he or she focuses on the unique contribution that individual staff members can make.

Tannenbaum and Schmidt (1983, p. 163) summarized the synthesis of personality and interpersonal relationships in leaders that result in success as follows: "The successful leader is one who is keenly aware of those forces which are most relevant to behavior at any given time [and] who is able to behave appropriately in the light of these perceptions."

# Leadership Styles

Leadership style comes from a variety of factors. Individual personality, life philosophy, and socialization in early life have a significant impact on the leadership style developed according to Baird (1982). External factors also contribute to the leadership style. An organization in which the product is the result of a group effort demands a style different from an organization in which individuals are responsible for separate products. The type of leadership valued by the organization and society also affects the style.

It should be apparent that managerial or leadership style cannot be appropriate for all occasions. In some cases it is essential that the manager encourage utmost participation, while in others the manager must assume a more dominant role. Often this shift of personality will depend on the work group. However, the goal of the department is for its manager to adopt a style of management that promotes a high level of work performance in a wide variety of circumstances as efficiently as possible and with little disruption.

Styles of leadership have been classified into many types. Tramel and Reynolds (1981) identified three general categories: tight, team, or loose rein. Likert (1967), however, delineated four leadership styles. The *exploitive* or *authoritative* style appears synonymous with the autocratic style espoused in the early 1970s. There is also the *benevolent-authoritative* style which is less autocratic. The third leadership style is termed *consultative* and the fourth style is known as *participative* leadership.

Participative leadership focuses attention on human aspects and building effective work groups. Interaction between manager and staff is open, friendly, and trusting. There is a mutual responsiveness to meeting group goals, and work-related decisions are made by the group. There are some decisions that do not permit the therapeutic recreation manager to exercise participative management, but use of the participatory process, when possible, permits each member to identify with the work setting by establishing challenging goals, providing opportunities to change or improve work methods, pursuing professional and personal growth, recognizing achievement, and helping personnel learn from their mistakes.

As has been noted, Tannenbaum and Schmidt (1983) emphasized three sets of forces that determine the leadership pattern that will be successful. The set of forces found within the leader such as personality, knowledge, and background are a primary determinant of leadership style because it is the closest force to the leader. The second set of forces has to do with the individuals involved within the relationship. These forces include motivation, knowledge, and understanding. The third set of forces that determines the style of leadership that will be successful is composed of forces within the environment.

Baird (1982) identified three factors that affect the leadership style that is used. The first factor is the assumption that a leader makes about people (good or bad). A second factor is how the leader uses or shares power (autocratic, democratic, laissez-faire, and situational). The last factor focuses on the way in which the leader communicates.

Fiedler's (1967) research on contingency theory identified three factors as noted earlier that influence the leader's effectiveness. While there will be further discussion in a practical sense regarding leadership behavior and leadership style, it is well to note that leadership is composed of a group of individual characteristics and behaviors that utilize a wide compendium of human relation abilities, management techniques, and power. The unique blend of these actions results in the movement of individuals toward goal setting and goal achievement. A successful leader is one who maintains a high batting average in accurately assessing the forces that determine what the most appropriate behavior at any given time should be and actually being able to behave accordingly while getting the individual to participate.

Most recently, two new leadership styles have emerged (Megginson, Mosley, and Pietri, 1992). One style called *transformational leader* incorporates three factors: charismatic leadership, individualized consideration, and intellectual stimulation. Of the three factors, charismatic leadership is the most important and is receiving considerable attention from the advocates of the trait approach. It focuses on the leader's "need to instill pride, respect, and esprit de corps and have a gift of focusing on what is really important as well as a true sense of mission" (Megginson, Mosley, and Pietri, 1992, p. 478). Other characteristics noted include self-confidence, a vision, ability to articulate the vision, strong conviction about the vision, and behavior that is out of the ordinary and is perceived as being a change agent (cited in Robbins, 1995). Individualized consideration focuses on delegating responsibilities to promote learning and development as well as giving personal attention to employees. The third factor, intellectual stimulation, is concerned with the leader having vision and rethinking old ideas in a new way.

Transformational leadership, in contrast to older management concepts (e.g., planning, organizing, staffing, directing, coordinating, reporting, and budgeting [POSDCORB]; management by objectives [MBO]) recog-nizes that there is more to a job than performing a set of functions no matter how effective. The new paradigm looks at relationships among the manager and practitioners. It values mutuality and affiliation; acknowledges complexity and ambiguity; advocates cooperation instead of competition; emphasizes human relations and process instead of task; accepts feelings; values networking instead of hierarchy; and values intuition and empowerment of all employees (Bass, 1985).

Tim Porter-O'Grady (1993), an international health management consultant, observes that the transforming leader as a manager during this period of healthcare system change gives attention to employees and assists in their adjustment to change. The manager in the healthcare system becomes "a change agent—challenging, questioning the status quo, and creating an atmosphere where self-directing activities, workplace partnerships and shared critical outcomes become the norm" (p. 52). In addition, the manager is a provider of information and resources.

The other leadership style is the transactional leader who identifies desired standards of practice, recognizes the rewards practitioners want from their practice, and rewards practice based on achieving standards of practice (Megginson, Mosley, and Pietri, 1992).

While a variety of leadership styles have been considered, numerous studies indicate that two styles consistently surface. They are *task-centered* and *people-centered* leadership. Robbins (1995, p. 329) defines these leadership styles as follows:

> *Task-centered leaders* emphasize the technical or task aspects of the employee's job. They let the employee know what is expected, define and structure the employee's tasks and give specific guidance as to how to accomplish the tasks. *People-centered* leaders emphasize good interpersonal relations. They show support for employees by being concerned for their needs, displaying trust, respecting employee ideas, and being sensitive to employee feelings. [Robbins' italics]

Is there a preferred style? No. Some studies have found that a people-centered style results in both higher employee production and personal satisfaction. While the task-centered approach is more effective for achieving high employee production only (Robbins, 1995). In addition, Robbins (1995, p. 335) notes that men appeared to "use a directive command-and-control style of leadership" and are task centered. Women on the other hand, "use a more democratic style" of leadership which resembles a people-centered approach.

From a follower's perspective Kouzes and Posner (1990) studied more than 7,500 workers to determine what followers look for or admire in a leader. The four crucial attributes that appear most often were honesty, competence, a forward-looking approach, and the ability to inspire others. Honesty was the most selected attribute and was measured by the leader's behavior, not by what he or she said. It is also important that the leader display a trust of others. The followers want the leaders to have competence and to be able to inspire, enable, and encourage. A forward-looking approach includes having a sense of direction and concern for the future of the organization as a whole. Finally, followers want a leader to be inspiring, enthusiastic, energetic, positive, and able to communicate a vision. Demonstrated consistently, these attributes lead to credibility.

# Leadership and Power

Several times in the previous section the word *power* was used. Fiedler (1967) used it to define one of his three leadership contingency dimensions. But what is power, and how can a first time manager learn to use power wisely?

The need to define the meaning of power becomes one of the most difficult aspects of approaching this subject. It is a word used continuously and yet if one asked what it is, like leadership, the variety of responses leads to an obvious conclusion; individuals define power in different ways.

Effective leaders understand the nature of power and how to use it. For one thing, they know that power is found in relationships, in connections and associations between and among people. They also know that power is based on formal relationships and informal relationships; that is, on what is given them by their formal position in the organization, as well as on what they are blessed with in terms of charisma and persuasiveness. Further, they know that power may be good or evil; good if used for positive purposes or evil if sought as an end in itself. The way in which leaders make use of power will determine greatly how effective they function as leaders (Hitt, 1988).

When trying to get to the substance of what *power* is, like other abstract concepts, it is best to seek its most universal definition. A consensus of most authors shows that the essence of power is the ability to affect something or to be affected by something (i.e., the ability to cause or prevent change). In addition, most authors agree that there are two aspects to power: the source of the power and the object of power (Claus and Bailey, 1979; Kotter, 1983; McClelland and Burnham, 1983).

Essential to establishing an understanding of power is the need to distinguish it between other related terms. One of the most difficult aspects of this topic is sorting out how power relates to a number of other management concepts, especially leadership, authority, and influence. If influence is presumed to be a substantial component of leadership, then influence has to do with a set of actions

and behaviors that the first time manager initiates to bring about change—change in the behavior and/or attitude of another individual or group. The therapeutic recreation manager brings about change by influencing others through the use of power and motivation.

Authority is a source of power which can be considered the right to command. It has implied legitimacy; those who are affected by the authority figure agree that the power vested in that person is legitimate. The structure of any organization delineates the hierarchy of power. Authority is intimately related to the *Chain of Command* or the *Organizational Chart* which tells employees where they fit in the organizational ladder. Job descriptions frequently define the level of authority; therefore, formal authority derives from the position.

In a broader concept, power is the capacity or ability to command. Power comes from the person and is the source of his or her strength, energy, and action. Strength includes the internal resources of a strong self-concept and an awareness of reality. But strength also includes tangible assets such as resources and information. Energy is composed of both internal and external energy. Most leaders possess high energy levels that are expressed as positivism, optimism, and enthusiasm. This element also includes the ability to obtain the cooperation of others. Initiating the cooperation of others leads to the final stage in the power relationship, the act. This is why power is frequently discussed in terms of results (Claus and Bailey, 1979).

If a person has power, he or she can act to influence outcomes. Influence has to do with the process as it relates to goals and outcomes. Power is an important source of an individual's influence. A leader leads by influencing. However, influence emphasizes the ability and energy elements more so than the action element of the power relationship.

## *Base of Power*

Generally speaking, organizations are made up of people who are consistently vying with one another for power, status, and prestige. Power is the ability to impose the will or desire of one person or group of persons on another individual or group of individuals to influence and alter behavior. However, one must keep in mind that power itself is neither good nor bad. It is how an individual or group uses or abuses power that ultimately colors its perception. Power is inherent in the ability to lead. How that power is used ultimately determines the effectiveness of the leader (Hersey and Blanchard, 1982).

French and Raven (1968) are credited with identifying five types of power. They explained the sources or bases from which power emanates and called these bases legitimate, coercive, reward, expert, and referent. The therapeutic recreation manager has legitimate power and authority based on his or her position. Reward and coercive powers are present, based on the right to hire, evaluate, promote, or discharge individuals. Expert power is derived from professional knowledge and demonstrated management skills. Referent power may also be present based on attractiveness and a pleasant, motivating personality. Hersey and Blanchard (1982) added information power and connection power to these five powers. Besides the sources of their own power, the therapeutic recreation manager needs to be aware and concerned with the power of others since the source of others' power can dilute his or her power.

While the seven types of power have been briefly described, they will be considered in a bit more detail here:

1. **Reward power** comes from the ability of the manager to give awards. The use of positive sanctions is the hallmark of a good manager. This is demonstrated through compensation, verbal praise, taking staff to lunch, etc. When monetary rewards are insufficient or nonexistent, then subtle forms of reward and acknowledgment assume special importance. One who can distribute rewards that others view as valuable will have power over them.

2. **Coercive power** is the opposite of reward power; a manager deliberately withholds rewards or punishes in order to promote compliance. Staff react to this power out of fear of the negative ramifications resulting from failing to comply. Withholding sanctions is clearly part of the system. For example, an employee whose performance is unsatisfactory does not deserve a merit increase. A caution here is that this type of power can be somewhat subjective.

3. **Legitimate power** relates to official position in the organizational hierarchy. Most people recognize this, but there is something peculiar that has to be faced in providing healthcare services that other businesses do not have to confront—the impact of physicians.

4. **Referent power,** sometimes called charismatic power, is the therapeutic recreation manager's ability to use influence because the staff identifies with the manager as a leader. Employees generally identify with a person who has the resources or personal traits they believe are desirable. If a manager's "leadership style" is working, staff practitioners will choose to emulate some of the manager's more attractive qualities. Thus, the greater the attraction, the greater the identification, and subsequently the greater the referent power.

5. **Expert power** is the influence a manager wields as a result of his or her expertise, special skill, or knowledge. Therapeutic recreation managers gain power through knowledge because respect and compliance from the people they interact with will follow. Managerial knowledge and knowledge of the organization, including its mission, goals, objectives, and operations will help a manager acquire power.

6. **Informational power** is the power which proceeds from the ability of an individual to gain and share valuable information.

7. **Connection power** becomes a reality when the manager is perceived as having close contact with other influential people.

The wise therapeutic recreation manager will use all sources of power while moving between the various sources as circumstances warrant. However, many authors (Fiedler, 1967; Moore and Wood, 1979; Stoner, 1982) contend that no other power source is as valuable as expert power. Having the knowledge and the ability to apply it will go a long way toward establishing the therapeutic recreation manager's credibility with superiors, peers, and subordinates. However, the manager is cautioned that having access to one or even all of these powers does not guarantee the ability to influence particular individuals or groups in a specific way. A manager may be widely accepted and admired as an expert but still may be unable to influence his or her staff to be more creative in their jobs or even get to work on time.

## Power Strategies

Assuming that one has the desire, ability, and will to be powerful, and occupies a management position, what are some of the other strategies used to assist in acquiring power? Benziger (1982) has noted several strategies designed to increase an individual's power. Although these strategies were formulated with women in mind, they are certainly applicable to this discussion. Benziger cited 12 organizational power strategies:

1. Learn to speak the organization's language and don't expect it to use the manager's.

2. Learn the organization's priorities and explain one's needs in terms of how it will aid in meeting the organization's needs.

3. Learn the power lines and who has the power. Time and energy can be wasted when the wrong people are contacted.

4. Become acquainted with those who are powerful. One may find that one shares an interest and discussion of that interest will enhance the relationship. This is a form of networking which at times takes some meticulous attention to details and patience.

5. Develop professional knowledge. Develop knowledge based on the needs of the organization.

6. Develop power skills. Develop one's bases of power remembering that they are additive in their effect.

7. Be proactive rather than passive or reactive. Not only does the person get the work done faster and better, but the person generates alternative solutions if something does not meet expectations. In addition, the person plans for the future.

8. Assume authority in one's dealings. Once power is activated, it either results in authority or force. Only when authority is disregarded, does an individual choose to use force over authority. An individual will not be seen as displaying authority if his or her power bases have not already been established.

9. Take risks. Men are introduced early to taking risks while women do not generally have the opportunity to practice this.

10. Be verbal with achievements. One may not like this approach and may feel uncomfortable, but it will move one into a more visible and powerful situation.

11. Meet one's supervisor's needs. Become knowledgeable about his or her goals because one's performance can give the supervisor credit. (More about this subject is found in Chapter 9.)

12. Take care of oneself. In the process of becoming powerful, remember to take care of oneself physically, emotionally, and socially.

A word of caution to the manager. In health and human service settings, issues of power according to Lewis and Lewis (1983) are often especially difficult because managers as supervisors tend to be wary of overcontrolling others' efforts. Professionals want to be mentors but might feel uncomfortable about evaluating and influencing other practitioners' progress toward effectiveness. The manager-supervisory relationship must recognize the existence of power while taking into account the unique aspects of the human service environment.

# Individual Relationships

Identifying the strengths and weaknesses of a therapeutic recreation practitioner is a difficult process. It is done through conversation, working together, and the intuition of the manager. The therapeutic recreation manager tries to provide opportunities for growth in the areas of programming and interpersonal and peer relations.

In order to provide professional growth, the therapeutic recreation manager must allow subordinates freedom to think and to try new techniques. At the same time, the manager must maintain control over the delivery of service. This is done by setting high performance expectations and standards of practice. These expectations and standards are conveyed to each therapeutic recreation practitioner at the time of employment. Standards of practice are reinforced on a daily basis through service, staff conferences, and individual discussions regarding quality service. Over time, standards of practice become the department norm. The manager expects it, looks for the plans, and provides positive rewards to staff members who meet the expectations. Recognition by the manager is another reward. The continuous quality improvement program is a mechanism that the leader can use to evaluate achievement of standards. Yearly performance reviews give the manager an opportunity to evaluate each individual's performance and to discuss areas for future growth (see Chapter 18).

One of the pitfalls every manager must avoid is that of encouraging dependency of the staff on each other. This inhibits individual growth on the part of the staff. The manager must focus on bringing each subordinate to his or her maximum potential. This means creating independent, secure practitioners of therapeutic recreation who act in the best interests of the consumer.

According to Wadia (1965) who developed a conceptual framework for management in which he incorporated the behavioral sciences into the management process of planning, organizing, directing, and controlling, managers who know how individuals generally behave, why they behave as they do, and the relationship between human behavior and the environment are better equipped to function in their role.

The following dichotomies by Skidmore (1995) concerning attributes significant for effective management in therapeutic recreation provide a conclusion to this brief discussion of leadership and individual relationships:

- *Trust versus Mistrust*
  Where trust exists between the manager and practitioners, morale is usually high. Effective managers are those who genuinely accept and trust those with whom they work. Even more important, managers should consistently let their staff know they accept them and believe their abilities are adequate to accomplish tasks.
- *Building versus Destroying*
  Effective managers compliment their staff when appropriate, show appreciation for their achievements, and let staff members know how important they are.
- *Support versus Abandonment*
  Competent managers support their staff. This does not mean they agree with everything the practitioner says and does. In fact, at times, they may need to disagree, even strongly. It does mean, however, that

when practitioners have been asked to do something and have done their best, the manager backs them up.

- *Consistency versus Inconsistency*
Effective managers are ordinarily consistent; when they say something, they follow through with appropriate action. They do not send conflicting messages at different times. When they make an assignment or a suggestion to a practitioner, they back it up with genuinely supportive behavior.

- *Caring versus Coldness*
Caring involves feelings. It makes a great difference if feelings expressed are positive and if a practitioner has the sense that the manager really cares. The essence of caring is giving. The most effective manager is one who gives enough of his or her time and self that practitioners feel that the manager cares.

Further consideration of qualities that promote individual and employee relations is found within Chapter 15 which is concerned with motivation.

# Group Relationships

The therapeutic recreation manager relates to a group of diverse individuals including volunteers in much the same manner as with individual relationships. Differences occur in gender, education, maturity, behavioral needs, and in cultural background. It is the manager's task to develop these individuals into an effective work group so that each member is able to experience the optimum of success and goal achievement. The manager builds on the desire to provide quality service to the consumer. The manager instills in the practitioners common values about consumers. Conflicts are brought out and dealt with so that the end result is a well-functioning group with similar principles and standards. Building an effective work group involves carefully planning and exerting power through leadership. How the manager accomplishes this is just as important as choosing the most appropriate leadership behavior in a given situation.

The therapeutic recreation manager who begins to develop an effective working group will need to meet regularly with the group to discuss programs and group interaction and to provide feedback to the group based on its success. The manager will need to become skilled in using conflict management techniques (see Chapter 11).

In conclusion the manager may want to consider the following attributes which constitute a positive work practitioner group according to Hitt (1988):

1. **Common agreement on expectations of group.** All practitioners have a will to excel.
2. **A commitment to common goals.** Goals provide practitioners with a common focus. All practitioners have a clear understanding of the goals, and they accept the goals.
3. **Assumed responsibility for work that must be done.** While each practitioner has a defined job, each also has a commitment to do anything that needs doing.
4. **Honest and open communication.** Authentic dialogue is the norm. Practitioners openly express their thoughts and feelings, and they feel free to ask questions with the confidence that they will receive honest answers. There are no hidden agendas.
5. **Common access to information.** Information is viewed as a vital resource to each practitioner, and it is the manager's responsibility to make certain that every practitioner has the information to get his or her respective job done.
6. **A climate of trust.** Each practitioner has an instinctive unquestioning belief in the other practitioners.
7. **A general feeling that one can influence what happens.** Each practitioner has a definite feeling that what one does will produce positive results in the consumer.
8. **Support for decisions that are made.** While there is general support for decisions once they are made, on key decisions practitioners are given an opportunity to express their thoughts and feelings on matters at hand. The practitioners have confidence in the sincerity of the manager in soliciting their input in decisions.
9. **A focus on process as well as results.** Practitioners focus both on results and how the results are achieved.

# Situation Leadership

A therapeutic recreation manager makes decisions and provides guidance to staff in a rapidly changing environment. Actions which are effective in one instance may not be in another. Therefore, the manager must assess each situation and the reactions of therapeutic recreation staff members to the situation before taking action. A manager's actions are always designed to obtain cooperation, collaboration, and support of the staff and to influence future actions of the staff.

Keeping this in mind, the manager analyzes the situation for the following criteria:

1. Importance to consumer service. Is it directly related to consumer service or does the situation involve staff?

2. Immediacy. When does the situation demand action?
3. The individuals involved in the situation. Are therapeutic recreation practitioners the only people involved or are other professionals or volunteers involved?
4. The thoughts, feelings, and reactions of the staff collectively as well as the individual feelings. The manager must keep in mind that the feelings of the group are not always the same as the feelings of the individuals making up the group.
5. The thoughts, feelings, and reactions of the therapeutic recreation manager. The therapeutic recreation manager is not immune to feelings such as anger or frustration at a given situation. It is essential that the manager never reacts to a situation out of anger or frustration.

The manager's actions and behaviors will vary based on the situation. However, the leader must be consistent in his or her approach to the individual and the group. This means the manager will always convey understanding and concern for the feelings and reactions of others. The manager will acknowledge the negative feelings and allow subordinates to express anger. The manager recognizes and expresses his or her own feelings but does not allow them to influence his or her actions or decisions. The therapeutic recreation manager must be able to admit when he or she is wrong. By having honest, open exchanges, the subordinate's respect for the manager will grow and with it the manager's ability to influence the group.

# Leadership and Supervision

If leadership is defined as the process of influencing human behaviors in the interest of achieving particular goals, it is a key factor in supervision. The supervisor is clearly interested in influencing the practitioner's behavior; therefore, some kind of "leadership event" must take place. The process of supervision involves helping practitioners increase their effectiveness in service delivery. The supervisor provides support and encouragement, helps build skills and competencies, and oversees the practitioner's work. The nature of the relationship depends to a large degree on the supervisor's leadership style, the practitioner's motivation and the department's needs.

Much of what has already been discussed can be related to the manager as a supervisor. However, it is important to highlight those factors that make the first-line manager, as a supervisor, a special case of leadership since the activity is associated with directing subordinates. The first-line manager functions in a situation that requires management of professionally knowledgeable practitioners—people who base their work activities upon a compendium of knowledge, skills, and abilities too extensive to be translated into a routine, standardized pattern of behavior.

Knowledgeable workers, it is well-known, are a difficult group in some respects. They expect more than mere wages from their work; they expect to derive a sense of satisfaction and self-esteem from work well-done. They do not require a great deal of externally based motivation. They are, in effect, practitioners who can be defined both as achievement motivated and as possessing high task maturity. They also may be quite determined about holding to internalized goals and values that dictate how they will proceed in work.

As first-line managers, supervisors must, by definition, occupy the only level of management charged with the responsibility of directing the work of nonmanagement personnel. As supervisors, managers are directly responsible for the daily, face-to-face, immediate, and operative activities of a group of personnel. Getting the most out of knowledgeable workers requires special managerial skills. Those who are enthusiastic and perform exceptionally well in their jobs usually feel challenged by their work itself and take responsibility for their own jobs. Managing professionals requires more than overseeing; managers serve as guides and teachers who provide information and set standards.

The uniqueness of being a manager or supervisor calls for the following abilities, but is not limited to:

1. **Heavy reliance on technical expertise.** Supervisors are required to know the job they supervise. They spend a large portion of their time directing and overseeing the activities of their subordinates. Because of the problems they face at this level—experienced and inexperienced personnel—they must have expert knowledge of jobs that their subordinates perform.
2. **Skills assessment.** After learning the skills required of each position, the manager must assess each practitioner's suitability for the varied positions in the department. It is up to the manager to identify areas of excellence, competence, and deficiency for every practitioner under supervision. It is important to differentiate between performance and ability.
3. **Facilitation of work.** The work environment needs to be monitored to identify barriers to accomplishments. Thus, the therapeutic recreation manager must look for barriers within the practitioner, the staff as a group, and the organization with its various support systems. One of the manager's most important tasks is the challenge of developing positive feelings of capability and potential achievement in each practitioner. In addition, the manager attempts to manage and facilitate change rather than regarding change as a threat to the status quo. As has been noted in earlier chapters, the external environment for any organization today is changing rapidly. The manager, therefore, should attempt to

lead practitioners to embrace change as a permanent way of life.

4. **Communication in two languages.** Communication is a problem at all levels of management. First-line managers are required to communicate in two distinct languages—that of management and that of workers. Differing educational backgrounds, value systems, and points of reference are just several of the major disparities between the two groups.

5. **Coping with role conflict.** Managers are neither fish nor fowl. They are not practitioners, and although they are officially classified as managers, they are not often accepted by other middle- or top-level managers. A first-line manager may be assumed to be like other managers, but the individual's activities, status, and security are at times quite different. The activities are associated with nonmanagement personnel, the status is "low person on the totem pole" when it comes to management, and security is not always solid if performance is not tops. Finally, managers who are promoted from within face the task of learning new behaviors when being subtly or not so subtly coerced to retain the behaviors of the past role as a practitioner.

6. **Coping with constrained authority.** Today managers must adapt to a less autocratic style than their predecessors. Managers must also adapt to the constraints imposed by internal and external factors such as the intricate appeals systems that most organizations provide for their workers. In addition, managers are required to interact in an authority relationship with two groups: subordinates and supervisors who are their superiors.

7. **Reinforcing employees' good performance.** On a day-to-day basis this reinforcement mainly takes the form of oral behavior with compliments and praise when a job has been well-done. For the longer term, a variety of rewards may be used to recognize good performance (e.g., material rewards). (Consideration of these factors in more detail will be found in Chapter 16.)

8. **The management's representative.** Rules, policies, procedures, and other dictates from above are implemented at the first-line manager level, so when practitioners think of management, their usual point of reference is their manager. This obviously places high responsibility on the managers to reflect accurately the vision, philosophy, and attitudes of the management, a task made even more difficult because they rarely have the opportunity to participate in major policy decisions that may affect the people they directly supervise.

# Integrative Leadership

A review of leadership theories and styles shows that there obviously is no one best leadership style. Managers are roughly either people- or task-oriented. Managers, followers, situations—all of these influence leadership effectiveness. Consequently, an integration of leadership theories seems appropriate. Although the contingency or situational theories of leadership can be helpful, it will take considerable practice before a manager will be comfortable in knowing what to do and when to do it.

Under normal circumstances the maturity of the therapeutic recreation manager will be a strong factor in determining leadership style. The manager's comfort level will also affect the style of interacting. Allowing others freedom will be easy if the manager is mature and comfortable in his or her role and relationship. The manager must recognize his or her own feelings and understand how they affect behavior and decision making. Individual differences of staff members, group characteristics, motivation, task structures, environmental factors, degree of power to do the job, and situation variables must also be noted so that the manager can adjust his or her leadership style accordingly. Leadership behavior must always be adaptive. If therapeutic recreation managers are relatively inflexible in their leadership style, they will function well only in certain situations.

Considering the theories presented in this chapter, the following descriptive statements offer general guidelines regarding leadership and the first-line manager:

- use a leadership style that is natural;
- use a leadership style appropriate to the task and the group;
- assess how one's behavior affects others and vice versa;
- be sensitive to forces acting for and against change;
- express an optimistic view about human nature;
- be energetic;
- be open and encourage openness so that real issues are confronted;
- facilitate personal relationships;
- plan and organize activities of the group;
- be consistent in behavior toward group practitioners;
- delegate tasks and responsibilities to develop practitioners' abilities, not merely to get tasks performed;
- involve practitioners in all decisions that are appropriate for them;
- value and use group practitioners' contributions;
- encourage creativity; and
- encourage feedback about management-leadership style.

Frank (1993) noted, after reviewing various theories and definitions of leadership as well as the types of power and their uses in addition to the above guidelines, that "...interacting with others is the foremost ability one needs to successfully lead" (p. 387). Other major characteristics of effective leadership suggested included assertiveness (not aggressiveness), personal and professional goal setting, time management coupled with the ability to delegate work, effective communication skills, negotiating abilities so that both sides feel they are a winner, knowing when and how to use power, and the ability to recognize and understand the stress that may be associated with leadership obligations. Specifically related to therapeutic recreation managers and practitioners, Peg Connolly (1994), Executive Director of the National Council for Therapeutic Recreation Certification notes the following leadership characteristics. A good leader:

1. communicates, allows input, is willing to listen;
2. is interested, appreciative, complimentary, supportive, humanistic, considerate;
3. displays honesty, integrity, trustworthiness;
4. is objective, open-minded, tolerant, rational, reasonable, fair;
5. delegates, trusts subordinates, allows room to achieve;
6. motivates, challenges, inspires; is team oriented;
7. is knowledgeable, experienced, competent, intelligent; has good judgment;
8. is available, approachable; provides feedback; trains, coaches;
9. is constructive, enthusiastic, positive, friendly, humorous;
10. is decisive, courageous; takes risks; is willing to commit;
11. is goal oriented, makes plans, clarifies expectations, follows through;
12. accepts responsibility, blame; admits errors; is respected, respectful;
13. is a doer, participates, sets example;
14. is open, candid, sincere, credible; and
15. is creative, resourceful; has vision.

# Summary

While leadership is a complex, multidimensional concept, it is at the same time a process of influencing a group to set and achieve goals. There are several major theories of leadership. One of the earliest theories of leadership is the trait theory. This theory has been succeeded by other leadership theories including behavioral, situational, and interactional; although none of these approaches has adequately defined successful leadership.

Even though overlapping of leadership theories can occur quite easily, careful consideration was given to a number of leadership styles and the forces that influence the development of these various styles.

It was noted that power and authority are closely related. Power is the capacity to influence others, whereas authority is the right to direct others. Authority is obtained through position power, but several other types or categories of power exist. Consideration was also given to several strategies designed to increase an individual's power.

This chapter concluded with a discussion of factors associated with behavioral or reality approaches to leadership including individual relationships, group relationships, situation leadership, manager-subordinate relationships, integration of leadership or putting it all together, and suggestions for effective leadership behavior in being a first-line manager.

# Discussion Questions

1. What do you see as the essence of leadership?
2. Do you believe there is an ideal leadership style? Explain.
3. "All managers should be leaders, but not all leaders should be managers." Do you agree or disagree with this statement? Support your position.
4. What are your major strengths as a leader?
5. Can there really be any transformational leaders in therapeutic management practice regardless of setting? Explain.
6. Which of the various leadership theories discussed in this chapter do you think is the most applicable in a therapeutic recreation setting? Support your position.

# References

Adorno, T. W., and others. (1950). *The authoritarian personality.* New York, NY: Harper & Row.

Baird, J. E., Jr. (1982). *Quality circles leader's manual.* Prospect Heights, IL: Waveland Press, Inc.

Bass, B. M. (1985). *Leadership and performance beyond expectations.* New York, NY: The Free Press.

Bass, B. M. (1981). *Stogdill's handbook of leadership* (rev. ed.). New York, NY: The Free Press.

Blake, R. R., and Mouton, J. S. (1964). *The managerial grid.* Houston, TX: Gulf Publishing

Benziger, K. (1982). The powerful woman. *Hospital Forum, 25(3),* 15–20.

Claus, K. E., and Bailey, J. T. (1979). *Power and influence in healthcare: A new approach to leadership.* St. Louis, MO: C. V. Mosby.

Connolly, P. (1994, May). *Leadership style analysis* (brochure). Mid-Eastern Symposium on Therapeutic Recreation, Atlantic City, NJ.

Fiedler, F. E. (1967). *A theory of leadership effectiveness.* New York, NY: McGraw-Hill.

Fiedler, F. E., and Chemers, M. M. (1974). *Leadership and effective management.* Glenview, IL: Scott, Foresman and Company.

Frank, M. S. (1993, Fall). The essence of leadership. *Public Personnel Management, 22:3,* 381–389.

French, J. R. P., Jr., and Raven, B. (1968). The base of social power. In D. Cartwright and A. Zander (Eds.), *Group dynamics* (3rd ed., pp. 262–268). New York, NY: Harper & Row.

Gibb, C. A. (1969). Leadership. In G. Lindsy and E. Aronson (Eds.), *The handbook of social psychology* (2nd ed., pp. 216–228). Reading, MA: Addison-Wesley Publishing Co., Inc.

Hein, E. C., and Nicholson, M. J. (1990). *Contemporary leadership behavior* (3rd ed.). Glenview, IL: Scott, Foresman and Company.

Hersey, P., and Blanchard, K. H. (1982). *Management of organizational behavior: Utilizing human resources* (4th ed.). Englewood Cliffs, NJ: Prentice Hall.

Hitt, W. D. (1988). *The leader-manager: Guidelines for action.* Columbus, OH: Battelle Press.

House, R. J., and Mitchell, T. R. (1974). Path-goal theory of leadership. *Journal of Contemporary Business,* Autumn, 81–97.

Kotter, J. R. (1983). *The general manager.* New York, NY: The Free Press.

Kouzes, J. M., and Posner, B. Z. (1990). The credibility factor: What followers expect from their leaders. *Management Review, 79,* 29–33.

Lewis, J. A., and Lewis, M. D. (1983). *Management of human service programs.* Belmont, CA: Brooks/Cole Publishing Co.

Likert, R. (1967). *The human organization.* New York, NY: McGraw-Hill.

McClelland, D. C., and Burnham, D. (1983). Power is the great motivator. In E. G. C. Collins (Ed.), *Executive success: Making it in management* (pp. 289–305). New York, NY: John Wiley & Sons.

McGregor, D. (1966). *Leadership and motivation.* Cambridge, MA: MIT Press.

Megginson, L. C., Mosley, D. D., and Pietri, P. H., Jr. (1991). *Management: Concepts and applications* (4th ed.). New York, NY: HarperCollins Publishers.

Megginson, L. C., Mosley, D. D., and Pietri, P. H., Jr. (1986). *Management: Concepts and applications* (3rd ed.). New York, NY: Harper & Row.

Mintzberg, H. (1989). *Mintzberg on management: Inside our strange world of organizations.* New York, NY: The Free Press.

Moore T., and Wood, D. (1979). Power and the hospital executive. *Hospital and Health Services Administration, 24,* 30–41.

Porter-O'Grady, T. (1993, April). Of mythspinners and mapmakers: 21st century managers. *Nursing Management, 24:4,* 52–56.

Prentice, W. C. H. (1983). Outstanding leadership. In E. G. C. Collins (Ed.), *Executive success: Making it in management.* New York, NY: John Wiley & Sons.

Robbins, S. P. (1995). *Supervision today.* Englewood Cliffs, NJ: Prentice Hall.

Robbins, S. P. (1980). *The administrative process* (2nd ed.). Englewood Cliffs, NJ: Prentice Hall.

Schein, E. H. (1970). *Organizational psychology* (2nd ed.). Englewood Cliffs, NJ: Prentice Hall.

Schreisheim, C. A., Mowday, R. T., and Stogdill, R. M. (1976). Critical dimensions of leader-group interactions. In J. G. Hunt and L. L. Larson (Eds.), *Cross-currents in leadership* (pp. 113–121). Carbondale, IL: Southern Illinois University Press.

Skidmore, R. A. (1995). *Social work administration* (3rd ed.). Boston, MA: Allyn & Bacon.

Stogdill, R. M. (1974). *Handbook of leadership: A survey of the literature.* New York, NY: The Free Press.

Stoner, J. A. F. (1982). *Management* (2nd ed.). Englewood Cliffs, NJ: Prentice Hall.

Tannenbaum, R., and Schmidt, W. H. (1983). Effective Leadership. In E. G. C. Collins (Ed.), *Executive success: Making it in management* (pp. 151–168). New York, NY: John Wiley & Sons.

Tramel, M. E., and Reynolds, H. (1981). *Executive leadership: How to get it & make it work.* Englewood Cliffs, NJ: Prentice Hall.

Wadia, M. (1965). Management and the behavioral science: A conceptual scheme. *California Management Review, 8(1),* 65–72.

Yukel, G. A. (1989). *Leadership in organizations* (2nd ed.). Englewood Cliffs, NJ: Prentice Hall.

# Chapter 5

# Vision, Mission, Philosophy, and Objectives

## Introduction

A statement heard most frequently in the workplace is: "Today we have got to get organized." Individuals who express this view are in many instances venting frustration about the fact that the workplace is not functioning in a smooth and systematic manner. A major reason for this is the lack of statements associated with the workplace vision, mission, philosophy, goals, and objectives.

Statements regarding the vision, mission, or purpose of the therapeutic recreation department in a healthcare facility or a division of a public park and recreation department that espouse the philosophy, beliefs, goals, and objectives are part of the planning function or process. These statements provide the framework for all plans and activities within the department. These statements evolve from and support those that have been developed by the top management of the organization. These statements are the blueprints for effective management, and they set the stage for smooth operations. They are also the reasons for being. They articulate the major tasks to be carried out and the kinds of technologies and human resources to be employed.

This chapter focuses on aspects of a vision statement which may incorporate a vision, mission, philosophy, goals, and objectives. A vision statement is like a cascade, a series or succession of statements which act upon the preceding statement—flowing from one component or statement to the next. Not all organizations, agencies, or therapeutic recreation departments have implemented a total vision statement into their management operation or planning process. Some organizations tend to have independent components such as a mission or philosophy, while others tend to be a mixture of values, purpose, philosophy, beliefs, goals, and operations. The concern here is to clarify those components of a vision statement with examples from various types of organizations and their respective departments of therapeutic recreation. Likewise, to give some consistency to the various components or statements, illustrations of various statements of vision, mission, philosophy, goals, and objectives have been used from the same organization and its department of therapeutic recreation where possible. One is cautioned that there is some variance in the content from one component or statement to another.

## Vision

Vision is the buzzword of the 1990s. In recent years many health and human service organizations such as hospitals and community-based leisure service agencies, like business and industry before them, have developed vision statements. Further, some therapeutic recreation departments have developed vision statements in consonance with their organization or agency. A limited random sampling of therapeutic recreation departments regarding vision, mission, and philosophy statements taken by the authors produced few vision statements but a large percentage of mission and philosophy statements were evident. However, a vision and a mission can be one and the same: "Vision refers to a future state (i.e., a condition that is better than what now exists), whereas mission more normally refers to the present" (Campbell, Nash, Devine, and Young, 1992, p. 32).

A vision is a dream of greatness (Block, 1987). It is a word picture—a description of the future that provides a focus for coordinating the efforts in an organization or agency. Its expression is to provide a unifying theme and a challenge to all organizational departments or units. The vision communicates a sense of achievable ideals, serves as a source of inspiration for confronting the daily activities, and becomes a contagious, motivating, and guiding force congruent with the organization's ethics and values (Hax and Majluf, 1984). "A vision is a target that beckons" (Campbell, Nash, Devine, and Young, 1992, p. 38). From another perspective, the vision must relate to the wants of the customers while being grand enough and imaginative enough to fuel the employees' spirit (Block, 1987). From still another perspective a vision statement indicates quality and "a benchmark for value measurement" (Russoniello, 1991, p. 26).

Russoniello (1991, p. 22) defines a vision statement as "a description of a desired state that an organization or therapeutic recreation department commits to." According to Silvers (1994–95, p. 11) a vision is a "statement of what an organization stands for, what it believes in, why it exists, and what it intends to accomplish." A vision focuses on end results but not necessarily on how to get there. Goals focus on the direction, while objectives focus on how to get there. "A powerful vision provides the sense of where one is going. It empowers people. It provides the force, or guiding principle, behind why we do what we do" (Turpel, 1992, p. 4). As noted by Schroll (1995a, p. 25):

> When the organization has a clear, widely
> shared vision of its purpose and direction,
> it empowers individuals and confers status
> upon them. They see themselves as part of
> a worthwhile enterprise in pursuit of a
> shared mission.

Martin Luther King espoused a vision in his "I Have a Dream" speech; President John F. Kennedy espoused a vision when he said the United States should put a man on the moon by the end of the 1960s (Sorensen, 1965). Kearns and Nadler's (1992) history of the Xerox Corporation in *Prophets in the Dark* describes the vision of that company through the decades. The articulations of King and President Kennedy involved hoped for future end results; the Kearns narrative is ongoing.

Although the vision is initiated and developed by top management, the practitioner working for the organization has to become an active collaborator in the pursuit of the organization mission or purpose; he or she must share the vision of the organization and feel comfortable with the

way in which it is translated or expressed in values. The behavior of practitioners is conditioned by this framework, and they must intimately sense that by following the vision, they are fulfilling a personal need for achievement. The vision of the organization becomes a personal drive for their own lives. Russoniello (1991) notes that a vision statement provides motivation while Turpel (1992, p. 74) comments: ". . . that the vision must be fertile. The vision must excite people. . . . Focused vision inspires, empowers, and generates the commitment needed for innovation and effective action."

While a vision statement in its development is usually confined to senior management, there is no reason that a therapeutic recreation department cannot form a vision that is relevant to its own department by building on the organization's vision, mission, and objectives. The development of a vision may improve department planning and performance. If the organization does not have a vision, the initiation of one by the therapeutic recreation department may stimulate the organization as a whole to think about a vision.

## Creating a Vision

In developing of a vision statement for the therapeutic recreation department, intense focus must be on the consumer and must describe something that is markedly better than the current state. The vision is based on the values and beliefs of the department and its practitioners; on knowledge of the department's capabilities; on technical, regulatory, and environmental conditions; and on consumer requirements. "A vision statement is the collective identification of those aspects of care that recreational therapists feel are critical in the quest for quality" (Russoniello, 1991, p. 23).

How does one create a vision statement? Silvers (1994–95) suggests incorporating four basic components into the vision statement including values and beliefs, purpose, mission, and goal. The foundation of the statement consists of core values and beliefs. Achievement may be one of the core values of the department. Consumer satisfaction may be the measure of that value. Purpose is the second aspect of the vision and is an outgrowth of the department's values and beliefs. "A statement of purpose should clearly convey the basic human needs which are fulfilled by the department" (Silvers, 1994–95, p. 12). Mission comes next and states what the department does. The last aspects of the vision are goals. Goals are built upon the previous three statements. Goals focus on the future and guide the efforts of the department. "The goals should have a long-range outlook and reflect lofty ideals" (Silvers, 1994–95, p. 12).

Once the statement is completed and approved, the manager needs to communicate it to staff and motivate them to embrace it. By enthusiastically communicating the vision to practitioners, the manager begins the process of motivating them toward achievement of the vision (Silvers, 1994–95).

Figure 5.1 illustrates the vision statement of Sheltering Arms Physical Rehabilitation Hospital, a freestanding rehabilitation hospital, while Figure 5.2 (page 64) is the vision statement of the Recreation Therapy Department at the Iowa Methodist Medical Center.

## Mission or Purpose

Every organization, public or private, has a fundamental mission or purpose. The mission defined by an organization identifies its basic thrust—its business. For example, Southern Health (1995, p. 67), a managed care organization states its mission as follows: "Southern Health's mission is to be the preferred manager of high quality, cost-effective health benefit services." In many instances this statement is drawn from the vision statement but is more concise or focused on the type of services provided. Hospitals exist to provide healthcare services to the community. Local public park and recreation departments exist to provide recreation and leisure facilities and experiences to meet individual needs within the community. Churches exist to minister to the spiritual needs of individuals. Each department or unit within an organization has a mission which contributes to the overall purpose of the organization. In a broad sense, the therapeutic recreation depart-

ment in a general medical hospital exists to provide quality therapeutic recreation to patients. In the therapeutic recreation division of a community-based park and recreation department, the same purpose is intended but directed toward individuals with disabilities who live in the community.

The mission states the reason this particular therapeutic recreation department exists and the intent that it serves. A mission influences the philosophy, scope of service, goals, and objectives as well as the policies and procedures of an organization. For example, if a therapeutic recreation department in a general medical hospital is responsible for providing services in a psychiatric unit and that unit prepares patients for community adjustment, it should be staffed with a therapeutic recreation specialist particularly skilled in leisure counseling or education. How broad or narrow a mission statement should be is a controversial question. There are advantages and disadvantages to both narrow and broad mission statements. A narrow statement carefully specifies the area within which the department will consider its service, whereas a broad mission statement widens the areas of service. Too narrow a statement can blind the department to significant threats and opportunities from other departments or service units. Too broad a statement, on the other hand, encourages the department to expand into services where it has limited expertise.

The mission of the department should be known and understood by other facility staff, consumers and their

---

### Figure 5.1   Vision Statement of Sheltering Arms Physical Rehabilitation Hospital

The Sheltering Arms vision is to set the standard for providing comprehensive rehabilitation services of such high quality that our patients, clients, families and payers will receive superior value, and our employees, partners and community will benefit from successful outcomes.

*Sheltering Arms seeks to achieve its mission and vision by:*
- Continually improving the delivery of effective, personalized rehabilitation services along a broad continuum of care at convenient locations to persons who need and will benefit from our services.
- Providing superior physical rehabilitation services to persons in financial need through prudent stewardship of our resources.
- Recognizing and addressing the needs of the whole person—mind, body and spirit.
- Developing partnerships with persons and their families who are experiencing physical disabilities so that they actively participate in determining and achieving high quality functional outcomes.
- Creating an environment in which employees effectively use their knowledge and skills in which personal satisfaction and growth may be experienced.
- Establishing and fostering viable relationships and alliances with other healthcare providers, funding sources, educational institutions, and providers of products and services who share our values.
- Developing educational and research programs to advance the knowledge and science of physical medicine and rehabilitation.
- Creating processes that allow for the rapid infusion of new technologies and the dissemination and retrieval of information.
- Promoting public awareness and position attitudes concerning the capabilities and needs of persons with disabilities.

Used by permission of Sheltering Arms Physical Rehabilitation Hospital, Richmond, VA.

**Figure 5.2    Vision Statement, Recreation Therapy Department, Iowa Methodist Medical Center**

The Recreation Therapy Department is dedicated to making a difference in the lives of our patients, the community, and other professionals. Through our actions we will provide efficient treatment, assessment, and evaluation of patients and provide educational options to meet specific needs of patients and their families. We will strive to be recognized as the premier recreation therapy department in Iowa.

We are in pursuit of a vision that will:
- provide leisure education of the highest quality with opportunities for building independent, healthy lifestyles through creativity and self-expression while retaining positive self-esteem.
- strive to share our diversified professional skills through publishing articles and sponsoring and coordinating professional workshops and seminars in an effort to stimulate professional growth statewide and nationally.
- actively seek ways to enhance the quality of life for those we serve by advocating on their behalf to community, state and federal organizations. We are advocates of a "barrier-free" environment for all.

Used by permission of Iowa Methodist Medical Center, Des Moines, IA.

families, and the community. "An individual feels a sense of purpose when the organization has a strong mission and its values are attractive to the individual" (Campbell, Nash, Devine, and Young, 1992, p. 65). A mission statement must be dynamic, giving action and strength to evolving statements of philosophy, objectives, and management plans. Statements of mission can be made dynamic by indicating the relationship between the therapeutic recreation department and consumers, personnel, and community. Above all, it must be realistic. As Schroll (1995b, p. 22) comments: "If wrongly formulated, mission can become a straitjacket that prevents a company from moving forward."

The worded mission statement may be given from several different perspectives. First, it may state the purpose of the therapeutic recreation department *qua* organization, that is, the desired *structure* that provides for and controls therapeutic recreation service. A second option is to word the mission so as to describe the *process* of therapeutic recreation service desired. Other mission statements are worded in terms of desired consumer *outcomes*. In this regard, Russoniello (1991) comments that the mission statement "should reflect . . . what the consumer can expect as a result of the [therapeutic recreation] service" (p. 25). Some statements of mission choose to include all of these perspectives: structure, process, and outcome.

According to the management style of the organization, its size, and its structure, the therapeutic recreation manager may have more or less leeway in developing the department's mission and in defining the boundaries of therapeutic recreation's role.

Like the organization's mission, the therapeutic recreation department's mission is elaborated into a number of specific objectives. Otherwise, they remain good intentions that are not operationalized.

Figure 5.3 shows the respective mission statements of Sheltering Arms Rehabilitation Hospital and its therapeutic recreation program. The mission statement of Iowa Methodist Medical Center is found in Figure 5.4. Figure 5.5 (page 66) notes the Cincinnati Recreation Commission, Division of Therapeutic Recreation, mission statement including its operating principles. Figure 5.6 (page 66) illustrates the mission statement of both the city of Los Angeles Department of Recreation and Parks and its Special Services Adaptive Division.

# Philosophy

Philosophy is a statement of beliefs and values that direct one's practice. It verbalizes the therapeutic recreation managers' and therapeutic recreation practitioners' visions of what they believe therapeutic recreation management and practice are. It states their beliefs as to how the mission or purpose will be achieved, giving direction toward this end. It creates a climate for achieving professional excellence by stressing high standards. If a philosophy is stated in vague, abstract terms that are not easily understood, it is useless. Practitioners are most likely to interpret a philosophy from the pronouncements and actions of others in the organization. Therefore, conformity of action to belief is important. In addition, William G. Ouchi (1981) argued in *Theory Z* that a philosophy is critical because it enables individuals to coordinate their activities to achieve a purpose even in the absence of direction from managers.

The advantages of a philosophy statement are twofold. The first is that it can be used to guide behavior and decisions. Values, which a philosophy statement expresses, by their very nature define what course of action and outcomes "should be." Thus the statement can help direct

---

**Figure 5.3   Mission Statement, Sheltering Arms Physical Rehabilitation Hospital**

Sheltering Arms' mission is to provide comprehensive physical rehabilitation of the highest caliber to all who can benefit and to enhance the quality of life of persons experiencing disabilities.  For over 100 years Sheltering Arms has provided needed healthcare with compassion and respect to each individual, regardless of his or her ability to pay.

**Mission Statement, Therapeutic Recreation Program, Sheltering Arms Physical Rehabilitation Hospital**
To provide a comprehensive, team-oriented Therapeutic Recreation Program which includes a specific plan of care for individuals with a variety of physical disabilities.  To develop attitudes and skills necessary for maximum independence of leisure lifestyles through assessment, goal-oriented treatment sessions, group interaction, community reintegration, and discharge planning. Treatment is pursued in conjunction with family, physician, and treatment team.  Families are invited and encouraged to attend treatment sessions and community reentry evaluations.  Participation is encouraged to increase the family's knowledge of the patients' disability and to learn the skills necessary to promote a healthy leisure lifestyle.

---

Used by permission of Sheltering Arms Rehabilitation Hospital, Richmond, VA.

practitioners' attention in some directions and not others. A second potential advantage is that it may contribute to organization and department performance by motivating practitioners or inspiring feelings of commitment.

One does not need to be a philosopher to express ideas underlying therapeutic recreation practice.  A philosophy simply represents the central beliefs and values of the department relative to therapeutic recreation and therapeutic recreation practice.  Philosophies are not right or wrong, and their content varies from organization to organization depending on what values are perceived as central to therapeutic recreation.  In some settings a value statement is expressed in lieu of a philosophy statement.

Figures 5.7 (page 67) and 5.8 (page 67) represent therapeutic recreation philosophy statements from a public healthcare facility and a public community-based leisure service agency.

Before proceeding it is important to note that a therapeutic recreation department's vision, mission, and philosophy statements usually complement those of the organization or larger divisions or departments within the organization.  In such situations, the therapeutic recreation statements would need to be consistent with the organization or division statement.  It is not unusual to begin the various statements with: "We concur," "We believe," or "We are committed."  The various statements do not repeat generalities that might be found in the organization or larger di-

vision statements.  Instead, it focuses on the uniqueness within the context of the therapeutic recreation department.

# Goals and Objectives

It is well to note that the two terms *goals* and *objectives* are in many instances used interchangeably and should be considered as ends towards which all activity is directed.  These terms suggest aspirations or the desired end that any organization or department of therapeutic recreation attempts to realize.  This discussion will consider them separately. A goal is a state or condition that the organization and department want to achieve; it offers direction.  An objective, on the other hand, is the result to be achieved to reach the goal; it is the action taken to achieve the goal.

The reader is also reminded that within some therapeutic recreation departments there may be a scope of care or service section before the goals and objectives section or as a part of the section.  Such a section may address the services provided and if within the goals and objectives section notes the goal of a specific service and how it will be met through various objectives.  Figure 5.9 (page 68) provides an example of a scope of service statement relative to therapeutic recreation services within a physical rehabilitation department of a general medical hospital. The service activities in the example could be expanded to include the types of activities or specific focus of the

---

**Figure 5.4   Mission Statement, Iowa Methodist Medical Center**

Improve the health of our communities through healing, caring, and teaching.

---

Used by permission of Iowa Methodist Medical Center of Central Iowa Health System, Des Moines, IA.

---

### Figure 5.5 Mission Statement, Cincinnati Parks and Recreation Department

**Division of Therapeutic Recreation**
**Mission Statement**

The purpose of the Division of Therapeutic Recreation is to provide recreational programs and support services for individuals with disabilities. These programs and services are designed to develop leisure skills and facilitate participation in general recreation activities.

Operating Principles:
- Programs and activities will be based on participant's expressed interests.
- Programs will provide opportunities for the acquisition of skills, knowledge and attitudes relating to leisure involvement.
- The therapeutic recreation staff will emphasize personal choice, encourage independence and inspire individual achievement through each activity.
- Whenever possible, programs will be conducted in an inclusive environment. Therapeutic recreation staff will promote opportunities for individuals with and without disabilities to participate together.
- The therapeutic recreation staff will advance the concept of inclusive programming through advocation and alliance with the general recreation staff.

Used by permission of Cincinnati Recreation Commission, Cincinnati, OH.

---

activities found in each service area depending on the department's or hospital's policies and procedures addressing rehabilitation care planning.

Goals and objectives state actions for achieving the mission and philosophy. They are specific statements that therapeutic recreation managers seek to accomplish. Performance standards, deadlines, budgets, "to do" lists, and work objectives are all examples of work goals. If the mission and philosophy are to be more than good intentions, they must be translated into explicit goals. A major characteristic of effective goal setting is the avoidance of ambiguity in determining the exact goal. Goals are central to the whole management process—planning, organizing, directing, and controlling. Planning defines goals. The or-

ganization is organized and staffed to accomplish goals. Directions stimulate personnel to accomplish objectives, and control compares the results with objectives to evaluate accomplishments.

## Goals

According to Richards (1986), goals serve four important purposes. First, they provide guidance and a unified direction for all people in the organization. Goals can help everyone understand where the organization is going and why getting there is important. Second, planning, as noted earlier, is facilitated. Goals and planning are highly interrelated. Third, goals can serve as a source of motivation and

---

### Figure 5.6 Mission Statement, City of Los Angeles Department of Recreation and Parks

We unify Los Angeles by providing diverse recreational opportunities, beautiful facilities, and innovative leadership for our residents' and visitors' universal enjoyment.

**Mission Statement, Special Services Adaptive Division, City of Los Angeles Department of Recreation and Parks:**
We encourage our consumers with disabilities to integrate into classes and programs that meet their recreational and leisure needs at their local community recreation centers. For those consumers who prefer, our unit provides specialized programs with certified therapeutic recreation specialists who will provide quality care and close staff to consumer ratios. Consumers with disabilities in our specialized programs will have an opportunity to develop, maintain and express a satisfying leisure involvement.

Used by permission of City of Los Angeles Department of Recreation and Parks, Los Angeles, CA.

---

**Figure 5.7   Philosophy Statement, Activities Therapy, Northern Virginia Mental Health Institute**

Recreation therapy supports a philosophy consistent with the stated mission of the Institute: to conduct a program of therapeutic activities designed to strengthen the patient's skills and confidence and to promote independent leisure functioning through educational and recreational experiences and activities.

Recreation therapy service is composed of three components designed to meet individual needs:

I. **Treatment Services**—Through this component recreation therapy focuses on the improvement of some functional or behavioral need of the patient. Individuals are assessed to determine their physical, cognitive, social and emotional abilities and deficits. Recreational and leisure activities that have goals related to these identified needs are selected.

II. **Leisure education services**—Focus is on the development of acquired skills, attitudes and knowledge related to leisure participation and development. Through the leisure planning group, there is an emphasis on teaching the patients the proper use of leisure time, through discussion, assisting with the planning and taking on a responsible role as a leader in recreation therapy groups. Through the areas mentioned, the program develops the clients' leisure experience and maintains these skills as a carry-over in the community.

III. **Recreation participation service**—It provides opportunities for patients to participate in structured groups for recreation experience, self-expression, confidence, social and verbal interaction with others, physical exercise, group cohesiveness and enjoyment. Diversified recreational activities are developed to meet identified needs, abilities and interests through individual assessments.

Used by permission of Northern Virginia Mental Health Institute, Falls Church, VA.

---

at times inspiration to the employees of the organization. Goals that are specific and moderately difficult can motivate people to work harder, especially if attaining the goal results in a reward. Last, goals provide an effective mechanism for evaluation.

Who sets goals? The answer is actually quite simple. All managers at all levels within the organization should be involved in the goal-setting process. Moreover, goal setting incorporates short, intermediate, and long-term goals. There tends to be more organizational long-term goals than short-term goals associated with top management, whereas first-line managers are usually responsible for short-term goals, and there tends to be a balance or mix of management regarding intermediate goals (Griffin, 1990). As a final note, all organizations and departments have a multiple set of objectives, all of which should be compatible.

## Making Goal Setting Effective

Goal setting is an important task. There are several guidelines reflected in the literature for making goal setting effective. The following five guidelines noted by Griffin (1990), are the ones most frequently mentioned:

1. **Understanding the purposes of goals.** The best way to facilitate the goal-setting process is to make sure that all managers and practitioners understand the four main purposes of goals as noted earlier: (1) source of guidance and direction, (2) catalyst for planning, (3) stimulus for motivation and inspiration, and

---

**Figure 5.8   Philosophy Statement, Recreation for Special Needs, Alexandria Department of Recreation, Parks and Cultural Activities**

The Recreation for Special Needs section's programs are based upon the foundations and philosophies of therapeutic recreation, normalization and community integration. It is our belief that individuals with disabilities greatly benefit from participation in the experiences and enjoyment of recreation programs in the community. Programs emphasize learning and developing recreational skills, fine and gross motor development, and increasing self-awareness, communication and socialization skills. Activities are geared toward providing a challenge to the participants while allowing them to test their own abilities and increase their self-confidence.

Used by permission of Alexandria Department of Recreation, Parks and Cultural Activities, Alexandria, VA.

---

**Figure 5.9  Scope of Service**

Therapeutic Recreation Services of Community Memorial Hospital serves all patients, both inpatients and out-patients, with services provided by certified therapeutic recreation specialists in a professional, effective, and efficient manner. Services are delivered, only when medically indicated, under the direction of physicians and in collaboration with the rehabilitation interdisciplinary team. The hours of service are between 8:30 a.m. and 4:30 p.m., Monday through Friday. Some services are scheduled in the evenings and on weekends when appropriate.

    The scope of services includes an initial assessment to determine patient needs. Based on this assessment, services are provided to achieve maximal rehabilitation or functional ability through the use of activities which focus on treatment, leisure education, community integration, and general recreative participation.

---

(4) mechanism for evaluation and control (Richards, 1986). Goal setting and implementation should be undertaken with those purposes in mind.

2. **Stating goals properly.** Making sure that goals are properly stated is another way to improve the goal-setting process. To the extent possible, goals should be specific, concise, and where necessary, time related.

3. **Goal consistency.** A third way to improve the goal-setting process is to be sure that goals are consistent throughout the organization. All goals must agree with one another—be compatible.

4. **Goal acceptance and commitment.** People, regardless of their place in the organization, need to have a high level of acceptance and commitment to work toward organization and department goals. Managers need to demonstrate their vision for the organization in everything they do in order to encourage goal acceptance and commitment by those who work for them. Moreover, managers should also allow for broad-based participation in the goal-setting process whenever appropriate, and they should make sure that goals are properly communicated. People are much more likely to accept and become committed to goals if they help set them or at least know how and why the goals were established.

5. **Effective reward systems.** Goal setting can also be improved if it is integrated with the reward system of the organization or department. People should be rewarded first for effective goal setting and then for successful goal attainment. However, since failure sometimes results from factors outside the manager's control, people should also be assured that failure to reach individual goals will not necessarily bring punitive consequences.

It is important also to recognize that while these guidelines are positive in nature, the reverse of these guidelines can disrupt things. An inappropriate goal would be one that is not consistent with the organization or department mission. Another obstacle would be goals so extreme that accomplishing them is virtually impossible. Overemphasis on quantitative or qualitative goals is another problem. And finally, improper reward systems act as a barrier to the goal-setting process.

Figures 5.10 and 5.11 illustrate goal statements from a community-based leisure service agency and a healthcare facility respectively.

## Objectives

Good objectives have two principal characteristics. They should be (1) specific and verifiable, and (2) attainable. Specific and verifiable means that, where possible, objectives should be stated in quantitative terms like goals. The more quantitative the goal, the more likely it is to receive attention toward its accomplishment and the less likely it is to be distorted. Unfortunately, it is not possible to quantify all objectives. Some objectives, because of the nature of the plan, will have to be qualitative. Nevertheless, even qualitative objectives should be made as specific and verifiable as possible.

Sometimes it is said that qualitative objectives are gauged by the standard of "how well," and quantitative objectives by "how much." To some extent this is true, but in the author's experience, a qualitative goal can be made highly verifiable by spelling out the characteristics of the programs or other objectives sought and a date of accomplishment.

The second important characteristic of a good objective is that it is attainable. Optimally, an objective should be fairly difficult but not impossible to reach. Goals that are too high tend to discourage managers and practitioners. Those that are too low have little motivational impact and may result in under accomplishment.

### Writing Objectives

The development and writing of objectives should not be a difficult undertaking providing that there has been a thorough collection of data, and a definition of the needs of the

---

**Figure 5.10 Goals Statement, Recreation for Special Needs, Alexandria Department of Recreation, Parks and Cultural Activities**

To expand knowledge of the leisure and recreational opportunities and resources available in the community.
To provide opportunities for social interaction through the use of leisure activities and programs.
To promote the physical, emotional, and social growth and development of the individual.
To motivate and encourage participation in recreational activities.

---

Used by permission of Alexandria Department of Recreation, Parks, and Cultural Activities, Alexandria, VA.

situation have been established. The essentials of developing and writing objectives are quite simple: set meaningful goals written in the form of objectives and evaluate how well the objectives have been met. In general, the objectives should begin with an action verb and describe an activity that can be measured or at least observed. Whenever possible, the objective should be specific, time bound if feasible, and state a measurable or observable end result in order to increase the objectivity of the evaluation done at the end point.

The objective should also be meaningful and either congruent with the goals of the organization or department or deliberately aimed at changing the goal. The time set for completing the objectives depends on the nature of the work being planned and other factors that will affect the speed with which the work can be completed. Time lines are particularly helpful in working out the specific objectives leading to a long-term goal. When the objective is complex, it may also be necessary to break it down even further into separate steps or components to have an adequate guide to work by and to evaluate the progress toward meeting the goal. Objectives and time estimates should be considered as flexible guides not unbendable demands.

## Objective Areas

Since organizations or departments have more than a singular objective, it is valuable to consider areas from which goals can emanate. Goals may be internal or external. They either relate to the direct needs of the organization or to the consumer and society it serves. Internal goals are primarily concerned with human, physical, and financial inputs and their transformation into desirable outputs. External goals focus on consumer satisfaction and social awareness. Every organization or department must satisfy the needs of consumers who have the power to curtail its livelihood.

The therapeutic recreation staff, specifically the therapeutic recreation manager, must decide where efforts will be concentrated to achieve results. A major objective area is evaluation of consumer service, or developing methods of measuring the quality of patient care. Certainly, the American Therapeutic Recreation Association's (ATRA) *Standards for the Practice of Therapeutic Recreation and Self-Assessment Guide* (1993) and the National Therapeutic Recreation Society's (NTRS) *Standards of Practice for Therapeutic Recreation Service and Annotated Bibliography* (1995) should be used as guidelines in the development and evaluation of consumer service and patient care.

---

**Figure 5.11 Goals Statement, Recreation Therapy, Iowa Methodist Medical Center**

**Recreation Therapy Goals**
To assist in the development of leisure awareness and the appreciation of the values and importance of participation in one's leisure.

To engage client in the acquisition of leisure interests and activity skills commensurate with his or her abilities, including socialization and interactive skills.

To assist in the development of health emotional functioning including improved levels of self-esteem, increased motivational level, and the identification and expression of feelings.

To provide an opportunity for community awareness and participation, and to facilitate a link with community programs.

To provide leisure services to patients as stated above, and also to families, employees, volunteers, affiliated students, and community interest groups.

---

Used by permission of Iowa Methodist Medical Center of Central Iowa Health System, Des Moines, IA.

In addition, the concepts of *appropriateness, quality assurance,* and *continuous quality improvement* should be incorporated.

Other internal objectives would include evaluation of personnel performance and staffing in accordance with practitioner's skill levels; educational program planning; requisition of supplies and equipment to facilitate consumer service; innovation to introduce new methods; and particularly, the application of new knowledge.

No organization can survive very long if it does not meet the needs of some constituency. When an organization no longer satisfies its consumers, it finds its charter rescinded, its revenues shrinking, and a lack of public support for its objectives. Therefore, all organizations must serve a constituency and satisfy the needs of consumers. The same is so for the therapeutic recreation department. As part of the health and human service delivery system, it must provide quality service.

## *Implication for Therapeutic Recreation*

Objectives are the fundamental strategy of therapeutic recreation since they are the end product of all therapeutic recreation activities. Objectives must be capable of being converted into specific targets and specific assignments so that therapeutic recreation personnel will know what they have to do to accomplish them. Further, objectives become the basis and motivation for therapeutic recreation work and for measuring therapeutic recreation achievement regardless of setting.

In therapeutic recreation, all objectives should be performance objectives. They should provide for existing therapeutic recreation services and for existing consumer groups. They should provide for abandonment of unneeded and outmoded therapeutic recreation services. They should provide for new services, for new consumers, and for standards of therapeutic recreation service and performance.

Objectives are the basis for work and assignments. They determine the department structure, key activities, and the allocation of staff to tasks. Objectives make the work of therapeutic recreation clean and unambiguous, the results are measurable, there are deadlines to be met, and there is a specific assignment of accountability. Objectives also give direction and make commitments that mobilize the resources and energies of therapeutic recreation for the future. Finally, objectives should be changed as necessary particularly when there is a change in mission or purpose or when they are no longer functional.

Figure 5.12 represents goals and objectives from the Activities Therapy Department, Northern Virginia Mental Health Institute of Falls Church, Virginia.

## Summary

It was noted that the development of a statement of the vision, mission or purpose, philosophy, goals, and objectives of an organization at the division or department level sets the stage for smooth operations. Moreover, all managers use such statements in their management operation and planning process to accomplish the work of therapeutic recreation.

The vision statement articulates what an organization and department considers important and what it hopes to achieve. The mission or purpose articulates the reason for the department's existence within the organization while the philosophy reflects the values and beliefs of the organization and the department. Goals and objectives state actions for achieving the purpose and philosophy and serve as a guide in planning work, setting priorities, and evaluating effectiveness. Objectives should be verifiable and attainable and are of a short-, intermediate-, and long-term nature. Guidelines for setting effective goals and the areas from which goals can emanate were given. This chapter concluded with the implications of objectives for therapeutic recreation.

## Discussion Questions

1. Make a list of goals you wish to achieve in the next five years. Are they verifiable? Are they attainable?
2. Write a concise vision statement (including mission, philosophy, values, goals, and objectives) for a department of therapeutic recreation with which you are familiar.
3. Interview the head of the parks and recreation department in your community or the director of therapeutic recreation at the local hospital to ascertain what the mission, philosophy, and objectives of his or her department are. Share findings with class.
4. In considering question three above, can the department, regardless of setting, accomplish its vision, mission, and objectives? Why or why not?
5. Develop a picture vision in your mind of a therapeutic recreation department regardless of setting. Put the picture in words.
6. Collect and critique vision, mission, purpose, philosophy statements and write statements according to guidelines presented in this chapter.
7. Develop a mission statement reflective of structure, process, and outcome per descriptions in this chapter.
8. Write objectives for the goal statements presented in Figures 5.10 and 5.11.

**Figure 5.12 Goals Statement, Activities Therapy, Northern Virginia Mental Health Institute**

**Goal 1**
To provide an individualized treatment plan for each patient that includes instructions and practice in areas of physical, social, emotional, cognitive, and recreational skills supportive of independent living.

*Objective A*
Recreation therapy staff will orient patients on the acute treatment unit to a schedule of supervised activities in which patients can participate to provide structure to their day. Staff will initiate weekly charting within 15 days.
*Objective B*
Recreation therapists will evaluate each patient's abilities, problems, and needs and develop goals and plans based on that evaluation within six to nine working days following admission.
*Objective C*
Recreation therapy staff will reassess patient's needs based on performance, and, in consultation with the patient, staff will select and design a schedule of activities targeted towards further improvement of independent living.
*Objective D*
Recreation therapy staff will review patient's progress weekly while on the acute care unit and revise as goals are met or new data indicates. Maintenance goals may be developed after 60 days if patient's level of performance in recreation therapy remains unchanged for one month.

**Goal 2**
To provide a therapeutic treatment program of recreation therapy services based on identified needs of patients during the day, evenings, weekends and holidays.

*Objective A*
Recreation therapy supervisor and clinical director will annually review the effectiveness of each activity program in meeting the needs of all patients and revise as indicated.
*Objective B*
Recreation therapy supervisor, in conjunction with administration, will ensure that there are sufficient, qualified, credentialed staff and volunteers and adequate space, budget, and equipment to meet program goals.
*Objective C*
Recreation therapy supervisors and all recreational therapy staff will incorporate community volunteers and resources in supporting treatment programs.

**Goal 3**
To maintain departmental and interdisciplinary communication in delineating goals for patient's treatment and co-ordinating delivery of service.

*Objective A*
At least one recreation therapy staff will attend one Client Treatment Plan (CTP) per week on each team. Recreation therapy staff will also serve as CTP documenters as assigned by Medical Records.
*Objective B*
Recreation therapy staff will meet weekly to plan coordinated activities, exchange information, and monitor patient care and quality assurance.
*Objective C*
Recreation therapy supervisor will participate in clinical services meeting each month.
*Objective D*
Recreation therapy personnel will serve on Institute committees as assigned by the Institute Director.

*Figure continues on page 72*

**Figure 5.12 Continued**

**Goal 4**
To provide education opportunities for Institute staff, students and volunteers, and interested members of the community.

*Objective A*
All recreation therapy personnel, students of affiliated colleges and universities, and volunteers will receive training at times of placement in policies and procedures as defined in orientation procedures.
*Objective B*
All recreation therapy staff will participate in continuing education as defined in staff development procedure.
*Objective C*
Recreation therapy department staff will provide orientation to activities program and expectations for other departmental staff of the Institute.
*Objective D*
Recreation therapy supervisor will provide information about the Institute program and needs to members of the community as requested.
*Objective E*
Recreation therapy supervisors will actively recruit educational affiliations, comply with contractual agreements to ensure close cooperation with the educational establishment, and provide a positive learning experience for the students.

**Goal 5**
To ensure compliance with established standards for quality of services provided and competency of activities staff and volunteers.

*Objective A*
All recreation therapists will ensure compliance with all hospital, federal, state, and local policy requirements and maintain standards needed for accreditation by professional agencies.
*Objective B*
Recreation therapy services will maintain a systematic, ongoing collection and analysis of data to ensure that services provided have the intended effect.
*Objective C*
All recreation therapists will review all objectives, goals, policies and procedures of the recreation therapy department at least biannually, and revise as needed when a change in organization or program occurs.
*Objective D*
Recreation therapy supervisor will ensure that the quality assurance plans are in place, implemented according to stated schedule and reported to the Quality Assurance Committee quarterly as scheduled.

**Goal 6**
To maintain safety of all patients and personnel involved in activities by monitoring safety of equipment and environment at all times in compliance with federal, state, and local regulations.

*Objective A*
Recreation therapy supervisor is responsible for developing infection control and safety policies and procedures for his or her respective service, as well as monitoring the personnel, equipment and environment in their related activities at all times.
*Objective B*
Recreation therapy director will ensure that all activities personnel and volunteers are aware of and responsible for safety procedures at all times.

# References

American Therapeutic Recreation Association (ATRA). (1993). *Standards for the practice of therapeutic recreation and self-assessment.* Hattiesburg, MS: Author.

Block, P. (1987). *The empowered manager.* San Francisco, CA: Jossey-Bass.

Campbell, A., Nash, L. L., Devine, M., and Young, D. (1992). *A sense of mission—Defining direction for the large corporation.* Reading, MA: Addison-Wesley Publishing Co., Inc.

Griffin, R. W. (1990). *Management* (3rd ed.). Boston, MA: Houghton Mifflin Co.

Hax, A. C., and Majluf, N. S. (1984). *Strategic management: An integrative perspective.* Englewood Cliffs, NJ: Prentice Hall.

Kearns, D., and Nadler, D. A. (1992). *Prophets in the dark.* New York, NY: HarperCollins.

National Therapeutic Recreation Society (NTRS). (1995). *Standards of practice for therapeutic recreation service and annotated bibliography.* Arlington, VA: National Recreation and Park Association.

Ouchi, W. G. (1981). *Theory Z: How American business can meet the Japanese challenge.* Reading, MA: Addison-Wesley Publishing Co., Inc.

Richards, M. D. (1986). *Setting strategic goals & objectives* (2nd ed.). St. Paul, MN: West Publishing Company.

Russoniello, C. V. (1991). "Vision statements" and "mission statements": Macro indicators of quality performance. In B. Riley (Ed.) *Quality management: Applications for therapeutic recreation* (pp. 21–28). State College, PA: Venture Publishing, Inc.

Schroll, C. (1995a). Strategic planning to strategic management: Incorporating vision and mission. *Virginia Parks and Recreation, 22:1,* Spring, 25–26.

Schroll, C. (1995b). Part two: Strategic planning to strategic management: Incorporating vision and mission. *Virginia Parks and Recreation, 22:2,* Summer/Fall, 22–23, 28.

Silvers, D. I. (1994–95, Winter). Vision—Not just for CEOs. *Management Quarterly, 35:4,* 10–14.

Sorensen, T. C. (1965). *Kennedy.* New York, NY: Harper and Row.

Southern Health. (1995, August 13). Who is Southern Health? *Discover by the Seasons* (Supplement to the *Roanoke Times*).

Turpel, L. T. (1992). Strategic management. In R. M. Winslow and K. J. Halberg (Eds.), *The management of therapeutic recreation service* (pp. 71–83). Arlington, VA: National Recreation and Park Association.

# Chapter 6

# Organizational Behavior

## Introduction

Therapeutic recreation managers can benefit from the study of organizational behavior because it helps them understand and predict human behavior within individual groups and teams in an organization—and at the department level—even though therapeutic recreation departments in health-care facilities and community-based leisure service agencies are relatively small in comparison to other organizational departments. Before considering the behavior of individuals, groups, and teams in an organization it is important to realize that organizations, regardless of size, have a culture and a climate which affect individual and group behavior throughout the organization.

## Organization Culture and Climate

Organizational culture is similar to societal culture in that both are pervasive and powerful forces that shape behavior. Every organization has a culture of values and behaviors. A culture consists of both the implicit and explicit contracts among individuals that include what is expected of them and the rewards or sanctions associated with compliance or noncompliance of these contracts. Further, a culture is based on a pattern of basic assumptions or behaviors that have worked in the past and are taught to new individuals as the correct way to perceive, to think, to feel, and to act.

One often assumes that everyone, particularly managers, are savvy about organizational culture just as one assumes everyone is politically savvy or "street smart." Indeed, culture smart is part of street smart or political savvy. Unfortunately, many managers and employees, regardless of setting, are naive about the concepts, application, or importance of organizational culture. Thus, a brief discussion is in order about this matter.

Organizational culture is the sum total of symbols, language, philosophies, traditions, sacred cows, and unspoken gestures that overtly reflect the organization's norms and values. For the most part, these shared, and unquestioned assumptions and behaviors have a profound effect on both the organization's decision making and the staff's performance (Wilkins, 1984).

Cultural norms and values are reflected in policies and practices, social decorum, physical environment, communication networks (formal and informal), status symbols, and in virtually every other aspect of the organization work life. Management style, whether authoritarian or participatory, is also part of organizational culture.

The basic assumptions that form the foundation of the culture are illuminated and understood through organizational tropes, metaphors, stories, myths, rituals, and ceremonies. A culture characterized by militaristic metaphorical expressions such as "we run a tight ship here" is quite different from one with family metaphors like "people care about each other here." Other metaphors identified by del Bueno and Vincent (1986) to characterize personalities and

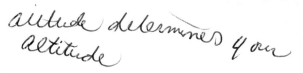

work styles include sports, anthropology, television, mechanics, and animals. The underlying culture of an organization can be determined by listening carefully to the tropes, metaphors, and other cultural indicators.

A successful therapeutic recreation manager identifies quickly and accepts the prevailing culture before attempting to bring about change. Organizational culture is difficult to change because it operates at the level of basic beliefs, values, and perspectives. Moreover, since change often involves revolution and conflict, it is a tough issue (Dyer and Dyer, 1986).

Organizational climate, as opposed to the values and behaviors of organizational culture, is the emotional state shared by members of the organization. More specifically, it is a "measure of whether people's expectations about what it should be like to work in an organization are being met" (Schwartz and Davis, 1981, p. 31). The climate can be formal, relaxed, defensive, cautious, accepting, trusting, and so on. A work climate that is set at the top management level impacts the first-line manager, and, in turn, this determines the behavior of the staff in the department.

Staff members want a climate that will give them job satisfaction, high salaries, good working conditions, and opportunities for professional growth that increase self-esteem through self-actualization. Therapeutic recreation managers can establish this type of climate by emphasizing tasks that stimulate motivation and by using discipline fairly and uniformly to provide opportunity for committee assignments, to promote participation in decision making, and to reduce boredom and frustration (Conway-Rutkowski, 1984). In addition, a successful manager will be not only professionally competent but also organizationally acculturated.

The organizational climate and culture is also supported directly and indirectly by work rules. In addition, these rules provide assistance in motivating the employee. Liebler, Levine, and Rothman (1992, p. 222) suggest that work rules serve several functions:

- they create order and discipline so that the behavior of workers is goal oriented;
- they help unify the organization by channeling and limiting behaviors;
- they give members confidence that the behavior of other members will be predictable and uniform;
- they make behavior routine so that managers are free to give attention to nonroutine problems;
- they prevent harm, discomfort, and annoyance to clients; and
- they help ensure compliance with legislation that affects the institution as a whole.

# Principles of Organizational Behavior

It is well-known that people differ in their work performance. Numerous factors have been identified as affecting individual performance in an organization. Factors that affect performance include (1) personality, (2) motivation, (3) perception, (4) group size, and (5) organizational support (Baron, 1983).

## *Personality*

Each person exhibits a unique combination of behaviors and characteristics that are relatively stable. All personalities exhibit demographic, competency, and psychological characteristics. A manager seeks to have a blend of personalities on staff, including volunteers, where possible, who will be able to interact not only with one another but also with a diverse consumer population. Persons of varied demographic characteristics (for example, a 24-year-old single male graduate practitioner and a 55-year-old female practitioner aide and grandmother) present different developmental concerns, societal role expectations, and past experiences. These differences may enrich the lives of both staff members, or they may present obstacles to their working together. Encouraging acceptance and respect for the uniqueness of each person and emphasizing what each person can contribute to the organization and department is an essential role of the therapeutic recreation manager.

Just as people vary in demographic characteristics, they also have individual competency differences. The abilities, aptitudes, and skills of each staff member must match the tasks they are expected to perform. Frustration grows quickly if one's capabilities are overused or underused. Continuing education or training activities can be practiced and/or adopted to develop or enhance job skills, but they cannot correct for the lack of a person's ability to perform the job.

Psychological characteristics also contribute to one's personality. Values, attitudes, interests, and traits provide other sources of differences among individuals. Attitudes are usually expressed by feelings of like and dislike or by thoughts and beliefs about something in the environment. Organized attitudes about a larger system are considered values. Individuals are most content when they feel that the attitudes and behaviors of everyone are balanced and consistent. Interests are based on likes and dislikes of different activities. Determining which activities are most relevant to the department's purpose helps the therapeutic recreation manager accurately describe the department tasks to prospective staff members. When the interests and the needs of the department's practitioners and the department's needs are congruent, work performance is enhanced. Traits are particular ways that people vary from one another; they are descriptors of the way people act or are perceived (i.e., sensitive, aggressive, self-starter).

Values, attitudes, interests, and traits predispose persons to certain behaviors. For therapeutic recreation managers an understanding of these characteristics can be useful in trying to improve individual performance and group behavior.

## *Motivation*

People employ certain behaviors to attain certain goals. Motivation derives from the needs and drives of a person. Needs are related to goals toward which behavior is directed. Staff practitioners with a high need for recognition will be most productive if their participation in department activities is recognized by the manager. If a staff practitioner is asked to coordinate a staff meeting for the purpose of clarifying patient goals and objectives because the manager is off that particular day, early recognition by the therapeutic recreation manager of this meeting and its contribution to the delivery of service will reinforce the staff practitioner's action.

Drives are directed energy. Some therapeutic recreation practitioners continually strive to be the most knowledgeable person in the department concerning the delivery of services to a particular group of consumers. If this drive is identified and responded to positively by the manager, the department can benefit from the expanded knowledge base of this practitioner. By supporting the practitioner's quest for continued education through attendance at conferences or additional course work, the therapeutic recreation manager can request that the practitioner share information with the rest of the staff through an in-service training program.

Motives cannot be directly observed; they can only be inferred. Motives may raise from curiosity, activity, or exploration. Since motives are often difficult to ascertain, therapeutic recreation managers need not focus on the reason for the behavior but rather on the behavior itself and its results.

Therapeutic recreation managers can motivate staff by setting specific expectations, providing prompt feedback, and giving plenty of encouragement. More about motivation is found in Chapter 15.

## *Perception*

People tend to organize the sensory input from their environment selectively into meaningful patterns. Past experience is related to the present situation. A certain amount of selective attention allows a person to fill in missing data or to simplify his or her response to a wide range of situations. Varied individual perceptions of a situation are evident when people are asked to describe an incident they witnessed. No two accounts of it will be exactly the same. There is also a certain amount of self-preservation in one's perception. The uniqueness with which each person perceives helps that person to create and maintain a sense of order and constancy in a complex and changing world by filtering some of the sensory stimuli.

The therapeutic recreation manager must remain aware of the fact that perceptions vary from person to person. To keep perceptions fairly uniform, the manager needs to: (1) update information, (2) use written rather than verbal methods of information giving, (3) repeat information periodically, (4) report information in group meetings, (5) encourage asking questions for clarification, (6) keep minutes of meetings, and (7) check the minutes for accuracy.

The more an individual disagrees with the sensory stimuli, the greater the chance for distortion of it. When a department policy is changed and announced at a staff meeting, the actual change is frequently lost. Some staff members, usually in favor of the change, may be able to articulate clearly the difference from the old and new policy requirements. However, other members, often those not in agreement with the change, may leave the meeting unable to describe the policy change and quickly forget that they are expected to change their behavior in accordance with the change in policy. To prevent this kind of discordance in perception, therapeutic recreation managers need to seek out ways to make staff perception uniform. For example, policy changes may be presented in writing.

## *Group Size*

Group size influences the possible relationships, communication patterns, and responsibility for participation in a group. Researchers have found that as the number of group members increases, so, too, does the number of possible relationships among the members. Thus, more group members means more avenues of communication and consequently the possibility that multiple communication difficulties will arise. Large groups may inhibit member participation and may result in domination by a few and the split into subgroups. These factors can have a negative effect on the attractiveness of the group and can contribute to greater turnover and absenteeism of its members. The larger the group, the more effort needed by the manager to coordinate and organize the collective potential of membership.

There are times, however, when a large group is advantageous. Increasing group size offers more human resources and helps accomplish the group task especially when the task is complex. Small groups tend to foster more personal discussion and more active participation, but fewer people exist to share in the work responsibilities. Problem solving is handled more efficiently in groups of five to seven members because there is less chance for differences between the leader and members, less chance of domination by a few members, and less time required for reaching decisions (Megginson, Mosley, and Pietri, 1992). Any size group can be well-managed and can achieve a high task level performance through attention to the group process, group dynamic, and with good decision-making strategies.

## *Organizational Support*

Work group dynamics significantly affect individual performance. This factor will be fully discussed in the following section.

# Groups and Organizations

People are born into a group (i.e., the family) and interact with others at all stages of their lives in various groups: peer groups, work groups, recreational groups, religious groups, etc. A group is a collection of two or more people interacting with one another over a period of time. People join groups for many reasons: security, proximity, goals that would be unattainable by individual effort alone, economics, social needs, and self-esteem needs. Much of a therapeutic recreation manager's or practitioner's professional life is spent in a wide variety of groups, ranging from *dyads* (two-person groups) to large professional organizations.

Groups and their performance are assuming today greater importance in modern organizations. The complexity and interactions of both technology and social systems are increasing. In various forms (e.g., matrix organizations, cross-functional teams), team effort and performance have taken on greater importance in organizational situations. Indeed, many organizations are consciously and deliberately moving toward organizational structures based on group concepts as a means of improving responses to an increasingly complex environment. The emphasis on quality circles and self-managed teams in various organizations provides excellent examples.

Groups usually form by the same process regardless of the type of group. Members develop a mutual acceptance of each other, discuss and experiment with decision, select a leader, develop motivation, and thus establish norms of operation. Each member influences, and is influenced by, the others with some degree of dependence on each other in respect to the attainment of one or more common goals.

Groups appear in various forms in the work setting of an organization. They are good for the organization and its members, making important contributions to organizational task accomplishments. Organizational groups can also influence work attitudes and behaviors. Schermerhorn, Hunt, and Osborn (1982) describe other effects of groups in organizations that include:

1. influence on an individual's choice of performance goals and work methods,
2. positive effect on productivity,
3. clarification of the rewards to be expected,
4. facilitation of members' learning of job skills and knowledge, and
5. establishment of expectations regarding the probability of success.

The first-line therapeutic recreation manager should view groups as an important phenomenon in organizations. Groups can have both positive and negative effects on an organization and its members since in some instances they have potential influence on the organization. The manager should recognize that groups in organizations or departments are human resources. An understanding of behavior and dynamics within the group can help reduce undesirable consequences while enhancing desirable consequences.

The following section describes three major groups found in organizations: formal, work group or committee, and informal.

## *Types of Groups*

### Formal Group

The formal group, as noted previously, is one created by the formal authority of the organization to accomplish specific goals. It is part of the formal structure of the organization and usually appears on formal organizational charts. The formal group has goals specifically created to achieve the goals of the organization and typically has clear-cut superior-subordinate relationships as opposed to meeting needs of group members. Committees and task forces are additional examples of a formal group.

Traditional features of formal groups include the following:

1. Authority is imposed from above.
2. Leadership selection is assigned from above and made by an authoritative and often arbitrary order or decree (fiat).
3. Managers are symbols of power and authority.
4. The goals of the formal group are normally imposed at a much higher level than the direct leadership of the group.
5. Fiscal goals have little meaning to the members of the group.
6. Management is endangered by its aloofness from the members of the work group.

7. Behavioral *norms* (expected standards of behavior), regulations, and rules are usually superimposed. The larger the turnover rate of members, the greater the structuring of rules.
8. Membership in the group is only partly voluntary.
9. Rigidity of purpose is often a necessity for protection of the formal group in the pursuit of its objectives.
10. Interactions within the group as a whole are limited, but informal subgroups are generally formed (Kaluzny, Warner, Warren, and Zelman, 1982).

## Work Group

The work or task group is created by the formal authority of an organization for a clearly defined purpose as opposed to a collection of people who congregate to see a play or a sporting event. Specifically, a work group is any number of people who (1) interact with one another, (2) are psychologically aware of one another, (3) perceive themselves to be a group, and (4) are motivated to participate in the group (Shortell, Kaluzny, and associates, 1988; Kaluzny, Warner, Warren, and Zelman, 1982). The work done by this group is goal and reality oriented. There are usually clear specifications of the procedures or methods needed to achieve the task. In community-based leisure service agencies and healthcare facilities this means providing quality service according to clearly defined therapeutic recreation standards. In addition to providing quality service, therapeutic recreation work groups have other reasons for forming: to hear reports, impart assignments, conduct direction-giving sessions, solve consumer problems, or engage in committee activities.

The work group enables organizations and their members to accomplish things that individuals cannot do alone. A group can pool resources, divide responsibility, represent more interest in a decision, and may provide better communication. Schermerhorn, Hunt, and Osborn (1982) describe the work group as created by a formal authority to transform inputs (ideas, materials, and objects) into outputs (report, decision, and service). Some of these groups are permanent (i.e., therapeutic recreation department, standing committees), while others are temporary (i.e., ad hoc or special committees) and usually dissolve after the group has accomplished its task. Permanent or standing committees are usually advisory in authority, but some may have collective authority to make and implement decisions.

According to Schermerhorn, Hunt, and Osborn (1982), an effective work group is one that achieves high levels of both task performance and human resource maintenance overtime. A number of forces or dynamics facilitate the effectiveness of the work group (e.g., purpose, norms, status, role). And group dynamics affect task performance and membership satisfaction as well.

Berne (1983) writes that effective work groups depend on sensitive leadership that elicits creative group participation. Therapeutic recreation managers, as has been noted, are involved in any number of work groups in their specific setting and should become as familiar as possible with the dynamics of groups in order to promote work group effectiveness and productivity. Managers will need to work hard in creating cooperative work groups from a staff that may not share cultures, ideals, and values.

While work groups or committees have advantages, they also have disadvantages. The division of responsibility may be considered a disadvantage in many situations because there is no place to assign blame. Groups may successfully avoid action. Most group decisions are compromises; therefore, they are neither the best nor the worst decision that could be obtained. Often a group assumes no responsibility for decisions or actions. A group may engender a false sense of democracy in the organization especially when it is dominated by a powerful chairperson. Last, groups within an organization may be in conflict. The limit to available resources, a difference in goals, a failure to clearly define tasks, and a false perception of the role of the group may lead directly to conflict within the group and between groups.

## Informal Group

The informal group is a group formed by coworkers to satisfy their own personal needs. Its major difference from the formal group is that the informal group is not created by the formal authority. In a strict sense, informal group activity constitutes those activities not officially sanctioned in any organization policy or manual. The informal group affords its members a sense of affiliation, emotional support, identification, belonging, and security. Moreover, the informal group develops its own communication network known as the "grapevine" which is outside the formal communication channel designed by management. As noted by Mayo (1933), research showed that the lack of opportunity for social contact resulted in employees experiencing a loss of self-esteem and perceiving their jobs as unsatisfying.

The informal group can serve to complement the formal organization by generating optimal task performance and productivity and by giving social values and stability to the workplace. The informal group can also have negative and more destructive effects on the organization when it works directly in opposition to the organization's goals and objectives and creates only negative conflict that affects group task performance and productivity.

The astute therapeutic recreation manager needs to become familiar with these effects in order to gain a better understanding of how the informal group operates in relation to the formal organization and to one's own department. In all cases, the formal structure must prevail; the informal group should always complement and assist the effort of the formal group.

## *Group Development*

B. W. Tuckman (1965) developed a model of small group development that incorporates four stages of growth: (1) forming, (2) storming (3) norming, and (4) performing.

### Forming

In this stage individuals first come together and form initial impressions. They begin by determining the task of the group although some purposes, objectives, and goals may already have been set by management. In addition, individuals try to determine role expectations of one another. Since group members are unsure of their roles, considerable attention is given to the leader in establishing the agenda.

### Storming

In the second stage individuals begin to express themselves about goal setting, who is responsible for what, a standard of behavior. It is not unusual for conflict among group members to arise. Since individual differences need to be resolved to the mutual satisfaction of all, this is good and should be allowed. However, conflict does have to be managed, and reorganizing is sometimes necessary.

### Norming

This stage is viewed as sharing group norms. In other words, teamwork begins to develop, there is a sense of group cohesiveness and openness of communications with information sharing. Trust and cooperation develop and goals and standards by which the group will operate are finalized. Decisions are made about what has to be done and who will do it. If problems continue to exist or are carried over from any of the earlier stages, progress to the next stage will be slow, if at all.

### Performing

The final stage occurs when there is a stable pattern of personal interaction, joint problem solving and shared leadership including achievement of goals and objectives. The performing group is much like a mature group that has been described by Bradford (1976) and Cohen, Fink, Gadon, and Willitis (1988). The characteristics of a mature group are as follows:

- a sense of ownership, or involvement, by the members is established;
- group difficulties become everyone's concern;
- leadership is shared by all;
- responsibility for one's own behavior and its effects on other members is assumed;
- trust and caring reduce the defensiveness within the group;
- self-awareness is heightened, and the group uses ideas more efficiently;
- more diverse resources are sought and used;
- different viewpoints are encouraged and exchanged;
- listening to one another becomes an active process;
- the group is able to examine its own method of operating with a minimum of defensiveness;
- solving problems can be experimented with by using different methods or approaches;
- task forces can be formed for certain tasks with open recognition;
- differences in perception, need, purpose, and contribution of all members can be explored;
- flight from a task by the group can be recognized and dealt with openly;
- new members can be incorporated and accepted; and
- hidden agendas can be allowed to surface in open discussion without disrupting the group.

A mature group develops over time with the careful interventions of the manager. Affirmative action on the part of the therapeutic recreation manager helps to develop the kind of member participation that ensures a high level of group productivity and member satisfaction.

## *Group Dynamics*

Shaw (1971) noted several dynamics that influence work group effectiveness are (1) group rank, (2) group status, (3) group role, (4) group norms, and (5) group cohesiveness.

### Group Rank

When an individual joins a group, he or she will be implicitly evaluated by the other group members. This is called group rank, or the position of a group member relative to the evaluation of other members of the group. The rank order can influence an individual's behavior in a group by affecting: (1) the member's interactions with other group members, (2) the individual's level of aspiration, and (3) the individual's self-evaluation. All of these can combine to affect the group member's ability to perform the task assigned to him or her in the group.

Group members rank each other on a variety of characteristics including intelligence, verbal performance, and popularity. The first-line therapeutic recreation manager as a group leader should be aware that all group members, including the group leader, will be evaluating each other throughout the life of the group and that this evaluation can affect the group member's and the group's work. It is important to note that the manager as group leader may rank a member high on a particular characteristic but that this member may not rank high on this same characteristic according to other group members. Being aware of the group rank dynamic can help the manager avoid communication problems that affect the group's work.

## Group Status

Group status is the prestige attributed to particular positions in the group. Cohen, Fink, Gadon, and Willitis (1988) describe status as a collection of rights and duties. A group member can bring status into the group from outside or can be assigned status as a result of behavior with the group. Status can be based on a number of characteristics such as age, work seniority, past positions held within the organization, performance in the group, and education. Status congruence occurs when a group member's standing in each factor is consistent with the standing in other factors. When standings vary among factors, status incongruity occurs. Status incongruity can affect individual and group performance because members that experience a range of status incongruities are not sure how to react to it. Status incongruities can pose challenges to department managers who want to assure group effectiveness. The following is an example of status incongruity.

An assistant therapeutic recreation manager position is available in a large staff therapeutic recreation department in a general medical hospital. One applicant has been working in the department for only a short time in the psychiatric unit. However, the applicant had leadership positions in two previous jobs in other hospitals. In addition, the applicant has advanced education. The incongruities among these factors can pose questions in the minds of the staff as to how best to react to these inconsistencies if a new (or different) applicant is appointed to this position. Some staff may find it is difficult to work with this. It might be helpful for the manager and/or the committee choosing the assistant to arrange an interview with some staff representatives and this applicant so that the staff can discuss with the applicant some of the questions or concerns.

## Group Role

A group role is the function or part a person assumes as a member of a group. It is often referred to as the part a person plays in a group. Role and status can be viewed as inseparable; role is the dynamic aspect of status that operationalizes the rights and duties granted by other group members. Role is often referred to as the set of expectations that group members share concerning the behavior of a person who occupies a given position in a group. A role acted out by a group member may or may not be useful for the task. Further, an individual in a group receives multiple role expectations and occupies multiple roles. It is important for all group members to develop role flexibility, skill and security in a wide range of roles as well as an awareness of those roles that negatively affect the work of the group.

A broad range of roles assumed in work groups have been described by Benne and Sheats (1984, p. 47). The following list contains a description of each of these roles that serve to enhance the group task and promote group functioning:

1. initiator-contributor—suggest new ideas;
2. information seeker—clarifies suggestions;
3. opinion seeker—clarifies values;
4. information giver—offers facts or generalizations;
5. opinion giver—states beliefs or opinion;
6. elaborator—spells out suggestions;
7. coordinator—clarifies relationships;
8. orienter—summarizes what has occurred;
9. evaluator-critic—evaluates the logic of group discussion;
10. energizer—prods group interaction;
11. procedural technician—does things for group;
12. recorder—writes down suggestions;
13. encourager—praises contributions of others;
14. harmonizer—mediates differences between members;
15. compromiser—offers compromise by coming "halfway";
16. gatekeeper—tries to keep communication channels open;
17. standard setter—applies standards to group;
18. commentator—keeps records of group process; and
19. follower—goes along with group movement.

On the other hand, Benne and Sheats (1984, p. 49) also list group roles which have a negative, inhibiting effect on groups which include:

1. aggressor—disapproves, deflates status of others;
2. blocker—is stubborn and negative;
3. recognition seeker—calls attention to self;
4. self-confessor—uses group as an audience to express personal feelings;
5. playboy—exhibits general lack of involvement;
6. dominator—tries to control groups;
7. help seeker—tries to provoke sympathy response from group members; and
8. special interest pleader—states biases in his or her own stereotypic fashion.

Since the group leader can assume any or all of these roles, the therapeutic recreation manager should become familiar with those roles that have a more facilitating or vitalizing effect on the group's task or functioning and should strive to assume more of those positive roles. If a therapeutic recreation manager has an awareness of the roles that inhibit a group's work and are irrelevant to the group task and functioning, the manager can begin to create some sort of harmony within the group.

## Group Norms

Group norms are the organized and largely shared, unwritten rules or ideas that evolve in every group and determine the behavior of the group. They also function to regulate the performance of a group as an organized department. The collective will of a group determines its group norms. Norms cannot be dictated. The norms adopted by the group are many and can be both positive and negative. A manager wants the group to acquire norms supportive of organizational goals.

The performance norm is especially important for the work group. Members of a group with a positive performance norm give the best they can to a task or project always striving for success. Group members with a negative performance norm may do just enough work to get by and may have an attitude of "not really caring" if they fail or if a project does not turn out well. Other group norms especially important for the work group include the adaptation or change norm, the interaction-communication norm, and the leadership-support norm. Researchers report that work groups with more positive norms tend to be more successful in accomplishing organizational objectives than groups with more negative norms (Heidman and Hornstein, 1982; Homans, 1961).

Conformity to norms is strongly influenced by group cohesiveness. In a highly cohesive group there is strong conformity to group norms. Therapeutic recreation managers as group leaders can help groups build positive norms. The following are ways to influence positive norm building as suggested by several sources: (1) emphasize positive role modeling, (2) reward desired behavior, (3) give regular feedback and performance reviews, (4) work with new group members to adopt desired behavior, (5) include desired behaviors in group member selection criteria, (6) hold regular meetings to look specifically at task performance and member satisfaction, and (7) utilize group decision making to agree on desired behaviors (Heidman and Hornstein, 1982; Homans, 1961; Napier and Gershenfeld, 1973).

## Group Cohesiveness

Group cohesiveness is the end result of all the forces operating in a group that motivate members to remain or leave the group. It is often referred to as group "we-ness" or the amount of "group-ness." Group cohesion can be viewed as an "organizing" force that contributes to overall group potency and vitality. This cohesive force increases the significance of membership for those who belong. When a person is attracted to a group, he or she is motivated to behave in accordance with the wishes of other group members. Important characteristics of high cohesive groups include the following: trust among members, high group productivity, group satisfaction with work, tasks accepted readily, more group energy for projects, commitment to group goals, high member interaction, low turnover, and promptness (Homans, 1950, 1961).

The therapeutic recreation manager can employ the following methods according to Homans (1950, 1961) to build a cohesive group: (1) induce agreement on group goals, (2) increase member homogeneity, (3) support member interactions, (4) introduce competition with other groups, (5) provide groups with individual rewards and praise, and (6) decrease group size.

On the other hand, examples of how the therapeutic recreation manager could help decrease group cohesion include:

1. induce disagreement on group goals,
2. increase member heterogeneity,
3. inhibit interaction among staff,
4. provide individual awards and praise,
5. remove physical isolation,
6. enlarge group size,
7. introduce a dominating staff member, and
8. disband the group.

When a group is highly cohesive, there is greater conformity to group norms. Also, when the performance norm of a highly cohesive group is high, there is a positive effect on task performance and productivity. In this case increased conformity to the group norm serves the organization well (Cartwright and Zander, 1968).

Sometimes a group will be congenial, agree on goals, and feel like a team yet fail in its mission. In such instances, what may have caused the failure is a phenomenon called *groupthink.* This factor is examined in the next section.

## *Groupthink*

The groupthink phenomenon occurs when highly cohesive groups lose criteria evaluative capabilities for one another's ideas and suggestions (Janis, 1982). The group no longer becomes willing to disagree or appraise alternative courses of action when problem solving. Loyalty and unity norms are weak when members become unable to challenge each other. Groupthink is often referred to in the literature as *negative cohesion,* and it has a negative influence on decision making in the group. Highly cohesive groups can be conducive to groupthink except when certain conditions are present, or special precautions are taken to counteract the group's push for unanimous agreement.

Irving Janis (1968) is known for describing eight main symptoms of the groupthink phenomenon:

1. the group experiences an illusion of invulnerability that promotes excessive risk taking, optimism, and confidence in the group's work;
2. the group makes collective efforts to rationalize its decisions stopping any warnings that might promote reconsideration of other assumptions;
3. the group unquestionably believes its morality and does not address ethical and moral consequences of the decision;
4. all group members look at any possible opposing factions in a stereotypical way as being too weak or stupid to challenge the group's decision;
5. group members put strong, direct pressure on any dissenters in the group, forcing a hard (or solid) loyalty norm;
6. each group member self-censors any of his or her own doubts or objections;
7. the group members share the illusion that all decisions and judgments are unanimous; the group relies on consensual validation versus individual thinking or reality testing.
8. "mindguards" emerge from the group who serve to protect everyone from thoughts that might present opposing views and that question the group's morality or effectiveness.

Therapeutic recreation managers as leaders of a variety of groups are in a key position to identify a group's movement toward the groupthink phenomenon. A manager can ask the following questions when suspecting groupthink according to Janis (1968):

1. Do I, as the group leader, cause members to "fall into line" with my way of thinking thereby strongly influencing their decision making?
2. Are there discussions of any opposing views or possibilities?
3. Is the group able to look at the advantages and disadvantages of any decision?
4. Are objectors or opposing views tolerated by the group?
5. Is decision making rushed or do group members take time to reach a decision?
6. Does the group feel overly confident with its decision making?
7. Are various ideas criticized or pulled apart?
8. Does the group look at the possible consequences of its decisions?
9. Does the group reach a decision too easily with a general consensus?

Several means to decrease groupthink by the therapeutic recreation manager have also been described in the literature by Janis (1982). They include the following:

1. Give priority to verbalizing objections while assigning each group member the role of critical evaluator.
2. Remain impartial about own preferences and expectations, especially at onset.
3. Encourage group members to discuss periodically the group's deliberations with two trusted associates and report back.
4. Invite outside qualified experts into the group periodically.
5. Continuously attempt to encourage critical thinking, open inquiry, while avoiding a "unity at all costs" thinking.

A final note about groupthink. It is important for the therapeutic recreation manager to understand that conflict is not always dysfunctional and dissent must be allowed if good decisions are to be made.

The next section addresses specific behaviors within groups and suggests both a philosophy and first-line manager activities to promote effective behavior within groups.

## Affirmative Action in Groups

Activities which are most beneficial in groups can be categorized as: (a) information gathering, (b) discussion, (c) problem solving, (d) making and implementing decisions, and (e) evaluating the outcome of the group's work (Cartwright and Zander, 1968).

The therapeutic recreation manager needs to monitor the information flow within the group—who introduces new information, how it is received by the staff, and what action follows it can be indicative of the maturity of the group. The manager can check the facts with the staff and supply missing or misconstrued data.

Closely related to information gathering is the kind and amount of discussion that takes place within the group. For example, are staff freely exchanging their ideas, or are they exchanging glances? Does discussion of a topic cease after one staff member speaks, or is a topic fully explored by those present? The manager can help the group become conscious of topic hopping if it continues for a few minutes.

Modeling behavior helps the group to become aware of its own behavior and to move on to address less obvious issues that are blocking the group.

Problem solving is a significant task of most work groups. The manager must be sure the group is given problems that it has the capability, capacity, and authority to solve. Groups will soon learn if their solutions are taken seriously. If they are not, the group will either stop participating in the process, or it will offer hastily considered solutions just to be done with the process. Decision making requires much forethought on the part of the manager before the group is asked to participate in the decision-making process. Managers must be willing to abide by the group's decision even if it is different from their own. Groups become frustrated when asked to participate in a decision only to find themselves trying to guess what their manager wants! This behavior promotes distrust and apathy in the group. Staff can learn to live with an autocratic therapeutic recreation manager more easily than a so-called participative manager who changes the decision after the staff is dismissed (Maier, 1967).

While a manager may not agree with the group's decision, if the manager has delegated decision-making responsibility to the staff, he or she must abide by the decision. Abrupt changes by the manager who favors a different approach will negate effective functioning of the group. If the decision presents a serious problem, the manager is bound by the group process to take the issue back to the group for further discussion. However, a wise therapeutic recreation manager will not use this mode of action too often, or the group will refrain from decision making.

Once a decision has been made, all staff should be aware of who, when, and how the decision will be implemented. When these details are left vague, confusion and a delayed implementation of the decision occurs at best. Poorly implemented decisions often lead group members to grumble that "nothing ever changes," or "I'm not going to waste my time in trying to make changes." Routine evaluations of the outcomes of the group's work helps everyone to see how the organization or department is developing, how they can learn from mistakes, and it will allow them to feel appreciated for fruitful efforts. Further discussion of decision making and group process will address some of the guidelines and factors facilitating group decision making (see Chapter 11).

In conclusion of this discussion about groups and their behavior, Table 6.1, offers a comparison between effective and ineffective groups.

## Group Meetings

The therapeutic recreation manager will participate in a variety of conferences, committee meetings, and department meetings. Conferences are usually one-time affairs, held for a limited time and dealing with a specific topic or problem. Committees are relatively permanent groups with organizational sanction. They are usually directed toward a specific purpose or task, have some mechanism for selecting members, and have authority to make recommendations or decisions. Both types of groups involve persons representing several units or departments.

A number of characteristics influence the nature and effectiveness of small group communication. For one thing,

the status and authority of each member in relation to the other, his or her past experiences together and current relationships both individual and as a group, and the expectations and preconceptions he or she have of each other will influence the communication patterns they use. Second, the structure of the group imposes certain patterns of interaction. Time and place characteristics are additional determinants of communication (see Chapter 14). A final characteristic is the expertise of each member in relation to the assigned task. Department meetings are similar to committee meetings. Most organizations expect their various departments to have staff meetings. These meetings are broader in scope than committee meetings and have authority to make recommendations and decisions concerning the function of the department.

Agendas are essential for conducting efficient meetings. They allow group members to prepare for meetings and ensure that all necessary items are addressed. Whether conducting a committee meeting or a department meeting the following steps are important:

- To prepare an agenda in advance and distribute it to those who will be attending. This enables participants to gather materials, if needed, and be prepared for any discussion.
- To state the purpose of the meeting at the top of the agenda.
- To state a definite start and stop time for the meeting and stick with it.
- To structure a content and process agenda and to determine the type of process and action desired on each agenda item. One is likely to have "information only," "decision only," and "decision required" items.
- To establish priorities by setting priorities for each agenda item so that group members focus on addressing the most important items.
- To determine the order of the agenda items. Place important items toward the beginning of the agenda.
- To establish time limits on items by deciding on an approximate amount of time to be spent on each agenda item. On "decision required" items acknowledge when the time limit has been reached; then ask the group to decide whether and how to continue with these items.
- To appoint a recorder who will take minutes and monitor time.
- To express concern if the group is straying from the agenda.
- To take a few minutes at end of meeting to "process" the meeting and discuss what went well, what problems came up, and what can be done about the ways in which the group works together.

## Table 6.1 Comparative Features of Effective and Ineffective Groups

| Factors | Effective Groups | Ineffective Groups |
|---------|------------------|--------------------|
| Atmosphere | Informal, comfortable, and relaxed. It is a working atmosphere in which people demonstrate their interest and involvement. | Obviously tense. Signs of boredom may appear. |
| Goal setting | Goals, tasks, and objectives are clarified, understood, and modified so that members of the group can commit themselves to cooperatively structured goals. | Unclear, misunderstood, or imposed goals may be accepted by members. The goals are competitively structured. |
| Leadership and member participation | Shift from time to time, depending on the circumstances. Different members assume leadership at various times, because of their knowledge or experience. | Delegated and based on authority. The chairperson may dominate the group, or the members may defer unduly. Members' participation is unequal, with high-authority members dominating. |
| Goal emphasis | All three functions of groups are emphasized—goal accomplishment, internal maintenance, and developmental change. | One or more functions may not be emphasized. |
| Communication | Open and two way. Ideas and feelings are encouraged, both about the problem and about the group's operation. | Closed or one-way. Only the production of ideas is encouraged. Feelings are ignored or taboo. Members may be tentative or reluctant to be open and may have "hidden agendas" (personal goals at cross-purposes with group goals.) |
| Decision making | By consensus, although various decision-making procedures appropriate to the situation may be instituted. | By the highest authority in the group, with minimal involvement by members; or an inflexible style is imposed. |
| Cohesion | Facilitated through high levels of inclusion, trust, liking, and support. | Either ignored or used as a means of controlling members, thus promoting rigid conformity. |
| Conflict tolerance | High. The reasons for disagreements or conflicts are carefully examined, and the group seeks to resolve them. The group accepts unresolvable basic disagreements and lives with them. | Low. Attempts may be made to ignore, deny, avoid, suppress, or override controversy by premature group action. |
| Power | Determined by the members' abilities and the information they possess. Power is shared. The issue is how to get the job done. | Determined by position in the group. Obedience to authority is strong. The issue is who controls. |
| Problem solving | High. Constructive criticism is frequent, frank, relatively comfortable, and oriented toward removing an obstacle to problem solving. | Low. Criticism may be destructive, taking the form of either overt or covert personal attacks. It prevents the group from getting the job done. |
| Self-evaluation as a group | Frequent. All members participate in evaluation and decisions about how to improve the group's functioning. | Minimal. What little evaluation there is may be done by the highest authority in the group rather than by the membership as a whole. |
| Creativity | Encouraged. There is room within the group for members to become self-actualized and interpersonally effective. | Discouraged. People are afraid of appearing foolish if they put forth a creative thought. |

Source: *Psychiatric nursing,* Second Edition, by H. S. Wilson and C. R. Kneisl. Copyright 1983 by Addison-Wesley Publishing Co. Reprinted by permission.

- To follow up by distributing copies of meeting minutes including reminders about assignments and deadlines to all persons who attended (Davis, Skube, Hellervik, Gebelein, and Sheard, 1992).

# Teams

Considerable emphasis in recent years has been placed on self-managed teams in the workplace. McHenry (1994) suggests that self-managed teams are a "tool for the 21st century workplace" (p. 801). It is argued that individuals working as a team can bring results that surpass in quantity and quality the contributions of individuals working independently. According to Katzenbach and Smith (1993) teams are the key to improving performance. They further comment that organizations cannot meet the challenges from total quality to customer service without teams. Robbins (1995) notes that "teams typically outperform individuals when the tasks being done require multiple skills, judgment, and experience" (p. 387). Last, "self-directed teams are an integral part of reengineering" in healthcare suggests Blancett and Flarey (1995). If teams are so successful, what constitutes a "team"? Elizabeth D. Becker-Reems (1994), director of human resources at Memorial Mission Hospital in Asheville, North Carolina, defines a self-managed team as a "permanent, self-managed group of employees who work together to produce a product or service" (p. 3).

The implementation of self-managed teams within health and human service organizations has been primarily associated with total quality management (TQM) and other employee involvement practices wherein the work relationships are interdependent (e.g., nursing service, psychiatric unit, physical rehabilitation unit). Therapeutic recreation managers and practitioners are involved as members of TQM or continuous quality improvement (CQI) teams which focus on improving quality and consumer satisfaction as well as being members of various unit treatment teams.

Robbins (1995) notes that teams fall into three categories depending on their objectives. These include teams used to *provide advice* (i.e., improve quality), teams that *manage* (i.e., run things), and teams that *do things* (i.e., handle administrative work).

While teams and groups are not necessarily the same thing, there appears to be some similarity between group development, as discussed earlier in this chapter and in the literature (Eggert, 1994; Smith and Hukill, 1994; Tuckman, 1965), and team development (see Table 6.2). Regardless, the literature (Becker-Reems, 1994; Katzenbach and Smith, 1993; Osburn, et al., 1990; Robbins, 1995) suggests there are several characteristics or elements associated with teams:

1. They are usually of small size—six to ten members—but this may vary depending on the volume of work to be accomplished. It is suggested that no team should consist of more than 18 members.
2. For a team to perform successfully, there should be a mix of skills, but not all team members should have all these skills: technical or functional expertise, problem-solving and decision-making skills; interpersonal skills (i.e., listening, risk taking, objectivity, feedback), and administrative skills.
3. A commitment to a common purpose relative to the responsibilities given to the team usually by management.
4. The development of specific performance goals which are measurable.
5. The development of a common approach to meeting the purpose and goals of the team.
6. Team accountability which is mutual among all team members.

The roles and responsibilities of team members vary depending on the nature of the work and the degree of empowerment given to them by the organization. Six functions have been identified by Becker-Reems (1994): planning, performing the work, measuring and improving performance, solving problems and making decisions, conducting meetings, and training other team members.

While self-managed teams have been successful in industry, their successful implementation in health and human service organizations is still a question mark. At the same time there is a downside to self-managed teams. A major concern noted by Megginson, Mosley, and Pietri (1992) as related to industry is that the reward systems (pay, promotion, career paths, etc.) do not support the team approach. Moreover, the United States has a strong political and personal tradition of individual freedom that, at times, runs counter to the collective nature of teamwork. For many employees, both managerial and nonmanagerial, an emphasis on team values threatens not only their traditional views of work, but also their approach to life (Sims and Lorenzi, 1992). Another concern, if implemented within a department, is that the department manager's responsibilities are absorbed within the team. However, the former manager can move into other positions such as team coach, technical advisor, trainer, multiteam manager, or transition planner (Becker-Reems, 1994). Although, in general, employees that have moved into the self-managed team concept are better satisfied and quality has improved, it is suggested that any organization develop a solid foundation for the change including the benefits of the change. Robbins (1995, p. 399) observes that teams perform poorly as a result of "a weak sense of direction, infighting, shirking of responsibilities, lack of trust, critical-skill gaps, or lack of

**Table 6.2    Summary of Stages of Team Development**

| Stage | Team behaviors | Leadership behaviors |
|---|---|---|
| Orientation | Uncertainty<br>Unfamiliarity<br>Mistrust<br>Nonparticipator | Directive style<br>Outline purpose<br>Negotiate schedules<br>Define the team's mission |
| Forming | Acceptance of each other<br>Learning communication skills<br>High energy, motivated | Plan/focus on the problem<br>Positive role modeling<br>Actively encourage participation |
| Storming | Team spirit developed<br>Trust developed<br>Conflict may arise<br>Impatience, frustration | Evaluate group dynamics<br>Focus on goals<br>Conflict resolution<br>Establish goals and objectives |
| Norming | Increased comfort<br>Identify responsibilities<br>Effective team interaction<br>Resolution of conflicts | Focus on goals<br>Attend to process and content<br>Supportive style |
| Performing | Clear on purpose<br>Unity/cohesion<br>Problem solve and accept actions | Act as a team member<br>Encourage increased responsibility<br>Follow up on action plans<br>Measure results |
| Terminating | Members separate<br>Team gains closure on objectives | Reinforce successes<br>Celebrate and reward |

Source: Smith, G. B., and Hukill, E. H. (1994). Quality work improvement groups: From paper to reality. *Nursing Care Quality, 8:4,* 1–12. Reproduced by permission of *Journal of Nursing Care Quality.* Aspen Publications.

external support." Last, Perley and Raab (1994) note that it takes three to five years to implement a self-managing work team with commitment of top management.

The different characteristics of groups and teams are shown in Table 6.3 (page 88).

## Summary

Initially it was noted that people differ in their work performance and that a number of factors affect individual performance. They include personality, motivation, perception, group size, and organizational work.

Also noted was that groups appear in various forms in the work setting of an organization. Three major groups are usually found in the organization: formal, informal, and work groups. The formal group is created by the formal authority of the organization, while the informal group is formed by people who work together mainly to meet the social needs of its members. The work group is created by a formal authority for a clearly defined purpose. It is goal

directed and reality oriented. Work groups can be permanent or temporary.

Several dynamics affect work group effectiveness. They include group rank, group status, group roles, group cohesiveness, and group norms. Characteristics associated with each group were identified by listing the roles that function to enhance the group task and promote group functioning as well as those roles that inhibit effective group task.

Consideration was also given to groupthink, a phenomenon that occurs when highly cohesive groups lose their ability to evaluate critically one another's ideas and suggestions. Symptoms of the groupthink phenomenon were identified.

It was noted that a mature work group has less need for the informal group. The mature work group is characterized by a shared sense of ownership of the group. The therapeutic recreation manager can encourage a high level of group productivity and staff satisfaction by engaging in affirmative actions which include information gathering,

### Table 6.3    Characteristic Tendencies of Groups and Teams

| Groups | Teams |
|---|---|
| Managed | Led |
| Perform best in stable situations | Perform best in dynamic situations |
| Members need to conform | Members need to challenge |
| Clear, hierarchical lines of management | Differentiated roles |
| Delegation of responsibility | Shared responsibility |
| Behavior can be learned | Behavior can be learned |

Source: Eggert, M. (1994, April 6). Team-playing. *Nursing Standard, 8:28,* 50–54. Reproduced with permission. RCN Publishing Co.

discussion, problem solving, decision making and evaluation of outcomes.

Last, consideration was given to self-managed teams which in the opinion of some authors surpass the contribution of individuals working independently. Characteristics associated with teams as well as the role and responsibilities of team members were identified. In addition, problems associated with teams were noted.

It may be concluded from this chapter that an awareness of behavior and its effect on an individual or a group within an organization or department helps the therapeutic recreation manager anticipate and predict reactions to particular activities and situations.

# Discussion Questions

1. Consider a setting wherein a therapeutic recreation department exists. What cultural factors lead to managerial effectiveness?

2. Compare and contrast formal groups with informal groups. Is leadership important in both types? Why or why not?

3. If groups have so many limitations (ineffective), why are they so popular?

4. As a therapeutic recreation manager for a division or department, regardless of setting, how would you deal with an informal leader in a work or task group who seems to be totally opposed to the objectives of the task group?

5. Identify conditions within a healthcare facility where self-managing work teams would not be the way to organize, and vice versa.

6. Identify some typical tendencies in perception. Does any one apply to you? What are the implications for your everyday life? How can you guard against perceptual fallacies?

# References

Baron, R. A. (1983). *Behavior in organizations: Understanding and managing the human side of work.* Boston, MA: Allyn & Bacon.

Becker-Reems, E. D. (1994). *Self-managed work teams in health organizations.* Chicago, IL: American Hospital Publishing Company and American Hospital Association Company.

Benne, K., and Sheats, P. (1984, Spring). Functional roles of group members. *Journal of Social Issues,* 42–49.

Berne, E. (1983). *The structure and dynamics of organization and groups.* New York, NY: Grove Press, Inc.

Blancett, S. S., and Flarey, D. L. (1995). Teams: The fundamental reengineering work unit. In S. S. Blancett and D. L. Flarey (Eds.), *Reengineering nursing and healthcare: The handbook for organizational transformation* (pp. 87–99). Gaithersburg, MD: Aspen Publishers, Inc.

Bradford, L. P. (1976). *Making meetings work: A guide for leaders and group members.* La Jolla, CA: University Associates.

Cartwright, D., and Zander, A. (1968). *Group dynamics* (3rd ed.). New York, NY: Harper & Row.

Cohen, A. R., Fink, S. L., Gadon, H., and Willitis, R. D. (1988). *Effective behavior in organizations.* Homewood, IL: Irwin.

Conway-Rutkowski, B. (1984, February). Labor relations: How do you rate? *Nursing Management,* 13–16.

Davis, B. L., Skube, C. J., Hellervik, L. W., Gebelein, S. H., and Sheard, J. L. (1992). *Successful manager's handbook.* Minneapolis, MN: Personnel Decisions, Inc.

del Bueno, D. J., and Vincent, P. M. (1986, May/June). Organizational culture: How important is it? *Journal of Nursing Administration,* 7–21.

Dyer, W. G., and Dyer, W. G., Jr. (1986, February). Organizational development: System change or culture change? *Personnel,* 14–22.

Eggert, M. (1994, April). Team-playing. *Nursing Standard, 8:28,* 50–54.

Heidman, M. E., and Hornstein, H. A. (1982). *Managing human forces in organizations.* Homewood, IL: Richard D. Irwin, Inc.

Homans, G. C. (1961). *Social behavior: Its elementary forms.* New York, NY: Harcourt Brace Jovanovich.

Homans, G. C. (1950). *The human group.* New York, NY: Harcourt Brace Jovanovich.

Janis, I. L. (1982). *Groupthink: Psychological studies of policy decisions and fiascos* (2nd ed.). Boston, MA: Houghton Mifflin.

Janis, I. L. (1968). *Victims of groupthink.* Boston, MA: Houghton Mifflin Co.

Kaluzny, A. D., Warner, D. M., Warren, D. G., and Zelman, W. N. (1982). *Management of health services.* Englewood Cliffs, NJ: Prentice Hall.

Katzenbach, A. E., and Smith, L. R. (1993). *Wisdom of teams: Creating the high performance organization.* Boston, MA: Harvard Business School Press.

Liebler, J. G., Levine, R. E., and Rothman, J. R. (1992). *Management principles for health professionals.* Gaithersburg, MD: Aspen Publishers, Inc.

Maier, N. R. F. (1967). Assets and liabilities in group problem solving. *Psychological Review, 74*(4): 239–249.

Mayo, E. (1933). *The human problems of an industrial civilization.* Cambridge, MA: Harvard University Press.

McHenry, L. (1994). Implementing self-directed teams. *Nursing Management* (Critical Care Management Edition), 25:3, 80I–80L.

Megginson, L. C., Mosley, D. C., and Pietri, P. H., Jr. (1992). *Management: Concepts and applications* (4th ed.). New York, NY: HarperCollins Publishers.

Napier, R., and Gershenfeld, M. (1973). *Groups: Theory and experience.* Boston, MA: Houghton Mifflin Co.

Osburn, J. D., et al. (1990). *Self-directed work teams.* Summertown, TN: The Book Press, Inc.

Perley, M. J., and Raab, A. (1994). Beyond shared governance: Restructuring care delivery for self-managing work teams. *Nursing Administration, 19:1,* 12–20.

Robbins, S. P. (1995). *Supervision today.* Englewood Cliffs, NJ: Prentice Hall.

Schermerhorn, J. R., Hunt, J. G., and Osborn, R. N. (1982). *Managing organizational behavior.* New York, NY: John Wiley & Sons.

Schwartz, H., and Davis, S. (1981, Summer). Matching Corporate Cultures and Business Strategy. *Organizational Dynamics,* 30–48.

Shaw, M. E. (1971). *Group dynamics: The psychology of small group behavior.* New York, NY: McGraw-Hill.

Shortell, S. M., Kaluzny, A. D., and associates. (1988). *Healthcare management: A text in organization theory and behavior* (2nd ed.). New York, NY: John Wiley & Sons.

Sims, H. P., Jr., and Lorenzi, P. (1992). *The new leadership paradigm.* Newbury Park, CA: Sage Publications, Inc.

Smith, G. B., and Hukill, E. (1994). Quality work improvement groups: From paper to reality. *Journal of Nursing Care Quality, 8:4,* 1–12.

Tuckman, B. W. (1965, May). Developmental Sequence in Small Groups. *Psychological Bulletin,* 384–399.

Wilkins., A. L. (1984). The creation of company culture: The soul of stories and human resource systems. *Human Resource Management, 23:1,* 41–60.

Wilson, H. S., and Kneisl, C. R. (1985). *Psychiatric Nursing* (2nd ed.). Menlo Park, CA: Addison-Wesley Publishing Co.

# Chapter 7
# Ethical Perspectives

## Introduction

All persons, whether in business, government, a hospital, or any other enterprise, are concerned with ethics. Webster (1971, p. 780) defines ethics as "the discipline dealing with what is good and bad and with moral duty and obligation." In *The Social Work Dictionary* (Baker, 1995, p. 124), ethics is defined as: "A system of moral principles and perceptions about right versus wrong and the resulting philosophy of conduct that is practiced by an individual, group, profession, or culture." As noted in this definition, professional organizations often choose to establish rules or standards governing the conduct of members of its profession. One attribute of a profession is its ethical code (Greenwood, 1957). By articulating standards in a code of ethics, professions establish expectations for every member of the profession and provide a basis for the evaluation of professional behavior. According to Levy (1982), social organizations and institutions also have ethical obligations. Organizational ethics are based on the selection and pursuit of organizational purposes and functions in consideration of the many people and groups the organization affects. Organizational ethics are put into practice by employees who are bound by those moral and ethical obligations in their role as employees. In addition, "once managers take action, they are deeply involved in ethics all the time, whether they are conscious of it or not" (Williams, 1991, p. 245).

Healthcare facilities, for instance, are ethically obligated to maximize patients' health. They also have obligations to their employees and communities. These ethical obligations are separate from, but may be reinforced by, legal, political, business, and other considerations.

From a professional and health perspective, ethics has been defined as follows:

- ethics is the study of rational processes for determining the best course of action in the face of conflicting [moral] choices (Brody, 1981, p. 24);
- ethics . . . [is] the systematic examination of the moral life [and] is designed to illuminate what we ought to do by asking us to consider and reconsider our ordinary actions, judgments, and justifications (Beauchamp and Childress, 1989, p. xii); and
- ethics . . . is concerned with doing good and avoiding harm (Bandman and Bandman, 1990, p. 27).

Often ethical standards are enacted into laws, but ethical behavior is just and fair conduct which goes beyond observing laws and government regulations. Ethical behavior is behavior which adheres to moral principles, and is guided by particular values.

While the above definitions capture the spirit of the ethics concept, ethics has three specific implications that warrant a brief comment. Ethics are individually defined. How the individual operates in a management role is influenced by his or her beliefs and values. Second, what constitutes ethical behavior can vary from one person to another. The manager is influenced by the experiences that form him or her as an individual and as a leader. Third, ethics are relative, not absolute. Thus, ethical behavior is in the eye of the beholder, but it is usually behavior that conforms to generally accepted social norms while unethical behavior does not conform.

Despite the magnitude of their presence in individual and societal existence, value and ethics are difficult and complex concepts to articulate. Yet, as society becomes more complex because of the increased sophistication of social and medical science and technology, the concern about practical limits on financial resources for healthcare and the growing emphasis on the autonomy of the individual, there are more alternatives, more choices to be made, and consequently ethical decisions seem to be necessary more frequently (American Hospital Association, 1985).

Only in the last ten years has there been serious discussion in journal articles and at professional conferences regarding the ethical aspects of therapeutic recreation practice. A first-line therapeutic recreation manager often receives the first level of inquiry from staff, volunteers, and interns as to what is ethical and legal. Since therapeutic recreation services include these dimensions, it is imperative that the therapeutic recreation manager has an understanding of them. Likewise, the therapeutic recreation manager is responsible for directing the ongoing professional growth and development of staff and interns. This task involves knowing how to recognize the ethical dimensions of therapeutic recreation and how to make ethical decisions in practice.

Initially this chapter will consider ethics as an integral part of therapeutic recreation management followed by a theoretical discussion of values and rights. An overview of several schools of ethical thought is presented thereafter. Consideration is also given to ethics as related to cultural and individual conflicts. Finally, a model for ethical decision making is presented. Please note, while the focus of the discussion will be health related, its application has no boundaries.

# Ethics and Therapeutic Recreation Management

How the therapeutic recreation manager operates in a management role is influenced by the beliefs, values, and experiences (i.e., family, peers, situations) that inform him or her as an individual and leader. In the language of Mark Pastin (1986), the individual's values are the set of "ground rules" for making what the individual considers to be a "right" decision. In addition to personal value, the therapeutic recreation manager is guided by values of the profession (i.e., responsibilities to consumers and to society). The American Therapeutic Recreation Association (ATRA) and National Therapeutic Recreation Society (NTRS) have each published a Code of Ethics (see Appendix A) in addition to several position statements and guidelines that seek to assist therapeutic recreation managers and practitioners in making ethical decisions in practice (e.g., see NTRS, 1994). In fact, not only should ethics be ingrained in staff to create a strong sense of professionalism, but also the codes should be the basis of a planned approach to all management functions of planning, organizing, directing, and controlling. Last, the manager, because of his or her role in the organization, is expected to further the organization's ethics and to assist staff and other practitioners in doing the same. Managers have special obligations to exercise their power—derived from their position, responsibility, and relationships—responsibly and ethically (Levy, 1982).

Spurred in part by recent scandals in both industry and healthcare, many organizations have increased their emphasis on ethical behavior (Carroll, 1987). Leaders of some organizations have initiated internal conferences on ethics (Lee, 1986). Others offer their employees training in how to cope with ethical dilemmas (Businesses Are Signing Up for Ethics 101, 1988). Organizations have also prepared detailed guidelines describing how employees are to deal with suppliers, competitors, and other constituents. Last, some organizations have developed a policy on ethics.

Of course, no code, guideline, or training program can truly replace an individual's personal judgment about what is right or wrong in any particular situation. Such devices may explain what people should do, but they often fail to help people deal with the consequences of their choice. To make ethical choices may lead to unpleasant outcomes—firing, rejection by one's colleagues, and so on. Thus, the manager must be prepared to confront his or her own conscience and weigh it against the various options available when making the difficult decisions that every manager must make (Cadbury, 1987).

However, the stress associated with ethical behavior in management can be reduced if therapeutic recreation managers attempt to practice management that realizes the highest good. The highest good may be found in the comments of Kenneth Blanchard (Fernicola, 1988). When translated into therapeutic recreation theory, Blanchard's comments can be summed up as follows:

1. Therapeutic recreation managers can influence the ethical behavior of therapeutic recreation personnel by treating them ethically.
2. Therapeutic recreation managers have a code of ethics that peers have agreed upon (see Appendix A). They enter into ethical dilemmas when they go against that code.
3. Therapeutic recreation managers fall into moral dilemmas when they go against their internal values.
4. While ethical and moral dilemmas differ, an ethical therapeutic recreation manager is a moral manager.
5. Ethical functions can be confronted by three questions:

5.1 Is it legal?

5.2 Is it balanced?

5.3 How will it make me feel about myself?

6. Therapeutic recreation managers with high self-esteem usually have the internal strength to make the ethical decision.

7. An ethical leader is an effective leader.

8. Therapeutic recreation managers should apply six principles of ethical power:

8.1 The manager promotes and ensures pursuit of the stated mission or purpose of the department, division, or unit since this statement reflects the vision of its practitioners. While the mission should be reviewed periodically, goals or objectives are set for yearly achievement.

8.2 Therapeutic recreation managers should build a division or department to be outstanding, thereby building self-esteem of staff through pride in the workplace.

8.3 Therapeutic recreation managers should work to sustain patience and continuity through long-term effect on the agency or organization.

8.4 Therapeutic recreation managers should plan for persistence by spending more time following up on education and activities that build commitment of personnel.

8.5 Therapeutic recreation managers should promote perspective by giving staff time to think. They should practice good management for the long term.

8.6 Therapeutic recreation managers should consider developing a department code of ethics expressed in observable and measurable behaviors.

# Values and Rights

## *Values*

To understand ethics and what influences ethical conduct, it is essential that the manager understand the nature of values, "the bedrock of ethics" (Hitt, 1990, p. 31). Values are a set of beliefs and attitudes about the truth, beauty, or worth of any thought, objective, or behavior. Values are those qualities that are intrinsically desirable to everyone. Every decision made, or course of action taken, is based consciously or unconsciously on such beliefs and values. In other words, what is really important, and what are the priorities in life, what is one willing to sacrifice or suffer in order to achieve, obtain, protect, or maintain are basic value issues for everyone. The majority of people in today's society have not had to answer these kinds of tough questions consciously. As a result, there is a lot of unnecessary confusion, inconsistency, and ambivalence exhibited in people's behavior. A person is frequently confronted with this confusion and ambivalence concerning his or her own values during a difficult decision-making time.

Values provide individuals with the ideological justification for roles and norms within society (Vustal, 1977). Without values, there are no standards and hence no moral code, no right nor wrong, and ultimately chaos results. When a person has at least a tentative idea of what is considered to be truth, beauty, and right or wrong, he or she is able to act in a manner consistent with those values. This behavior is more organized and predictable not only for the individual but for society as well. Jourard (1964, p. 27) wrote: "That until an individual knows his values he cannot know himself. Until one knows what he values or what lines in life he is going to cross, an individual doesn't know himself very well."

Values are both simple and complex and vary in the degree to which they are believed to be important to the person. Raths and associates (Raths, Harmin, and Simon, 1966) identified three processes that individuals go through as they attempt to clarify their values. The first process is the choosing process. Values are considered completely unique to each individual. Although two people may share the same value, they each arrived at that value individually. Theoretically, the choice of these values is made freely without indoctrination or coercion. Since values involve choosing, it is explicitly assumed that alternative values exist simultaneously. Because alternatives exist and because all decisions have consequences, the individual considers the consequences of all choices in making the ultimate decision.

The second process in the value clarification process is labeled prizing. This occurs when the individual acknowledges first to him or herself and then publicly what choice has been made and how he or she feels about it. Generally, the individual is proud of his choice. In addition to publicizing his values, the individual will also actively support his values (Raths, Harmin, and Simon, 1966).

The third process in value clarification according to Raths (Raths, Harmin, and Simon, 1966) is called *acting.* It is at this point that the individual has truly internalized the value. In this aspect, the individual's behaviors are a direct reflection of that value. Likewise, as an integral part of the individual's behavior, the value is then expressed not just episodically, but repeatedly.

As an individual grows, develops, and matures, values are defined and clarified, tested and revised, and gradually become all pervasive to the individual's existence. As such, the individual becomes an agent of value or, more commonly, a moral agent. The terms value and moral frequently are used interchangeably because they both deal with human behavior and values (Vustal, 1977).

When individuals have developed values, generally their decisions are made in terms of those values. Thus, it is easy to understand the magnitude and extent of the effect that values have on lives. Values have significance for people as individuals and collectively as societies. Values are useful because they provide order and predictability. Values can be considered as a means to a good end. Inherently, values can make an individual feel good inside. Finally, values contribute to social order and societal maturation.

## Values Clarification

Because every person holds individual and shared values, both consumer and therapeutic recreation managers and practitioners hold wide ranges of values. Given this reality, it is apparent that often therapeutic recreation managers and practitioners and their consumers will hold dissimilar values. Dissimilar values can contribute to misunderstanding or even to serious conflict. If therapeutic recreation specialists are going to give service, they will need to find ways to accommodate these differences. This accommodation must be achieved both for the sake of the consumer and for the sake of therapeutic recreation specialists' own personal and professional well-being. Understanding one's own values can be a first step that helps a therapeutic recreation manager or practitioner to identify, understand, and learn strategies that accommodate these differences.

Values clarification, is, as the name suggests, clarifying what values are important to a person. It is a self-awareness process that not only identifies what values are "me" but also asks the individual to prioritize or rate different values to determine which are most important.

The following values clarification exercise is associated with professional values:

- How much do I value therapeutic recreation as a commitment to a lifelong career of learning and competence?
- Do I like to provide service for some kinds of consumers and not others?
- Do I prefer working with healthy consumers to working with ill ones? young to old? physical to psychological disabilities?

A first step in accomplishing the preceding exercise is to reflect on such questions privately. A second and more enlightening step is to participate in values clarification with one's classmates.

More specific reasons exist for potential therapeutic recreation managers to examine their value systems:

- some inconsistencies in personal values are not apparent until consciously examined;
- some inconsistencies may cause problems if conflicting values are caught in the decision-making process;
- personal value may conflict with certain professional practice responsibilities;
- examining values can guide ethical choices in professional practice; and
- values clarification contributes toward functioning at a higher level of moral reasoning.

## *Rights*

Individuals struggling to clarify their values do not always identify rights as values. However, as values are peeled away to their basic layer, the rights of humans usually become clear.

Individuals have the human right to existence and therefore have the right to choose or to make decisions concerning themselves as long as they are willing to accept the consequences. The concept of self in this respect refers to an individual's body, life, property, and privacy. Nevertheless, because individuals exist within societies, the actions associated with these choices cannot infringe on another person's right. Within the concept of human rights is the associated concept of duties and responsibilities. Rights equate with responsibilities. If one has a right to his or her existence, other persons and society have a duty or obligation not to kill him. Moreover, in the opinion of the authors, health professionals, because of the roles they assume within society, assume additional responsibilities toward others that other individuals do not assume.

Scholars suggest the existence of six conditions that are associated with the fundamental rights of individuals. In some respects Thomas Hobbes and John Locke developed early rights theories in the 1600s. First, there is an accompanying condition of the freedom to exercise the right or not to exercise the right if the individual so chooses. Second, rights are associated with duties for others to facilitate, or at least not to interfere with, the exercise of those rights. Third, rights are usually defined or defended in basic terms that equate with the principles of fairness, impartiality, or equality. A fourth condition is that a basic fundamental or significant right is considered enforceable by society. Fifth, is the right to express oneself without fear of punishment. The final condition is also the result of societal maturation because this condition concerns compensation due an individual whose rights have been violated (Cavanaugh, Moberg, and Velasquez, 1981).

In decision making the rights of the individual need to be respected. The decision maker need only avoid violating the rights of the individual affected by the decision. As an example, firing an employee for wrongdoing on the basis of hearsay evidence would violate that person's right to due process. Of course, there are many situations where the issue is clouded. For instance, to what degree does a therapeutic recreation manager have the right to interfere with a staff member's right to privacy if that member's use of drugs or alcohol is affecting his or her job performance?

One must remember that human beings have rights because they are unique creatures that possess the ability to know and think. What a person knows about himself or herself and what he or she defines as unique becomes the source of human right. As a unique, self-contained human, an individual possesses certain needs in order for that existence to continue. Humans have a common origin which results in having common needs and a subsequent interdependence on one another. Because of these principles human needs exist whether they are recognized or not.

Specifically, defined sets of rights have developed in society as a result of the increased attention being devoted to the field of moral and ethical issues. For instance, the American Hospital Association (1985) has a Patient's Bill of Rights. Nursing homes are another example. In order for nursing homes to participate in Medicare and Medicaid programs, they have been required by the federal government to establish residents' rights policies. The Universal Declaration of Human Rights of the United Nations claims "everyone has a right to a standard of living adequate for the health and well-being of himself or his family, including . . . medical care . . ." (as quoted in Beauchamp, 1982, p. 38). These policies focus on the right to respectful and considerate care and treatment, right to information about treatment and cost, informed consent about procedures and outcomes, patient autonomy, right to refuse treatment, and right to privacy and confidentiality. Other health-related organizations and even particular facilities have developed "sets of rights" which contain many of the same basic elements noted above. As a result, today's consumers are appropriately aware of what is being done to and for them.

# Ethical Theories

Examination of societal values and moral issues has led to the study of ethics. Ethics is a branch of philosophy that deals with questions of human conduct, the values and beliefs that determine human conduct and how these elements change over time. Metaethics focuses on the study of moral judgments to determine if they are reasonable or in some way justifiable. As the study of ethics has developed, ethical theories have been proposed to identify, organize, and examine as well as justify human behavior through the application of the concepts and principles of human rights and values. The ultimate goal of ethics is to be able to determine what is right or good to do in a given situation.

## *Teleology*

Philosophical ethics is divided into two primary theories or systems—teleology and deontology. The outstanding example of teleological approach is utilitarianism. It is sometimes called "end-result ethics" (Hitt, 1990). Teleology gauges the rightness or wrongness of actions by their ends or consequences. The Greek *telos* means end, so it may not be surprising that one way of summarizing the utilitarian approach is that the end justifies the means. The approach is pragmatic: it is a practical approach to problems and affairs, it focuses on consequences, and it appeals to one's common sense (Hitt, 1990). In healthcare, for example, a shot may hurt but it prevents a crippling disease; the pain is for a good cause. This perspective has its critics.

Another summary of the utilitarian position is the aphorism, "The greatest good for the greatest number." The founders of modern utilitarianism, Jeremy Bentham and John S. Mill, were concerned with the greatest good, or maximizing the good. The good is sometimes identified with happiness or pleasure and the absence of pain (Bentham, 1969). Pleasure may be reading a good book, eating a good meal, and so on. Mill defined happiness on a broader level to mean social utility. Human actions contain a moral aspect, an aesthetic aspect, and a sympathetic aspect. All of these aspects contribute to the rightness or wrongness of an action and its ultimate worth to society (Mill, 1950).

The "greatest number" may sound democratic unless one belongs to a minority (i.e., Afro Americans, women, disabled). The greatest number may be simply those in power or those with the ability to pay which is not an unusual situation in healthcare. This concept of the greatest good for the greatest number appears to be the ethical basis of the various proposed national healthcare policies. On a large scale it is difficult to consider the individual. For this very reason, some would say utilitarianism is an inadequate ethic for healthcare because of its lack of concern for the individual patient.

## *Deontology*

The Greek *deon* means rule or principle. Deontology focuses on duties and obligations and holds that the features of actions themselves determine whether they are right or wrong. However, there is an overlap here with moral rules which is why some do not make the distinction between morals and ethics. The Ten Commandments of the Judeo-Christian tradition are a familiar example of moral rules.

Theoretically, there is no limit to the number of ethical principles. The Golden Rule, "Do unto others as you would have others do unto you" or "Do not do unto others that which is hurtful to thyself," is common to many of the religions of the world. Deception is commonly seen as immoral or unethical; it violates the principles of truth telling. The relief of pain or suffering is a major principle in healthcare. The law of double or secondary effect says that if the primary aim is good a negative side effect may be acceptable. The hair falls out, but the cancer is cured (Beauchamp, 1982).

Beauchamp and Childress (1989) have suggested that many ethical principles can be organized under larger umbrella units. They posit four of these: autonomy, do no harm (nonmaleficence), do good (beneficence) and justice. These principles, according to the authors reflect strong values, are universalizable and are framed in terms of the welfare of others. To a large degree these four principles provide the foundation for the principles of biomedical ethics.

Under the first is personal autonomy, "being one's own person, without constraints either by another's action or by psychological or physical limitations" (Beauchamp and Childress, 1989). Autonomous people are self-governing; they exercise control over their actions and circumstances. As an ethical principle, autonomy guides one to respect others as autonomous and to enhance, support, or restore autonomy insofar as possible (Beauchamp and Childress, 1989). Other writers would include informed consent, privacy, and confidentiality as part of personal autonomy. Regarding this principle, the therapeutic recreation manager or practitioner, in attitudes and actions, shows respect for the self-governing of consumers by recognizing their diverse abilities and viewpoints while respecting their prerogatives to make independent decisions and take actions accordingly.

*Primum non nocere* comes from the famous Hippocratic oath which says do good, or at least no harm. This ethical principle is so obvious that it is often overlooked or taken for granted. This principle is reflected by a therapeutic recreation practitioner who discourages a consumer from seeking involvement in a specific activity which involves risk of harm.

The third category includes beneficence, the doing of good. In many respects, it is not unlike the principle of nonmaleficence. The distinction between the two comes in the degree of activity required to act. Beneficence requires action that contributes to the welfare of others. It is a principle that underlies the goals of many social and healthcare organizations. Beauchamp and Childress (1989) point out that in healthcare facilities this principle is often expressed in the form of paternalism. Paternalism is doing what one believes is for someone else's good without necessarily having obtained the other person's knowledge or consent. Justice is usually considered an umbrella term and has to do with how people are treated when their interests compete and are compared with the interests of others.

Most often, justice is equated with fairness or merit. In addition, justice incorporates just allocations of scarce resources (Beauchamp and Childress, 1989).

Three types of justice are of concern to managers: distributive justice, procedural justice, and compensatory justice. Distributive justice requires that differentiated treatment of individuals not be based on arbitrary characteristics (i.e., men and women doing the same job should be paid equally). Procedural justice requires that rules be fair to all concerned and be administered consistently and impartially (although mitigating circumstances should be considered). Compensatory justice is concerned with compensating people for past harm or injustice (Gray and Smeltzer, 1989).

Another major approach to deontology was outlined by Immanuel Kant. He summed up previous thoughts by saying that every human being is unconditionally required to obey universal laws regardless of consequences. Kant insisted one is to do one's duty whether one likes it or not. This approach to ethics is governed by rules. Rules are essential to survival of a community, an organization, or a society. He also raised up a series of principles such as autonomy, freedom, dignity, self-respect, and respect for individual rights. One of the most important of these is that human beings are an end in themselves and not a means to someone else's end (Baier, 1978).

Kent Baier (1978) devised yet another deontology theory. He proposed the theory of intuitionism. Intuitionism says one simply knows. It is a matter of feeling or intuition. This is sometimes related to natural law, either as part of nature or as part of human creation by God. It is sometimes compared to or identified with conscience (Beauchamp, 1982).

Another form of ethical deontology is the human nature perspective. Unique to human nature is the ability to think, reason, and understand. Therefore, right or wrong are determined by rational thinking. This approach recognizes the complexities of human behavior and the existence of conflict between an individual's self-interests and the interests of others (Beauchamp, 1982).

The last theory to be offered is the justice as fairness theory proposed by Rawls (1971). Rawls' position is that social and economic inequalities are to be arranged so that they are the greatest benefit to the least fortunate of society. More important, each person is to have equal rights to the maximum liberty for all. Included in his concept is the idea that the disadvantaged have a priority claim to healthcare.

Anderson and Glesnes-Anderson (1988) note that both utilitarianism and deontology are flawed and can be subject to misuse. Imperfect as they are, however, these are the two predominant models of analysis available for thinking through ethical problems. There are others and even combinations of these two, but the most useful and important ideas needed for clear ethical thinking can be found in these two.

# Ethics: Cultural and Individual Conflicts

Though one of the primary goals of therapeutic recreation is to provide the best service for each consumer, it is not always clear what is "best" for whom. The consumer's definition of best may conflict with that of the therapeutic recreation manager's, agency administrator's, or the family's definition.

One source of conflict is the difference in cultures. Historically, cultures have dealt with the disabled in a variety of ways. Even in modern society questions are raised about the way the elderly are "warehoused." At times it appears that society does not follow the ethical views of Kant regarding the treatment of people—the aged, neonates and those in between—with respect and dignity.

The population of the United States and even Canada is a mixture of many ethnic groups and cultures. While there are differences in the ethics between cultures, there are also universal elements. Many, if not all, cultures have some form of the Golden Rule ingrained into their system. While different cultures have different perspectives on health and illness care service, the common ethic calls for respect of their differences. Native Americans, for example, tend to value harmonious relations with the world around them. Each rock, tree, animal, flower, and person is equally respected, and all are seen to coexist in harmony. A state of health exists when a person is in total harmony with nature. Illness, on the other hand, is seen as an imbalance between the person who is ill and the natural or supernatural forces around the person rather than an altered physiologic state (Spector, 1985).

Understanding other cultures takes time and communication. It also takes knowledge and requires a personal investment and commitment to learning. It is not always easy to know or understand how another will respond to health or illness. However, such knowledge is important for ethical decision making.

Another or related source of conflict is the differences in values. Value clarification helps individuals explore what it is they believe in and how to put those beliefs into daily practice. Such clarification may be vital to the provision of ethical service not only in the healthcare setting but also in the community-based leisure service arena. Therapeutic recreation practitioners' need to be aware of value differences so that they can avoid the unconscious imposition of either their personal or professional values on consumers. Likewise, if practitioners know what con-

sumers value, these values can be respected in daily service whenever possible.

In many settings it is assumed that it is all right for professionals to impose their values on clients because the professional "knows best." However, the current scene calls for informed consent and support of self-determination by consumers capable of such participation in decision making. The therapeutic recreation manager or practitioner may agree or disagree with the consumer's choices and values but may also choose to support them.

Providers of service to the ill and disabled work in an environment oriented toward ethical situations. To ignore this is to ignore reality. Williams (1991) notes that the three most important factors in personal and organization ethics are "integrity, purpose, and responsibility" (p. 245). The two main group providers of therapeutic recreation have recognized the ethical essence of their work and have developed professional codes of ethics. Both the ATRA and NTRS Codes of Ethics contain principles or statements that recognize human rights. The responsibility of providing quality service and concern for the dignity of the consumer are noted. Confidentiality and privacy are also recognized as ethical issues. Besides the positive actions of these provisions, the manager or practitioner prevents harm from occurring by safeguarding of the consumer from incompetent providers. Honesty is another ethical principle embraced by the code for therapeutic recreation specialists. Other professional associations especially health-related associations and individual facilities have developed similar ethical guidelines or principles. These statements are intended to serve daily practice as well as to provide a basis for dealing with more complex ethical dilemmas. One of the most difficult aspects of professional therapeutic recreation practice is the daily source of conflict. For the therapeutic recreation specialist these conflicts usually are associated with allocation of resources and practice respectively.

Resource allocation, including staff, supplies and equipment, is given considerable attention because of the commonalities between economics and ethics. The need for more staff or supplies and equipment to provide better service is not an infrequent dilemma. The clinical area in healthcare facilities provides ground for ethical dilemmas. Some of this conflict is territorialism, a power struggle for influence and space. Some conflict may also reflect differences in value systems. When professionals disagree, ethical practice requires time, listening, respecting, and sharing the sources of conflict to seek jointly an acceptable solution.

The therapeutic recreation manager as a first-line manager may be the first source of help when therapeutic recreation staff find themselves in conflict with other professionals. The manager then needs to be able to sort out the reasons for the conflict and determine which values are involved. Conflicts over power and territorialism will be handled with different approaches. The therapeutic recreation professional remains mindful that the primary goal of any professional practice is an ethical concern for the best service possible.

Individual conflicts involving unethical or illegal practice of a peer or other professional staff are probably the most difficult for the therapeutic recreation manager. Clarity of thought, responsiveness, listening, and data collection are needed. Support networks for substance abusers, consultation for legal concerns, and confidentiality in handling these difficult situations are vital. Likewise, knowing when to take what action is crucial. All are learned through experience and support from other colleagues.

## Ethical Decision Making

Ethical decision making is a process. It is theoretically based on moral reasoning, decision theory, moral development, values and valuing, and evaluation. It differs from traditional decision making in that the step-by-step process focuses on the moral or ethical dimensions of therapeutic recreation service. The reasoning process concludes when a decision of a morally acceptable action to be taken in a given situation is reached. Knowledge of ethical theories and principles helps a manager to identify the ethical issues or dimensions of the situation while providing the moral justification for the final selection of action to take.

The authors have developed a ten-step model for ethical decision making based on moral reasoning:

1. identify the problem including decisions needed, ethical components, and key individuals;
2. gather additional information to clarify the situation;
3. identify the ethical issues of the situation;
4. define personal and professional moral positions of the problem;
5. identify moral positions of key individuals involved in the situation;
6. identify value conflicts;
7. determine who should make the decision;
8. identify the range of actions with anticipated outcomes;
9. decide on a course of action and carry it out; and
10. evaluate and review the results of the decision or action including monitoring the situation over time.

This kind of feedback helps put the entire process into perspective.

Therapeutic recreation managers are in key positions regarding ethical decision making. One of the major responsibilities of the therapeutic recreation manager is to encourage as well as to guide ethical decision-making efforts. Such decisions take time and effort, and both should

be encouraged among staff members. Ethical dilemmas arise as a result of conflict in values. Difficult ethical dilemmas (consumer abuse, practitioner substance abuse) which go unnoticed and/or unresolved may lead to unethical (unprofessional) service as well as job dissatisfaction and apathy on the part of staff. If therapeutic recreation practitioners wish to be accorded professional status, they must also accept responsibility for decision making. All daily decisions have an ethical dimension which requires ethical decision making. Many of these are relatively minor; some are major. One of the greatest challenges of management is making right, good decisions.

## Summary

Ethics involve an individual's personal beliefs about what is right and wrong or good and bad; however, ethical behavior varies from person to person and is relative. In addition to personal beliefs and values the therapeutic recreation manager is governed by the values of his or her profession. Eight ethical suggestions to reduce management stress were noted.

How individuals develop values and rights was considered. It was noted that without values, there are no standards and hence no moral code. The concept of rights generally include the existence of six conditions: (1) free consent, (2) privacy, (3) freedom of conscience, (4) free speech, (5) fairness, and (6) due process.

The major ethical theories of utilitarianism and deontology were presented. Utilitarianism holds that plans and actions should be judged in terms of their consequences. On the other hand, deontology theories take the perspective that existing rights require certain duties, behaviors, and obligations among individuals. A number of ethical principles were also outlined.

This chapter concluded with a discussion of cultural and individual ethical conflicts faced by practitioners and the presentation of a model of ethical decision making associated with ethical conflict.

## Discussion Questions

1. What ethical dilemmas do you feel most therapeutic recreation managers face? Why? How would you handle one of the ethical dilemmas presented?
2. What are some types of behavior that would be unethical for students? What are some that would be ethical? Compare your responses with those of other students. Are these unethical and ethical behaviors carried over into the work environment?
3. Do you think you will be able to solve an ethical dilemma you might face in the future by applying one of the two primary theories presented? Explain.
4. List and discuss some codes of ethics associated with

professionals, organizations, university students, and your family. How should these codes be enforced?

5. Can a therapeutic recreation manager act in a way that is legal but unethical? Illegal but ethical? Why or why not?

6. Do you think a therapeutic recreation manager has a responsibility to disclose illegal or unethical conduct by others within the organization? Why or why not? If the manager may lose his or her job does the same responsibility exist? Why or why not?

# References

American Hospital Association. (1985). *Values in conflict: Resolving ethical issues in hospital care.* Report of the Special Committee on Biomedical Ethics. Chicago, IL: The Association.

Anderson, G. R., and Glesnes-Anderson, V. A. (1988). *Healthcare ethics: A guide for decision makers.* Rockville, MD: Aspen Systems Corporation.

Baker, D. L. (1995). *The social work dictionary* (3rd ed.). Washington, DC: National Association of Social Workers.

Baier, K. (1978). Deontological theories. *Encyclopedia of bioethics,* 413–417.

Bandman, E. L., and Bandman, B. (1990). *Nursing ethics through the life span* (2nd ed.). Norwalk, CT: Appleton & Lange.

Beauchamp, T. L. (1982). Ethical theory and bioethics. In T. Beauchamp and L. Walters (Eds.), *Contemporary issues in bioethics* (2nd ed.). Belmont, CA: Wadsworth Publishing Co.

Beauchamp, T. L., and Childress, J. F. (1989). *Principles of biomedical ethics* (3rd ed.). New York, NY: Oxford University Press.

Bentham, J. (1969). *A Bentham reader.* M. P. Mack (Ed.). New York, NY: Pegasus.

Brody, H. (1981). *Ethical decisions in medicine* (2nd ed.). Boston, MA: Little, Brown and Company.

Businesses are signing up for ethics 101. (1988, February 15). *Business Week,* 56–57.

Cadbury, A. (1987, September–October). Ethical managers make their own rules. *Harvard Business Review,* 69–73.

Carroll, A. B. (1987, March–April). Search of the moral manager. *Business Horizons,* 7–15.

Cavanaugh, G. F., Moberg, D. J., and Velasquez, M. (1981, July). The ethics of organizational politics. *Academy of Management Review, 6:3,* 363–374.

Fernicola, K. C. (1988, May). Take the high road . . . to ethical management: An interview with Kenneth Blanchard. *Association Management,* 60–66.

Gray, E. R., and Smeltzer, L. R. (1989). *Management: The competitive edge.* New York, NY: Macmillian Publishing Co.

Greenwood, E. (1957, July). Attributes of a Profession. *Social Work, 2,* 45–55.

Hitt, W. D. (1990). *Ethics and leadership.* Columbus, OH: Battelle Press.

Jourard, S. (1964). *The transparent self: Self-disclosure and well-being.* New York, NY: Van Nostrand Reinhold Co.

Lee, C. (1986, March). Ethics Training: Facing the Tough Questions. *Training,* 30–33, 38–41.

Levy, C. S. (1982). *Guide to ethical decisions and actions for social service administration: A handbook for managerial personnel.* New York, NY: Haworth Press.

Mill, J. S. (1950). *On Bentham and Coleridge.* New York, NY: Harper & Row.

National Therapeutic Recreation Society (NTRS). (1994). *Code of ethics and interpretive guidelines.* Arlington, VA: National Recreation and Park Association.

Pastin, M. (1986). *The hard problem of management: Gaining the ethics edge.* San Francisco CA: Jossey-Bass.

Raths, L. E., Harmin, M., and Simon, S. B. (1966). *Values and teaching.* Westerville, OH: Charles E. Merrill Books, Inc.

Rawls, J. (1971). *A theory of justice.* Cambridge, MA: Harvard University Press.

Spector, R. E. (1985). *Cultural diversity in health and illness* (2nd ed.) New York, NY: Appleton-Century-Crofts.

Vustal, D. B. (1977). Searching for values. *Image, 9:1,* 15–17.

*Webster's Third New International Dictionary.* (1971). Springfield, MA: G. and C. Merriam Company.

Williams, L. R. (1991). Ethics in management. In G. S. Fain (Ed.), *Leisure and ethics* (pp. 244–246). Reston, VA: American Alliance for Health, Physical Education, Recreation and Dance.

# *Chapter 8*

# Working with Higher Management

## Introduction

Most successful managers acknowledge that their success is dependent on their ability to manage people: for the most part, staff that reports to them. Much has been published about how to motivate, get more from, create a bond with, and lead those who work for or report to a manager or executive. A manager's success is often gauged by how well those relationships are developed and how well they support the department or organization. Perhaps even more important, however, is the managing of one's supervisor, or rather, managing the relationship between oneself as a manager and one's supervisor, for it is through this relationship that the manager acquires the authority to act. To manage upward the manager must remember that the relationship requires participation by both the manager and the boss. The manager will know when he or she is managing upward successfully because power and influence will be moving in both directions.

It may strike therapeutic recreation managers as odd to consider managing their supervisor or "boss." However, since it is through this relationship that work is accomplished and goals achieved, allowing the relationship to flounder without direction, support, and guidance is neglecting a critical resource. In reality, the relationship is of more consequence to the junior manager. The success of the relationship is dependent on the consistent effort applied toward development, the thoroughness of the understanding of the needs, goals, pressures, and work styles of the parties, and the willingness to suspend one's personal agenda in favor of the organization's goal. Managing the relationship clarifies one's job and enhances effectiveness (Gabarro and Kotter, 1980).

This chapter explores the foundations of a good relationship, the political climate in the relationship, and how one goes about establishing that relationship, reflecting that superior, getting what is needed, working with a difficult boss, and dissolving the relationship. In conclusion, dealing with physicians is discussed.

## Foundations of a Good Relationship

A relationship is usually considered as a logical and natural association between two or more things. Close relationships between two people are often built on strong bonds of trust. The foundation for a boss-subordinate relationship is not unlike the foundation for a relationship with a good friend. This is not to suggest that the boss should be a friend, but rather that the same factors that characterize a friendship—trust, respect, and good communication—should be fostered in the relationship with the boss. Moreover, in many instances the management concepts related to dealing with subordinates also can be applied to the relationship with a superior.

Three fundamental components are critical to setting the foundation for a solid relationship. First, the parties in any relationship must be viewed as fallible, with strengths and weaknesses. Second, both parties must make a good faith effort to establish the relationship. It is best to proceed from a positive position. Third, the mutual dependence between superior and manager must be recognized (Gabarro and Kotter, 1980).

Just as first impressions are important in forming a lasting opinion, the initial development of a relationship is vital to its continued strength. In most agencies or organizations, the initial development of a working relationship is a joint effort that takes place during the orientation or adjustment period of the newer employee. This introduction period offers an opportunity for one to assess the superior's managerial and interpersonal style. The superior's ethical and personal values are important points for discussion. In addition, it is important to observe the superior's interactions since they will form the context for further relationships. As part of this introduction personal and professional goals for the division or department should be shared.

## Managerial Style

A therapeutic recreation manager will be more successful if he or she makes information easily accessible to his or her superior. Understanding the superior's managerial style will help one to be more supportive. Drucker (1967) identifies two types of managers, the readers and the listeners. The reader is one who studies volumes of background information before making a decision. The listener, on the other hand, prefers the information delivered orally, followed by a brief written summary of what has been discussed. This aspect of style is often overlooked. Subordinates frequently submit information in the style that is most comfortable for them, without looking for cues from their superior. It is important to address the issue with the superior, either by asking for direction or by watching for cues.

Drucker (1967) mentions two other styles of management that are particularly prevalent. One style is held by those superiors who prefer to stay close to the front line and who are active in the decision-making process. The second type of superior prefers that the person closest to the situation has complete responsibility. Those who prefer to be close to the decision-making process require ongoing, detailed communication. Those who allow one to have complete responsibility usually require summary information of what is going on with notes on decisions as they are made. A wise manager, taking into account his or her own style, will be attentive to, and thus supportive of, the boss's style of management.

A corollary to knowing about oneself and one's superior is recognizing that neither possesses all encompassing knowledge. Working toward the same goal does not guarantee that each is always aware of the other's activities. A manager should never assume that the superior knows what he or she is doing. An aside to this point is that there is information at times that one need not know. While styles dictate the manner of communication, it is essential to keep the superior informed of activities, progress, obstacles, and when assistance is needed. Assumptions are always dangerous.

## Ethical and Interpersonal Skills

Honesty is the essence of a good working relationship with one's boss. A climate of trust and honesty must be built and developed over time. A dishonest relationship is quickly discovered. Much of the dishonesty that is generated within agencies and organizations arises from the manager's need to appear knowledgeable on all topics. Regardless of the reason—power, manipulation, or recognition—the impulse to provide a supervisor with potentially incorrect information must be resisted. Blanchard (Blanchard and Peale, 1988, p. 19) says, "There is no right way to do the wrong thing." Personal integrity, principles, and commitment to the truth will facilitate and enhance all other aspects of the relationship.

Robert Fulghum's (1988) popular book, *All I Really Need to Know I Learned in Kindergarten,* discusses the real importance of treating one another with courtesy, kindness, and tact. This advice could easily include being punctual, polite, and nonjudgmental. These courtesies are as applicable to the boardroom and the administrative suite as they are to the kindergarten classroom.

## Goals

In order for the health and human services world to function at all, especially complex healthcare facilities, critical choices must be made. These choices, expressed as vision, mission, purpose, and goals, are the cement that solidifies and strengthens the relationship between superior and subordinate. Success requires effort and thought, an awareness of one's strengths and weaknesses (as well as those of one's boss), astute observation, and a willingness to adapt in order to reach a goal. Each will have separate goals surrounding specific issues. However, these specific goals should be gathered under mutually held general goals that guide the superior-subordinate relationship. At the outset of any relationship, goal consensus is critical. It serves as a bridge between manager and superior while creating consistent expectations and the means to measure progress.

## Communications

Communication is often viewed as the life's blood of a good relationship. Meaningful communication does not occur without a certain amount of risk. The risk is small at first, but it becomes greater as one allows a superior to see beneath one's outer surface. Below the surface personal and professional goals and ethical beliefs are hidden; however, still deeper lies the inner self.

One of the real difficulties in communication is that the superior and the department manager may define terms or matters in different ways. Thus, they appear to be communicating but really do not understand one another at all. It is important that a manager and his or her superior get together to define the terms used in their communication.

Not all superiors and managers will be comfortable or able to communicate about things below the surface, and they may choose not to expose inner thoughts and feelings. However, such communication is worth the risk of exposure because the knowledge gained will allow a boss to better understand a manager and his or her motivation, needs, and style. Sharing the responsibility of a deeper communication can result in an increased interdependence and mutual satisfaction. This should be an important goal for the manager.

# Establishing a Relationship

When one is new to an agency or organization, establishing a relationship with the boss is relatively easy—after all, one was probably selected for the job by that person. It is imperative that the positive qualities and abilities revealed during the interview process be demonstrated. One will be "on trial" as one begins to familiarize oneself with the agency or organization; although, most organizations allow a "honeymoon" period with leeway for exploration of the organization.

If a superior is new to the agency or organization, the principles of establishing a relationship remain intact. However, there are distinct and important differences. A incumbent has a history with the organization and may have a history with the supervisor's predecessor. This may or may not be viewed positively by the supervisor. Considerable finesse and sensitivity may be required in order to provide insight into the organization without creating the impression that the new supervisor is suspect or unwelcome. No matter what the relationship was like with the previous supervisor, the new person must be viewed with an open mind and a willingness to create a new and positive relationship. At some point, no matter how knowledgeable one is of the organization's history, the new supervisor will appropriately assert a new agenda. Wise therapeutic recreation managers will recognize this and move toward putting the past behind them.

A truly close working relationship, built on trust and reinforced over time, is often a friendly one. This does not mean that a supervisor is a friend, nor does it give one license to allow familiarity. Each supervisor and manager will have to decide whether or not a relationship outside the workplace is acceptable. The capacity for mixing business and a personal relationship varies according to the individual's philosophy, experience, organization expectations, and energy. Relationships that compromise organization and department goals ultimately destroy the working relationship, and the wise therapeutic recreation manager will avoid them.

Establishing a professional relationship with organizational board members or commissioners, regardless of setting, is largely an indirect process. Creating a good working relationship with one's supervisor and working toward the organization's or department's goals will give one a reputation for trustworthiness, which can then be enhanced with direct interaction. This interaction requires the same direct communication, understanding, and feedback utilized in forging a relationship with one's own supervisor. Once a relationship is established, free and open communication will sustain and nurture that relationship.

Just as it is essential to let a supervisor know what one is doing, it is equally important to transmit information about what is going on in the organization. This does not mean that a manager reports detailed stories and comments overheard in the cafeteria or at social gatherings. The therapeutic recreation manager should consider whether the supervisor *needs* to know a detailed account of an incident. At the same time, it is important to give an accurate sense of employee attitudes, liability risks, widely held concerns, and potential conflicts.

Sometimes a manager tries to protect the boss from bad news. No one likes to be the bearer of bad news. However, withholding negative information makes a supervisor less powerful in dealing with issues in the agency or organization as they arise. This affects not only the supervisor's credibility and ability, but also one's own. In this case, bad news is better than no news (Fulghum, 1988).

Finally, it is important to communicate recognition of work done well. Therapeutic recreation managers are admonished to provide positive feedback to their department staff and should also provide feedback to their supervisors. Like staff members, they need the warmth of positive strokes.

Progress and stability in an organization depends on, among other things, a uniform approach to meeting goals, completing projects, and allocating resources. One of the cardinal rules of management is that a commitment to a direction or goal must be supported by all. This does not mean that everyone always agrees. Sometimes this is difficult to do; perhaps one believes that the decision was unwise or unjust. It is important that a way to support the decision without compromising one's values is found. If, on the other hand, the decision or occurrence violates one's moral or ethical code, one may wish to consider leaving the environment.

# The Political Climate

The word *politics* brings a grimace to the face of many therapeutic recreation practitioners. It is cited as a reason for leaving positions and not seeking others. It is often given as a reason for failure or unearned success. It is a word often spoken with skepticism and sometimes as though it were slightly obscene. It is seen as manipulative and not quite respectable. Politics is not a four-letter word. In fact, politics is in the eye of the beholder. What is politics to one is very likely characterized by another as effective management. One cannot escape the fact that it is highly unlikely that an organization is free of politics.

Politics is often defined as the art of influencing others so that the events move toward a desired outcome. In a positive sense, it connotes "campaigning, lobbying, bargaining, negotiating, concurring, collaborating, and winning votes" (Kanter, 1983, p. 213). Politics is associated with leadership and the exercise of power. To be politically successful is to be able to move smoothly through the environment, exerting one's influence in an attempt to accomplish goals. The successful manager understands that this ability is equally important in the management of one's relationship to one's supervisor.

To be sensitive to a political environment implies the understanding of power and its source. This environment is like a body of water on which one must sail a boat. Understanding the wind direction and velocity is critical to plotting a course. One has a choice to try to maneuver against the wind, with the possibility of being stalled, or working with the wind by choosing the appropriate tack, so that progress can be made and the destination is reached.

A supervisor, as the captain, may be depending on a manager to employ his or her understanding to win a race or achieve a goal. If one is stalled, has misread the political winds and has capsized due to turbulence, the skipper may be called upon for rescue. While that rescue may be forthcoming, one should not grow dependent on it. If one keeps getting thrown overboard because one has not learned the winds, one may expect to stay in the water. No matter how the supervisor feels about the manager, the race cannot be won if he or she continually needs to be pulled out of the water. At some point the rescue will interfere with the goal.

The sooner a therapeutic recreation manager becomes involved in the political aspects of a job, the sooner that manager will find that results begin to impact his or her position. A manager will win some and lose some, but win or lose, he or she must always be ready to return and play the game again. Involvement in the politics of a job is a do-it-yourself endeavor. In reality, waiting around for others to invite one into the arena is a passive posture that signals powerlessness. Edmunds and Scott (1981) state

that "playing the game" is sometimes as important as doing the work. In actuality, playing the game is the work.

To develop and improve political skills Robbins (1995, pp. 423–425) suggests the following:

1. frame arguments in terms of organizational goals,
2. develop the right image,
3. gain control of organizational resources,
4. make oneself appear indispensable,
5. be visible,
6. get a mentor,
7. develop powerful allies,
8. avoid "tainted" members, and
9. support the boss.

# Reflecting One's Supervisor

Effective managers realize the importance of activating the strengths of their supervisors. Drucker (1967, p. 116) states, "Contrary to popular legend, subordinates do not, as a rule, rise to the position and prominence over the prostrate bodies of incompetent bosses."

For better or worse, bosses in any organization are perceived and judged not only on their own merits and accomplishments, but also on the merits and accomplishments of those who report to them. This means that work, attitudes, and values reflect on the supervisor in the same way that staff's work and attitudes reflect on the manager. Of course, the reverse is also true; a manager is also seen in the light of the supervisor (Drucker, 1967).

In an organization the manager's appearance and attitude communicate the attitude of the supervisor. To the extent that the picture is positive, the employee's work and effort will be enhanced and the employee will feel valued. The wisdom of making others look good, whether they are supervisors or subordinates, is clearly demonstrated in the creation of a positive atmosphere where accomplishments are recognized.

Part of the benefit and expectation of being a manager is participation in activities outside the organization. Whether it is serving on a committee of another organization, serving on citizen committees, or merely appearing at a public hearing, a manager will be perceived as a representative of the organization, even if the service is of purely a personal interest. Behavior and image will be as much a reflection of the boss and the organization as it is of one personally. For the most part, this external visibility does not become an issue of importance unless the values expounded on the community are in conflict with the values of the organization. It might be wise to give thought to what might be said in certain situations rather than having to face the many small decisions about expressing or not expressing a point of view.

# Getting What One Needs

One of the lures of being a manager is the autonomy and ability to influence change in the direction one thinks it needs to go. However, that autonomy is not absolute. At some point, the supervisor's approval will be required to proceed with a project. Further, in a collegial relationship with the supervisor, the opportunity to use each other as resources should be taken frequently.

When approaching a supervisor, one should have already carefully defined what one wants or needs from the encounter. If approval is needed, it should be asked for. If a listening ear or a sounding board is needed, it should be requested. It is disconcerting to get the "go ahead" for a new program when one only wanted to talk about the idea and was not prepared to pursue it.

Once a manager's purpose is clear, he or she must carefully prepare for the meeting with the supervisor. This preparation is no less important than preparing for a meeting with staff. The "homework" must be done. Facts, figures, ramifications, and potential results must be in hand. Most importantly, a recommendation must be developed. It is naive to expect that any purpose can be achieved without these items in place.

Preparation is only part of the effort, however. Presentation is at least as important. Understanding of the issue and the supervisor's style is essential. Putting oneself in the boss's position and visualizing his or her frame of reference may make it easier to prepare the proposal. If one has been observant, it will be clear whether the supervisor responds best to a written document or an oral report, a detailed analysis or a digest highlighting important points. Although a positive response is not solely dependent on the presentation, communicating in a style that is comfortable to the supervisor can make a manager's task much easier.

Even if one is well-prepared and the project is well-presented, the premise might not be accepted. Perhaps the goal for a new program is at variance with the supervisor's goal, or one is competing with resources of another peer or interest. In that event, negotiations may have to take place. Negotiation, that sometimes artful give-and-take, may be a reasonable technique for getting part of what is needed. One should consider whether approval for part of a request will be helpful and what part could be given up. The federal government does this quite frequently in providing grants so as to allow more grants. One should prepare for this ahead of time; otherwise, one runs the risk of loosing it all.

In seeking to persuade, one of the most pertinent skills a manager can have is knowing when "the sale is made." There are few things more irritating to a supervisor than to give approval and then to have persuasive arguments from

the manager continue. This behavior, according to Gabarro and Kotter (1980), can create questions in the supervisor's mind about the wisdom of the decision to approve and may result ultimately in a negative decision. At the very least, it calls into question the manager's attentiveness and willingness to listen.

Therapeutic recreation managers want to be able to create situations in which a supervisor agrees with their point of view, their ideas can be advanced, and their proposals are approved. Some people think of this as gamesmanship, others as manipulation. Both of these terms have negative, somewhat unsavory, connotations. It is more helpful to think of these skills in terms of the ability to define strategies. The manager tries to plan sequential moves to ensure that the desired outcome is achieved with as little disruption, furtive energy, or backtracking as possible. Administrative strategy, as it applies to the relationship with a supervisor, is simply the foresight to anticipate the opportunities for and obstacles to success and to plan to meet or avoid them. This strategy is respectful of the supervisor's time and energy, and when done well, is indicative of a manager's acumen and insight.

There will be times when approval from the supervisor is not forthcoming, despite a manager's best efforts and most persuasive arguments. At those times, one will have to decide how to proceed. One may believe that the goal is so important that one needs to seek the approval of the supervisor's supervisor. In that event, one should be aware that "going over the supervisor's head" entails some risk—disapproval, anger on the part of the supervisor, or other negative reactions. There is also the risk that the individual at the next level will also disapprove. Whatever decision a manager makes about proceeding to the next level, it is always appropriate to inform the immediate supervisor of the intentions, but one should never propose that option as a threat. If a manager tells the supervisor of plans to go to the next level, he or she should do it. If one decides not to do so, it will enhance one's credibility to inform the supervisor of the decision and the reasons for that decision.

Even in the best of relationships, managers and supervisors sometimes disagree. Conflict created by disagreement must be resolved, and it is important to assess the risks before choosing a course of action to resolve them. Only the therapeutic manager will know whether the issue is important to achieving his or her goals, how it will affect staff, and whether there is a potential impact on ethics and morals. Whether one decides to stand fast or give in, one must act graciously, maintaining one's self-esteem.

When the decision is made to "go all out," in other words, when an ultimatum is issued, a manager should do so with great care. This is an extreme action that cannot be taken back. One must be prepared to act on it, so it should only be used if one is absolutely willing to have it accepted.

Figure 8.1 gives guidelines that may help the manager achieve success in influencing the boss.

# The Difficult Boss

This chapter is predicated on establishing a relationship with an excellent supervisor, but not all supervisors are ideal. A therapeutic recreation manager may have to find ways to work with a "difficult" boss.

It is hard, if not impossible, to manage the incompetent boss. Competence cannot be taught. In this situation, Kiechel (1984) advises that one perform to the best of one's ability while continuing to communicate with others in the organization. This will allow others to distinguish between one's level of competence and the supervisor's level of incompetence.

Many therapeutic recreation managers have had the experience of dealing with explosive individuals, whether staff, physicians, or other managers. In dealing with or managing these individuals, it is sometimes helpful to use the principle of disengagement; that is, exiting the situation and letting the individual know that one will return at a time when the matter can be discussed less emotionally. If the outbursts continue, it will be necessary to tell him or

---

## Figure 8.1 Guidelines for Influencing the Boss

Capitalize on the boss's strengths:
- What strengths and limitations does he or she have?
- What information do you have that he or she needs?
- What help can the boss provide personally and organizationally?

Be prepared:
- Do you know your boss's overall professional priorities or goals?
- What concerns or difficulties may he or she be facing?
- What excites your boss? What turns him or her off?

Cite benefits:
- What's in it for the boss if he or she supports your idea, proposal, or plan?
- How will the organization benefit?
- What are the short-term and long-term advantages?

Build a strong case:
- What policies, precedents, or procedures support what you want to do?
- Which of your supporters are valued by the boss for their opinions?
- How can you trade on your own expertise or credibility?
- What will the consequences be if the proposed idea is not accepted?
- What will have to be done later as a result?

Avoid surprises:
- Do you need to lay some groundwork with a brief memo or phone call explaining the purpose and importance of the meeting?
- What are the risks or advantages of hitting the boss cold with your idea, proposal, or plan?

Anticipate resistance:
- What aspects of your plan are likely to prompt resistance, such as "costs too much," "takes too long," or "too risky"?
- How can you minimize or eliminate potential resistance by the way you manage the meeting?
- What data do you need to help overcome resistance?
- How will your idea affect morale, turnover, and absenteeism? These cost money.

Separate needs from "nice to have":
- What tradeoffs or compromises are you prepared to make?
- What part of your proposal is essential, what part merely desirable?
- "Half a loaf is better than none"; which half do you want?

Persist:
- How far and how hard are you willing to push to get your idea accepted?
- What does past experience tell you about the best timing or sequence for your attempts to influence your boss?
- Remember: The best ideas or changes seldom are accepted the first time they are proposed. If you learn from previously unsuccessful efforts and try again, you improve your chances of acceptance.

---

Adapted from Development Dimensions International, *Leadership and influence, part 3,* (Pittsburgh, PA: Development Dimensions International, 1986). Reprinted with permission.

her any observations and concerns with the communication difficulty.

The indecisive boss is not an impossible boss. Before taking an action, it is important that one accurately assesses the management style to identify that one is working with an individual who cannot make decisions. It is important to distinguish between a boss who lacks decisiveness and one who lacks accessible information (Kiechel, 1984).

There are a number of tactics that may be employed when working with an indecisive boss. The first is perseverance. The manager may need to address an issue a number of times, varying the style of request, before a decision is made. The second solution is more risky. It consists of addressing the boss by memo requesting a decision and stating that if no answer is forthcoming by a given date, the suggested recommendations will be pursued.

If a boss lacks knowledge about what therapeutic recreation is, one has a responsibility to inform him or her about the service or field. This can be done through appointment meetings or taking the boss to lunch.

## Dissolving the Relationship

At some point, it may become necessary to dissolve or change the existing relationship with the supervisor. If the relationship has been a positive one, it may continue on different terms. If a manager is promoted, for example, it is likely to be the result of a favorable recommendation from the supervisor. The straightforwardness, honesty, and respect that characterized the former relationship will be equally essential in the new position.

Should one move on to another organization, goals will change, and one will undoubtedly have to accommodate a new supervisor. The suggestions outlined throughout this chapter regarding the relationship with a new supervisor should prove effective.

It is desirable that a relationship ends positively, but there are instances when this is not possible. Unless his or her morals or ethics are compromised, a manager should make every effort to leave while ensuring the smooth continuation of work in progress including making it as comfortable as possible for those who remain.

## Managing Physicians

As a last note in this chapter it is well to consider how to "manage" physicians. It is not unusual for the authors to have heard about the experience of therapeutic recreation practitioners with physicians. The same laments can be heard from managers and practitioners that were heard a decade or two ago. In addition is the fact that the profession of therapeutic recreation has a majority of female practitioners. While the emergence of the women's movement has reduced the female therapist-physician conflict, the problems still exists.

While therapeutic recreation managers and practitioners in healthcare facilities are taught to be team players, physicians are encouraged to develop their individuality even though there has been a significant change in attitude in recent years. Individualistic attitudes are acquired during undergraduate and medical school. Medical students are conditioned to be in control which is imperative in life-threatening situations. In addition, they may develop other common traits, such as omnipotence, dominance, and authoritarianism. Another possible factor may be the differences in the structure of medical practice and therapeutic recreation practice. The intensity and extensity of each practitioner's relationship with consumers differ. The physician usually has a long-term relationship with the consumer and deals with that consumer individually. The therapeutic recreation practitioner, on the other hand, is usually involved with several consumers and for only a short time. Last, medical students probably buy into stereotypes and public images of what is recreation or therapeutic recreation. To compound the problem, hospital administrators simply do not have the time and energy to create the kind of in-service training or environment to educate physicians or other personnel about therapeutic recreation.

The following are guidelines the authors have found successful in dealing with physicians:

- consider oneself and the physician equal partners of a healthcare team;
- focus on the task to be accomplished or the problem to be solved, not personal differences;
- maintain the improvement of consumer service as the goal of all collaborative efforts;
- establish clear roles and responsibilities for the physician, oneself, and one's staff;
- always be prepared with *facts* when talking with physicians;
- respect the physician as a person—not as "just a doctor"; and
- serve as a role model to one's staff exemplifying the above behaviors.

The therapeutic recreation manager is in a key position to influence therapeutic recreation practitioner-physician relationships. As a manager one has frequent contact with physicians and can help both physicians and therapeutic recreation practitioner staff to deal with each other.

One approach the manager can use is to use every opportunity to include therapeutic recreation practitioners in meetings that include physicians. The view of many physicians is that the work of the practitioner is "invisible." Thus, the more the physician has the opportunity to interact with the practitioner, the more positive effect on the relationships between the two professionals. A successful event reported frequently to the authors which has fostered knowledge about therapeutic recreation is Therapeutic Recreation Week which usually occurs in July.

The manager also serves as a role model for the staff. When therapeutic recreation staff see the manager collaborating with physicians, they may tend to emulate that behavior. An attitude of cooperation and collaboration rather than an adversarial one of *we versus they* encourages a similar response in staff practitioners. A similar attitude should also be taken regarding interaction with other disciplines (e.g., occupational therapists, music therapists).

The therapeutic recreation manager may need to be mediator in a conflict between a practitioner and a physician. The reader is referred to Chapter 11 on dealing with conflict for specific skills in conflict resolution.

In an effort to improve collaboration between physicians and therapeutic recreation practitioners, the manager must remember that his or her staff need support to participate in collaborative effort. They must be assured by words and actions that they will be supported by their therapeutic recreation manager, who is "on their side." This is critical for the manager's success with staff and success in the organization.

## Summary

Managing the relationship between manager and supervisor requires skill, insight, patience, and perseverance. It requires self-knowledge, careful observation, analysis, and the ability to take risks. The effort required is great, but the reward for success is equally great. Mutual growth, mutual success, and mutual satisfaction are the rewards in the well-managed supervisor-manager relationship.

Initial consideration was given to those factors which underline the foundation of a good relationship. Thereafter, attention was focused on how one goes about establishing a working relationship with one's supervisor followed by a discussion of politics and its meaning in the work environment. Steps were outlined as to how to present one's needs to the supervisor as well as noting the risk involved when the request is not forthcoming. Consideration was also given to handling a difficult boss and how a relationship is dissolved. This chapter concluded with a discussion of factors associated with managing physicians including guidelines for successful interaction.

## Discussion Questions

1. What is your attitude toward the concept of politics as being manipulative? Discuss.
2. Outline a plan that you would use to "sell" a new program to your supervisor in a physical medicine unit or in any organization.
3. Do you support the idea that a supervisor should receive recognition for work you have done?
4. Why should the therapeutic recreation manager, regardless of setting, be aware that political behavior may be going on within the organization? What might occur if he or she were not aware?
5. Describe a person who is successful at using organizational politics. What makes that person successful?
6. Do you think a therapeutic recreation manager should have the opportunity to regularly appraise (i.e., evaluate) his or her boss? Why or why not?

# References

Blanchard, K., and Peale, N. V. (1988). *The power of ethical management.* New York, NY: William Morrow & Co.

Drucker, P. F. (1967). *The effective executive.* New York, NY: Harper & Row.

Edmunds, M. W., and Scott, J. D. (1981, August). The name of the game is politics. *Hospitals, 55,* 67–71.

Fulghum, R. (1988). *All I really need to know I learned in kindergarten.* New York, NY: Harper & Row.

Gabarro, J. J., and Kotter, J. P. (1980). Managing your boss. *Harvard Business Review, 58:1,* 93–102.

Kanter, R. M. (1983). *The change master.* New York, NY: Simon & Schuster.

Kiechel, III, W. (1984). How to manage your boss. *Fortune, 110:6,* 206–210.

Robbins, S. P. (1995). *Supervision today.* Englewood Cliffs, NJ: Prentice Hall.

# Part 3

# Operational Management

# Chapter 9

# Financial Management and Budgets

## Introduction

The therapeutic recreation manager today who believes that it is not necessary to be aware of the financial side of delivering health and human services is very much like the proverbial ostrich that sticks its head in the sand and hopes that what it cannot see will not hurt it. Given the choice, it is likely that the majority of first-line managers would relinquish the budgetary aspects of their jobs. However, as noted by Powell (1984), the survival of therapeutic recreation service in healthcare systems may be dependent on effective fiscal management and therapeutic recreation specialists having "at least minimal fiscal management competency" (p. 40).

In the past, financial management, to a large degree, was associated with the complex and technical work of accounting. It was viewed as a specialized area delegated to a number of individuals who were separated and apart from general management and operation. This has changed dramatically. Today the role of the therapeutic recreation manager with respect to the costs of providing therapeutic recreation service in health and human services, especially in healthcare facilities, has changed. In the healthcare arena budgeting has not only become increasingly decentralized with managers taking on a growing role, but also resources for healthcare are more limited, and consumers bear more responsibility for payment. In the community-based leisure service agencies and organizations there is a climate of fiscal austerity.

As a final note, therapeutic recreation managers need to look at money matters and budgets philosophically as well as pragmatically. They also need to recognize and maintain a realistic attitude toward obtaining and dispensing funds. Managers, and to a lesser degree staff, can be appreciative or critical towards funds allocated to them, and the position they take does make a difference. Managers are likely to achieve better results in the delivery of services if they are realistic about the money available. Managers who overemphasize the value of money in their department may have morale problems with staff and difficulties with supervisors that surpass financial realities. Likewise, managers and practitioners who are constantly critical about budgetary matters will eventually hurt their program delivery of services and lessen the contributions they make. This does not mean financial questions and concerns should not be raised or addressed and budgetary suggestions should not be made. In fact, managers and staff should have input in making suggestions about the budget and help maintain efficiency and effectiveness in implementing financial plans.

This chapter makes no pretense of covering the complexities of financial management and budgeting in detail; initially its purpose is to provide a brief historical overview of sources of revenue to support services coupled with why there is a need for proper fiscal management. This is followed by a discussion of the various revenue sources that organizations presently use. Thereafter, there is a review and consideration of the basic concepts of financial management including budgeting, budget process, types of budgets, and budget review. The role of the first-line manager in the fiscal management process concludes this chapter.

# Historical Overview

Financial management and budgeting were common practices in public community-based leisure service agencies before their use in private sector planning. In the 1950s budgeting began to be seen as a planning tool, and planning was increasingly adopted as a management tool. Subsequent to the enormous investments of the Great Society era, the concern for better leisure resource allocation and program evaluation gave rise to the concept of cost-effectiveness evaluation and cost-benefit analysis (Anthony and Herzlinger, 1980), zero-based budgeting (Cheek, 1977), and social accounting (Melton and Watason, 1977). Other factors that have contributed to fiscal stress within the park and recreation field outside of the severe economic recession include forced reduction in the size of the work force, growing interdependency of the public and private sector, increasing complexity of the law coupled with new legislation (i.e., Americans with Disabilities Act [ADA]), and an increase in the gross value of publicly owned park and recreation resources.

The current crisis in the United States relating to the cost of healthcare has been brought about by increased use of healthcare facilities, inflation, population increase, increasing numbers of elderly, focus on illness care, cost reimbursement, fee for service reimbursement, technology, indigent care, malpractice, and recently the impact of various catastrophic diseases (e.g., AIDS). These cost factors have been further complicated by hospital competition, redesigned care delivery service (e.g., freestanding clinics, home care, outpatient surgery, and other ambulatory services that focus on preventive or rehabilitative healthcare and service), and marketing of healthcare services.

Depending on the source, there are various approaches to explaining the high cost of healthcare. Hospitals in the early 1900s had a basic mission to care for the sick and poor. In many cases the family was surprised by a patient's discharge, not by a patient's death. Hospitals were financially supported by philanthropy, and there was no hospitalization insurance (Rosenberg, 1987). However, when an individual did pay, it would be on what is now called an all-inclusive rate. That is, hospitals charged all patients the same daily rate. This single rate covered all services that the hospital provided.

By the 1920s it was not unusual for patients to be charged a regular daily service and special service charges for specific techniques in surgery, anesthesia, X-ray, laboratory services, drugs, physical therapy, and so forth. The intent of the special service charge system was simply to maintain equity between patients who used particular services and those who did not (Berman, Weeks, and Kukla, 1990).

During the late 1920s an inclusive rate system was applied to certain admissions according to diagnosis such as tonsillectomies and maternity service. In the 1930s all-inclusive rates were established by many hospitals for all inpatients. These rates varied only as to the length of stay of the patient and the type of accommodations (ward, semi-private room, private room). Also during the 1930s the federal government became involved through the Children's Bureau in hospital care reimbursement. As opposed to full hospital costs, the Children's Bureau only paid the cost per day that was applicable to patient care, excluding costs that were not for direct patient care such as administrative and benefits costs (Berman, Weeks, and Kukla, 1990). During this same period Kaiser Permanente in California developed the forerunner of today's health maintenance organizations (HMO); payment and delivery of healthcare were merged into a single system.

Meanwhile in 1929 Dr. Justin Ford Kimball, the executive vice president of Baylor University, found that the University Hospital in Dallas, Texas, was in serious financial trouble because of the large amount of outstanding accounts receivable. It was noted by Dr. Kimball that a large number of delinquent debtors were teachers. As a result, he initiated a prepayment plan for teachers to aid in hospital care costs. The teachers who joined the plan could pay a fixed sum (i.e., fifty-cents-a-month premium) and be assured of up to 21 days of hospital care in a semiprivate room at Baylor University Hospital. The Baylor prepayment idea caught on in other parts of the country where other hospitals faced a problem of collecting unpaid bills. Eventually, these various plans came together under the term *Blue Cross* (Berman, Weeks, and Kukla, 1990).

Throughout the next four decades, with the exception of the period in the 1930s when Blue Cross plans were getting started and a flat rate system was used, a variety of retrospective, prospective, incentive, and disincentive systems were used to pay hospital bills (Berman, Weeks, and Kukla, 1990).

The end of World War II brought a demand for more beds to care for the injured. The passage of the Hill-Burton Act provided funding for construction to expand existing hospitals and build new ones. The Hill-Harris Hospital and Medical Facilities Amendments were enacted in 1964. They dealt with modernization grants, areawide planning, and long-term care facilities (Tillock, 1981). In 1966 the Medicare and Medicaid programs were initiated to improve access for the elderly to health services and facilities. By 1970 medical care costs began to escalate at an astonishing rate with no end in sight (Rosenberg, 1987).

In the early 1970s managed care came more into existence as the result of the Health Maintenance Organization Act (PL 93–222) of 1973. HMOs are characterized as independent plans that offer comprehensive medical service through a group of medical practitioners, often in one location. The subscriber to an HMO pays a set monthly premium, and physicians and other health professionals employed by the HMO typically are paid on a salaried, rather than fee-for-service basis. HMO's are not the only managed care plans available. Others include competitive medical plans (CMP), hospital-physician organizations (HPO), preferred provider organizations (PPO), and direct agreements between the employer and providers.

The rapid expansion of healthcare services and the corresponding escalation in healthcare cost coupled with a significant increase in premiums for malpractice insurance prompted numerous cost containment efforts during the 1970s and into the 1980s (Rosenberg, 1987). Government regulations were expanded and, for the first time, provided limits on cost. Utilization review was introduced as a program designed to place limits on consumer stays in hospitals. An attempt to control the expansion of hospital physical facilities and technological equipment was done through a certificate-of-need program. At the urging of the American Hospital Association (AHA), hospitals developed programs to control health expenditures. By the end of the seventies, third-party payers were paying two-thirds of all hospital care costs (American Hospital Association, 1983). According to Jonas (1992), the vast majority of third-party payments are for services provided in medical rehabilitation and psychiatry.

Third-party payers include the federal government Medicare program, state government Medicaid programs, Blue Cross and Blue Shield (BC/BS) plans (i.e., separate statewide or substatewide area operation coordinated through the BC/BS Association), commercial insurance companies (e.g., Prudential, Travelers), HMOs, PPOs, and third-party administrators (i.e., for-profit general business corporations which provide all services of a BC/BS plan or a commercial insurance company with the exception of the insurance underwriting). Blue Cross and Blue Shield plans are the market leaders. Most operate as not-for-profit health service corporations although there is a trend to convert to for-profit organizations. In addition, people are now making higher copayments for insurance than ever before.

The most significant change in health cost containment took place in the early 1980s with the initiation of the Prospective Payment System (PPS) through the Tax Equity and Fiscal Responsibility Act (PL 97–182). This system provided payment to most hospitals at a predetermined specific rate for each Medicare discharge based upon the consumer's diagnosis. Under this system, discharges are classified into diagnosis-related groups (DRG), with 24 major diagnostic categories (MDC) organized by organ system and disease etiology, and 470 DRGs applicable to Medicare. The PPS system provided hospitals the opportunity to realize a direct savings for the first time in providing services. This system not only provided a savings for hospitals, but it assisted greatly in the development of fixed payment plans with employers, HMOs, PPOs, and other health provider organizations. Moreover, the PPS provided a strong incentive for hospital management to organize its operations and to provide services to consumers in the most cost effective and efficient manner (American Hospital Association, 1983). In 1985, the Consolidated Omnibus Budget Reconciliation Act was passed. This act and various amendments to it in succeeding years have modified the reimbursement provisions of PPS.

The challenge to therapeutic recreation managers in the current economically constrained and competitive environment, regardless of setting, is to have an understanding of the relationship among agencies and organizations, the environment, and the evolving social, political, and economic trends. Therapeutic recreation managers must be responsible for the effective, efficient financial management of their departments. Thereafter, the manager must be accountable for monitoring the budget. Efficient, high quality service will prevail only through accountable monitoring.

# Revenue Sources

Health and human services are funded through a variety of sources: appropriations; grants and contracts; contributions; fees, charges, and reimbursement; or a combination of two or more of these sources. The nature of the organization, public or private, not-for-profit or for-profit determines the funding sources as well as the implications for the planning and budgeting process to a large degree.

## *Appropriations*

The major source of funds for most public health and human service organizations come from tax-based revenues in the form of appropriations or grants. These tax-based funds may be federal, state, or local allocations. Then too, a community, freestanding, leisure service center for the disabled which is part of a local department of parks and recreation may get a fixed-dollar allocation from the city budget through the department in addition to possible federal or state funds that supplement the allocation by a grant. This may further be supplemented by a grant from a foundation or a large contribution from a private donor.

Public state agencies (e.g., institution for the mentally ill) receive appropriations through the legislative branch of state government, usually on a yearly basis. These funds may also be supplemented by specific organizations or programs with other government and nongovernment grants.

It is not unusual, in some state institutions, for profits from concessions or the institution's canteen to be allocated to the activity therapy department.

Normally, a public entity can expect support on a long-term basis, with yearly appropriations primarily affecting the level of increment or decrement. This continuity, however, can sometimes limit the flexibility of the organization and its program units attempt at innovation. Many functions of public health and human service organizations and the services they offer are prescribed by legislation. As a result, this leaves little room for deviation even when outside funds are available to support growth and change.

Dependency on tax-based revenue and legislative appropriations also means that a public health and human service organization is subjected in a direct way to changes in funding level brought about by broad economic and political changes. Governmental bodies are immediately affected by economic stress and shifting political tides; consequently the level and allocation of resources becomes a focal point for political processes. Agencies or organizations that do well in times of economic stress tend to have strong, cohesive, and politically active consumer groups. Public agencies cannot lobby, but citizen support groups can.

Funding by appropriation has strong impact on the budgeting process and on the nature of agency or organization accountability. Ongoing use of public funds does tend to allow for continuity and consistency in meeting organizational missions and goals. There still appears to be a strong tendency, however, for accountability to be measured in terms of traditionally understood services, regardless of setting, rather than in terms of community or individual impact. Because public health and human service organizations are held accountable for the means they use rather than the ends they seek in so many situations, they tend to have difficulty reforming budgetary processes or attempting innovations in service delivery unless these innovations have gained political acceptance.

## Contributions

Contributions to health and human service agencies (e.g., Easter Seal self-supporting therapeutic recreation service agencies) can run the gamut from $5.00 donations by individuals to multimillion-dollar endowments. The process of fund-raising can mean anything from direct mailings, to knocking on doors of corporate offices, to sponsorships, to mounting campaigns, to special events (e.g., walk-a-thons), to arts and crafts sales, and even to garage sales. Some agencies depend on professional fund-raising or development specialists which also encourages the fund-raising efforts of board members.

The implications of contributed funds for the budgeting process depends more on the type of contribution than on its size. Unrestricted donations can be used to carry out

any of the normal agency functions; thus, they become part of the operating budget. Sometimes, however, contributions are restricted to use for specific purposes. These funds earmarked either for specific current activities or for specified future use. Endowment funds may be restricted or unrestricted in terms of activities supported but involve the use of only the income earned from assets. An agency depending on various types of large contributions that include endowments must either develop or purchase investment expertise. In addition, an agency depending on contributions for a major portion of its revenue must also develop mechanisms for recording pledges or bequests.

For small agencies, participation in consolidated fund-raising efforts is the norm. Contributions are received indirectly through participation in such programs as United Fund, United Way, or local community chests. In some respects, receiving funds from such campaigns is more similar to obtaining grants than it is to mounting direct campaigns for donations. Agencies that apply for funding indicate the objectives to be met by the funds, follow specified reporting procedures and must fit the program's funding priorities.

## Grants and Contracts

Grants involve the obtaining of funds from governmental agencies, particularly the federal government, and from private corporations and individuals. The process of funding can be both enriching and overwhelming. Applications for funds are usually made in accordance with printed guidelines supplied to help applicants define their objectives and describe their framework and methodology. The applications also include a systematized, built-in evaluation procedure to help the applicant. Still, the process can be daunting because of the many details and decisions that must be included and made.

Books and pamphlets have been written providing guidelines and suggestions for those who apply for grants. Workshops and seminars are conducted at conferences and at universities to train people in how to apply for and get grants. This is an area that requires much knowledge, and managers who are interested in obtaining grant money should increase their understanding of it.

The best source for learning about private foundations is the Foundation Center (79 Fifth Avenue, New York, NY 10003). The center will send a publication catalog that describes major sources of information about foundations. Among major publication and computer services of the Foundation Center are the following: *The Foundation Directory, Foundations Grants Index, Foundation Center National Data Book*, Comsearch printout, and Sourcebook profiles. To obtain information on smaller foundations one should contact the local office of the Internal Revenue Service (IRS) or nearest Foundation Center Library for the latest Form 990FF. Small foundations must submit this form annually to the IRS on which they list all their grantees, finance details, funding interest and restrictions, and application procedures and deadlines.

Tracking government funds may be even more challenging than searching for grants from foundations. Despite a general decline in support, the federal government is still the largest resource of external funding. Information on government funding may be obtained from the following major sources: *Federal Register, Catalog of Federal Domestic Assistance,* and *Commerce Business Daily.* All documents can be obtained through the Superintendent of Documents, (U.S. Government Printing Office, Washington, DC 20402). Relative to federal agency priorities and applications, the program officer who is responsible for the grant in one's regional office or in Washington, DC, can be contacted as can the person whose name and number are listed in the *Federal Register.* The program officer will be able to provide criteria for selection and an application packet for the grant program which includes forms, rules and regulations, and guidelines. Most grants in therapeutic recreation are obtained through the Rehabilitation Services Administration, U.S. Department of Education and the National Institute on Disability and Rehabilitation Research.

Obtaining grants is usually dependent on the following: (1) a clear understanding of the guidelines and specific instructions, (2) careful formulation of the application, and (3) effective submission of the application to the funding agency and its representatives. Careful reading of the announcements and guidelines is essential in the grants process. The clearer the understanding of what is suggested and what is possible, the more likely it is that the application will be on target. The better the preparation for the proposed action, the more likely its acceptance.

The application needs both to be well-organized and related to the objectives of the funding agency. Governmental proposals have a highly structured format while proposals for foundations are less structured. Regardless, the more the application touches on specific areas, the more likely it is to be approved. Since many applications are ordinarily reviewed for most grant programs, the more unique and ingenious the application the better. Whenever a new approach can be introduced with anticipated pragmatic results, the more likely it is to be accepted. Creativity and organization are paramount.

The following format is offered as a guide to be modified if the funder requests a different outline:

1. summary statement,
2. statement of need,
3. goals and objectives,
4. components of the program (activities and tasks),
5. evaluation,
6. capability of the organization (ability to implement project),
7. continuation of the program,
8. dissemination plan,
9. budget, and
10. appendices (letters of support, affirmative action policy, etc.).

If the application does meet the funding organization's goal, it will be considered, in most instances, on the basis of the following questions:

- How well does the applicant demonstrate that there is a real need for the proposed project?
- How clear and attainable are the project's objectives?
- Does the proposal spell out a plan of action that suits project goals and objectives?
- Is the applying agency likely to be able to carry out the proposed project and meet the specified goals within the suggested time frame?
- Is the budget clearly thought out and appropriate for the scope of the project?
- Are the plans for evaluation well-documented, feasible, and appropriate?

In addition to routine answering of questions and following of suggestions outlined, if personal contacts can be made, the more likely a grant may be obtained. Contact, especially with private agencies, allows enthusiastic interest and comprehensive knowledge of the program area being considered to be expressed. Person-to-person contact before and during the grant preparation is desirable and may make the difference.

As the result of the ADA, more therapeutic recreation practitioners are developing small corporations to provide services to consumers with disabilities on a contractual basis. In fact, more and more public park and recreation departments are contracting for specific services because of a more conservative economic and political climate (Kraus and Curtis, 1986).

*Contracts* are more specific than grants. They usually specify an outcome to be accomplished or a procedure to be followed or performed before the recipient of the funds is selected. When a funding source utilizes a performance contract or subcontract as a funding mechanism, its own personnel might spell out the specific activities to be performed and then select, as the recipient of the allocated funds, the individuals or organization deemed most likely to be successful in carrying out the specified functions.

## *Fees, Charges and Reimbursement*

Nearly all private community-based leisure service agencies and organizations charge a direct fee for their services.

As noted earlier, some public community-based leisure service agencies may receive appropriated funds as well as charge a direct fee for their services. For therapeutic recreation service in these various community-based settings, a regular fee may be charged, or fees may be based on a sliding scale with the consumer paying differing amounts depending on his or her financial status. In freestanding public or private recreation and leisure centers for the disabled there may be a membership fee or a combination membership and special fee or charge for specific courses or activities. Again, these types of fees and charges may be offset by grants, corporations, civic organizations, individual contributions, or gifts.

Sometimes these fund-giving organizations can have the same kind of effect on agency practices as other funding sources might have. "Strings" attached to funding can provide restrictions on an organization's activities. Likewise, fee-based services sometimes have difficulty moving into innovative service areas when their funding depends almost completely on the number of consumers personally served.

Another implication of the use of fees as a funding base is the inherent difficulty in predicting income. The therapeutic recreation manager must be able to estimate very accurately the number of consumers likely to be served in a given time period. Estimations become more complex when sliding scales mean that not all consumers generate the same amount of revenue.

Within healthcare facilities, and to a lesser degree in school systems and other community cooperatives, organization agreements exist where a majority of consumers are charged direct fees for services rendered. These fees are paid through a third party. For reimbursement, an agency acts on behalf of an organization or consumer to reimburse the provider for all or some portion of the provider's cost or charges of providing services. In such an arrangement the consumer is called the *first party,* the healthcare organization is the *second party* and the agency acting on behalf of the consumer is the *third party.* Thus, the third party is a highly important factor in the operation of a hospital or any healthcare agency (e.g., home healthcare agency). Although there are a number of different governmental reimbursement sources, the major ones at present are Medicare and Medicaid. Medicare is federally administered while Medicaid is administered by the individual states. Other third-party providers include the various Blue Cross plans, commercial insurance carriers, HMOs, PPOs, and self-insurance by the employer.

The rules and regulations involving Medicare and Medicaid reimbursement are voluminous, and any discussion of the respective reimbursement programs is beyond the scope of this chapter or even this book. Likewise, a discussion of the various Blue Cross plans and other health insurance policies is impossible. One thing is certainly clear regarding health insurance policies—policies are no longer simple contracts providing hospital care coverage for subscribers as noted in the Historical Overview section of this chapter. Today insurance companies will usually pay up to a certain fixed amount for various procedures. This amount is specified in the contract between the first party and the insurance company. The difference is usually *written off* or paid directly by the consumer. Changes taking place in reimbursement design make it essential that an organization have accurate data on what costs are actually incurred by individual consumers and separate departments.

Therapeutic recreation within healthcare facilities or clinical settings, as a reimbursable revenue source, varies nationwide among Blue Cross plans, commercial insurance companies, workers compensation, and Medicare and Medicaid. Van Hyning and Teaff (cited in Reitter, 1989, p. 250) found the financing for therapeutic recreation service:

> to be through diverse sources, including direct third-party payments, per diem rate allocations, public allocations, private support and the facility overhead, as well as indirectly, through other hospital departments such as physical therapy.

However, these sources include only inpatient services and the present trend of healthcare services, in general, is toward outpatient services that do not always include a per diem room rate. Berman, Weeks, and Kukla (1990) commented that between 1985 and 1990, inpatient hospital days dropped more than 25 percent while outpatient days raised by about the same percentage.

A 1994 survey conducted by O'Morrow (1995) for the National Therapeutic Recreation Society (NTRS) reported that only 22 percent of the respondents (N = 840) indicated that therapeutic recreation received reimbursement within their employment site. The percentage may be even lower since the survey did not consider multiple responses from practitioners working in the same setting. Moreover, the survey did not consider whether the reimbursement was in association with inpatient service, outpatient service, or home care. The major sources of reimbursement in the survey in rank order were Medicare and Medicaid, private insurance, Blue Cross, and consumer pay.

An earlier study (1989) conducted by the American Therapeutic Recreation Association (ATRA) (Skalko and Malkin, 1991) found that slightly over 27 percent of the respondents (N = 101) charge for therapeutic recreation service. In addition, over one-half of the respondents (57 percent) indicated that their services were billed as therapeutic recreation service while other services (e.g., occupational therapy, physical therapy) and departments (e.g., nursing, psychiatry) are used to bill therapeutic recreation service. The study also noted that approximately 40 percent of the respondents received reimbursement for inpatient service from Medicare and Medicaid and 50–60 percent from various commercial insurance carriers. The investigators also noted that 23–30 percent of respondents received reimbursement for outpatients from Medicare and Medicaid while 40–60 percent received reimbursement from commercial carriers. Last, nearly 40 percent received reimbursement from workers compensation for outpatient and inpatient services respectively.

## Charges and Rate Setting

Therapeutic recreation services in healthcare facilities, primarily acute care hospitals and HMOs are classified as either routine services or ancillary services. Routine services are those services that are provided to the consumer as part of basic services. These services are usually incorporated into the operating cost or overhead of the facility. Ancillary services are services that are prescribed or ordered by the physician to meet a specific consumer need (i.e., treatment). The consumer is charged directly for these services, and the hospital or facility is reimbursed for these services in part or whole by a third party.

Charges or rate setting for unit of service vary from one facility to another and are relatively complex. A unit of service is a statistical measure for output of service consumed. There are various methods or techniques used for determining the rates applicable to the provided services. Environmental service departments use square footage, the dietary department uses meals served, the emergency room uses consumer visits, nursing care units use consumer days. The one most frequently used method in association with therapeutic recreation services is the hourly rate method. The method is based on consumer use in terms of rate per hour. These rates may be broken down into fractions of an hour. The rate usually incorporates therapist cost and time and could be further affected by adding material cost. In some settings, depreciation of equipment cost and other overhead costs such as electric, phone, and administrative costs could be added to the rate. Hourly rates or units of service cost are based on past and present trends and changes in the services provided. Unfortunately, the nationally used Medicare reimbursement system does not use a time-dependent unit. The reimbursement is per consumer which is not a natural measurement. For example, some consumers may participate in a treatment procedure or activity program for one hour while others may be involved only for 15 minutes.

Reimbursement for any one of the illustrated services may be the same as the actual cost, or it may be lower. Some commercial insurance carriers will pay actual cost while Blue Cross and Medicare usually pay a lower cost based on an arrangement agreed upon by the provider of the services and the third party.

A recent study commissioned by the National Council for Therapeutic Recreation Council (NCTRC) (Connolly and Garbarini, 1996) regarding pricing and cost of therapeutic recreation services in healthcare facilities noted the following:

1. Charges for services vary depending on "type of facility, the area, staff time, staff qualifications, individual versus group rates, and direct and indirect costs."
2. Cost may vary by diagnostic group to include individual or group services to a package of services—recreation therapy, physical therapy, and occupational therapy for a specific amount. This process can be found primarily in managed healthcare services. On the other hand, the cost may vary by services provided (e.g., aquatics therapy, wherein the cost to provide is based on the service as opposed to a community outing which takes longer and may include more staff).
3. Cost varies by how often the consumer is seen coupled with whether the treatment is individual or in a group. This cost is compounded by consumer stay and what insurance companies will pay for the treatment.
4. A key element in the cost is having qualified therapeutic recreation personnel (e.g., certified therapeutic recreation specialist [CTRS]).

In the conclusions reached, the study noted that: "In harmony with agency practices and client diagnostic needs, the qualified CTRS can provide effective, cost-efficient services in healthcare today" (p. 3).

In conclusion, charges and rate setting are very complicated procedures that incorporate the philosophy behind third-party payment contracts, economics, political factors, local managed care arrangements, and whether the hospital is for-profit or not-for-profit. Additionally, the therapeutic recreation manager needs to realize that whether the facility is for-profit or not-for-profit, the facility administrators are concerned with the amount of revenue that can be expected from the department so as to balance facility financial needs and income.

The history of therapeutic recreation service being reimbursable through government or commercial insurance carriers has been uneven. It is difficult to determine to what extent therapeutic recreation service is being reimbursed for inpatient or outpatient service due to the limited number of studies conducted (Esneault, Malkin, and Sellers, 1992; Malkin and Skalko, 1992; Teaff and Van Hyning, 1988) and the lack of clarity among factors within the studies (e.g., consumers treated, respondents). The reimbursement problem is further compounded, according to West (1995), by a lack of understanding and recognition of therapeutic recreation as treatment on the part of the Health Care Financing Administration [HCFA], which monitors and reviews financing of healthcare services in the United States. While all investigators above concluded from their studies a need for additional research in all factors associated with reimbursement, West (1995, p. 169) noted:

> [that] . . . financing therapeutic recreation by third-party reimbursement (especially workman's compensation) is beginning to expand to some community-based treatment and home healthcare agencies, particularly pain clinics and traumatic brain injury agencies that have programs. These programs have demonstrated to clients, physicians, and insurance carriers that therapeutic recreation intervention can be a cost-effective service that can positively affect the functional capacity, health status, and the quality of life of individuals with disabilities or illnesses. As the value of therapeutic recreation services is further documented, there should be increasing opportunities for expanding reimbursement of therapeutic recreation programs and services in a wide variety of settings.

For additional information on the topic of financing and reimbursement relative to therapeutic recreation including a short annotated bibliography on third-party reimbursement see the NTRS's *Understanding Financing and Reimbursement Issues* (1996).

# Financial Management

In commercial enterprises the objective of management is not difficult to identify. It is basically that of maximizing owner's profits. In the case of a hospital, whether for-profit or not-for-profit, the *bottom line* profitability is not easily definable. Hospitals, like other public health and human service organizations and agencies are vital community resources. As such they must be managed for the benefit of the community. The objective of hospital management, for example, must be to provide the community with the services it needs at a clinically acceptable level of quality, a publicly responsive level of amenity, and at the least possible cost (Berman, Weeks, and Kukla, 1990). The same can be said for a community-based leisure service agency.

The financial management of the organization affects many aspects of work in the organization. It affects program services, salaries, staffing, quality of services, and quality and quantity of equipment and supplies available. The notion that competent financial management is necessary for efficient and effective organization operation is by any standard an accepted truism.

Financial management requires planning and predicting how much money the organization will bring in during the next year and how much it will need to spend in order to continue operating. The people who prepare the organization's budget must look ahead and consider such trends as economic inflation, recession, community needs, public demands, availability of quality staff, changes in service delivery, and competition from other organizations. Failure to consider these factors and others can result in an inadequate budget and eventual depletion of resources.

Budgeting is a management responsibility. In authoritarian-style organizations, the process is highly centralized so that only a few people at the higher levels of administration are involved in preparation of the budget. This top-down approach leaves the implementors of the budget without autonomy or the right to appropriate or control expenses. In others, budgeting may be widely decentralized, involving all managers at all levels within the organization, who in turn seek input from their staff. In fact, more and more organizations are recognizing the value of having budgets prepared by those who must implement them. For the first-line therapeutic recreation manager this bottom-up approach has distinct advantages:

1. the therapeutic recreation manager has a more intimative view of his or her needs than do those at the top;
2. the manager can provide a more realistic breakdown to support requests;
3. there is less likelihood of overlooking vital needs;
4. morale and satisfaction are usually higher when the manager and staff participate actively in making decisions that affect them; and
5. there is room for more flexibility and quicker action.

Whichever way is used, the final authority for the organization-wide budget rests with the governing board and chief executive office (CEO) since they are in a position to study population changes; consider any changes, such as closing or opening of facilities or services; and take account of any regulating changes that might result in policy change or legislation.

# Prerequisite to Budgeting

Before the actual process of budgeting can occur, several prerequisites need to be met. If the organization desires commitment to its goals and budget, it is essential that the therapeutic recreation manager be involved in budget development. Budget development begins at the top management level with the vice president, finance, chief financial or fiscal officer (CFO), sometimes called the comptroller, who provides the information on past budgets and expenses that is needed to begin the process of preparing a new budget. In some organizations a *budget calendar* is prepared to indicate when specific budget activities are to be carried out and completed. A set of guidelines is also prepared to assist managers in completing their portion of the budget. These guidelines include explanations of the budget forms and reporting procedures and, of course, the deadlines for submitting budget requests. Procedures for review, revision, and approval of budgets are usually provided.

An example of a hospital budgeting organization structure is illustrated in Figure 9.1 (page 122). The structure notes the accountabilities of the various management levels. Therapeutic recreation's place in the structure would obviously differ from one hospital to another although more than likely it would be at the department or section manager's level.

In some hospitals the creation and use of a staff level budget committee is an optional component of the budget preparation. Its place in Figure 9.1 represents a logical extension of the principles of participatory management and provides a vehicle that can yield operational as well as political dividends. Ideally, the committee would be multidisciplinary in nature.

In the decentralized, participative approach to budgeting, every department head and manager is responsible for preparing his or her section of the budget. Likewise, these same managers are also responsible for defending the budget. Because it may not be possible to implement all goals and projections, the manager must be prepared to discuss the relative priority of budget items and the potential impact of implementing or not implementing them. The therapeutic recreation manager needs to be consciously aware of the department's goals and objectives. It is also important that the needs and goals of the department be congruent with the organization's goals. Although decisions and approvals on budget proposals are the responsibility of top management, these proposals are influenced many times by the information presented through the negotiation process. Compromise invariably has to play a part in working out differences; the manager who is too rigid will ordinarily end up with fewer funds. Finally, if the manager is new, it is essential that the budget process be understood. Even managers who have had previous budget experience will need an orientation to the format or process utilized in a specific organization.

Data must be available to facilitate forecasting or projecting activity. Revenue and expense data, such as income from services and cost of services, may be provided with the budget information compiled by the CFO. If not, it is the manager's responsibility to gather such information. In addition, nonmonetary statistical information, such as number of services provided and number of consumers participating, is needed for planning the budget.

It is well to recognize at the prerequisite stage that negotiations usually take place regarding each department's budget. Further, one should be aware that power and influence enters into budget negotiations. The therapeutic recreation manager must be willing to devote time and energy to the budgeting process.

It is also well to recognize that the wise therapeutic recreation manager does not "pad" his or her requests in anticipation of having them cut thus ending up with what is needed. This action often backfires to the detriment of the department. At the same time, it is advisable to request that a limited contingency fund be available for emergencies and unexpected developments.

# Budgets and Budgeting

A manager may become directly involved in preparing and monitoring a budget in the various organizations that provide health and human services. This has come as a surprise to many new therapeutic recreation managers, especially those in healthcare facilities, who are left to learn by trial and error how to prepare a good working budget in many instances.

The process of budgeting has gained importance in recent years. Traditionally, budgeting has been the process of asking for a percentage increase over what was offered the previous year with specific justification for innovative requests. However, this is no longer acceptable because of the rising service costs and the emphasis on cost containment. Today, budgeting should be looked upon as a living process with a reasonable degree of flexibility, fluidity, and mobility to meet changing conditions and unforeseen exigencies. If the position is taken that budgeting is a dynamic rather than a static process, one must be prepared to adjust to changes in demand for services, changes in the cost of services or supplies, and changes in a variety of other conditions that force adjustments in budgeting projections.

Using data from budgets to guide decision making is important for every level of management regardless of setting. It is essential that budgeting be accomplished in such a way that it facilitates goal achievement. Further, it is important that therapeutic recreation managers, even at the first-line management level, participate in the development of the budget.

Consideration of therapeutic recreation budgets and budgeting will be focused primarily within healthcare facilities. Even here there is much variation in budgets and fiscal management. No attempt is purposely made to ignore therapeutic recreation budgets and budgeting in profit and nonprofit community-based leisure service agencies or organizations. To a large degree there is considerable similarity and overlapping. On the other hand, healthcare facilities have the following unique characteristics that are

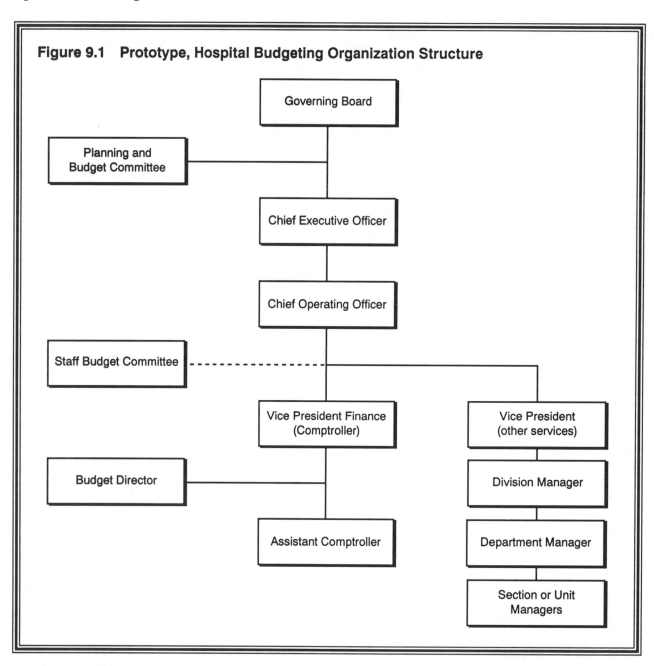

**Figure 9.1   Prototype, Hospital Budgeting Organization Structure**

not found in community-based leisure service agencies: cost-based reimbursement programs and private expenditures, shared hospital expenses and other multihospital arrangements, HMO and PPO models of service and large administrative structures.

## Budgets

The word *budget* derives from an old French term *bougette* which means a "little bag," a sack or pouch:

> The British adopted the word to describe the motion engaged in by the chancellor of the exchequer when he presented his annual financial statement to Parliament. He was said to open his 'budget' or bag which contained the various financial documents. (United Way of America, 1985, p. 3)

A budget is an operational management plan for the allocation of resources and a monitor and control for ensuring that results comply with the plans. Results are expressed in quantitative terms. Although budgets are usually associated with financial statements such as revenues and expenses, they also may be nonfinancial statements covering output, materials, and equipment. Budgets help coordinate the efforts of the agency by determining what resources will be used by whom, when, and for what purpose. Budgets are frequently prepared for each organizational unit and for each function within the unit.

Every budget starts with a plan. Planning is done for a specific time, usually a fiscal year but may be subdivided into monthly, quarterly, or semiannual periods. In order to work, the plan and the resultant budget(s) are formulated in the context of the overall objectives of the therapeutic recreation department and the short- and long-range goals of the organization. In setting objectives for the department, resource requirements need to be built-in. Budgeting translates objectives to be accomplished into financial terms. The budget should help to guide first-line managers in their decision making. The future is unknown, and so any plan has to be flexible enough to allow for changing conditions. For example, an unexpected shortage of therapeutic recreation personnel will adversely affect the staffing budget resulting in more overtime or a reduction in services. There are four purposes of budgeting according to Kaluzny, Warner, Warren, and Zelman (1982, p. 113):

> One of the major purposes is to force managers to plan. Second, as a by-product of the planning and budgeting process, it helps develop coordination and cooperation within the organization. Plans made by various departments have to be coordinated.... Third, within any particular department, budgeting can help staff members become aware of their role in the organization and bring to the fore the extent to which their jobs require resources. A fourth purpose ... is communication. By documenting the plans for the coming year[s], a budget can help communicate the goals and objectives, the types and levels of services to be delivered, the resources needed, and the income generated for a particular program.

Although one thinks of budgets in a positive way, there are disadvantages to budgeting. One major problem is that budgets convert all aspects of an agency or organizational performance into monetary values for a single comparable unit of measurement. Consequently, only those aspects that are easy to measure may be considered, and equally important factors such as development and research efforts may be ignored. Another problem may arise when budget goals supersede agency or organization goals which in turn affect department goals. Budgets may also be applied too rigidly affecting innovation and change. Last, budget development is time consuming (Bart, 1988). However, careful planning provides an opportunity for examining options and alternatives in a calm, rational setting. The result is generally a more satisfactory outcome, with fewer crisis situations arising.

## Types of Budgets

There are numerous types of budgets used to express the plans and to meet the goals and objectives of health and human service agencies and organizations. They are powerful instruments since they serve as a guide to therapeutic recreation performance and allocation of personnel, supplies, support services, and facilities. The format of these budgets is usually of the *line-item* type. This type of budget procedure notes specific expenditures and revenues for specific items. It does not present the organization or department goals, targets, programs, or results. This text will consider only those budgets that are prepared and used most frequently by first-line managers.

### Revenue and Expense Budget (Operating Budget)

By far the most common budgets are the revenue and expense budgets. Combined, they are frequently referred to as the *operating budget*. This budget spells out the plans for day-to-day operating revenue and expenses in dollar terms for a period of one year. In other words, this budget projects the services to be provided, the revenue which will be generated from these services, and the expenses associated with providing the services (see Figure 9.2, page 124). In many agencies the operating budget is usually based on the previous year's budget. This practice is sometimes referred to as historical or incremental budgeting. Another practice is program budgeting and zero-based budgeting which will be discussed shortly.

Some may wonder about for-profit and not-for-profit organizations as related to the operating budget. In general, if the budget shows an excess of revenues over expenses, it means that the organization expects to make a *profit* from its activities for the year. If the organization is a for-profit company, some of the profits can be paid to the owners of the company in the form of a dividend. Even not-for-profit organizations, such as hospitals and community-based leisure service agencies need to earn profits. These profits are used to replace worn-out equipment and old buildings or to expand the services available to the community.

Returning to budget development, in some organizations, based upon an analysis of the organization's past budget and future plans, dollar figures are assigned to all departments and to all categories on both income and expenditure sides of the budget. In other organizations, individual departments are given some flexibility in requesting or allocating funds for various categories. However, in

---

### Figure 9.2   Components of the Operating Budget

Expenses (Cost):
- Payroll: salary, vacation, holidays, social security, education, other fringe benefits
- Supplies: office supplies, program supplies, etc.
- Equipment (dollar limits): program and office equipment
- Overhead: building maintenance, water, electric
- Other: mortgage, interest, loans, insurance, maintenance service contracts, contractual arrangements, education materials, transportation, marketing, etc.

Revenue (Income):
- Consumer services: fees and charges, Medicaid, Medicare, other insurance
- Contributions: philanthropic, grants-in-aid, research and program grants
- Other: interest, rent, contract

---

many other organizations, departments are restricted to using funds only as designated by the CFO unless a justification is offered and approved. In some instances, the manager may be required to balance the budget (i.e., expenses equal income). Considering present cost containment efforts, more demands for balanced budges may be seen in the future.

Expense factors that the therapeutic recreation manager might consider in the operating budget would be personnel salaries, employee benefits, insurance, activity programs, special events, supplies and equipment for both activity programs and office, laundry service (if personnel are required to wear uniforms), repairs and maintenance, depreciation and replacement of supplies and equipment, travel, education, books, periodical subscriptions, dues and membership fees, legal fees, and contractual services. In freestanding recreation centers for the disabled, one would have additional expenses of depreciation on the center, insurance, utilities, mortgage interest or rent, and possibly bad debts. Depending on the budget system of the hospital or agency, some of the previously mentioned expenses such as cost of utilities, postage, mortgage rate and rent, and maintenance are considered overhead expenses. These expenses are allocated to all areas by the accounting department according to a specific formula.

In some organizations, salaries, benefits, and insurance would be provided by the CFO when budget guidelines and budget forms are forwarded to various departments. In other organizations, a formula is provided to assist the manager in determining benefits and insurance. In addition, many organizations require a written justification for each expense or category of expenses.

The next step in developing the operating budget is to determine the revenues associated with the provision of services. As noted earlier, revenue development varies from organization to organization. In some organizations such as healthcare facilities, therapeutic recreation is reimburs-

able through various insurance programs. However, other similar organizations make therapeutic recreation part of consumer cost by incorporating it into the consumer's bill. Other sources of revenues include general donations, donations and grants for specific programs, United Fund, investment revenues, and funding from various tax levies in the form of budget appropriations from governmental units.

In an organization where a program budgeting approach is used, projected service revenue is determined by multiplying the projected volume of service by the price charged for the service. The volume estimates are derived in the planning process when the number of consumers using a service or program is projected.

Figures 9.3 through 9.8 represent a number of operating budgets. Figure 9.3 shows the expense budget of the Recreation Therapy Department of Iowa Methodist Medical Center of Central Iowa Health System. Line-item code number 83610 may be misleading in the sense that it makes reference to medical and surgical supplies. However, this is the line-item name used within the center with reference to all departments and their supply needs. In the Recreation Therapy Department it refers to items such as games and arts and craft supplies. Line-item code number 90010 Recreation is associated with out trips and parties.

The Therapeutic Recreation Region 4, Cincinnati Recreation Commission line-item operating budget is illustrated in Figure 9.4 (page 126). A revenue budget of Region 4 is shown in Figure 9.5 (page 128), while Figure 9.6 (page 129) represents a budget summary for Region 4. In this figure, Services (i.e., 7200 sum) refers to bus transportation, trips, printing, and seasonal program guides. Materials and Supplies (i.e., 7300 sum) refers to equipment and supplies of various kinds while Fixed Costs (i.e., 7400 sum) includes such items as rental charges, heat, electric, and postage.

Another community-based leisure service agency expense and revenue budget is shown in Figure 9.7 (page 130).

## Figure 9.3  Expense Budget

ACCOUNT CODE LEVEL BUDGETER
CIHS (HC)—CENTRAL IOWA HEALTH SYSTEM
BUDGET 1996

Cost Center: 52410 RECREATION THERAPY

| | | BUDGET 1996 |
|---|---|---|
| EXPENSE ACCOUNTS | | |
| SALARY AND WAGES | | |
| 70040 | Salary—Professional | $118,567 |
| | | |
| SUPPLIES AND OTH EXP | | |
| 79062 | Food | $ 167 |
| 80320 | Paper Goods | $ 144 |
| 83610 | Medical/Surg Supplies | $ 1,786 |
| 83620 | Office Supplies | $ 229 |
| 83900 | Minor Equipment | $ 148 |
| 84500 | Phone | $ 319 |
| 85000 | Equipment Repairs | $ 262 |
| 90000 | Miscellaneous | $ 200 |
| 90010 | Recreation | $ 2,290 |
| 90400 | Postage/Freight | $ 186 |
| 90475 | Meeting And Travel | $ 1,311 |
| | | $ 7,042 |
| | | |
| | Subtotal Sal/Sup/Exp | $125,609 |
| | | |
| FRINGES | | |
| 74220FB | Other Fringes Allocation | $ 3,466 |
| 74500FB | Pension Expense Allocation | $ 2,529 |
| 75400FB | Health Insurance Allocation | $ 9,380 |
| 74100 | Fica Tax Expense | $ 9,097 |
| | | $ 24,472 |
| | | |
| DEPRECIATION | | |
| 8857*0010 | Bldg Depr—Powell | $ 1,484 |
| 8857*0017 | Depr Exp N. Parking Ramp Extra | $ 82 |
| 8858*0001 | Amort Lshld-Woodland Parking | $ 22 |
| 8859*0001 | Powell Fixed Equip Depr | $ 2,733 |
| 88500 | Moveable Equipment Depr | $ 1,448 |
| 88560 | Depre Exp—Land Improvements | $ 349 |
| | | $ 6,119 |
| | | |
| | Total Expense Accounts | $156,199 |

Used by permission of Iowa Methodist Medical Center of Central Iowa Health System, Des Moines, IA.

The Recreation for Special Needs Division, City of Alexandria, Virginia, budget also notes its need for positions. Line-item code number 1108 is in reference to summer seasonal employees. Number 2102 refers to contract for services (e.g., bus drivers), money for theater and sport events, and staff training. Recreational supplies (e.g., board games, arts and crafts) are in item number 2306 and 2502 is for bus rentals for day trips. Figure 9.8 (page 132) reflects the explanations given for the 1995 budget.

## Figure 9.4  Operating Budget

CARS    REC         CFSFB202

**CINCINNATI AGENCY REPORTING SYSTEM**
**ALL FUNDS EXPENSE BUDGET REPORT**
**FOR FISCAL YEAR 1996**
AS OF 02/29/96

DEPARTMENT: 190   DEPT OF PUBLIC RECREATION
ORGANIZATION: 6000   THERAPEUTICS

FUND: 323   RECREATION SPECIAL ACTIVITIES
AGENCY: 194   REGION 4

BUDGET PSONS:.00

| ORG OBJ OBJ | SUB | DESCRIPTION | CURRENT BUDGET | EXPENDED | ENCUMBERED | PREENCUMBERED | PERCENT UNCOMMITTED | COMMITTED |
|---|---|---|---|---|---|---|---|---|
| 6000 7111 | | REGULAR HOUR | 110.00 | .00 | .00 | .00 | 110.00 | .000 |
| *OBJECT CAT 7100 | | | 110.00 | .00 | .00 | .00 | 110.00 | .000 |
| 7211 | | POSTAGE | 920.00 | 192.25 | .00 | .00 | 727.75 | .209 |
| 7212 | | TELEPHONE | 210.00 | 74.10 | .00 | .00 | 135.90 | .353 |
| 7213 | | LOCAL TRAVEL | 2,300.00 | 130.77 | .00 | .00 | 2,169.23 | .057 |
| 7214 | | NONLOCAL TRV | 740.00 | .00 | .00 | .00 | 740.00 | .000 |
| | 51 | TRAVEL NOC | .00 | 23.25 | .00 | .00 | -23.25 | .000 |
| 7219 | | COMMUNICATIO | 750.00 | .00 | .00 | .00 | 750.00 | .000 |
| 7221 | | PREPARE MEAL | 4,400.00 | 1,182.75 | .00 | .00 | 3,217.25 | .269 |
| 7232 | | PRINTING SRC | 2,490.00 | 22.00 | 1,530.49 | .00 | 937.51 | .623 |
| 7234 | | LEGAL ADVERT | 1,410.00 | .00 | .00 | .00 | 1,410.00 | .000 |
| 7252 | | OFFICE MACH | 210.00 | .00 | .00 | .00 | 210.00 | .000 |
| 7289 | | EXPRT SV-NOC | 4,770.00 | .00 | .00 | .00 | 4,770.00 | .000 |
| | 54 | ADMISSIONS | .00 | 684.00 | .00 | .00 | -684.00 | .000 |
| 7297 | | TEMP SERVICE | 9,290.00 | .00 | .00 | .00 | 9,290.00 | .000 |
| 7299 | | OTHR SERVICE | 1,840.00 | .00 | .00 | .00 | 1,840.00 | .000 |
| | 51 | SUNDRY NOC | .00 | .00 | 1,925.00 | .00 | -1,925.00 | .000 |
| *OBJECT CAT 7200 | | | 29,330.00 | 2,309.12 | 3,445.49 | .00 | 23,565.39 | .197 |
| 7311 | | OFFICE SUPPL | 2,210.00 | 116.69 | .00 | .00 | 2,093.31 | .053 |
| 7313 | | PHOTO SUPPLY | 700.00 | 288.57 | .00 | .00 | 411.43 | .412 |
| 7316 | | COMP PERIPH | 430.00 | .00 | .00 | .00 | 430.00 | .000 |
| 7329 | | FOOD PRODUCT | 2,480.00 | .00 | .00 | .00 | 2,480.00 | .000 |
| 7341 | | MEDICAL SUPL | 220.00 | .00 | .00 | .00 | 220.00 | .000 |
| 7354 | | CHLORINE | .00 | 96.00 | 204.00 | .00 | -300.00 | .000 |
| 7361 | | PLANT SUPPLY | 180.00 | .00 | .00 | .00 | 180.00 | .000 |

**Figure 9.4  Continued**

CARS REC

| | | | CINCINNATI AGENCY REPORTING SYSTEM | | | | | |
|---|---|---|---|---|---|---|---|---|
| | | | ALL FUNDS EXPENSE BUDGET REPORT | | | | | |
| | | | **FOR FISCAL YEAR 1996** | | | | | |
| | | | AS OF 02/29/96 | | | | | |

FUND: 323 RECREATION SPECIAL ACTIVITIES  
AGENCY: 194 REGION 4  
DEPARTMENT: 190  
ORGANIZATION: 6000  
DEPT OF PUBLIC RECREATION THERAPEUTICS  
CFSFB202

| ORG OBJ | SUB OBJ | DESCRIPTION | CURRENT BUDGET | EXPENDED | ENCUMBERED | PREENCUMBERED | PERCENT UNCOMMITTED | COMMITTED |
|---|---|---|---|---|---|---|---|---|
| 7364 | | CLOTHES | 6,020.00 | .00 | .00 | .00 | 6,020.00 | .000 |
| | 51 | APPAREL NOC | .00 | 245.71 | .00 | .00 | -245.71 | .000 |
| 7366 | | TRAINING AID | 600.00 | .00 | .00 | .00 | 600.00 | .000 |
| 7369 | | TECH SUP NOC | 160.00 | .00 | .00 | .00 | 160.00 | .000 |
| 7371 | | CLEANING SUP | 100.00 | .00 | .00 | .00 | 100.00 | .000 |
| 7374 | | RECREATIONAL | 5,320.00 | .00 | .00 | .00 | 5,320.00 | .000 |
| | 51 | RECREAT. NOC | .00 | 152.05 | .00 | .00 | -152.05 | .000 |
| 7375 | | CONCESSION | 290.00 | .00 | .00 | .00 | 290.00 | .000 |
| 7379 | | OTHER SUPPLY | 1,850.00 | .00 | .00 | .00 | 1,850.00 | .000 |
| 7381 | | OFF FURNITUR | 710.00 | .00 | .00 | .00 | 710.00 | .000 |
| 7399 | | PARTS-NOC | 190.00 | .00 | .00 | .00 | 190.00 | .000 |
| | 51 | MISC. PARTS | .00 | 9.69 | .00 | .00 | -9.69 | .000 |
| *OBJECT CAT 7300 | | | 21,460.00 | 908.71 | 204.00 | .00 | 20,347.29 | .052 |
| 7419 | | RENT-NOC | 1,670.00 | .00 | .00 | .00 | 1,670.00 | .000 |
| 7452 | | SUBS-MEMBERS | 170.00 | .00 | .00 | .00 | 170.00 | .000 |
| 7459 | | FIXED CH-NOC | 930.00 | 100.00 | .00 | .00 | 830.00 | .108 |
| *OBJECT CAT 7400 | | | 2,770.00 | 100.00 | .00 | .00 | 2,670.00 | .036 |
| *ORGANIZATION 6000 | | | 53,670.00 | 3,317.83 | 3,659.83 | .00 | 46,692.68 | .130 |
| *FUND 323 | | | 53,670.00 | 3,317.83 | 3,659.83 | .00 | 46,692.68 | .130 |
| *AGENCY 194 | | | 347,794.00 | 30,752.55 | 3,659.49 | .00 | 313,381.96 | .099 |
| *DEPARTMENT 190 | | | 347,794.00 | 30,752.55 | 3,659.49 | .00 | 313,381.96 | .099 |
| *TOTAL BFY 96 | | | 347,794.00 | 30,752.55 | 3,659.49 | .00 | 313,381.96 | .099 |

**Figure 9.5   Revenue Budget**

```
CARS                        CINCINNATI AGENCY REPORTING SYSTEM
REC             ALL FUNDS CURRENT MONTH AND YTD REVENUE BUDGET REPORT
                               FOR FISCAL YEAR 1996
                                  AS OF 02/29/96

   DEPARTMENT:  190 DEPT OF PUBLIC RECREATION      AGENCY:  194      REGION 4
                                              ORGANIZATION:  6000    THERAPEUTICS
```

| REVENUE/SUBREVENUE CODE-DESCRIPTION | CURRENT MONTH | | YEAR TO DATE | | | | |
|---|---|---|---|---|---|---|---|
| | REVENUE RECOGNIZED | CASH COLLECTED | REVENUE RECOGNIZED | CASH COLLECTED | REVENUE BUDGET | UNRECOGNIZED BUDGET BALANCE | PERCENT UNRECOGNIZED |
| FUND        :319  CONTRIBUTIONS FOR RECREATION | | | | | | | |
| REV. CATEGORY  :86  CHARGES FOR CURRENT SERVICES | | | | | | | |
| 8673  57 THERAPEUTIC | 525.00 | 525.00 | 525.00 | 525.00 | .00 | -525.00 | .000 |
| *TOTAL RCAT 86 | 525.00 | 525.00 | 525.00 | 525.00 | .00 | -525.00 | .000 |
| *TOTAL FUND 319 | 525.00 | 525.00 | 525.00 | 525.00 | .00 | -525.00 | .000 |
| FUND        :323  RECREATION SPECIAL ACTIVITIES | | | | | | | |
| REV. CATEGORY :98  CHARGES FOR CURRENT SERVICES | | | | | | | |
| 8673  54 PROGRAM FEE | 2,967.00 | 2,967.00 | 3,086.00 | 3,086.00 | .00 | -3,086.00 | .000 |
| *TOTAL RCAT 86 | 2,967.00 | 2,967.00 | 3,086.00 | 3,086.00 | .00 | -3,086.00 | .000 |
| *TOTAL FUND 323 | 2,967.00 | 2,967.00 | 3,086.00 | 3,086.00 | .00 | -3,086.00 | .000 |
| *TOTAL ORG 6000 | 3,492.00 | 3,492.00 | 3,611.00 | 3,611.00 | .00 | -3,611.00 | .000 |
| *TOTAL AGY 194 | 3,492.00 | 3,492.00 | 3,611.00 | 3,611.00 | .00 | -3,611.00 | .000 |
| *TOTAL DEPT 190 | 3,492.00 | 3,492.00 | 3,611.00 | 3,611.00 | .00 | -3,611.00 | .000 |

**Figure 9.6   Operating Budget Summary**

Request Year: 1996

Date: 1/17/96

Fund:     ALL
Agency:  194   Region 4
EXPB Org./Program:  6000   Therapeutic Recreation

BUDGET SUMMARY FOR THE PROGRAM

| Object | Object Category | Requested Budget | REB Recommend | Change from Request | EBC Recommend | Change from Request | Approved Budget | Change from Request |
|---|---|---|---|---|---|---|---|---|
| 7100 sum | Personnel | 294,234 | 294,234 | 0 | 294,234 | 0 | 294,234 | 0 |
| 7200 sum | Services | 29,330 | 29,330 | 0 | 29,330 | 0 | 29,330 | 0 |
| 7300 sum | Materials & Supplies | 21,460 | 21,460 | 0 | 21,460 | 0 | 21,460 | 0 |
| 7400 sum | Fixed Costs | 2,770 | 2,770 | 0 | 2,770 | 0 | 2,770 | 0 |
|  | Sub Total | 53,560 | 53,560 | 0 | 53,560 | 0 | 53,560 | 0 |
| 7600 sum | Office/Tech Equip. | 0 | 0 | 0 | 0 | 0 | 0 | 0 |
| 7615 sum | Motorized Equipment |  |  |  |  |  |  |  |
|  | Total | 347,794 | 347,794 | 0 | 347,794 | 0 | 347,794 | 0 |
|  | Employee Benefits | 78,718 | 78,718 | 0 | 78,718 | 0 | 78,718 | 0 |
|  | Gen Fund Overhead | 8 | 8 | 0 | 8 | 0 | 8 | 0 |
| 7700 sum | Debt Service | 0 | 0 | 0 | 0 | 0 | 0 | 0 |
|  | Total Budget | 426,520 | 426,520 | 0 | 426,520 | 0 | 426,520 | 0 |
| Full-Time Equivalent |  | 17.5 | 17.5 | 0.0 | 17.5 | 0.0 | 17.5 | 0.0 |
| Positions |  | 69 | 69 | 0 | 69 | 0 | 69 | 0 |

**Figure 9.7  Operating Budget**

REPORT ID: BPR155  
DATE: 06/24/93

CITY OF ALEXANDRIA  
EXPENSE AND REVENUE BUDGET DETAIL

PAGE: 701  
TIME: 15:06:59

| DEPARTMENT | 80 | RECREATION & CULTURAL ACTIVITIES |
|---|---|---|
| DIVISION | 05 | RECREATION FOR SPECIAL NEEDS |
| SECTION | 00 | *** UNASSIGNED TITLE *** |
| FUND | 01 | GENERAL FUND |
| INDEX CODE | 121723 | RECREATION SPECIAL NEEDS |

POSITIONS BY SUB-OBJECT

CHARACTER 02 POSITION CLASSIFICATION

| | | | CURR YR BUDGET | PROPOSED | APPROVED | PERCENT CHANGE |
|---|---|---|---|---|---|---|
| FR11 | 06 | RECREATION LEADER II | | 1.00 | 1.00 | |
| FT18 | 20 | THERAPEUTIC RECR SUPV II | | 1.00 | 1.00 | |
| FT21 | 16 | THERAPEUTIC REC SUPV I | | 1.00 | 1.00 | |
| PR11 | 06 | RECREATION LEADER II | | .60 | .60 | |

TOTAL CHARACTER 02

TOTAL POSITIONS    3.60    3.60

EXPENDITURES BY SUB-OBJECT

CHARACTER 10 PERSONNEL SERVICES

| | | CURR YR BUDGET | PROPOSED | APPROVED | PERCENT CHANGE |
|---|---|---|---|---|---|
| 1101 | SALARIES FULL-TIME EMPLOYEES | 80,605 | 85,621 | 90,279 | 6.22 |
| 1102 | PART-TIME EMPLOYEES | 16,926 | 17,993 | 17,993 | 6.30 |
| 1108 | SHORT-TERM SALARIES | 35,756 | 44,267 | 44,267 | 23.80 |
| 1200 | SOCIAL SECURITY | 10,454 | 11,806 | 11,806 | 12.93 |
| 1201 | RETIREMENT CONTRIBUTIONS | 10,630 | 11,037 | 11,037 | 3.82 |
| 1202 | GROUP LIFE INSURANCE | 555 | 315 | 315 | 43.24- |
| 1203 | GROUP MEDICAL | 8,277 | 8,347 | 9,414 | .84 |
| 1211 | LONG-TERM DISABILITY | 421 | 458 | 458 | 8.78 |

TOTAL CHARACTER 10    163,624    179,844    185,569    9.91

**Figure 9.7 Continued**

```
REPORT ID:  BPR155                          CITY OF ALEXANDRIA                    PAGE:   702
DATE:       06/24/93                EXPENSE AND REVENUE BUDGET DETAIL             TIME:   15:06:59
```

```
DEPARTMENT   80       RECREATION & CULTURAL ACTIVITIES
DIVISION     05       RECREATION FOR SPECIAL NEEDS
SECTION      00       *** UNASSIGNED TITLE ***
FUND         01       GENERAL FUND
INDEX CODE   121723   RECREATION SPECIAL NEEDS
```

| | CURR YR BUDGET | PROPOSED | APPROVED | PERCENT CHANGE |
|---|---|---|---|---|
| **EXPENDITURES BY SUB-OBJECT** | | | | |
| **CHARACTER 20 NONPERSONNEL SERVICES** | | | | |
| 2102  FEES FOR PROFESSIONAL SERVICES | 5,436 | 6,786 | 6,786 | 24.83 |
| 2105  OTHER EQUIPMENT MAINTENANCE | 515 | 515 | 515 | |
| 2204  PHOTOCOPYING CHARGES | 400 | 200 | 200 | 50.00- |
| 2205  PRINT SERVICES | 500 | 251 | 251 | 49.80- |
| 2301  OFFICE SUPPLIES | 300 | 500 | 500 | 66.66 |
| 2302  FOOD SUPPLIES | 800 | 800 | 800 | |
| 2306  OPERATING SUPPLIES & MATERIALS | 1,000 | 1,000 | 1,000 | |
| 2308  UNIFORMS & WEARING APPAREL | 150 | 150 | 150 | |
| 2482  REGIONAL TRAVEL | 500 | 500 | 500 | |
| 2502  RENTAL VEHICLES | 1,350 | | | 100.00- |
| TOTAL CHARACTER 20 | 10,951 | 10,702 | 10,702 | 2.27- |
| TOTAL EXPENDITURES | 10,951 | 10,702 | 10,702 | 2.27- |
| | | | | |
| REVENUES BY SUB-OBJECT | | | | |
| TOTAL EXPENDITURES | 174,575 | 190,546 | 196,271 | 9.14 |
| | | | | |
| TOTAL REVENUES | | | | |
| BALANCE:  NET TO CITY | 174,575 | 190,546 | 196,271 | 9.14 |
| PERCENT CITY SHARE (%) | 100.00 | 100.00 | 100.00 | |

131

---

### Figure 9.8   Budget Explanation

**Nonpersonnel Services Explanations:**

**2102:**
Costs for direct service field trips admissions, staff reimbursement for trip admissions, in-service training costs for staff, fees for specialists to teach classes, cost for summer buses and drivers (the charge for this service from the Alexandria School system is estimated $4,000).
FY '94 under 121723 total spent was: $5749 (school bus bill was less than expected)

**2105:**
Office equipment maintenance as follows: Xerox 1020 copier $596
FY '94 under 121723 total spent was: $578

**2205:**
Special Needs Newsletter that is printed now three times a year. Each time printed is about $60.
FY '94 under 121723 total spent was: $116

**2301:**
Supplies needed to support daily operation of the Special Needs Office and Programs which include writing materials, typewriter ribbons, computer supplies, folder, etc.
FY '94 under 121723 total spent was: $640 (upgraded some out-of-date equipment such as a paper cutter, electric stapler, etc.)

**2302:**
Purchase of food for cooking sessions, special event activities, snacks, and other cooking-related needs for programs serving persons with mental health conditions or mental retardation.
FY '94 under 121723 total spent was: $737

**2306:**
Purchase of games, puzzles, sports supplies, craft supplies, adaptive equipment and any other supplies needed for the direct service programs.
FY '94 under 121723 total spent was: $2006 (made some large ticket purchases such as a button machine, new radio, replenished many craft supplies)

**2308:**
ADD IN AGAIN FOR—
Staff shirts for three full-time staff, year around part-time staff and summer staff. Jackets, sweatshirts for three full-time staff and permanent Recreation Leader II, 24 hours.
FY '94 under 121723 total spent was: $147

**2482:**
Reimbursement for Recreation for Special Needs staff (TR Supervisor II, TR Supervisor I, Full-time Recreation Leader II, 24 hr Recreation Leader II)
Travel for the following reasons:
Business at Lee Center, Administration Offices. Various recreation center site visits for programs or meetings.
Local professional meetings (VRPS, NTRS, Volunteer Coordinators meetings, Commission meetings) Cooperative program-related meetings (with Dept. of Special Education, Department of Mental Health, Mental Retardation and Substance Abuse, Social Services or other related type of agencies). Public relations type of meetings for participant recruitment and/or volunteer recruitment.
FY '94 under 121723 total spent was: $403 (Rec. Leader II failed to turn in his mileage for the first half of the year.)

Used by permission of the Alexandria Department of Recreation, Parks and Cultural Activities, Alexandria, VA.

---

## Capital Expenditure Budget

Capital expenditure budget is usually related to long-range planning that spans a three- to five-year period. The capital budget looks at a capital investment to determine whether the expenditure is economically feasible over the lifetime of the asset. As a result of this time period, more expansive "vision" on the part of the manager is required to identify needs. The capital budget can go beyond simply dollars and cents and look at costs and benefits in a broader sense. The general service provided to the community or to the consumer can be considered. Capital expenditures include physical changes such as replacement or expansion of the facility, property, and equipment.

It has been well-established that the health and human service industry is operating in an era of limited resources and increased cost. Thus the capital budget process in this industry will become more critical. In most settings, the agency or organization administrator establishes a ceiling for capital expenses. Therefore, it is important that the therapeutic recreation manager recognize and be prepared to identify capital needs on a priority basis and defend those needs when the capital budget is considered.

In brief, the manager should begin development of the capital budget by conducting a thorough review of all capital equipment and fixtures which are presently in use. Once this process is completed, the manager needs to review goals and objectives of the department for the next several years so as to identify new programs of service which may require new equipment or property. This procedure may also identify programs that will be phased out or will need equipment replaced.

The manager should now be prepared to construct a capital budget. The budget should include a description of each item needed, a statement of whether it is a new or replacement item, and an estimate of the item cost. The manager will need to justify the item and will likely be required to prioritize the entire budget. Depending upon the agency or organization, the names of manufacturers and suppliers, trade-in credits, and estimates of delivery, installation, and maintenance costs may be required.

As a final note, the therapeutic recreation manager should remember that the individuals making the decisions regarding this budget may not be familiar with many of the areas or aspects of therapeutic recreation service. Therefore, it is the manager's responsibility to make the justification, whether orally or in writing and to be very clear about what is needed.

## Program Budgeting

This budget focuses on specific programs to meet specific goals and objectives. It is a means for providing a systematic method for allocating resources in ways most effective to meeting specific goals. The program may be an existing one that the department is considering expanding, contracting, or adding. While most budgets focus on department revenues and cost, program budgets compare revenues and expenses for an entire program over its lifetime. In doing this, the program budgeting method identifies costs and benefits of different programs aimed at the same purpose or of different approaches to one program. By emphasizing goals and programs, program budgeting overcomes the common weakness of many budgets that are tied to a time-frame. Also, it does away with the line-item approach to budgeting. In other words, a program budget is constructed by regrouping all line-item expenditures into their respective program area. For example, the line items of personnel and/or utilities would be regrouped according to some rational formula of direct and indirect cost factors to reflect the various programs that these resources support.

## Zero-Based Budgeting

Zero-based budgeting (ZBB) is designed to require even more justification than is found in an operating or capital expenditure budget. With ZBB no service or program is taken for granted. This approach is based on the idea that no expense should be assumed to be absolutely necessary. The goal of ZBB is to reorient the manager's thinking and to reevaluate all programs. For example, just because a program received funds in the past does not mean that the program should again be funded or at least funded at the same level in the future. In theory, at least, ZBB begins with a blank slate every year.

The use of the *decision package* is the core of the ZBB process and is the feature that particularly distinguishes it from the traditional historical budgeting process (Pyhrr, 1973). In brief, a decision package is a description of one or more activities, services, or programs, the cost and justification of the activities, and the ramifications of including or excluding them from the budgets. After decision packages are developed, they are ranked in order of decreasing benefits to the agency or organization. They can be divided into high, medium, and low categories and reviewed in order of rank for funding. Resources are allocated based on the priority of the decision package.

A major advantage to ZBB is that it forces the manager to set priorities and justify resources. Unfortunately, the process is complex and time consuming.

## Flexible Budgeting

In recent years, flexible budgeting or variable budgeting as a managerial tool has been introduced into health and human service organizations. A flexible budget, as opposed to a fixed budget (one which remains the same regardless of the activity level such as a program budget), is defined "as a statement of expected performance that can be adjusted to reflect the effects of operating at different levels of volume" (e.g., number of participants) (Berman, Weeks, and Kukla, 1990, p. 499). In other words, flexible budgeting allows department management to adapt to changes in the volume once the fiscal year has started. From another perspective, a flexible budget is a series of fixed budgets covering a specified range of volume alternatives (Berman, Weeks, and Kukla, 1990). To a large degree, flexible budgeting is limited in application to expense budgets such as therapeutic recreation routine services and therapeutic recreation services provided in community-based leisure service organizations.

A flexible budget takes into account per unit of service costs of personnel, equipment, supplies, and overhead per unit of service and compares that to the actual units of service. Variance results are then compared to a flex standard rather than a budgeted standard. Figure 9.9 (page 134) and the following discussion concerning supplies used in a large therapeutic recreation department for one month are an example of flexible budgeting.

The supply budget illustration is based on 100 consumers with a disability participating in an arts and crafts program over one month. The budgeted expense is $250.

---

**Figure 9.9   Flexible Budgeting**

**Supplies:**

| Actual Expense | Budget Expense | Flex Budget | Variance to Actual |
|:---:|:---:|:---:|:---:|
| $260.00 | $250.00 | $187.50 | $72.50 |

---

The supply cost per consumer (unit of service) is $2.50 ($250 per 100 consumers). However, during this month, instead of 100 consumers, 75 consumers attended. Thus, the expected supply cost (flex budget) would be $187.50 (75 times $2.50). The actual dollars spent were $260. In this example, actual supply costs were $72.50 (negative variance) over what was expected (flex budget). Any variance, positive or negative, needs to be investigated by the therapeutic recreation manager. In this example the manager spent more than $2.50 per consumer.

# Performance Reporting

A good budget can only be effective if it is used as a tool for managing in a person's area of responsibility. This means that the budget must be regularly used to measure the effectiveness of actual performance in comparison to the goals that were established in the budget process.

The therapeutic recreation manager can expect to receive several types of financial accounting reports of the department's operation on a periodic basis from the budget office or the department responsible for monitoring the cost of programs or services within the organization. These reports, which are generated by a computer system and are usually provided monthly, include expenditures, income, and, perhaps, depreciation costs. If the department receives funds through special funds accounts (i.e., grants), a separate report is provided for each account. These reports not only include the current month's performance but also the year-to-date performance. Some reports may include percentage of budget spent by line item or category.

The monthly report will show the actual bimonthly or monthly annual salary and hourly employee expenditures. In relation to hourly employees, it should include the scheduled hours for each employee and an analysis of the hours which were actually paid. It should also identify any hours or days for which the employee was paid but did not work, such as vacation, holidays, illness, education, jury duty, or funeral leave.

This report will also include expenditures for supplies and equipment in comparison to the budget. It is important that a careful review of this information be undertaken for two reasons. The first is to catch possible errors made by the accounting department. For example, expenditures made by other departments may erroneously be charged to one's department. It is important that these errors are spotted and called to the attention of the accounting department. Second, since the report identifies both the budget amount and the amount actually spent for each item or category, any differences between these two figures should be checked.

The results of these financial analyses frequently can be used to support the manager's arguments in favor of needed improvements, more staff, and increased recognition of the contribution of therapeutic recreation to the overall success of the agency or organization. While financial management is time consuming, it often provides persuasive data to support any request for changes in the budgets or management of the division, department, or unit. A budget is only as good as the effective use which one makes of it. The amount of management responsibility the therapeutic recreation manager is willing to assume and the careful use of information and data contribute to how the administration will react to the agency or organization budget as a whole.

# Cutback Management

In a period of economic instability, increasing fund competition and resource scarcity, it is not unusual for program changes and downsizing to be taking place in health and human service organizations. Cutting back or downsizing on the part of the organization involves making hard decisions about who will be let go, what programs or services will be scaled down and/or terminated, and what consumers will be effected. At the same time, quality must be maintained.

There is no easy answer to these problems. If therapeutic recreation managers are requested to present a plan for scaling down programs and practitioners, they must examine the department's mission, recognize programs of limited utility, use rational mechanisms for making choices, encourage the active participation of department practitioners, and retain department openness.

# Summary

Initial consideration was given to a historical overview of the need for financial management in both community-based leisure service agencies and healthcare facilities. As a result of this need, therapeutic recreation managers must be more responsive in the fiscal management of their division or department.

Various revenue sources (appropriations, grants and contracts, contributions, fees and charges, and reimbursement) were discussed. These need to be considered when doing any kind of planning. The budget is a plan for the allocation of resources and, over a specific time period, a control for ensuring that results comply with the plans. There are advantages and disadvantages to budgeting.

It was noted that prior to developing the budget there are several prerequisites that need to be met which include participative approaches to budgeting. While there are many types of budgets, first-line managers are primarily associated with operating or revenue-and-expense budgets and capital expenditure budgets.

Most operating budgets are based upon the previous year's budget and reflect day-to-day operations for the department. They include both revenues and expenses. Examples of items found in these respective budgets were provided. Unlike the operating budget, the capital budget is usually prepared for a longer period of time and incorporates major expenditure items. Another budgeting approach considered was program budgeting which focuses on specific programs to meet goals. Revenues and expenses are budgeted for each program. Another budget tactic used frequently is zero-based budgeting which is based on objectives for the coming year and demands that every expenditure, no matter how basic, be justified. The use of a decision package is the core of zero-base budgeting. Consideration was also given to a fixed budget which is developed on the basis of a single estimate of expected volume.

This chapter concluded with a discussion of the importance of reviewing the budget periodically in association with financial accounting reports and downsizing.

# Discussion Questions

1. Ask permission to photocopy an annual operating budget, regardless of setting, for a therapeutic recreation division, department, or unit. (The budget should not include individual salary figures to protect confidentiality.) Compare the budgeted distribution of available funds to the agency's or organization's goals. Then try to work out a different distribution assuming 20 percent more available funds and 20 percent less available. What effect would the difference in funding have on the quality of the therapeutic recreation service given?

2. Develop a personal operating budget for a period of two weeks including justifications. Compare it with what actually happened.

3. Regardless of setting, critique the value of a day-to-day operating budget with zero-based budgeting for a therapeutic recreation department, division, or unit.

4. If you were a therapeutic recreation manager of a therapeutic recreation department in a rehabilitation unit of a general medical hospital what kind of information would you need concerning income and expenditure? Expand this question to any type of setting.

5. Do you think it is possible for a therapeutic recreation department in a healthcare facility to maintain its commitment to the central mission or purpose when its services are not reimbursable?

6. Review a grant proposal and outline the contents.

7. Compare and contrast a grant proposal or process of government agency with foundation requirements and procedures.

8. Study the directories mentioned in the chapter to ascertain funding preferences and procedures.

9. Visit with a development or fund-raising specialist and discuss strategies for securing external funds.

# References

American Hospital Association. (1983). *Managing under Medicare prospective pricing.* Chicago, IL: The Association.

Anthony, R. N., and Herzlinger, R. E. (1980). *Management control in nonprofit organizations.* Homewood, IL: Richard D. Irwin, Inc.

Bart, C. K. (1988, November). Budgeting gamesmanship. *The Academy of Management Executive,* 285–294.

Berman, H. J., Weeks, L. E., and Kukla, S. F. (1990). *The financial management of hospitals* (7th ed.). Ann Arbor, MI: Health Administration Press.

Connolly, P., and Garbarini, A. (1996). *Healthcare management and recreation therapy: Cost benefits.* Thiells, NY: National Council for Therapeutic Recreation Certification.

Cheek, L. M. (1977). *Zero-base budgeting comes of age.* New York, NY: AMACOM.

Esneault, C., Malkin, M. J., and Sellers, L. (1992). Third-party reimbursement for outpatient therapeutic recreation service. *Annual in Therapeutic Recreation, 3,* 90–95.

Jonas, S. (1992). *An introduction to the U.S. healthcare systems.* New York, NY: Springer Publishing Co.

Kaluzny, A. D., Warner, D. M., Warren, D. G., and Zelman, W. N. (1982). *Management of health services.* Englewood Cliffs, NJ: Prentice Hall.

Kraus, R. G., and Curtis, J. E. (1986). *Creative management in recreation, parks, and leisure services* (4th ed.). St. Louis, MO: Times Mirror/Mosby College Publishing.

Malkin, M. J., and Skalko, T. (1992). Third-party reimbursement survey. *Expanding Horizons in Therapeutic Recreation, 14,* 23–51.

Melton, J. W., and Watason, D. J. A. (Eds.). (1977). *Interdisciplinary dimensions of accounting for social goals and social organizations: A conference of the department of accountancy.* Columbus, OH: Grid, Inc.

National Therapeutic Recreation Society (NTRS). (1996). *Understanding Financing and Reimbursement Issues.* Arlington, VA: National Recreation and Park Association.

O'Morrow, G. S. (1995). *Therapeutic recreation practitioner analysis, 1994.* Arlington, VA: National Recreation and Park Association.

Powell, L. G. (1984). Fiscal management in therapeutic recreation: A perspective on educational preparation. *Therapeutic Recreation Journal, 28:4,* 37–41.

Pyhrr, P. A. (1973). *Zero base budgeting: A practical management tool for evaluating expenses.* New York, NY: John Wiley & Sons.

Reitter, M. S. (1989). Third-party payers: Are we getting our share? In D. M. Compton (Ed.), *Issues in therapeutic recreation: A profession in transition* (pp. 239–256). Champaign, IL: Sagamore Publishing, Inc.

Rosenberg, C. E. (1987). *The care of strangers.* New York, NY: Basic Books, Inc.

Skalko, T. K., and Malkin, M. J. (1991, May/June). ATRA third-party reimbursement survey: Preliminary feedback. *ATRA Newsletter 7:3,* 7–8.

Teaff, J. D., and Van Hyning, T. E. (1988). Third-party reimbursement of therapeutic recreation services within a national sample of United States hospitals. *Therapeutic Recreation Journal, 22:2,* 31–37.

Tillock, T. C. (1981). Cost containment in the healthcare industry. *Aging and Leisure Living, 2,* 5–15.

United Way of America. (1985). *Budgeting, A guide for United Ways and not-for-profit human service organizations.* Alexandria, VA: Author.

West, R. (1995). Management of therapeutic recreation in clinical settings. In M. J. Carter, G. E. Van Andel, and G. M. Robb (Eds.), *Therapeutic Recreation: A Practical Approach* (2nd ed., pp. 157–188). Prospect Heights, IL: Waveland Press, Inc.

# Chapter 10

# Computer and Information Systems

## Introduction

Use of the computer is a relatively recent addition to therapeutic recreation management, although computers have been used in health and human service agencies and organizations for many years. Those who ignore this technologic revolution will be left behind. The computer can organize, analyze, and store various kinds of information in a fast, accurate, and easily retrievable manner. It is a tool that transforms the individual, groups, and organizations that think and interact with each other. It is a tool that the therapeutic recreation manager should master.

In years past it was thought that to be a successful computer user, a knowledge of programming was necessary. A user had to have a solid background in mathematics to work with the computer's "logic." That situation simply is no longer true. Instead, a commitment to learn how computers can enhance productivity is essential. The more a user can learn about how the machine can be used to accomplish more work faster, better, and cheaper, the more value the use will be to the therapeutic recreation department.

In general, the computer systems found in health and human service organizations are designed to support user practices such as work, data, and information. Computers can assist therapeutic recreation managers in the decision-making process relative to two major categories: practice and management information systems. The former category is concerned with all matters associated with the development, implementation, and evaluation of consumer programs and services. The latter focuses on program and staff scheduling, supplies and materials management, financial management, policy and procedure matters, statistical reports, and management reports.

Computerized record systems are a by-product of computers that can improve the usability of consumer information. Data from one source or from a chart, if in a hospital, can be rearranged and made available to various other professionals via the computer network. Computer networking also allows for interdepartmental communication which makes the delivery of therapeutic recreation service more efficient and effective.

The purpose of this chapter is to help the reader become more acquainted with computer applications so that he or she can appreciate the broad range of these applications and use this knowledge to work intelligently with computer experts in planning the computer needs of a therapeutic recreation department. To this end, a brief introduction of basic terms and types of computer hardware and software, including the computer operating system, is provided and followed by a discussion of several computer applications for therapeutic recreation management. This chapter concludes with positive and negative issues associated with computers. A glossary of commonly used computer terms can also be found at the end of this chapter.

# Computer Hardware and Software

## *Hardware*

Computers are devices that accept numerical or alphabetical characters, otherwise known as *data,* process these data in some way, and then record the processed data. Data that have been processed or manipulated is called *information.* Information is stored temporarily in the computer's memory. For permanent storage it is recorded on magnetic tape or disk. The stored information or *database* is used as a source for decision making by the therapeutic recreation manager. Data is processed by the computer at the request of the user.

Hardware comes in two major types. The large *mainframe computer* is the systems controller, and the small *personal computer* (microcomputer) is a self-contained unit that fits on the top of a desk and is capable of running departmental subsystems. In between these two types of computers are minicomputers; however, these are being replaced by powerful microcomputers. Regardless of size, all computers must perform three functions: input (i.e., getting information into the computer), processing (i.e., manipulates information), and output (i.e., display results in some meaningful format) (Borner, 1984).

In large health and human service agencies or organizations, the mainframe computer runs the information systems and may be connected to or interfaced with personal computers in different departments. Communication is achieved by way of the terminals within each division or department using the computer system. The terminals usually resemble a television-type screen (monitor) and a typewriter-like keyboard. It is also possible to be connected with a mainframe computer in a different building or different city through the use of special telephone lines or other equipment. A *modem* is a device that allows one to connect a computer or terminal to a remote computer via telephone lines (Borner, 1984).

Personal computers can be either completely self-contained or connected to larger computers. The components typically include the hard drive, a keyboard, monitor, and a printer. These computers come in a variety of styles, sizes, and program capacities (i.e., word processing, spreadsheets, and file or database management capability). Communication with the personal computer is done by typing in data, and it responds with messages on the screen or prints out information on paper (hard copy). Any work that is on the screen can be stored in the computer's memory bank; however, it is up to the user to decide what information will be used occasionally and should be stored on tapes or disks and what will be used constantly and must be available in the computer's active file (or hard drive) for immediate retrieval. Regardless, if the work is not saved, it can be lost when one leaves (exits) the program or turns off the computer (Long, 1984).

## *Software*

The most important thing to remember about any computer is that, by itself, it is worthless. The computer chips, disks, monitor, and keyboard provide power, but without software they are as useless as a car with no engine. In other words, software is what makes the computer run. It is the intelligence of a system and tells the hardware what to do. The development of "user friendly" software has made the personal computer an extremely valuable tool. Software is described as user friendly if it leads the user through the system (e.g., prompting with questions and providing "menus" of choices) and is easy to operate without extensive training (Long, 1984).

The computer is a machine that uses a very simple language that is quite different from complex written and spoken languages. Communication between the computer and its user is done through intermediaries or translators called programs (*software* in contrast to the equipment or hardware). It is through these programs that one communicates with the computer, telling it what's to be done and receiving the results.

There are many general purpose programs available that can be used to meet therapeutic recreation needs such as spreadsheet programs, word processing programs, database management programs, and graphics programs.

Word processing, for example, is the manipulation of words and special characters to produce a printed document. A word processor can save time for the typist by eliminating the need to retype an entire document if only a few changes need to be made. The typist can also insert a block of text, and the computer will automatically repaginate and reprint the entire document. Only the new or changed paragraphs need to be proofread since the remainder of the text has not changed. Errors can be corrected by simply typing over the error. Thus, the bottle of whiteout may soon become a dinosaur. Last, word processing packages have options for enhancing the quality of the finished document such as various sizes of type, a variety of type fonts, and printing in *italics,* **bold,** and outline form (Christensen and Stearns, 1984). Examples of printed documents include memorandums, letters, policies and procedures, forms, and labels.

File or database management programs are the computer counterpart to the standard file cabinet and its contents. These electronic files are used to store data and are manipulated for information much like paper files. Once a database is created, one can add, update, display, or delete information as well as generate printed reports. For example, a therapeutic recreation manager could have last year's budget retrieved and last year's figures replaced with this year's figures without typing a whole new form (Christensen and Stearns, 1984).

In association with budget development, the manager might want to incorporate a graphic that allows numerical data to be displayed visually as pie charts or bar graphs. The old axiom about a picture worth a thousand words is nearly an understatement when it comes to computer-generated graphics, charts, and diagrams. Present day spreadsheets produce a wide variety of charts and graphics. This is valuable because often the essence of a quantitative analysis is captured more quickly and easily when depicted in the condensed form of a visual display than when presented in tabular form. Therapeutic recreation managers can also use graphics or charts to show progress toward achieving goals, number of participants in activity programs and demographic trends such as an increase in the number of elderly entering a particular program. Some current database programs can interact with spreadsheet programs and even some graphics programs to create charts and graphs.

Other modern word processing programs can be used to check for spelling errors and can suggest alternative word choices if they contain a thesaurus. Most programs also have *Help* messages that can be used to call for assistance if one has difficulty with the program. Some programs can even help one write new programs.

At the present time there are no specialized therapeutic recreation application programs for personal computers. On the other hand, there are application programs appearing in the park and recreation field which are being used in community-based leisure service agencies. Such programs are RecWare Pro[2], and RMS3[3]. Each year the December issue of Parks and Recreation usually provides a computer directory to the different products and services offered to park and recreation professionals and facilities. In addition, there has been a computer use institute during the past several years sponsored by the National Recreation and Park Association (NRPA) and Oglebay Department of Continued Education held at Oglebay Park, Wheeling, West Virginia.

Before one rushes out to get a specific program one should be sure to define the criteria of use. A major consideration among many is flexibility. Other factors incorporate validity, reliability, ease of use, comparability, conformity, performance target, action orientation, sensitivity, and timeliness (Batchelor, 1985).

## Operating Systems

The operating system manages the resources of the computer, such as the storage unit or printer, and provides a special command language for directing the computer to

[2]Sierra Digital, 937 Enterprise Drive, Sacramento, CA 95825.

[3]Programmed for Success, Inc., 503 Vista Bella, Suite 700, Oceanside, CA 92057–7007.

perform useful tasks. It is generally written by the computer's manufacturer and comes with the personal computer. An operating system is usually developed for a specific brand of personal computers; however, some operating systems are universal or generic in that they can run on several brands of computers (Long, 1984).

The operating system controls the input/output functions of the computer. No work involving disk memory files can be done on the personal computer until the operating system is loaded into the computer's memory. Once loaded, this system allows a number of basic tasks to be performed. For example, an operating system can be used to prepare disks for use and to determine what files are located on a specific disk. All of the other software purchased for use with a personal computer must be compatible with the specific operating system or systems for that personal computer (Long, 1984).

If the therapeutic recreation manager is given the opportunity to purchase a personal computer, he or she should try to anticipate the system's application and inquire specifically of vendors about the system's capabilities. Newman (1975) suggests three guidelines to assure that a computer is meeting the needs of the user:

1. The system must be related to the immediate and long-range goals of the user.
2. The system should not constrain the user. It must be flexible enough to allow the user to be creative and not force him or her to think in a restricted manner.
3. The system should allow for upgrades to meet both individual and organization needs as these needs change.

# Electronic Office Communication

How long is required for the messages or articles deposited in the out-basket to make it to the right in-basket? Some managers have relinquished precious documents to the pneumatic tube system only to find out later it was jammed. All managers have played seemingly endless games of telephone tag at one time or another. Electronic office communication systems enable the user to send text of any type electronically. The receiving location can view the information on a video screen or print it. Electronic mail (e-mail) services can transfer messages to sites around the world. Some electronic mail systems also include *electronic calendars* and ticklers (reminders) as substitutes for paper calendars, sequentially dated folders, notes on slips of paper, and the like. More recently, technology has advanced to allow communication through *voice mail*. Instead of using a keyboard for data entry, voice messages are digitized so they can be transmitted and stored by the recipient's voice mail system. Last, there is *facsimile* (or *fax*) equipment for the electronic transmission of copies of documents from one location to another.

# Information Systems

Information systems existed before computers; however, the process was turtle-slow, costly, and far from timely. Today, a computer-based information system (CBIS) has become a necessity in all health and human service organizations and should be an integral part of the therapeutic recreation manager's job.

A system is a set of related components (i.e., inputs, processes, and outputs) that collectively form a unified whole. A CBIS is composed of people, hardware, software, data, and procedures. A CBIS can provide operational efficiency, functional effectiveness, and quality service to customers. Although information systems had their initial beginning in 1951, it was not until the late 1960s that they became commonplace in industry and elsewhere. During the 1960s and 1970s the term management information system (MIS) came into being. The term was used in a very limited way to apply to the set of programs that generated periodic printed reports for the purpose of helping managers with decision making.

An MIS today refers to a system that provides individuals with either data or information related to an organization's operation, e.g., information to assist in program evaluation or to assist in performance and quality control. An MIS supports the managerial activities of managers at different levels within the organization's environment. The characteristics of information needed to support the managerial activities changes with each management level. In fact, these management levels correspond with the management levels discussed in an earlier chapter—top management, middle management, and lower level management. First-level managers are concerned mainly with day-to-day operations. The information they receive and provide is more routine, specific, and incorporates a short time frame. An MIS in practice may exist in a variety of combinations with other CBIS and address transaction processing (data processing) systems (TPS), management reporting systems, decision support systems (DSS), work group support systems, and office information systems (Parker and Case, 1993).

The information systems found in healthcare facilities can be classified into two general categories. They are the administrative information system (AIS) and the clinical information system (CIS). CIS is sometimes called the medical information system (MIS). In a hospital these systems may be subsystems under a hospital information system (HIS). In addition, one may have further subsystems such as a nursing information system (NIS) (Austin, 1988).

The AIS collects and uses data from and for admissions, discharges, and census; facilities utilization and scheduling; accounting; materials handling; payroll; personnel; budgeting; and financial planning. The CIS and MIS, as the titles indicate, are focused on the clinical care and service to consumers and are likely to include information from and for medical records, physicians' orders, clinical laboratory, radiology, EKG and EEG, and pharmacy (Austin, 1988). The therapeutic recreation treatment plan including progress notes would be data found in CIS or MIS. In addition, information generated in either of these systems would be useful in budgeting and financial planning which is found in AIS.

The use of computers or information systems in nonhealthcare facilities has followed the same pattern of use as that in healthcare facilities. The early use was in the development of financial and accounting records. Over time, computerization has facilitated the management of staff as well. Schedules can be developed that will make programming easier. Also, managers have begun to use these systems to track staff and volunteer performance. This has reduced the need for close monitoring. In addition, computers have been used more recently to keep uniform notes on participants thus providing a more reliable record of participation and behavior. Computerization has also assisted in making a base of information for reference, the capability to communicate with other professionals, and access to extensive training packages.

# Application to Therapeutic Recreation Practice and Management

As noted in the beginning of this chapter there are many areas where computers can assist therapeutic recreation functions. Such areas include consumer records, program standards, program and staff scheduling, report writing, budget development, policy and procedure development and change, inventory, announcements, research, and communication with other departments about the consumer, as well as accessing information outside the facility. All of these functions, of course, require that the information be communicated to the computer and that the computer be programmed to sort and categorize the information.

## *Consumer Records*

Most consumer recordkeeping can be computerized. Although the degree to which consumer charting in a health and human service facility is standardized varies from one facility to another, most have uniform procedures by which information about consumers is recorded and stored for later reference. However, to identify those therapeutic recreation charting functions that may readily lend themselves to charting in any particular system, a complete analysis of the various components of therapeutic recreation charting will be needed (Christensen and Stearns, 1984).

The computerized recordkeeping system may be very simple, merely listing categories under which information is classified, or it may be comprehensive and very detailed. In a healthcare facility, the latter would include an entire therapeutic recreation treatment protocol or plan including assessment, goals and objectives, activity interventions, progress notes, and discharge plans. Computerization also allows for the constant monitoring and evaluation of the treatment plan once it is designed and implemented. Moreover, computers allow for more uniformity on monitoring, which provides more reliable observation records.

One advantage of computers relative to consumer records is that the computer becomes an electronic reminder to therapeutic recreation staff of what information should be recorded and where gaps exist. If properly formatted, the information should be retrievable for measures of quality control. Further, accrediting bodies such as the Joint Commission on Accreditation of Healthcare Organizations (JCAHO), the Commission on Accreditation of Rehabilitation Facilities (CARF), and quite possibly state codes and regulations, dictate some of the kinds of information that must be charted. Automating that type of content can be relatively easy (Christensen and Stearns, 1984).

Another advantage of computer recordkeeping is that therapeutic recreation staff can be quickly made aware of changes in the consumer's condition that may require a different intervention plan because information from another department is sent to all care providers. From still another perspective, the consumer record contains valuable information that permits easy periodic reevaluation of the effects of service or treatment on the consumer as well as providing data for therapeutic recreation research. With the increase in outpatient therapeutic recreation service, the computer can provide periodic reminder information to both consumer and practitioner on the need for follow-up review and service. Last, the record can also provide information for the therapeutic recreation manager that meets the data and statistical demands of regulatory agencies (Christensen and Stearns, 1984).

As a final note, securing the confidentiality of consumer and personnel records by carefully locking up the system on diskettes or by constructing a password system is very important.

## Therapeutic Recreation Management

Effective managers must have timely, accurate, and comprehensive information to perform their responsibilities. The application of information systems to therapeutic recreation management is broad and varied depending upon the health and human services setting. Computers are well-suited to store and manipulate the range of data required for planning, budgeting, decision making, monitoring and scheduling of staff and facilities, purchasing, and materials management. An MIS or AIS applied to operational planning is a case in point since such planning is a typical function of first-line managers. Either system can effectively generate periodic preplanning reports as well as process data to assist in accounting and clerical functions.

Budget development and revision is another case in point. If one has ever produced a budget by hand, he or she knows that changing just one figure means that many other figures must be changed. This frequently leads to errors in calculation that can be prevented by automatic recalculation done within a computer program called an *electronic spreadsheet*. A spreadsheet manipulates numbers much as word processing packages manipulate words. The program cannot make budgeting decisions, but it can assist in evaluating alternatives and in keeping individual figures and totals accurate as one tries out various budgetary allocations. Electronic spreadsheet programs can also format the completed budget for presentation.

The advantages as provided by fiscal resource application relate to the speed with which the computer is able to organize, summarize, and retrieve stored data. The information generated can be used to monitor past performance or to predict future performance. Accumulated data can be analyzed for the development of trends that can be extrapolated to project future expenditures. Necessary reallocations and budgetary adjustment can then be made on the basis of these projections. In an era of demand for accountability and cost containment (while still providing quality service), health and human services are acutely aware of the importance of sound financial planning and management.

Efficient utilization of staff and facilities is a *sine qua non* of effective management. While there will always be some decisions that call for the judgment of the therapeutic recreation manager at any particular moment, most of the work of preparing a weekly or monthly program and staffing schedule can be computerized. Over the years, managers have invested an incredible amount of time in developing programming and staffing schedules. Instead of getting easier with experience, manual scheduling has become increasingly difficult as more variables must be addressed by the therapeutic recreation manager. Alterations made necessary by a change in the consumer's condition, demands for specific services, professional development for staff, or by last minute emergencies (e.g., contingency plan) are easily made on the computer. Managers are also able to plan program and staff schedules in advance with considerable time savings. Staff are informed well-ahead of time, and the computer is generally more able to meet their individual needs for time. All of these factors result in improved financial planning and permit the therapeutic recreation manager to plan and allocate resources better.

Over the last decade or so, quality service has become a major concern regardless of setting with its focus on specific standards of practice and immediate quality for the consumer. Of special note has been the concept of quality assurance (QA) and continuous quality improvement (CQI), and most recently, improving organizational performance (IOP). These sophisticated programs have been implemented in response to increased consumer awareness regarding healthcare, more stringent accreditation guidelines, and rising healthcare industry costs. When one considers the wealth of data that is involved in developing standards to meet the guidelines of these programs and their periodical review to ensure they are consistent with standards, the role of computers becomes readily apparent.

Chapter 11 will consider decision making in depth. However, it is well to note here that gathering data, whether internal or external to make a decision, developing decision criteria or standards that will be used to compare data solutions, establishing goals and objectives, deciding how to allocate resources, and developing a variety of solutions to a problem are all possible through a computerized information system.

Computers aid more effective management of materials and physical facilities. Examples include inventory control, monitoring and scheduling of preventive maintenance, and purchasing of supplies and equipment. Requisitions can be entered into the computer and matched against budgetary authorization for financial control.

Another application of computer-based information is in the area of staff training and education (see Chapter 17). Staff development and continuous learning are a major responsibility of the therapeutic recreation manager. The manager, for example, might want to use an old treatment plan as a training exercise in assessment with a new staff member or with old staff members if assessment procedures have changed. In addition, educational software consisting of programs designed to teach a skill, such as improvement in analytic abilities, or cover a specific body of knowledge or any aspects of administration are becoming more readily available. Computers can also be used with consumers in leisure education and can store and provide a list of leisure resources.

In freestanding independent community-based leisure service centers for the disabled a personnel information system can be important in assisting the therapeutic recreation manager. There are several important functions such a system can perform, including:

1. maintaining and updating the practitioners permanent records file;
2. retrieving information from this file upon demand;

3. producing reports for analyzing personnel problems, such as absenteeism and turnover;
4. maintaining an inventory of special skills and certification of practitioners; and
5. providing information on practitioner productivity and quality service.

A modification of this system can be used to produce similar information to be used within a therapeutic recreation department of healthcare facilities or community-based leisure service organizations if the department maintains its own staff records.

Last, the prediction of future trends will become an important concern of therapeutic recreation managers working in both healthcare facilities and community-based leisure service agencies. In hospitals for example, as a result of hospital mergers, therapeutic recreation managers may stay in the corporate hospital and direct the activities of practitioners in the multihospital system. In the community-based department of parks and recreation, therapeutic recreation managers will increasingly be asked to forecast the effects of the Americans with Disabilities Act (ADA) on the availability and demand for recreation and leisure services. Linkages from one agency to another will allow for communication about programming and where various programs exist. Consumers will be able to shop for leisure activities with the help of the latest consumer guide available on personal computers (PC) networks for access at home.

In summary, the use of personal computers in therapeutic recreation management is still in its infancy to a large degree. However, computers are beginning to establish themselves as useful in areas such as program development, staffing, scheduling, and operational budgeting. File management systems can be used effectively to monitor a variety of systems.

# Positive and Negative Aspects of Computerization

A number of issues have been raised about using computers. After conducting a thorough needs assessment for a computer, introducing the computer system into the therapeutic recreation division or department, regardless of setting, may cause some problems. First-line managers and practitioners need to be aware of and participate actively in the selection, implementation, and evaluation of computers into their department. The manager must be cognizant of the changes in procedures and functions that will result and must develop management approaches that will promote therapeutic recreation user acceptance.

Therapeutic recreation acceptance of the computerization can be facilitated by preparing practitioners for automation and soliciting their participation in the implementation process. Successful implementation can be facilitated by anticipating the potential reactions of practitioners. One strategy to ease into change is to focus on the rewards of the computer. When rewards are perceived to outnumber drawbacks, acceptance will usually occur. Another strategy is to involve practitioners concerned with and affected by the change in the change process. As noted by Youker (1983, p. 39): "Participation increases the potential intrinsic rewards and results in ownership and commitment." True participation means that the practitioners can influence the direction of the installation, and the manager must be prepared to respond to the concerns of the practitioners.

Naturally there is no success in computerization if an education and training program does not exist or is poorly managed. A consultation service is needed to provide ongoing user support. This may be provided through a hotline service, library, newsletters and bulletins, technology and research reports, individual consultation, and networking. In brief, consideration must be given to the needs of the department as a whole, concerning the consumers' rights of privacy and security, and the needs of those learning how to use the computer for the first time.

## Positive Benefits

A major advantage of computers is that both therapeutic recreation managers and practitioners will spend less time being clerks and more time being professionals. The practitioner's and manager's job will change as a result of computerization. For example, the manager will not need to spend as much time on program scheduling or deciphering illegible handwriting; hence he or she will have more time and energy for improving the efficiency and effectiveness of the department relative to quality service and better in-service training programs (Christensen and Stearns, 1984).

Computer systems, including the personal computer, have total and instant data and, for all practical purposes, unlimited capacity to store it. Moreover, they are accurate, reliable, and provide speedy delivery of information that cannot be matched by a manual system (Long, 1984).

In addition to those already mentioned, the following items can evolve from a computer system:

1. clear, concise consumer program and treatment plans including evaluation if input properly;
2. development of self-learning modules for training and educational purposes that are extremely useful to staff; and
3. automatic storing and printing of management data from disk to paper (e.g., budget planning, and policy and procedure manual).

Tonges and Lawrenz (1995) note that all indications point to a great potential in the use of information technology to improve the delivery of hospital services. Multimedia charts, for example, will enable therapists to observe a consumer's gait and listen to his or her speech, rather than just read another's description. Electronic medical records will streamline the collection and analysis of clinical information for quality improvement, and extensive paper trails will give way to paperless reviews (Wasden, 1991). Improved computerization will lead to improving the efficiency of communication among different professions (Trends, 1993).

## Negatives

### Depersonalization

Is it depersonalizing to talk with a computer about one's personal problems or to type one's leisure interest into a computer terminal instead of telling it to a social worker or therapeutic recreation practitioner? Is it less depersonalizing to talk with a practitioner who is typing information into a personal computer? These two questions and many others not associated with the consumer are concerned with the computer's possible dehumanizing effects. On the other hand, the computer cannot be surprised, shocked, or embarrassed by personal revelations. It lacks feelings, and this may be an advantage in some instances. In other instances, however, this is a characteristic to be avoided. Regardless, many programs now use bright colors and animated graphics to make computing more personal (Christensen and Stearns, 1984).

### Privacy and Security

It is easy to imagine the scenario in which a consumer's right to privacy as well as personal data on practitioners are violated when records are computerized. A break in consumer confidentiality can be a catastrophe, not only for the consumer, but also for the therapeutic recreation manager, the department, and quite possibly for the organization. It also can create an environment where general confidence in the system plummets. In many large healthcare facilities with comprehensive computer systems, terminals are distributed throughout the facility or personal computers are left unattended so there is easy access for most employees as well as curious volunteers. In addition, the system can be vulnerable to hackers who break into the system in order to scramble data. Consumer data is also threatened by systems that "go down," viruses, and even "acts of God." In reality, such a violation of privacy is possible with written charts as well.

Computerized records can be safeguarded to some extent through the use of identification numbers and passwords. These numbers indicate a person's status in the facility and determine the information to which that person may have access. In other words, it is possible to allow access to only certain specified parts of a record on a need-to-know basis (Christensen and Stearns, 1984). Other threats to data integrity noted by Immel (1984) are error and omission of information by employees, purposeful mistakes by disgruntled employees, dishonest employees, and natural disaster.

### Overdependence

Can one become too dependent on the computer? Will computers be responsible for one's loss of manual skills or, for example, one's not being able to remember what an assessment should include without referring to a screen? Does one assume that the computer is always right and that one's mental calculations are wrong even when the computer produces questionable results? Overdependence on the computer and its capability can cause serious problems in the workplace. Disruptions in work flow can occur when the central computer or personal computer is down (i.e., temporarily out of service). Tapes or disks can be damaged or inadvertently erased and the data irretrievably lost unless backup copies were made. A backup system is essential and should be automatic rather than dependent on human intervention. The existence of alternate methods for any essential operation should be planned in advance (Long, 1984).

A much more subtle problem is the assumption that when there is a discrepancy between expected outcome and the computer's output, the computer must be right. This is a dangerous assumption. The well-known *garbage in, garbage out* (GIGO) maxim about computers is true and explains one reason why output from a computer can be as wrong as it appears to be. In other words, if one puts garbage (erroneous data) in, the results one gets will also be garbage (erroneous results). Computers do not get bored or distracted as humans do. Errors are rarely the fault of the computer system. Most errors can be traced to a mistake in program logic or erroneous data. In other words, computer errors result from human errors (Gray and Smeltzer, 1989).

A final negative to consider is the perceived complexity of computers. The key word is *perceived*, because computers have become extremely easy to use over the past few years. This fear is so widespread that a term has been coined for it: *technophobia*. However, this fear should change soon as more people are taught to use them at an earlier age. One indication that efforts are being made to overcome technophobia is that most computer companies are now advertising their machines as user friendly (Gray and Smeltzer, 1989).

## Summary

The intent of this chapter was to provide an overview of computer application to therapeutic recreation. In doing so, initial consideration was given to both hardware (equipment) and software (programs) of a computer system and its operation. A brief introduction to computer-based information systems was provided. The application of information systems to therapeutic recreation practice and management in areas such as consumer records, charting treatment plans, monitoring, recordkeeping, budget development and revision, and education were highlighted. Important issues in computerization that focus on dependency, maintenance of privacy, avoiding depersonalization, and the overall benefits of the computer were discussed.

## Discussion Questions

1. Speculate on how you might use a computer as a first-line therapeutic recreation manager in either a community-based leisure service agency or a healthcare facility.
2. Visit a community-based leisure service agency that is using a computer within its therapeutic recreation division and a therapeutic recreation department or unit in a healthcare facility that is using a computer and compare likes and differences in their functions or operations.
3. Can you add one new concept to the information system of the future that will benefit the therapeutic recreation manager? Try to be futuristic and creative in your response!
4. What reasons can you offer that information systems assist in operational planning. Do not use those reasons noted in this chapter.
5. How does an information system assist the contingency theory of management?
6. Prepare a list of desirable information system qualities.
7. Discuss the application of computers to a therapeutic recreation protocol or treatment plan.
8. How can computers assist the therapeutic recreation manager in achieving more efficient management operations?

# Glossary of Commonly Used Computer Terms

**ABEND:** abnormal end of task.

**Algorithm:** a prescribed set of rules for the solution of a problem in a finite number of steps.

**Bar Code Reader:** an optical scanning unit that can read documents encoded in a special bar code; a laser scanner.

**Bit:** the smallest unit of data, a binary digit of 0 or 1.

**Buffer:** intermediate storage that is used in input/output operations to temporarily hold information.

**Bug:** a mistake or error in a computer program.

**Byte:** a set of eight adjoining bits thought of as a unit.

**Canned Program:** a program that has been written in advance to meet the needs of a group of users.

**Cathode-Ray Tube or Cathode-Ray Terminal (CRT):** the computer monitor or input station.

**CD-ROM Drive:** a piece of hardware that reads data files stored on a compact disk.

**Central Processing Unit (CPU):** the part of the computer that contains the circuits that calculate and perform logic decisions based on a set of instructions.

**Command:** an instruction from the user for the system to perform a certain function.

**Compact Disk:** a type of disk storage that uses magnetic optical recording and lasers.

**Data:** representation of information in a form suitable for processing.

**Database:** an electronic storage structure similar to a file.

**Debugging:** testing a program and changing it to get rid of bugs or faults.

**Disk Drive:** a piece of hardware that transmits information from a disk into the computer.

**Disk Storage:** a storage device that uses magnetic recording on flat rotating disks.

**DOS:** disk operating system.

**Downtime:** the elapsed time when a computer is not operating, which may be scheduled for maintenance reasons or unscheduled because of machine or program problems.

**Field:** a unit of information within a record.

**File:** an electronic storage structure for related records.

**Floppy Disk:** a flat, flexible, plastic disk that is magnetically coated for recording information for permanent storage.

**Gigabyte:** 1,024 megabytes.

**Hard Copy:** printed computer output such as reports, listings, and documents.

**Hard Drive:** a large-capacity data storage device.

**Hardware:** the physical computer equipment.

**Input/Output (I/O):** the transfer of data between an external source and internal storage.

**Interactive:** a program that carries on a conversation, whether by voice or screen prompt, with the individual who is entering information.

**Interface:** the point at which independent systems or computers interact.

**Internet:** a system of interconnected networks of information.

**Keyfield:** a field within a record that makes that record unique with respect to other records in a file.

**Kilobyte:** 1,024 bytes or characters.

**Load:** transferring a program from tape or disk where it is stored into the temporary memory (RAM) of the computer to be readily used.

**Mainframe Computer:** a large computer capable of being used and interacted with by hundreds of users seemingly simultaneously.

**Management Information Systems (MIS):** a system designed to manipulate information to assist in management decision making.

**Megabyte (MB):** a unit of measurement equal to 1,024 kilobytes used to measure the storage capacity of hard drives and disks.

**Microcomputer:** a small, desktop computer built around a microprocessor.

**Minicomputer:** a medium-sized computer smaller than a mainframe but larger than a microcomputer.

**Modem:** a device that converts computer signals into signals for transmission over a telephone line.

**Number Crunching:** the process of taking huge quantities of numbers and performing mathematical functions on them.

**On-Line Processing:** a form of input processing where information is added and updated at that time.

**Operating System:** an organized collection of techniques and procedures combined into programs that direct a computer's operation.

**Optical Disk:** same as a compact disk.

**Printer:** a terminal that produces hard copy or printed output.

**Printout:** the hard copy of computer output.

**Program:** a set of computer instructions directing the computer to perform some operation.

**Random Access:** a storage technique whereby a record can be addressed and accessed directly at its location in the file.

**Record:** a group of related fields of information treated as a unit.

**Scanner:** a device that optically reads a two- or three-dimensional image and converts it into digital form.

**Sequential Access:** a storage technique whereby a record can only be addressed and accessed after all those before it have been.

**Software:** a program or set of programs written to tell the computer hardware how to do something.

**Spreadsheet:** a specialized type of software for manipulation of numbers.

**Table:** a collection of data in a form suitable for ready reference.

**User Friendly:** software made easier to use because of menus and help facilities.

**Window:** the section of a spreadsheet or word processing text that is displayed on the screen at any one time.

**Word Processing:** the manipulation of words within documents by a computer.

**Word Processor:** a specialized type of software for manipulation of printed material.

**Worldwide Web (WWW):** a system of interconnected networks of information.

# References

Austin, C. J. (1988). *Information systems for health services administration* (3rd ed.). Ann Arbor, MI: Health Administration Press.

Batchelor, G. (1985). Computerized nursing systems: A look at the marketplace. *Computers in Health Care, 6,* 55–58.

Borner, E. B. (1984, May). What every manager should know about computers. *Supervisory Management, 13:5,* 16–23.

Christensen, W. W., and Stearns, E. I. (1984). *Microcomputers in healthcare management.* Rockville, MA: Aspen Systems Corporation.

Gray, E. R., and Smeltzer, L. R. (1989). *Management: The competitive edge.* New York, NY: Macmillan Publishing Co.

Immel, A. (1984). Data security. *Popular Computing, 3:7,* 65–68.

Long, L. (1984). *Introduction to computers and information processing.* Englewood Cliffs, NJ: Prentice Hall.

Newman, W. H. (1975). *Constructive control: Design and use of control systems.* Englewood Cliffs, NJ: Prentice Hall.

Parker, C., and Case, T. (1993). *Management information systems* (2nd ed.). Watsonville, CA: McGraw-Hill.

Tonges, M. C., and Lawrenz, E. (1995). Reengineering: The work redesign-technology link. In S. S. Blancett and D. L. Flarey (Eds.), *Reengineering Nursing and Healthcare.* Gaithersburg, MD: Aspen Publishers, Inc.

Trends. (1992). *Hospitals, 66:13,* 5.

Wasden, D. (1991). Quality assessment: From paper shuffle to paperless review. *Comp Health Care, 12:9,* 29–30, 32.

Youker, R. (1983). Implementing change in organization. *Project Management Quarterly, 6,* 55–58.

# Chapter 11

# Decision Making, Problem Solving and Conflict Management

## Introduction

Decisions, choices, problems, conflicts—therapeutic recreation managers, just as everyone else, face these on a daily basis every day. To function successfully the therapeutic recreation manager must demonstrate consistent decision-making, problem-solving, and conflict management skills. In this chapter the most basic of the decision-making and problem-solving processes along with how to manage conflict will be considered.

Before beginning the discussion of decision making and problem solving one major difference between them should be noted. Decision making may or may not involve a problem, and it requires the selection of one choice from several, each of which could be appropriate in certain circumstances. Problem solving, however, involves selecting the one correct solution for a problem.

## Decision Making

Decision making, according to Parker and Case (1993, p. 137), "has been called the essence of management because it is the most basic function that managers are paid to do." Decisions are made in isolation as well as within the context of individuals and groups. As a result, therapeutic recreation managers need to develop decision-making techniques that will enable them to make the right, effective, and successful decisions.

One is reminded that decision making is linked closely to the planning function discussed in Chapter 3; however,

decision making is also part of organizing, directing, and controlling. In fact, decision making is a major component of management regardless of setting. Because organizational and department life is characterized by an environment of competing values, the decision-making requirements in the position of therapeutic recreation manager are complex. The choices that confront managers daily are rarely choices between something that is good and something that is bad. If this were the case, the job of managers would be relatively easy. Although rationality is the goal of managers, many decisions are affected by such nonrational factors as emotion, attitudes, and individual preferences and needs.

### Decision Making Defined

Decision making may be defined as the act of choosing one alternative among a set of alternatives (Griffin, 1990). The essence of decision making is choice. However, the decision-making process is much more than this. For example, the person making a decision must somehow recognize that a decision is necessary and identify a set of feasible alternatives before selecting one. Hence, the decision-making process includes recognizing and defining the nature of a decision situation, identifying alternatives, choosing the "best" alternative, and putting it into practice (Harrison, 1987).

Decision making can be active; that is, a choice is made to do something different. Although this is what comes to mind when most people think of decision making, the definition also encompasses passive decisions. Passive decisions are "deciding not to decide," or maintaining the status quo. When a health and human service agency determines to maintain the size of its staff merely because the decision was never made to expand, a passive decision is made. The decision to do nothing is, in actuality, a decision to keep doing what is being done (Robbins, 1980).

## *Types of Decisions*

Therapeutic recreation managers must make many different types of decisions. In general, however, most decisions fall into one of two categories: programmed and unprogrammed (Huber, 1980). Decisions are programmed to the extent that they are repetitive and routine and to the extent that a definite approach has been worked out for handling them so that they do not have to be treated as new or unusual each time they occur. Given a certain known situation, the manager need only evoke a learned and appropriate response. Consideration of an alternative step in the decision-making process is minimal or nonexistent. In many situations it becomes decision making by precedent; that is, the manager simply does what the manager or others have done in the same situation. Objectives, standards, procedures, rules, and policies all represent examples of programmed decisions (Huber, 1980).

Occasionally, decisions must be made concerning a situation that is relatively unstructured or different. No cut-and-dried solution exists because the matter has either never arisen before—its structure is vague, ambiguous, or complex—or it is so important that it deserves a custom-tailored approach (Huber, 1980).

Unprogrammed decisions usually include the large and dramatic. Managers faced with these situations must treat them as unique by investing blocks of time, energy, and resources into exploring the situation from all perspectives. While top managers are usually involved in unprogrammed decisions, therapeutic recreation managers may very well be involved if the situation focuses on a new facility, legal issues, programs, or budgets.

Clearly, the greater the proportion of programmed knowledge and programmed application used, the simpler the job of the first-line therapeutic recreation manager. However, the manager has a particular responsibility when an unprogrammed situation arises. It is his or her responsibility to chart a course of action, to problem solve, in these circumstances. This does not mean that the manager will make all unprogrammed therapeutic recreation service or activity decisions. Indeed, the wise manager will use his or her best resource people for this purpose. Resource people can include experienced staff practitioners, personnel from other departments, or practitioners from other organizations who have special expertise. While it is not up to the first-line therapeutic recreation manager to make all

decisions, it is clearly the responsibility of the manager to be creative and effective at finding the best resource people for each unprogrammed situation.

An aside to types of decisions as related to programmed knowledge is that it is also the responsibility of the manager to document new approaches and new theories of service as they are tested or used in the environment. Whenever satisfactory results are obtained from a new approach, it is important that the findings be preserved and shared with other therapeutic recreation practitioners. Results obtained in any given situation are shared so they may be tested again. In this way programmed therapeutic recreation knowledge grows and is verified.

## *Decision-Making Conditions*

Just as there are different kinds of decisions, there are also different conditions in which decisions must be made. Managers sometimes have an almost perfect understanding of conditions surrounding a decision, but at other times they have few or no clues about these conditions. Decision theorists have identified three general circumstances that exist for the decision maker: certainty, risk, and uncertainty (Huber, 1980).

### Certainty

In theory, *certainty* means that a manager, when faced with a decision, knows the exact outcome of each alternative that is being considered. In reality, when managers have to make a decision, absolute certainty never exists.

### Risk

A more common decision-making condition is a state of risk. Essentially a *state of risk* implies that the manager knows the probabilities associated with the possible outcomes of the alternative under consideration. The probability may be based on statistical or recorded experience, or on subjective judgment. Subjective probability estimates are the product of the manager's experience and judgment. In decision making under condition of risk the level of risk is moderate. However, the ability to recognize and take a calculated risk is a skill required of all managers.

### Uncertainty

The final condition is *uncertainty*. In this situation, the manager does not know all of the alternatives, the risks associated with each, or the consequences each alternative is likely to have. This condition is the most ambiguous for managers. According to Ayert and De Groot (1984), the key to effective decision making under the condition of uncertainty is to acquire as much relevant information as possible and to approach the situation from a logical and rational perspective. Intuition, judgment, and experience play a major role in this condition as well.

Certainty, risk, and uncertainty may be viewed as a conceptual continuum that helps managers visualize and think about the decisions that face them. Although therapeutic recreation managers face decisions every day, they are more inclined to make decisions that fall between certainty and risk.

## Policies, Procedures, and Rules

While there is a decision-making process, decision making is made easier by policies, procedures, and rules. In fact, these factors are essentially the guidelines of the organization (Robbins, 1995). They are associated with planning, contributing to goals and objectives, budgeting, programming, purpose or mission, and thinking and action in decision making. In many organizations they are considered standing plans since they focus on programmed decision making which was discussed above (Megginson, Mosley, and Pietri, 1986).

First-line managers rarely make polices and procedures. Rather, they interpret and apply them. Department policies and procedures, when initiated, must be within the boundaries and guidelines established by organizational policies and procedures. All policies and procedures should be clearly written; that is, they should be precise and concise. Policies and procedures that are not intelligible are not likely to be followed. They should not only be documented, but also be periodically updated and revised or abandoned if no longer usable or outdated. Policies and procedures are usually found within a policy and procedure manual. A copy of the manual should be in each department of the organization. In some organizations the department may have a separate manual with reference to the organizational manual. To a great degree, the type of manual will be influenced by the sheer number of policies and procedures, and that, in turn, is influenced by the size of the organization.

Even when policies and procedures exist, staff are not always as familiar with them as they should be. To ensure that policies and procedures are followed, orientation and training sessions for old and new employees should be an integral part of employee development. Further, all policies and procedures should be accessible; employees should know where to go to obtain specific information.

Policies and procedures usually develop over time, incrementally, as situations arise where decisions have to be made. These informal policies and procedures usually become a working part of the department. Longtime employees feel there is no need, or they do not have the time, to document what they are doing. However, as departments and organizations grow larger, and as employee turnover becomes more of a factor, documentation of policies and procedures becomes necessary to ensure the continued efficiency and effectiveness of the department.

## Policies

Policies explain how goals will be achieved and serve as guides that define the general course and scope of activities permissible for goal accomplishments. They serve as a basis for decisions and actions, help coordinate plans, control performance, and increase consistency of actions by increasing the probability that different managers will make similar decisions when independently facing similar situations. Megginson, Mosley, and Pietri (1986) define policies as ". . . broad general statements of expected actions that serve as guides to managerial decision making or to supervising the actions of subordinates."

Policies establish the boundaries or limits within which a specified type of decision should be made. Within these boundaries, judgment must be exercised. The degree of discretion permitted varies from policy to policy. Some policies are broad in scope and permit much latitude and at the same time allow various departments to develop supplemental policies. Others are narrow and leave little room for interpretation.

Policies emerge in several ways. As noted above, they may be originated by top management, but they can be generated at the department level. At times, policies may be formulated simultaneously from both directions. Policies are usually prepared through committee action and circulated for comments on potential effect before final approval. Thereafter they are embodied in the organization's policy manual.

The second way policies come about is through appeal. When a manager does not know how to solve a problem, disagrees with a previous decision, or otherwise wants a question reviewed, he or she appeals to a higher authority for a decision. As appeals are taken up the hierarchy and decisions are made, precedents are set which guide future managerial actions. According to Gray and Smeltzer (1989), such action in many instances does not take into consideration its broader implications.

Finally, policies may be externally imposed. In many instances, health and human service organizations must conform to governmental laws, practice standards of professional associations (i.e., practice standards of the American Therapeutic Recreation Association [ATRA] and the National Therapeutic Recreation Society [NTRS] respectively) accreditation standards in healthcare facilities (i.e., Joint Commission on Accreditation of Healthcare Organizations [JCAHO] and Commission on Accreditation of Rehabilitation Facilities [CARF]), and in the foreseeable future, the community-based agency accreditation program of the National Recreation and Park Association (NRPA) and the American Academy for Park and Recreation Administration (AAPRA).

Policies relative to therapeutic recreation are usually associated with delivery of services, personnel, external factors, and, quite possibly, with interdependent and intradependent relationships. Following are several simple guidelines for establishing a therapeutic recreation policy manual:

1. If possible the title of every policy should use the most common terminology (for easy location).
2. A brief description of the policy should be set out at the top of the document so that the reader can rapidly tell if it contains the desired information without having to read the entire procedure.
3. Objectives (purposes) for the policy should be stated. This facilitates periodic manual review. If the policy no longer meets the original objectives, it will be apparent.
4. A code system should be used to enable the reader to find related policy and procedural statements.
5. All policies should be authenticated by date and by either the therapeutic recreation manager or his or her supervisor.

Examples of the tables of contents of therapeutic recreation policies and procedures are found in Figures 11.1 and 11.2. Figure 11.1 is an example of a therapeutic recreation department policy and procedures manual table of contents in a medical rehabilitation unit. The policy and procedures manual table of contents for the Recreation for Special Needs of Alexandria, Virginia, Department of Recreation, Parks, and Cultural Activities is shown in Figure 11.2 (page 152).

## Procedures

Procedures are guides to action or execution. They detail an exact chronological sequence of steps to be taken in performing specific duties. They are used in communication, understanding, standardization, teaching, coordination, and evaluation. Procedures are intradepartmental or interdepartmental and consequently may not affect the entire agency or organization to the extent that policy statements do. They usually become more exacting and numerous in the lower levels of the organization because of the necessity for more careful control while reducing the need for discretion in making a decision. In some instances, procedures provide a means for implementing certain organizational policies.

A procedure manual, like a policy manual, provides a basis for orientation and staff development and is a ready reference for all personnel. The manual should be well-organized with a table of contents, and an index. Each

procedure should be easily replaceable with a revised one. It is important to review and revise the procedure manual periodically.

Megginson, Mosley, and Pietri (1986), note the following advantages of procedures:

1. conserve management effort;
2. facilitate delegation of authority;
3. improve efficiency;
4. standardize activities;
5. increase performance while reducing cost; and
6. assist in evaluation.

Figure 11.3 (page 153) illustrates a combined pet therapy program procedure and infection control policy found in the policy and procedure manual of the therapeutic recreation department at Iowa Methodist Medical Center. The therapeutic recreation procedure associated with behavior management which is found in the table of contents (Figure 11.2, page 152) of the Alexandria Department of Recreation, Parks, and Cultural Activities, Recreation for Special Needs is shown in Figure 11.4 (page 154).

## Rules

Rules are specific statements of what must or must not be done in a given situation. Unlike policies, rules leave no room for discretion. Robbins (1995) notes that rules "are frequently used by managers when they confront a recurring problem because they are simple to follow and ensure consistency" (p. 40).

## The Decision-Making Process

Over the years a large number of decision-making models have been developed. Traditional theory holds that decision making requires a logical thought sequence, commonly called the rational decision-making process. Today recent advances in the field of cognitive science indicate that decisions made based on intuition (if verified on the basis of logic) by experienced managers can also be quite rational. Researchers further suggest that intuition and the rational decision-making process do not have to be a completely independent process; rather, both can be integrated components in an effective decision system (Simon, 1987).

Although intuition can be an important aid to decision making, managers understand the importance of following a logical thought sequence in making decisions according to Gray and Smeltzer (1989). However, it is well to review the research of Herbert A. Simon (1987) regarding how decisions are often made. According to his findings, managers often make decisions by using incomplete and imperfect information that is limited by their values, skills, or habits, and they tend to search only until an alternative that meets some minimum standard of efficiency is identified.

## Figure 11.1 Therapeutic Recreation Department Policies and Procedures Manual Table of Contents in a Medical Rehabilitation Unit

**Table of Contents**

**Therapeutic Recreation**
Introduction
Organizational Chart
Scope of Service
Mission and Philosophy of Therapeutic Recreation
Standards of Practice (see Appendix)
Structure Standards—Therapeutic Recreation Department
Treatment Programs
- Therapeutic Recreation Treatment and Descriptions and Definitions
- Program List

*Policies and Procedures*
- Adaptive Aquatics Footwear
- Aquatics Program
- Day Program Referral
- Discharge Planning
- Employee Health
- Evacuation Procedure—Rehabilitation
- Hazardous Materials
- Infection Control
- In-Service Education
- Isolation Procedures
- Therapeutic Community Outing with Therapist
- Community Outing Goal Sheet
- Medical Direction
- Patient/Staff Incidents
- Pet Therapy
- Plan of Care
- Professional Staff Development
- Referral
- Research Activities
- Safety Precautions
- Short-Term Pass
- Sick Leave
- Supply Requisition
- Team Conference
- Therapeutic Leave of Absence
- Transporting the Patient
- Travel and Other Business Expenses
- Treatment—Acute Care
- Treatment—Outpatient
- Treatment—Rehabilitation Unit
- Therapeutic Recreation Treatment Forms

*Staffing*
- Staffing
- Staffing Patterns
- Therapeutic Recreation Supervisor
- Therapeutic Recreation Staff Therapist
- Therapeutic Recreation Volunteer
- Orientation of New Employees
- Rehab Services Orientation and Skills Review
- Therapeutic Recreation Orientation Checklist
- Manager Clinical Orientation/Skills Checklist
- Staff Orientation Skills Checklist
- Rehab Bus Driver Orientation Checklist
- Dress Code
- Certification

*Documentation*
- Medical Records
- Inpatient—Medical Records
- Day Patient—Medical Records
- Folder
- Therapeutic Recreation Initial Assessment Form
- Leisure Interest Finder
- Initial/Discharge Evaluation
- Weekly Progress Note
- Daily Procedures
- Treatment Record Procedures
- Therapeutic Recreation Treatment Form
- Functional Independence Measure
- Functional Independence Measure Form

*Protocols*
- Cardiac Protocol
- CVA Protocol
- Brain Injury Protocol
- Spinal Cord Injury Protocol
- Chemical Spills Protocol
- Chronic Pain Protocol
- Fall Prevention Protocol
- Hypoglycemia
- Seizure Protocol
- Suicide Protocol
- Wandering Precautions

*Quality Assurance*
- Continuous Quality Improvement (CQI)/Quality Assurance (QA) Plan
- CQI/QA Monitors
- CQI/QA Reporting Form
- Chart Review Audit and Form
- Peer Review Audit and Form
- Postdischarge Evaluation and Form

*Student Education*
- Student Internship/Fieldwork
- Field Placement Guidelines
- Orientation of Students
- Orientation Checklist
- Student Safety Review
- University Contracts

*Appendix*
- American Therapeutic Recreation Association Code of Ethics
- National Therapeutic Recreation Society Statement of Professional Ethics
- American Therapeutic Recreation Association Standards for the Practice of Therapeutic Recreation
- National Therapeutic Recreation Society Standards of Practice for Therapeutic Recreation Services
- National Therapeutic Recreation Society Guidelines for the Administration of Therapeutic Recreation Services
- Abbreviation List

**Figure 11.2  Policy and Procedures Manual Table of Contents for the Recreation for Special Needs**

Used by permission of Recreation for Special Needs of Alexandria, Department of Recreation, Parks, and Cultural Activities, Alexandria, VA.

Why the latter? The decision maker may be unable to weigh and evaluate a number of alternatives at the same time. Also, subjective and personal considerations often intervene in decision situations.

A manager who really wants to approach a decision rationally and logically should try to follow certain steps. It is important to recognize this step format as a thought process, as thinking in a specific directional pattern in order to arrive at a satisfactory solution. However, it is also important to recognize that at times several steps may be going on simultaneously. Nevertheless, this approach should clarify what is meant by *the decision-making process*.

## Problem Identification

The decision-making process begins by determining that a problem exists; that is, there is an unsatisfactory condition. This is frequently expressed as a disparity between what is and what should be. In other words, when a person perceives a discrepancy between what is and what should be, a problem exists, at least in the mind of that person.

Problems arise from many different sources. Internal reports may indicate areas of unsatisfactory performance on the part of the staff. Pressures may be exerted by consumers, regulator organizations, or pressure groups to initiate a new service or improve services. Then too, managers may see the opportunity to emulate a successful program from another agency.

The key to good problem recognition is to define precisely what the problem is. This is easier said than done, however, because it is frequently difficult to distinguish the problem from its symptoms. The therapeutic recreation manager identifies the problem by analyzing the situation completely including the specific objectives to be accomplished by the solution. All too frequently, as noted by Herbert A. Simon (1987, p. 58), "decisions are made and implemented before all the facts have been gathered."

To avoid this the manager should have a questioning attitude. What is the desirable situation? What are the presenting symptoms? What are the discrepancies? Who is involved? When? Where? How? With answers to these questions the therapeutic recreation manager can develop tentative hypotheses and test them against what

## Figure 11.3 Pet Therapy Program Procedure

Iowa Methodist Medical Center
Des Moines, Iowa

Infection Control Policy
Recreation Therapy Department
Pet Therapy Department

DATE OF INITIAL APPROVAL: 06/13/90
DATE OF REVISION/REVIEW: 10/09/91; 09/08/93; 07/12/95

PURPOSE:
To provide guidelines for the human/animal bond program at Iowa Methodist Medical Center.

I.   Animal Resources Used for the Program

   A.  The Animal Rescue League puppies and kittens are selected for their positive behavior qualities and appeal to the target audiences. They have received the proper immunizations and are bathed, brushed and visually inspected before coming to the hospital. This option is used less frequently than other components of the program and is restricted to the Powell II recreation area.
   B.  Family pets—restricted to visiting patient who owns the pet. Arrangements are made for the pet and patient to meet and visit in the Recreation Department on Powell II. Other options are determined after initial screening, possibly a move to Lynn Cutler Park or pet riding around various parts of the hospital if the pet sits on the patient's lap and is well-controlled. A staff therapist is in attendance in the general area of activity. Exception: family pets may be brought into the oncology unit at the discretion of the nursing staff. This option is possible on other nursing units on a case by case basis and should be arranged with the nursing staff and pet therapy coordinators by calling 5902 or 6280.
   C.  Pet owners volunteering with their personal pets—owner and pet are interviewed and pet is screened by Recreation Therapy personnel to determine suitability for the program. Owner must provide proof that pet's immunizations are current. Volunteers are also registered with Iowa Methodist Medical Center volunteer services.
   D.  Special visits (i.e., litters of puppies or kittens)—Patients are brought to the area a few at a time. Special visitations to patient floors are mutually arranged through Recreation Therapy and the nursing staff. (See precautions and special patient concerns sections in this policy.)
   E.  Zoo mobile—zoo animals are brought in by trained Blank Park Zoo staff and volunteers for education programs. They are brought exclusively to the Recreation Therapy department on Powell II. Patients and visitors come to the area a few at a time.

II.  Patient Safety and Infection Control

   A.  Precautions for special patient concerns

      1.  Recreation therapy personnel check with nurses and charts regarding the potential of allergic conditions and possible infection issues.
      2.  Recreation Therapy personnel work closely with nurses to determine other specific concerns which would prevent a patient from being near the animals, i.e., Pediatric Oncology. Animals are always seen in the Blank playroom with the exception of a specific nursing request for animals to visit patient rooms. These situations are closely monitored by nursing and Recreation Therapy personnel.
      3.  Recreation Therapy personnel work closely with nursing in the rehabilitation area regarding the timing of room visits in order to avoid any contact with food or interference with patient procedures.
      4.  In the event that a patient or employee is bitten or scratched by an animal, the area of injury will be cleansed with an approved skin antiseptic and the physician notified.

   B.  Special animal considerations

      1.  Animal excretions are removed and surfaces washed with soap and water by the Recreational Therapy personnel.
      2.  Lynn Cutler Park—animal fecal excretions are gathered in a plastic bag and disposed of in garbage containers.

Used by permission of Iowa Methodist Medical Center of Central Iowa Health System, Des Moines, IA.

---

### Figure 11.4 Behavior Management Procedure

**Behavior Management**

It is essential that there is a well-thought-out plan for behavior management at the onset of the programs. The participants need to know what the rules and limits are, and what is expected of them. This plan should be agreed upon by all staff and must be **consistent** among all staff. The following guidelines are offered to assist staff members in developing a consistent plan of action for behavior management:

1. Have a well-planned program of activities that provides interesting opportunities for involvement and enjoyment. Keeping participants active and busy alleviates behavior problems.
2. Set a good example and always be a positive role model.
3. Request input from the participants when establishing rules.
4. Consequences should be relevant to the inappropriate behavior.
5. Consequences should occur immediately following the inappropriate behavior, so the participant understands the reason he or she is being disciplined.
6. A change of leaders may provide a new outlook on the situation if the leader is unable to redirect participant.
7. If behavior problems persist, notify the Assistant Director. Parents/guardians/teachers may need to be notified to offer input and suggestions for managing disruptive behaviors.

---

Used by permission of Recreation for Special Needs of Alexandria, Department of Recreation, Parks, and Cultural Activities, Alexandria, VA.

---

he or she knows. Progressive elimination of hypotheses that fail to conform to the facts reduces the number of causes to be considered. Feasible hypotheses should be further tested for causal validity. Once the cause or causes of the problem have been identified and available information analyzed, the manager begins to explore possible solutions.

As a final note in problem diagnosis, the managers may need to be aware of limits within which the solution may fall. Normally, problem analysis reveals the conditions that limit solutions. These limits may include budget constraints, agency or organization policy, organizational behavior, the individual characteristics of top managers, and just plain time (Simon, 1987).

## Exploring Alternatives

Once the problem has been identified and the objectives and boundaries of an acceptable solution have been determined, the manager must explore and identify alternative courses of action. If various alternatives are not explored completely, the course of action is limited. Griffin (1990) suggests that it is useful to develop both obvious, standard alternatives and creative, innovative alternatives. However, he cautions that creative solutions run the risk of various kinds of constraints such as legal restrictions, moral and ethical norms, and authority constraints.

Typical sources for initiating alternatives are experience, practices in other agencies and organizations, other managers, and other interested parties. There is no harm in obtaining input from others who are respected in decision making. Rarely can important decisions be made without input from others including those who may be affected by the decision. They may generate or identify other ways of looking at the problem. In addition, soliciting input from others shows respect for others' opinion and fosters open communication.

One may also generate alternatives from professional meetings, review of pertinent literature, continuing education, and correspondence with others. Inductive and deductive reasoning are both appropriate. Last, doing nothing (that is, maintaining the status quo) and postponing the decision to a later date, as noted earlier, are also alternatives (Griffin, 1990).

### Felt Need

It is during this process that creative solutions to problems may be developed. The creative process has steps similar to the problem-solving process, but the emphasis is different. Decision making stresses the choice of a solution, while the creative process emphasizes the uniqueness of the solution. Creativity is a latent quality which is activated when a person becomes motivated by the need for self-expression or by the stimulation of a problem situation. Thus the first phase of the creative process is a felt need. Similarly, when a decision maker is confronted with a problem, the maker starts seeking a solution (Summers and White, 1976).

## Preparation

The second phase of creative problem solving is a work stage known as preparation from which creative ideas emerge. Innovation is partially dependent on the number of options considered. By exploring relationships among potential solutions, one may identify additional solutions. Many decisions are made with little preparation and therefore result in commonplace solutions. Superficial analysis of obvious information does not facilitate creative answers. For example, extensive use of libraries for data collection is helpful. The creative person may take notes on readings, develop them into files with other clippings and ideas, review these materials, and combine the most appropriate aspects of old solutions into new answers (Summers and White, 1976).

## Incubation

Incubation, the third phase, is a period for pondering the solution. Repetition of some thoughts with no new ideas or interpretation is a sign of fatigue and indicates that it is a good time to start the incubation period. Switching one's attention provides a necessary respite, and yet the unconscious mind continues to deal with the problem. A time should be set to reexamine the situation and review the data collected during the preparation phase (Summers and White, 1976).

## Illumination

Illumination is the discovery of a solution. It may come to mind in the middle of the night or during the performance of another task. It is recommended that the idea be written down so the details can be preserved regardless of when the illumination occurs (Summers and White, 1976).

It is rare for an illumination to be ready for adoption. *Verification*, the fifth and final phase of creative decision making, is the period of experimentation when the idea is improved through modification and refinement. The advantages and disadvantages of each alternative must be weighed, resources and constraints have to be evaluated, and potential technical and human problems must be considered. By comparing the advantages and disadvantages of options, the manager can choose the most desirable alternative (Summers and White, 1976).

## Evaluating Alternatives

This step is a continuation of the previous step including the creativity process. Consideration in this step needs to be given to the feasibility of the alternative, its satisfaction, and its consequences (Griffin, 1990).

The first question to ask is whether or not an alternative is feasible. Is it within the realm of probability and practicality? Limited human resources may preclude the initiation of a new program. A manager may want to write down the pros and cons for each alternative and analyze this information to make his or her decision.

When an alternative has passed the test of feasibility, it must next be examined to see how satisfactory it would be. Satisfaction refers to the extent to which the alternative will satisfy the conditions of the decision situation. For example, the therapeutic recreation manager wants to increase programming in the community sector by 50 percent. One alternative is to hire a new practitioner. If closer examination reveals that the employment of the practitioner would only expand programming by 35 percent, it may not be satisfactory. Depending on the circumstances, the manager may go ahead and employ a new practitioner and search for other ways to achieve the remaining 15 percent expansion. Or the manager may simply drop the consideration until another day (Griffin, 1990).

Finally, if the alternative is both feasible and satisfactory, its probable consequences must be assessed. From a practical viewpoint however, one cannot project every possible consequence for every alternative. Still, questions need to be addressed. To what extent will a particular alternative influence or stress other parts of the agency or organization? What will the cost be to implement the alternative? Even when an alternative is both feasible and satisfactory, the consequences might be such that it must be eliminated from further consideration (Griffin, 1990).

## Selecting an Alternative

The next step in the decision-making process is to select an alternative course of action to make a decision. In many situations the decision is obvious from the analysis, although managers should remember that it may be possible to have two or more acceptable alternatives.

Empirical studies indicate that managers' perceptions are colored by their personal values and that their decisions can be influenced by these values, either directly or through their perceptions (Badr, Gray, and Kedia, 1982). Of course, the manager is influenced by many other things such as staff acceptance, morals, cost, and risk of failure.

Before implementation, managers may want to test the soundness of the decision depending upon the situation and solution. Several techniques may be employed. Herbert and Estes (1977) suggest that a person assume the role of "devil's advocate." Another possible method is to project the decision into detailed plans thereby revealing any serious flaws in the prospective course of action. Another answer is to ask others in similar managerial roles to give constructive feedback concerning the potential solution (Newman, 1964). Decisions may also be tested by trying them out on a limited basis such as pilot testing. Last, the manager may want to review and take a second look, just as a second opinion can determine the ultimate success or failure of a solution. The manager should go back to the basics and ask: Will this decision accomplish the stated objectives or answer the needs? Is it workable and efficient? Will it prove effective as a long-term investment? When these questions and others have been answered to the manager's satisfaction, it is time to implement the solution (Griffin, 1990).

Once a decision has been made, the manager should be aware of the natural postdecision reaction called "cognitive dissonance" (Festinger, 1975). Very simply, cognitive dissonance means that once a person makes a decision, he or she is likely to develop second thoughts because of the favorable characteristics of some of the rejected alternatives. Moreover, the manager may talk to others about the positive aspects of the decision. In doing so the manager is attempting to convince himself or herself, as well as others, of the wisdom of the decision.

In general, the more desirable the characteristics of the rejected alternatives and the faster the decision had to be made, the greater the cognitive dissonance (Brehm and Cohen, 1962). Awareness of this natural human tendency should give therapeutic recreation managers greater objectivity in testing and evaluating their choices. Moreover, it should provide the manager with a helpful perspective in discussing with staff the merits of the decisions.

## Implementing the Decision

After a decision has been reached, it needs to be implemented. In some decision situations implementation is easy; in others, it will be difficult. In the change process there are usually two types of resistance: that incurred by the nature of the change, and that incurred by misperceptions of what the change might mean. Some individuals resist change which is usually the result of insecurity, inconvenience, and fear of the unknown. Thus, the manager needs to communicate to appropriate staff in a manner that does not arouse antagonism. The decision and procedures for implementation can be explained in an effort to win cooperation. A major decision requires a plan of action when communicating to staff and implementing the decision. Anticipating most questions helps the manager to explain the changes in ways that will alleviate groundless fears (Griffin, 1990).

The therapeutic recreation manager should not let himself or herself be tricked into making premature and ineffective responses to resistance as it develops. These ineffective responses include self-justification, advice giving ("What I would do if I were you"), premature persuasion ("Later, you'll see it my way"), censoring (meeting opposition with disapproval), and punishing behavior. As will be noted later, there are ways to evaluate decisions.

## Evaluating the Decision

Evaluation, the final step, is a matter of analyzing the positive and negative aspects of a solution that was derived by using a specific thought process. Depending upon the solution being evaluated, suggested methods to use alone or in combination include interviews, individual observations, surveys, quality assurance scales, audits, and various types of questionnaires. The bottom line is evaluating whether or not the alternative chosen has served its original purpose.

Evaluation examines both the objective and subjective result. Was the result the one expected, and was the result desired positive or negative? If the alternative appears not to be working, the manager can identify the second or third choice for adoption. The manager might decide to give it more time to work or begin the decision-making process all over again.

Evaluation can occur in relation to application for future problems, or it can occur in terms of the entire decision-making process incurred for this particular situation. Which steps were performed adequately or inadequately? What did the therapeutic recreation manager learn as a result of the process? Finally, evaluation allows for the identification of serendipitous findings.

## *Group Decision Making*

At present, participative management is receiving considerable attention as a motivator of staff. Decision-making literature notes that, in certain types of situations, it appears decisions made by groups can be superior to those made by individuals. However, a manager must carefully assess the situation or problem and take into consideration all possible consequences as though the decision was being made by the manager alone (Griffin, 1990; Robbins, 1995).

A number of reasons are given to support this theory. First, groups consume more resources so their effectiveness is greater (Rose, 1975). Second, unprogrammed decisions appear to be more effectively made by groups, providing group members have heterogeneous backgrounds and experiences (Harrison, 1975). Errors frequently have a greater impact on unprogrammed decisions; therefore, these decisions can often most benefit from the collective judgment of a group. Last, if the decision is to be major, participation in the process increases the commitment and motivation of those who will carry out the decision (Maier, 1963). Some individuals are more reluctant to fight or undermine a decision which they helped to develop.

For this theory to be facilitated and successful, Lippitt (1978) suggests that attention needs to be given to the following factors:

1. clear definition of the problem;
2. clear understanding as to who has the responsibility for the decision;
3. effective communication within the group for idea production;
4. appropriate size of group for decision making; and
5. means for effective testing of different alternatives relative to the problem.

The manager can promote effective group decision making by rewarding behavior that focuses on and values the uniqueness of each individual's ideas and feelings. Through communication of concern for, and trust in, others' ideas and feelings positive norms are established. When the therapeutic recreation manager engages in promoting conformity to others' ideas and feelings, antagonism or mistrust results, and group development and decision-making ability are hampered. To avoid such problems when involved with a group making a decision in a staff meeting or committee meeting, the therapeutic recreation manager can request a member to record all the ideas as they are expressed. It is often useful to have a blackboard or large pad and easel for recording these ideas so that each member can read them. The manager can then focus on encouraging all members to participate rather than seeking opinions from the same few people. The usefulness of each person's ideas should be stressed rather than the weaknesses. The use of "yes, but" should be avoided as it may foster conformity to the manager's way of thinking at the expense of creative group decision making.

One should also recognize the disadvantages to group participation in decision making. Group decisions may result from social pressures. The subordinate may be influenced by a desire to be accepted by the group or to appease the manager. Hierarchical pressures can lead the subordinate to acquiescence to the manager's desires. Formal status is likely to inhibit interaction when the manager has less expertise than the staff. A competent manager is more likely to possess self-confidence and allow interaction. It is not always easy to determine another's competence, and one cannot expect the level of expertise to match the degree of participation (Langford, 1981).

Group participants change and so do the problems. A minority may rule if an individual or a few people dominate the group. Members may become more interested in winning an argument than in determining the best alternative. Choosing the most acceptable solution may produce consensus which is not necessarily the optimal alternative and may simply foster the status quo (Langford, 1981).

Other disadvantages to group participation in decision making may include the following: every problem situation is not automatically a group issue; some groups are not functioning at a level where they could produce a usable solution; sometimes information about a problem can-

not be shared with the staff, and the manager must make an independent decision; some managers work best when they retain responsibility for all decisions because they are unable to share responsibility with a group; and finally, in a crisis situation, there may not be time for a group to convene and produce a solution, and the manager must do so.

## Forms of Group Decision Making

### Interaction Group

One of the most common and popular forms of group decision making is an interaction group (Griffin, 1990). The format is simple; an existing or a newly designated group is asked to make a decision about something. Existing groups might be department staff or standing committees. Newly designated groups can be ad hoc committees, task forces, or teams. The group members talk among themselves, argue, agree, argue some more, form internal coalitions, and so forth. Finally, a decision is made. While there is value in this type of group such as sparking new ideas and promoting understanding, the disadvantage is that it is open to political pressures.

### Brainstorming

Another popular form of group decision making is brainstorming. Although it is similar to the above form, it is different in that the setting is usually away from the problem area or site. Environment is the key to successful brainstorming and participants must be comfortable within the setting. These brainstorming sessions may be called "retreats" if they last for a number of days. Such a group form takes considerable planning. Time should be structured for the sessions as well as for relaxation and recreation. The major disadvantage with this form is cost and arranging a time that can accommodate everyone. Brainstorming is also a technique used in total quality management (TQM) and continuous quality improvement (CQI). However, time is not spent away from the setting.

### Nominal Group Technique

In some settings and depending upon the situation, the nominal group technique (NGT) might be appropriate. Nominal groups are used most often to generate creative and innovative alternatives or ideas. In the NGT process, the manager presents a problem to a group that usually consists of no more than ten people, and each member silently lists what he or she believes to be the best solution or alternative. After a brief period of time each participant is asked to give his or her idea which is written down on a flip chart or blackboard. This process continues without discussion, except for simple clarification, until all ideas have been recorded. Then an open forum takes place. After each idea is openly discussed, the participants privately rank the various alternatives from least acceptable to the one solution they believe to be the best. The decision idea that receives the highest overall rating is the first choice and is presented as the decision of the group. Unfortunately, the manager may retain the authority to accept or reject the group's decision.

### Delphi Group Method

The final group participative method is the Delphi group method. The basic format is very similar to the NGT process. The major difference is that the group membership is anonymous. Only the manager who has selected the participants knows the group mix. All information gathered about the problem and all of the suggested ideas and solutions proposed by the participants are given in writing to the manager only. Personal feedback is provided by the manager to each member with regard to all written suggestions. All members of the group are made aware of the other responses and reactions being generated. The selection process is handled in a similar fashion as the NGT, but communication remains confidential and identities anonymous. When a final decision is reached, it is presented as a group decision, but participants are not identified. The time factor associated with this form rules out routine, everyday decision use. However, its use with large numbers of participants is extensive.

According to Shaw (1981), the manager who uses any of the more popular participative techniques described above is advised to consider a number of factors which include the quality of the issue and the decision to be made, the time allotted for a solution to be found, the importance of the solution being accepted by those it will affect, the accuracy of the information provided by the manager, the capabilities of the participants, the harmony of the work group, the group's ability to rethink the problem with objectivity if the solution fails, and the manager's willingness to accept the decision the group arrives at and supports.

## Personal Qualities for Effective Decision Making

Are there qualities that differentiate good decision makers from poor ones? Four qualities appear to be important to effective decision making according to Stephen P. Robbins (1980): experience, good judgment, creativity, and quantitative skills. This is not to say that other qualities may not be helpful. For example, computers and MISs are other important tools. However, the therapeutic recreation manager is going to have to become familiar with the decision-making software before the system can be of value. This section will consider the four qualities stated previously. These four appear to be the most critical requirements in decision making.

### Experience

It is intuitively logical to assume that experience increases one's ability to perform a job. Personnel selection traditionally places a premium on an individual's experience especially if the open position is at the management level. Past successes and failures form a basis for future action. Having learned from past mistakes, it is believed that the potential for future mistakes is reduced. Further, it is hoped that the intelligent individual can assess why certain actions in the past succeeded and then attempt to repeat them (Robbins, 1980).

Experience plays an important role in decision making. When confronted with a situation, the manager draws from past experience to solve the problem in a way that has worked previously. Experience leads to the development of specific responses which are demonstrated by habit, without hesitation, in a particular situation. For situations requiring a programmed response, the advantage of experience is obvious (Robbins, 1980).

When a situation requires an unprogrammed response, experience can provide both disadvantages and advantages. A major disadvantage is that the lessons of experience may be entirely unsuited to the new problem which results in a poor decision. However, experience can be a positive force when it provides insight into differing situations. For instance, experience helps the decision maker recognize that a situation requires an unprogrammed rather than programmed response (Robbins, 1980).

### Judgment

Sound judgment is a skill considered by managers to be most important (Davis, Skube, Hellervik, Gebelein, and Sheard, 1992). Judgment is the ability to evaluate information wisely. It is made up of common sense, maturity, ability to reason, and experience. Those who have good judgment demonstrate it by their ability to perceive critical information, weigh its importance, and evaluate it. In a decision-making context, judgment allows one to draw a conclusion based on past experience and the information that is available (Kaplan and Schwartz, 1977).

### Creativity

Why is creativity important in decision making? Why do successful managers need this skill? According to Maier (1970, p. 73) the answer is:

> to formulate adequate problem definition, develop alternatives, enrich possibilities, and imagine consequences. Creativity means a talent for unique combination or unusual association of ideas.

It is not easy to be creative—to see things that others do not see. It is not easy to be in an environment that supports and encourages homogeneity. Maier (1970) notes that creativity should be viewed as an attribute that, to some degree, all people possess. However, certain people have inherent abilities that make them more successful than others in utilizing this potential.

Some organizations influence creativity while others stifle it. Characteristics found associated with stifled creativity include narrowly defined jobs, clearly defined authority relationships, formal sets of rules and procedures, and impersonal relationships. On the other hand, creativity is probably fostered best in a permissive atmosphere where mutual respect prevails and people are encouraged to express their views and ideas even if they are at variance with current policies and practices. A free interchange of ideas with considerable borrowing and adaptation fosters creative ideas (Cummings, 1965).

### Quantitative Skills

Quantitative skills refer to tools used by the manager to make more effective decisions (Robbins, 1980). Some of these tools have been noted in the previous discussion on group decision making, others would include probability theory, decision trees, program evaluation and review technique (PERT), critical path method (CPM), and various simulation, models, and games to name a few (Robbins, 1980). The manager is reminded that by no means can these tools replace sound judgment in the decision-making process.

The need for experience and good judgment appears to permeate the limited research that focuses on the entire decision-making process. When confronted with a unique situation, the manager with extensive experience may seek an old solution to a new problem.

## Pitfalls of Decision Making

Carlisle (cited in Skidmore, 1995, p. 74) suggests numerous restrictions to problem solving, four of which are especially important:

1. people have limited rationality and knowledge;
2. lack of time often prevents intensive analysis;
3. goals sought are generally not maximal; and
4. pressures brought by others are often more significant than the "facts" collected to support each alternative.

Other pitfalls as noted by Simon (1961, p. 79) include procrastination, oversimplification, subjectivity, and complexities of the problem. The latter is associated with Carlisle's number one (see above). In this regard, Simon (1961) comments as follows:

it is impossible for the behavior of a single, isolated individual to reach any high degree of rationality. The number of alternatives he must explore is so great, the information he would need to evaluate them is so vast that even an approximation to objectivity is hard to conceive. (p. 79)

As a final note, the therapeutic recreation manager needs to keep in mind that poor decisions will be made from time to time and will have to be lived with. Even when the best decision-making techniques are used, errors occur because of the complexity of situations. A competent manager realizes no one is perfect, or even nearly so, and that an accepting attitude is paramount in management.

In summary, decision making is defined as the selection of a preferred course of action from two or more alternatives. There are two types of decisions. Those that are standardized or programmed responses and those that are unique responses to situations which are complex. These are called unprogrammed decisions. These two types of decisions are made under varying conditions referred to as certainty, risk, and uncertainty. The decision-making process is made up of six main steps. Group decision making takes on various forms which include interaction groups, brainstorming, nominal group technique, and the Delphi group method. The section closed with consideration given to the four personal qualities that contribute to better decisions coupled with pitfalls in decision making.

## Problem Solving

Problem solving is not the only skill needed by the first-line manager, but it is certainly a primary one. To oversimplify, management is the successful balance of two behaviors: solving problems and achieving goals. As noted at the beginning of this chapter, problem solving involves diagnosing a problem and solving it which may or may not mean deciding on the one correct solution. Managers usually associate problem solving with the conflict that stems from antagonistic interaction among individuals. However, problems can develop from unfinished paperwork, delays and interruptions, complaints from staff and consumers, lost or damaged supplies and equipment, excessive time spent on an activity, and absenteeism or turnover of staff. Simply put, its an obstruction, mental or physical, that presents itself to the individual—some undefined situation that keeps one from moving on. It is important, therefore, that the first-line manager be a resourceful problem solver. The manager must recognize when a problem exists and accept responsibility for its resolution.

## *Problem Solving Defined*

Problem solving can be defined as a process used when a gap is perceived between an existing state and a desired state. Problem solving, like decision making, is a series of steps designed to help one organize available information in order to come up with the best possible solution. It is a deliberate, thoughtful way to deal with an immediate situation that is creating some kind of difficulty for which there is no ready-made solution. Instead of reacting to a problem without thinking it through, problem solvers try to sort out the complexities of the situation first and then bring some thought and organization to their actions to resolve the problem (Golightly, 1981).

## *Problem-Solving Purpose*

Problem solving itself does not supply answers. It is only a process by which one arrives at an answer. Its major usefulness is in providing guidelines or structures when one is faced with a problem. As shown in Table 11.1, problem solving consists of steps that are quite similar to the therapeutic recreation process the reader is already familiar with.

Therapeutic recreation process refers to the use of these steps in relation to the consumer or group, while problem solving refers to any kind of problem, whether it is related to the consumer, coworkers, or disorderliness in the department. In other words, it might be said that problem solving is a generic process that can be applied to any number of problems.

## *Problem-Solving Process*

### Step 1A. Assessment: Collect Data

This first step is critical. The therapeutic recreation manager should insist on knowing all relevant facts. One should list as much information concerning the problem as possible. One may not have all the data needed to complete the process; one can and should seek more as needed as one proceeds. One should not rely on a single source of information in seeking the facts. If data are unreliable or too incomplete to define the problem, more will have to be gathered before proceeding. Sometimes a manager can include gathering more data as one of the selected strategies for resolving the problem. It should be remembered, however, that one is gathering data for a specific purpose and that when one has sufficient information to confirm or delete the hypotheses about the situation, one should proceed to the next step and not continue to gather unnecessary information.

It is important to state the data as objectively as possible, saving interpretation for the next step. One can do this by describing observed behavior instead of one's interpretation of that behavior. The following statements illustrate the difference between interpretative and objective data statements:

> **Interpretative:** The therapeutic recreation manager does not like the way I chart.
>
> **Objective:** The therapeutic recreation manager frowned when reading my chart notes, but said nothing.

It was noted in the previous section that soliciting input from others may be an appropriate approach in decision making. It is also appropriate in problem solving. A manager may involve everyone in every phase or engage different people in each, depending on the problem to be solved and input needed. Options for obtaining input may include one-to-one conversations, group discussions, memos requesting input, and electronic mail discussion.

When interviewing others to gain information for problem solving, open-ended questions and active listening should be used. The manager needs to take care not to judge others' suggestions or to convey, verbally or nonverbally, that he or she disapproves of their ideas. If the manager does not remain open to the information he or she solicits, others will sense that their input is not really important and will stop communicating with the manager

---

**Table 11.1   Comparison of the Problem-Solving and Therapeutic Recreation Process**

| Steps | I | II | III | IV |
|---|---|---|---|---|
| **Problem Solving** | Collect data | Select strategies | Take action | Evaluate |
| **Therapeutic Recreation Process** | Assessment (including problem identification) | Planning (including goal setting, activity, plan, and evaluation criteria) | Implementation | Evaluation |

## Step 1B. Assessment: Define the Problem

Once a reasonably adequate amount of data has been collected, one can begin to analyze it. Is it a problem in its own right, or is it merely a symptom of a problem that is broader in scope? It is important to look especially for patterns in the data as well as for clues to the underlying dynamics of the situation, remembering that there are often multiple rather than single factors at work when a problem arises. Then a summary statement of the situation should be prepared in which the problem is defined as specifically and objectively as possible. This summary should not include the solution to the problem. Jumping to the solution is tempting, especially when urgently needed, but it keeps one from exploring new avenues and selecting the best alternatives. It also prevents one from ensuring that the problem identification is correct before applying a solution.

Sometimes it is not possible to immediately define the problem, but only to come up with several alternative hypotheses. If this occurs, it is necessary to gather more information on each hypothesis before selecting one to follow through in the planning stage.

## Step 2. Plan: Select Strategies

Every alternative solution or appropriate action for any given problem that one can think of should be written down. None of these strategies should be discarded until all the possibilities have been considered. The identification of alternative solutions is a step that is needed to keep the problem solver flexible and open to the potentialities present in each situation. This action is a form of individual brainstorming.

Failure to generate enough alternatives is not the only possible defect at this stage of problem solving. Some situations simply offer an insufficient range of feasible solutions. Thus a lack of alternatives may reflect the environmental circumstances, or it may reflect a lack of creative thought on the part of the manager. The manager must consider the second of these explanations honestly before concluding that the first applies.

An even more complex situation is one in which there are unlimited potential alternatives. In this instance the problem solver must use categorization in order to select a representative but workable number of alternatives for consideration.

After having listed all of the possible actions, strategies should be selected that will be the most appropriate and effective strategies for the situation—select the strategies most likely to work. One's management skills and experience will help one make the decision.

## Step 3. Implementation: Take Action

Now one is ready to act. The manager has selected the strategies that in his or her judgment are most likely to be effective and appropriate for resolving the problem. As a plan is put into action, the verbal or nonverbal responses to it will indicate whether to proceed or to go back and think through the process again.

## Step 4. Evaluation: Evaluate Results

At each step one needs to analyze critically the data being collected, evaluate the responses that are gathered, or both. Thinking about what one is doing and what results one is gathering should be a continuous process so that one can revise one's plan where needed as one goes along. The evaluation can be subjective as well as objective, including not only the measurable results but also any feeling of accomplishment or satisfaction from having resolved the problem successfully. This evaluation should also provide clues for future action. For example, would one proceed the same way next time? Was a better way found?

## *Approaches to Problem Solving*

Individual or group approaches to problem solving vary little from what was discussed in the previous section. For example, long ago Benjamin Franklin described his personal method for solving a problem: list all factors for or against a particular matter, assign weights to each factor, sum these weights for each list, and then see whether the pros or cons weigh more.

Franklin's method bears a great deal of similarity to modern day problem solving. In fact, some research has indicated that people generally use one fundamental, perhaps even innate, approach that does not change easily even after they are taught a different method (Elstein, Shulman, and Sprafka, 1978). One extensive study found that people generate hypotheses early in the problem-solving process and do not wait until all the facts are in before coming up with some solutions. These researchers also found that different people are best at solving different types of problems (Colgrove, 1985). For example, one person may be particularly adept at solving problems with recalcitrant equipment, while another is particularly good at developing creative programs. Along these same lines, Holzemer (1986) has suggested that professions seem to affect how one problem solves; a therapist may focus on different aspects of a solution from those of a physician. As noted earlier people have a tendency to oversimplify or to choose a solution that has worked in the past. This desire for simplicity is strong enough that people will try to make new facts fit old facts in order to avoid having to redefine the problem (Elstein, Shulman, and Sprafka, 1978).

While each step of the problem-solving process can be approached by the individual, input from a group can promote the probability of more complete data collection, creative planning, successful implementation, and evaluation indicating problem resolution. Brightman and Verhoeven (1986, p. 26) state:

> a team of problem solvers has greater potential resources than an individual, can have a higher motivation to complete the job, can force members to examine their own beliefs more carefully, and can develop creative solutions.

The various group techniques outlined and discussed in the previous section for decision making can be applied in group problem solving such as Delphi and nominal group techniques, task forces, and so forth. Quality circles is another form increasingly being used to solve problems.

In summary, the therapeutic recreation process and the problem-solving process are based upon the same progression of events. Problem solving is particularly helpful in bringing a sense of order and manageability to a problem. However, some people have a tendency to try to define the problem quickly or to oversimplify it before they have all the facts.

# Conflict Management

Conflict is inevitable and can be constructive or destructive. It may offer an individual personal gain, provide prestige to the winner, be an incentive for creativity, and serve as a powerful motivator. According to researchers, there seems to be an optimal level of conflict or anxiety necessary for effective functioning (Bach and Goldberg, 1983; Liebler, Levine, and Rothman, 1992). Conflict that is managed instead of avoided, ignored, or suppressed can be used effectively. Winslow and Brownell (1992, p. 60) note the following constructive consequences of conflict:

1. conflict can identify problems and the need for solutions;
2. it can promote change as employees work to resolve their problems;
3. it can bring people together as the group seeks to deal with areas of concern and frustration; and
4. it can stimulate new ideas and creativity.

As a general rule, conflict is neither to be avoided nor stimulated, but managed. The ideal way of handling conflict is to lessen the perceptual differences so that the outcome is fair to everyone involved (Griffin, 1990). If conflict, on the other hand, goes beyond the invigorating stage, it becomes debilitating. Conflict is a warning to the manager

that something is amiss. When conflict is not recognized, it tends to go underground. It then becomes less direct but more destructive and eventually becomes more difficult to confront and resolve. Thus, the therapeutic recreation manager needs to learn the causes and types of conflict and how to manage them so as to minimize stress on staff while maximizing effectiveness.

## *Conflict Definitions*

Conflict is a disagreement between two or more individuals. According to Albanese (1981, p. 458):

> . . . it is a perceived condition that exists between parties (e.g., individuals, groups, departments) in which one or more of the parties perceive (a) goal incompatibility and (b) some opportunity for interfering with the goal accomplishments of others.

Liebler, Levine, and Rothman (1992, p. 230) define it as "basically a state of external and internal tension that results when two or more demands are made on an individual, group, or organization." Given this definition, what then is conflict management? It obviously includes the activities involved in resolving conflict or resolving it to a manageable level.

## *Causes of Conflict*

When people work together in an agency such as a community-based leisure service agency or a complex organization like a hospital, there are numerous causes of conflict. Further, conflict increases with both the number of organizational levels and the number of specialties. Conflict is greater as the degree of association increases and when some parties are dependent on others (Langford, 1981). In addition, conflict has an effect on both the psychological health of persons involved and the efficiency of organization performance. Unhealthy conflict relationships tend to involve feelings of low trust and low respect which in turn are reflected in performance. As a result, the individuals involved are so consumed by plans for counter strategies that little time will be left for fruitful performance (Walton, 1970).

Competition for scarce resources coupled with ambiguous jurisdictions plus the need for consensus contribute to conflict. A manager depends on the allocation of money, personnel, supplies and equipment, and physical facilities or space to accomplish objectives. Inevitably, one department, division, or unit receives fewer resources than another, and this of course, can lead to perceptions of inequity and conflict (Gray and Smeltzer, 1989).

Individuals may have different value systems and different perceptions of a situation. The differences may lead to conflict. For example, top management may perceive information provided by a report from first-line managers as valuable. But the first-line managers may view the time in preparing the report and the report itself as busy work and may in the future resist completing such reports.

Different managerial or personality styles can also result in conflict. For instance, one person's style may be to discuss problems thoroughly before taking action, whereas another prefers immediate action and becomes extremely impatient with lengthy discussions. In such a situation decision-making styles can cause conflict.

Associated with the previous example is conflict from interpersonal dynamics. In other words, the so-called personality clash when two persons distrust each other's motives, dislike one another, or for some other reason simply can't get along. Although standardized policies, rules, and procedures regulate behavior, make relationships more predictable, and decrease the number of arbitrary decisions, they impose added controls over the individual. Men and women who value autonomy are likely to resist such controls (Griffin, 1990).

From a psychoanalytical personal conflict perspective, Liebler, Levine, and Rothman (1992, p. 232) note that "Freud, Jung, and Erikson all agree that unresolved conflicts remain with the person, appearing again and again throughout life in a variety of forms." Likewise, small group conflict can be explained by studying group behavior from various theoretical perspectives (e.g., psychoanalytical, developmental, and systems).

Other conflicts arise from cultural differences, beliefs, language, education, experience, skills, professional values and norms, status, and pay differences. Work may be seen as a means to an end or as satisfying in itself. Change may be seen as progress or as an unfortunate disruption in the present order of things. Coupled with this is change as the result of a merger or "take over of an organization by another organization." Revealing personal feelings may seem natural to some people but inappropriate to others. Some people perceive teamwork as a threat to their professional identity and to the territorial rights of their profession.

Off-the-job problems can bring about on-the-job conflicts. These include marital discord, alcoholism, drug use, financial problems, and mental stress. Clearly, the sources of conflict are endless, and the number of conflicts increase as the number of unresolved differences accumulates.

Richard Mayer (1995, pp. 7–8) in his publication *Conflict Management* makes note of the following predictable factors associated with conflict:

1. When significant conflicts arise, each person involved typically believes he or she knows its cause (usually centered on other person or persons).

2. Actually, the protagonists in a conflict almost never know its cause; their diagnoses are almost always in error. More often than not, the cause they ascribe has little or no bearing on the conflict.

3. Conflicts perceived to be rooted in action and content are in reality often caused by communication failures, particularly in listening.

4. In spite of beliefs to the contrary, deliberate workplace attempts by one person to harm another in any way are extremely rare.

5. The need to be right—a strong drive in most men and women—is, almost invariably, a primary contributor to any conflict.

6. Many conflicts are fed by one's belief in the primacy of rational thinking and a one-to-one correspondence between words (especially written words) and their meanings. One tends not to recognize that everyone interprets reality subjectively and that the meanings of most words are rooted in individual experience. This leads to overreliance on words and insensitivity to nonverbal communication.

7. By the time a conflict has attained the proportions most people are willing to—or feel they have to—deal with, the apparent conflict is actually an accumulation of numerous half-forgotten, relatively minor incidents leading to a blowup over the last straw. Because of this underlying complexity, often coupled with faulty communication patterns, third-party assistance may be required for resolution.

8. Most interpersonal conflicts involve a dance—a series of moves and countermoves by each of the protagonists—with *no one to blame.*

In the final analysis, causes of conflict according to Walton (1970) can be divided into categories: emotional issues and substantive issues.

## Conflict Intervention and Resolution

Conflict resolution begins with preventive measures to reduce the number of conflicts within the division or department, between parties from different departments or units, or between internal and external parties (e.g., a therapeutic recreation university fieldwork supervisor has a conflict with the therapeutic recreation agency supervisor). Even before a conflict arises, a manager can take certain actions to prepare for conflict resolution.

It is especially helpful to create a climate in which individual differences are considered natural and acceptable. Although this does not sound difficult, there are strong pressures for conformity to counteract in establishing this climate. Encouraging open and honest communication, stressing to staff that department goals must take precedence over any individual or group goals, and having clearly defined tasks and areas of responsibility all help to reduce or avoid conflicts. A manager's effort to meet the needs of staff before a conflict arises can help reduce the occurrence of conflicts.

The existence of a conflict within the department or with another department or unit within the same facility should not be interpreted as a symptom of serious malfunction but rather as a sign of a problem that needs to be resolved. It is helpful to maintain a realistically optimistic attitude that the conflict can be resolved. However, it is not unusual for those inexperienced in conflict negotiation to expect unrealistic outcomes. When there are two parties or more with mutually exclusive ideas, attitudes, feelings, or goals, it is extremely difficult, without the commitment and willingness of all concerned, to arrive at an agreeable solution and to meet the needs of both parties.

While one usually attempts to resolve conflict, a moderate level of interpersonal conflict according to Walton (1970) may have the following positive effects:

1. it may increase the motivation and energy available to do tasks required of the situation;
2. it may increase the innovativeness of individuals because of the diversity of the viewpoints and a heightened sense of necessity;
3. each person may develop increased understanding of his own position, because the conflict forces him to articulate his or her views and to bring forth all supportive arguments; and
4. each party may achieve greater awareness of his or her own identity.

Conflict resolution begins with a decision regarding if and when to intervene. The therapeutic recreation manager should make sure the parties know when he or she is likely to intervene. Failure to intervene can allow the conflict to get out of hand, while early intervention may be demotivating to the parties causing them to lose confidence in themselves and reduce risk-taking behavior in the future. On the other hand, some conflicts are so minor, particularly if they are between two people, that intervention is not necessary and may be better handled by the two people. This may provide the positive effects noted above. However, where there is potential for considerable harm to result from the conflict, the therapeutic recreation manager must intervene.

If the manager decides to intervene, he or she must make decisions as to when, where, and how the intervention should take place. Routine problems can be handled in the manager's office, but serious conflicts should take place in a neutral location agreeable to both parties. The time and place should be one where distractions will not interfere and adequate time is available. Since conflict resolution takes time, the manager must be prepared to allow

sufficient time for all parties to explain their points of view and arrive at a mutually agreeable solution. A quick solution often resorted to by inexperienced managers is to impose positional power. This could lead to feelings of elation and eventual complacency on the part of the winner(s) and loss of morale on the part of the loser(s) (Walton, 1970).

Other management techniques besides personal intervention can be used to resolve conflict. Some of these include changing or clarifying goals, developing subordinate goals, appealing to the hierarchy, providing cooling off periods, and establishing liaison persons. The latter approach is effective to reduce conflict between departments or units. It provides a way of units not dealing directly with each other, in effect isolating the conflicting parties from each other (Klein and Ritti, 1984).

## Approaches to Conflict Resolution

Despite everyone's best intentions, conflict is inevitable. There are several widely accepted approaches to the resolution of conflict which are noted here.

### Active Listening

A manager may very well be involved at some time in conflict with a member of his or her staff or with other personnel outside his or her department. Too often, according to Davis, Skube, Hellervik, Gebelein, and Sheard (1992) individuals involved in an argument spent most of their time talking instead of listening. When one person is speaking, the other is busy preparing a rebuttal or thinking of additional ways to support his or her viewpoint rather than listening to what is being said.

In addition, most people immediately judge the statements of others—either to agree or disagree. Frequently, the listener judges a statement from his or her point of view without consideration of the other person's perspective. Thus, true listening is not occurring; people hear what they expect or want to hear, rather than what the speaker intends to communicate.

Both of these behaviors can cause disagreement to escalate into arguments. When neither person stops to listen, there is a good chance that agreement will be delayed or prevented altogether. Moreover, when emotions run high, people may say or do things they later regret. The following are techniques suggested by Davis, Skube, Hellervik, Gebelein, and Sheard (1992) to improve the effectiveness of active listening:

- Listen carefully to what the speaker is saying; giving full attention without thinking about how one intends to respond and without judging the speaker's statements.

- Get the speaker to clarify his or her position by asking open-ended questions starting with phrases such as: Tell me about . . . , Explain . . . , How do you feel about . . . , Describe . . . , and What. . . .
- Periodically paraphrase what the speaker has said to ensure that one understands.
- Determine whether one's interpretations are becoming more accurate as the discussion progresses.
- Avoid interrupting the speaker.

Further consideration of this topic is found in Chapter 14.

## Problem Solving

Problem solving, also known as confrontation or interpersonal problem solving, seeks resolution of disagreement through face-to-face confrontation of the conflicting parties. Confrontation requires a reasonable degree of maturity on the part of the participants, and the manager must structure the situation carefully. Rather than accommodating various points of view, this approach aims at solving the problem. It does not determine who is right, who is wrong, who wins, or who loses. It is also not concerned with power. Conflict stemming from semantic misunderstanding can be quickly and effectively alleviated by this method. But problem solving is inherently weak in resolving more sophisticated conflicts, especially those based on different value systems of individuals or groups (Baker and Morgan, 1986; Robbins, 1980).

## Avoidance

One method of dealing with conflict is to avoid it. The conflict is simply not addressed: "If we don't talk about it, the problem will go away." Avoidance does not offer a permanent way out of resolving conflict, but it is an extremely popular short-run solution. However, if the problem is avoided for a period of time, the conflict situation may be taken to a higher authority. This method has obvious limitations, but it has nonetheless been described as "society's chief instrument for handling conflict" (Baker and Morgan, 1986). Unfortunately, avoidance does nothing except create a stumbling block for the manager who would act.

## Smoothing

Smoothing can be described as the process of playing down differences that exist between individuals or groups while emphasizing common interests. It is a diplomatic way of dealing with conflict. Differences are suppressed in smoothing, and similarities are accentuated. Since most conflict situations have points of commonality between them, smoothing represents a way in which one minimizes differences. In many instances, smoothing strategy will be short lived because strife will emerge in one form or another and must eventually be handled (Baker and Morgan, 1986; Robbins, 1980).

## Compromise

This particular technique makes up a major position if resolution approaches. Compromise is a middle-of-the-road solution. Each party gives up something of value. While there is no clear winner, there is also no clear loser. Compromise has an advantage over restrictive and suppressive methods, since conflicting persons or groups are less likely to feel hostility over the resolution of the problem. In a democratic society compromise is the classic method in which conflicts can be resolved (Baker and Morgan, 1986; Robbins, 1980). From a management perspective according to Hellriegel and Slocum (1986), compromise is a weak resolution method because the process usually fails to reach a solution that will best help the organization achieve its goals. Instead, the compromise solution reached will be the one that the individual(s) will have to live with.

## Authoritative Command

In an agency or organization context probably the most frequently used method for resolving opposing conflicts interacts with the use of formal authority. This kind of behavior uses intellectual and managerial power and strength to affect the actions of others. Organizational values, cooperation, and teamwork are emphasized. While highly successful in the short-term, its major weakness is the same as avoidance (Robbins, 1980). Another weakness is that individuals may comply to the letter regarding responsibilities and fail to use their own initiative and judgment at times when independent action is desirable or necessary.

## Collaborating

This resolution conflict approach focuses on both parties finding a mutually acceptable solution. This method integrates insights from both parties with the commitment through participation to resolve the problem. Unfortunately, this approach may take considerable time and effort. A manager must ask if it is worth it (Baker and Morgan, 1986).

## Altering of the Human Variable

The final technique considers changing the behavior of one or more of the conflicting parties. As one may imagine, this is a difficult method of conflict resolution. Although this approach is slow and can be costly, the results can be substantial (Robbins, 1980).

Other techniques that may be used in conflict resolution include accommodating, cooling off periods, majority rule, negotiating, withdrawal, forcing, and suppression (Baker and Morgan, 1986; Hunger and Stern, 1976).

## *Strategies for Conflict Resolution*

Filley (1975) identifies three ways of dealing with conflict: the win-lose, lose-lose, or win-win strategy. *Win-lose* methods include the use of position power, mental or physical power, failure to respond, majority rule, and railroading a minority position. Win-lose outcomes often occur between groups. A potential negative consequence of this strategy is that frequent losing can lead to the loss of cohesiveness within groups and can diminish the authority of the manager. *Lose-lose* strategies include compromise, bribes for accomplishing disagreeable tasks, arbitration by a neutral third party, and resorting to the use of general rules instead of considering the merits of individual cases. If one uses this strategy neither side wins. Moreover, using a third-party arbitrator can lead to a lose-lose outcome. Since an outsider may want to give something to each side, neither gets what is desired.

In win-lose and lose-lose strategies, the parties often personalize the issues by focusing on each other instead of on the problem. Intent on their personal differences, they avoid the more important matter of how to mutually solve their problem. Solutions are emphasized instead of goals and values. Rather than identifying mutual needs, planning activities for resolution, and solving the problem, each party looks at the issue from his or her own point of view and strives for total victory.

By contrast, *win-win* strategies focus on goals and attempt to meet the needs of both parties. They emphasize consensus and integrative approaches to decision making. The consensus process demands a focus on the problem (instead of on the other), on the collection of facts, on the acceptance of the useful aspects of conflict, and on the avoidance of averaging and self-oriented behavior. Integrative decision-making methods focus on the means of problem solution rather than the ends and are most often useful when the needs of the parties are polarized. Using integrative decision-making methods, the parties jointly identify the value needs of each, conduct an exhaustive search for alternatives that could meet the needs of each, and then select the best alternative. Both methods focus on defeating the problem, not each other.

In bringing this section and chapter to a close, it is well to note that managers need to be realistic in their conflict resolution expectations. When two or more individuals hold mutually exclusive ideas, attitudes, feelings, or goals, it is difficult to arrive at an agreeable solution that meets the needs of everyone without the commitment and willingness of all parties involved. If the reader is interested, he or she may want to read Sun-tzu's (1993) classic text *The Art of War* which is a guide to conflict resolution without battle.

A final consideration affecting conflict as associated with therapeutic recreation managers and practitioners, especially in health-related facilities is the external environment. Since change is less important in stable environments, conflict is more likely to be functional in uncertain and dynamic environments where adaptation to change is more important.

# Summary

This chapter addressed three major issues of concern to therapeutic recreation managers: decision making, problem solving, and conflict management.

Decision making is the process through which choices are made. Managers make two distinct types of decisions: programmed and unprogrammed. Decisions may be made under states of certainty, risk, and uncertainty. Decision making is assisted by policies, procedures, and rules. The rational decision-making process follows a five-step sequence: (1) problem identification, (2) exploring alternatives, (3) evaluating alternatives, (4) selecting an alternative, and (5) implementing the decision. There are also a variety of techniques available to the manager for testing the soundness of a decision. There are two basic criteria to consider in evaluating managerial decisions: (1) the objective quality of the decision, and (2) the acceptance of the decision by those who must implement it.

The problem-solving process is similar in nature to the therapeutic recreation process: collect whatever data are needed and identify the problem, select appropriate strategies for dealing with the problem, take action, and evaluate results. It was noted that many individuals try to identify the problem without gathering all the facts or oversimplify the problem to make it more manageable. Various techniques were suggested for group problem solving.

Conflict was defined as a disagreement between two or more individuals. Conflict management includes those activities which attempt to resolve it. Possible causes of conflict include differences in perception and goals, scarce resources, nature of work activities, and other circumstances. Techniques and strategies for resolving conflicts were suggested. As a final point, it was noted that managers must be realistic in their conflict resolution expectations.

# Discussion Questions

1. Which step in the decision-making process would be the most difficult for a therapeutic recreation manager in a healthcare facility? In a community-based leisure service agency? Why?
2. What are the pros and cons of decisions made by groups such as a committee or task force as compared to decisions by one person or the manager?

3. Under what conditions, either in a healthcare facility or a community-based leisure service agency, would you expect group problem solving to be preferable to individual problem solving, and vice versa? Why?

4. Why do people resist change and what can be done to lessen this resistance?

5. How would conflict in either a healthcare facility, therapeutic recreation department, or a community-based leisure service therapeutic recreation division agency be beneficial to the department.

6. Think of an important decision you have made, such as choosing a university or this major or concentration. How did you make this decision? Write out your response, supplying as much detail as possible. Did you follow a natural decision-making process or use intuition? Was it some combination of the two?

# References

Ayert, R. M., and De Groot, M. H. (1984). The maximization process under uncertainty. In P. D. Larkey and L. S. Sproull (Eds.), *Information processing in organizations* (pp. 47–61). Greenwich, CT: JAI Press, Inc.

Albanese, R. (1981). *Managing: Toward accountability for performance.* Homewood, IL: Irwin.

Bach, G. R., and Goldberg, H. (1983). *Creative aggression: The act of assertive living.* New York, NY: Doubleday Publishing Co.

Badr, H. A., Gray, E. R., and Kedia, B. L. (1982). Personal values & managerial decision making: Evidence from two cultures. *Management International Review, 22*(3), 65–73.

Baker, H. K., and Morgan, P. I. (1986, February). Building a professional image: Handling conflict. *Supervisory Management,* 24–29.

Brehm, J. W., and Cohen, A. R. (1962). *Exploration in cognitive dissonance.* New York, NY: John Wiley & Sons.

Brightman, H. J., and Verhoeven, P. (1986, January–March). Why managerial problem-solving groups fail. *Business,* 24–29.

Colgrove, M. A. (1985). Stimulating creative problem solving: Innovative set. *Psychological Reports, 22,* 1205–11.

Cummings, L. (1965, September). Organizational climates for creativity. *Academy of Management Journal,* 220–227.

Davis, B. L., Skube, C. J., Hellervik, L. W., Gebelein, S. H., and Sheard, J. L. (1992). *Successful manager's handbook.* Minneapolis, MN: Personnel Decisions, Inc.

Elstein, A. S., Shulman, L. S., and Sprafka, S. A. (1978). *Medical problem solving: An analysis of clinical reasoning.* Cambridge, MA: Harvard University Press.

Festinger, L. (1975). *A theory of cognitive dissonance.* Stanford, CA: Stanford University Press.

Filley, A. C. (1975). *Interpersonal conflict resolution.* Glenview, IL: Scott, Foresman and Company.

Golightly, C. K. (1981). *Creative problem solving for health professionals.* Rockville, MD: Aspen Systems Corporation.

Gray, E. R., and Smeltzer, L. R. (1989). *Management: The competitive edge.* New York, NY: Macmillan Publishing Co.

Griffin, R. W. (1990). *Management* (3rd ed.). Boston, MA: Houghton Mifflin Co.

Harrison, E. F. (1987). *The managerial decision-making process* (3rd ed.). Boston, MA: Houghton Mifflin Co.

Harrison, E. F. (1975). *The managerial decision-making process.* Boston, MA: Houghton Mifflin Co.

Hellriegel, D., and Slocum, J. (1986). *Management* (4th ed., pp. 573–574). Reading, PA: Addison-Wesley Publishing Co., Inc.

Herbert, T. T., and Estes, R. W. (1977, October). Improving executive decisions by formalizing dissent: The corporate devil's advocate. *The Academy of Management Review, 2*(4), 662–667.

Holzemer, W. L. (1986). The structure of problem solving in simulation. *Nursing Research, 35,* 231–235.

Huber, G. P. (1980). *Managerial decision making.* Glenview, IL: Scott, Foresman Company.

Hunger, J. D., and Stern, L. W. (1976, December). An assessment of the functionality of the superordinate goal in reducing conflict. *Academy of Management Journal, 19*(4), 591–605.

Kaplan, M. F. and Schwartz, S. (1977). *Human judgment and decision processes in applied settings.* New York, NY: Academic Press, Inc.

Klein, S. M., and Ritti, R. R. (1984). *Understanding organization behavior* (2nd ed.). Boston, MA: Kent Publishing Co.

Langford, T. L. (1981). *Managing and being managed.* Englewood Cliffs, NJ: Appleton & Lange.

Liebler, J. G., Levine, R. E., and Rothman, J. (1992). *Management principles for health professionals* (2nd ed.). Gaithersburg, MD: Aspen Publishers, Inc.

Lippitt. G. L. (1978). Improving decision making with groups. In L. P. Bradford (Ed.), *Group development* (pp. 136–143). LaJolla, CA: University Associates.

Maier, N. R. F. (1970). *Problem solving and creativity.* Belmont, CA: Wadsworth Publishing Co.

Maier, N. R. F. (1963). *Problem-solving discussion and conferences.* New York, NY: John Wiley & Sons.

Mayer, R. J. (1995). *Conflict management.* Columbus, OH: Battelle Press.

Megginson, L. C., Mosley, D. C., and Pietri, P. H., Jr. (1986). *Management: Concepts and applications* (2nd ed.). New York, NY: Harper & Row.

Newman, W. H. (1964). *Administrative action.* Englewood Cliffs, NJ: Prentice Hall.

Parker, C., and Case, T. (1993). *Management information systems* (2nd ed.) Watsonville, CA: McGraw-Hill.

Robbins, S. P. (1995). *Supervision today.* Englewood Cliffs, NJ: Prentice Hall.

Robbins, S. P. (1980). *The administrative process* (2nd ed.). Englewood Cliffs, NJ: Prentice Hall.

Rose, G. L. (1975). Assessing the state of decision making. In J. W. McGuire (Ed.), *Contemporary management.* Englewood Cliffs, NJ: Prentice Hall.

Shaw, M. E. (1981). *Group dynamics—The psychology of small group behavior.* New York, NY: McGraw-Hill.

Simon, H. A. (1987, February). Making management decisions: The role of intuition and emotion. *The Academy of Management Executives,* 57–63.

Simon, H. A. (1961). *Administrative Behavior* (2nd ed.). New York, NY: Macmillan.

Skidmore, R. A. (1995). *Social Work Administration* (3rd ed). Boston, MA: Allyn & Bacon.

Summers, I., and White, D. E. (1976, April). Creativity techniques: Toward improvement of the decision process. *The Academy of Management Executives, 1*(2), 101–111.

Sun-tzu. (1993). *The art of war.* New York, NY: Quill.

Walton, R. E. (1970). *Interpersonal peacemaking: Confrontations and third-party consultation.* Reading, MA: Addison-Wesley Publishing Co., Inc.

Winslow, R., and Brownell, E. (1992). Conflict management. In R. M. Winslow and K. J. Halberg (Eds.), *The management of therapeutic recreation services* (pp. 59–70). Arlington, VA: National Recreation and Park Association.

# Chapter 12
# Marketing

## Introduction

Health and human services are big business. Marketing is a necessary management task of first-line therapeutic recreation managers. Health and human services operate in a competitive, resource-constrained, quality-controlled service environment. Therapeutic recreation managers are challenged to articulate the unique strengths and to create strategies which will ensure that therapeutic recreation services remain integral to the organization's future target markets. Strategic market planning is one avenue to ensure survival of the division or department. This process is similar to the therapeutic recreation process (i.e., assess, plan, implement, evaluate). The intent of this chapter is to explore marketing processes and the exchange relationships established as the first-line manager develops a marketing plan.

Consumers have become "hot commodities" as a result of the growth of alternative health and human service systems aimed at improving the efficiency and effectiveness of services. Marketing in health and human services came to the forefront in the 1980s. Competition was created by service providers who offered quality services to increasingly sophisticated clients. A number of factors have resulted in marketing becoming a significant management function. These forces and the nature of marketing in health and human services are introduced in the first section of this chapter.

Marketing is a dynamic process that involves using strategies in clinical and community therapeutic recreation settings to achieve specific outcomes. Initially, environmental assessments are taken to become aware of influences affecting the internal and external audiences. A marketing plan is designed to facilitate relationship building over an extended time. Marketing strategies are implemented with each target audience or market segment. Last, evaluation is undertaken to ensure quality and service efficacy. This marketing process is presented in the next chapter sections.

Health and human services operate between hard-sell marketing (e.g., automobiles) and soft-sell marketing (e.g., education). Therapeutic recreation managers provide services to enhance consumer well-being while operating at the margin of the market economy. Balancing market factors with client needs can leave therapeutic recreation vulnerable. These managers have traditionally not used marketing strategies. Ethical issues result as managers attempt to secure a fair share of client time and/or programming resources. Closing sections of this chapter examine the trends, issues, and roles of first-line managers as they develop and monitor marketing programs.

## Marketing in Therapeutic Recreation

Therapeutic recreation managers can no longer assume consumers will come to programs and services on their own and/or through referral. As the pressure to reduce healthcare costs mounts, consumers seek alternatives to quality efficient care. This creates incentives, as described by Chilingerian (1992), to reduce unnecessary ancillary services and length of stay. As a consequence, in clinical settings first-line managers scramble to secure reduced amounts of consumer time. In community settings reductions in social service and welfare monies and an influx of transitional client populations have contributed to fewer resources available to serve a greater number of individuals with increasingly complicated health and well-being needs.

Thorn (1984) noted that marketing can enhance therapeutic recreation services especially when healthcare agencies are experiencing increased competition; consumer sophistication and comparative shopping; and, payment systems are significantly different from cost-based reimbursement. In clinical and community settings therapeutic recreation is competing for dollars spent. Consumers are becoming more sophisticated in their ability to differentiate quality performance.

According to Chilingerian (1992) the federal government and corporate America are the two biggest buyers of healthcare services. The federal deficit and slow economic growth have created significant reductions in such reimbursement programs as Medicare. At the state level Medicaid payments have been reduced while eligibility criteria have been constricted. This action results in consumers seeking alternative assistance to meet fundamental needs through community social service agencies.

One trend that is currently impacting reimbursement is the shift toward managed care. Chilingerian (1992) predicts that during the 1990s corporate America is likely to see 60 percent of all employees and their dependents enrolled in managed care plans. In a managed care environment therapeutic recreation practices focus on quality outcomes through interdisciplinary strategies that minimize resource usage. Services are broadly packaged along consumer-related paths. To remain a vital part of the service package, therapeutic recreation managers will be required to articulate their contributions to specific facets of client well-being.

## Marketing Service Relationships

Marketing is a tool a manager uses to benefit the department, consumers, employees, and the profession. As suggested in a professional publication (NTRS, 1994), marketing promotes professional values, gains resources to meet programming needs, and accomplishes department goals.

Marketing is a broad concept that consists of a number of activities designed to identify the needs of consumers and to encourage consumers to establish a long-term relationship with the service provider. As described by Winslow (1992), the intent is to achieve specific outcomes which may include increases in consumers, revenue, programs, service visibility, department recognition, and good public relations with internal and external audiences.

O'Sullivan (1991a) outlines the evolution of marketing that has resulted in the present focus on exchange relationships along service lines. Originally, marketing dealt with manufacturing products or increasing output while reducing costs. Marketing has become a matter of convincing consumers to purchase particular products. With this orientation, marketing became synonymous with sales and advertising. Socioeconomic focus on health and human services during the 1980s caused marketing to emphasize customer needs. The aim of marketing, according to O'Sullivan (1991a), is to investigate and understand consumers in order to design a service specific to their needs. Relationship marketing intends to attract, maintain, and enhance customer relationships through exchange of quality services that satisfy specific health and well-being needs.

The trend toward total quality management (TQM), an outgrowth of socioeconomic demands for efficiency and effectiveness, has given impetus to the service-management-marketing marriage. A service is an intangible output produced at the time of delivery. Barber (1989) suggests that the service is delivered wherever the consumer is and that the value placed on the service depends on the consumer's experience. Three service dimensions are described by Barber (1989). A *fix-it* service dimension helps people deal with deficiencies; *help-me* services focus on skill acquisition; and *value-added* services aim to give the consumer more than is expected. The manager operating in the framework of TQM aims to reduce or eliminate any discrepancies that might exist between customer service expectations and perceptions of the services received. Delene (1992) suggests that an improvement in service design or processes reduces differences between expected and experienced service levels. With improved service levels, satisfaction is enhanced, quality appraisals result, and customers continue to use the service provider.

Marketing cultivates exchange relationships. The focus is on the quality of the experience and the retention of the consumers. Winslow (1992) notes that quality services garner internal and external support. O'Sullivan (1991b) suggests that quality of service will dictate which departments survive the competitive edge. Each service contact adds to or detracts from the user's view of service credibility and satisfaction. Customized services attract and retain users while reducing operational costs. To promote exchange relationships the manager supports those environmental processes that create perceptions of client well-being. The environment in which the experience occurs is as significant to the assessment of quality and return of the consumer as the experience itself.

## *Strategic Market Planning*

Strategic planning and marketing evolved as closely linked processes in the 1980s (Nestor, 1992). The socioeconomic factors that contributed to reduced work forces and resources and increased consumer demands also redirected planning to focus on impacts of change in the service environment. Change has become and will continue to be a factor in the health and human service environment. Crompton (1983) writes that strategic planning is a process that relates all resources to meeting client needs. Strategic planning is the overall direction-setting process, while, according to Nestor (1992), marketing is one strategy that guides service decision making.

Barber (1989) notes that quality service departments are identified by three distinguishing characteristics. First a clearly defined mission targets specific services, audiences, outcomes, and future directions. Second, a customer-friendly environment is founded on resources and processes that meet client needs. Finally, employees exhibit a consistently high level of concern for consumer needs. Crompton (1983) describes strategic market planning as the road map that guides service delivery. A first-line manager is the central figure in designing department management tools such as marketing and staff development plans. Also, the environment in which services are delivered is crafted and monitored by the therapeutic recreation manager. The manager is the active link between a department mission and the service quality that promotes exchange relationships.

# Marketing Process

The marketing process is similar in nature to the therapeutic recreation process. Four major steps organize the manager's tasks: assessment, planning, implementation, and evaluation. Strategic market planning targets specific population segments and attempts to provide services based on preplanned outcomes through the design of a marketing plan. A marketing plan, like a consumer treatment and/or program plan, guides the managers and practitioners in meeting objectives. Crompton (1983) suggests that market plans are developed to guide long-term (e.g., three years) and short-term (e.g., one year) actions toward goal achievement. The design of these plans commences by considering the people who will enter into exchange relationships through service provision to achieve department mission and goals. Assessments of the external and internal audiences, department, and environment are completed prior to design of an action plan. Information from assessments is brought together in order to define the department mission, marketing goals, and action plans with particular target markets. While writing a marketing plan, the manager considers the marketing mix variables and outlines specific

implementation strategies suited to each particular target audience. A marketing plan actually becomes a reality during service implementation. Ultimately, evaluation determines if the selected marketing strategies have been effective in facilitating exchange relationships with specific audiences or market segments.

## *Step 1: Assessment*

Needs assessments identify target markets, service needs of targeted markets, department strengths and weaknesses, and the opportunities and/or threats (e.g., competition) from the service environment. Whose needs should be served by the department?

### Target Marketing

Target marketing involves (1) identifying clients and related consumer groups likely to use and/or benefit from therapeutic recreation services, and (2) determining which particular types of services will be used currently and in the future by various target markets. A number of descriptors characterize the audiences the department is trying to reach. O'Sullivan (1991a) identifies five descriptors of targeted audiences: service needs and interests, geographic location, sociodemographics, behavioral, and synchronographics. Market segments have specific health and leisure needs precipitated by the etiology and manifestations of illness, disability, or trauma. Geographic location considers not only primary place of residence but also distance to service sites, access to and within service sites, and availability of usable transportation. Sociodemographics considers population profiles and available support and resources. For example, specific needs have been associated with particular age groups such as cardiac rehabilitation of older adults and physical rehabilitation of younger people with spinal cord and head injuries. Future marketing strategies might target these age groups through lifestyle management services and preventative strategies.

Market segments are also characterized by behavioral tendencies such as motivation, readiness, lifestyles, skill levels, and value orientations. People who value work may perceive the benefits of therapeutic recreation only as they relate to their ability to return to a productive lifestyle. The degree to which participants are motivated to engage in therapeutic recreation is influenced by their adjustment and acceptance of their functioning abilities. Further, the value placed on health and well-being will influence readiness to respond to prescribed treatments and lifestyle management.

O'Sullivan (1991a) describes the last factor, synchronographics, as those time-related factors affecting user groups. The length of time available to consumers to benefit from therapeutic intervention is decreasing. The time of the year also affects the census in behavioral medicine.

Consideration of the five descriptors helps the manager determine which population segments are likely to be attracted to therapeutic recreation services.

A number of target markets, other than consumers, are primary and/or secondary benefactors of therapeutic recreation services. These audiences directly or indirectly interact with clients. Internal audiences refer to persons within the work environment that interact with the therapeutic recreation department and the client. Primary internal target markets, therefore, include agency professionals, support staff, and committee and board members. External audiences provide resources and support while benefiting from department services. Caregivers, family members, the general public, insurers, managed care providers, policymakers, community health and human service agents, professionals in recreation and therapeutic recreation, and resource providers (e.g., transportation and medical supply vendors) comprise external target segments.

Each of the internal and external audiences has a unique need in relationship to the department. Customized marketing strategies attract and retain appropriate service clientele or target markets. Internal audiences must understand the nature of therapeutic recreation interventions, the standards and relationships of the organization's personnel, and the mission of the organization. External audiences (like internal audiences) need education, information, access to resources, support, and research and evaluation (e.g., efficacy). Proper identification of target markets allows the manager to amass the support and resources essential to develop an environment in which quality services are provided.

## Service Environment

The service environment is examined to help the manager establish the department's position in relationship to existing services, service gaps, and potential service markets. During this environmental scan, the manager becomes familiar with department strengths and weaknesses and the opportunities and threats currently facing the unit and likely to affect the unit. This process allows the manager to make the most of current resources while preparing for the future (Winslow, 1992). The research conducted allows the manager to find and establish a unique role or position upon which a reputation is built and reinforced through marketing. As described by one professional source (NTRS, 1994), this position reflects a unique service offering to which target markets tend to refer and associate. The perceptions people in various target markets have of the department influence whether or not they are attracted to the services provided. Viability of the service is dependent upon an image created through marketing strategies.

An inventory of department resources and marketing strategies currently in use helps the manager become familiar with the assets and liabilities of the department or past and present approaches. The manager must determine if the environment is consumer friendly, the employees are consumer oriented, and the mission is relevant. The tangible and intangible resources of the department are studied as the manager becomes aware of the qualitative aspects of current services and the potential for future service relationships. Past and current marketing processes are evaluated to determine which strategies were effective in attracting and retaining specific service groups in the past. The manager realistically identifies areas where a reputation can be built and gaps where department efforts require changes. Ultimately, mission and vision statements are reviewed and/or revised to reflect current and future service trends and market shifts.

As part of the department analysis, the manager ascertains the status of existing and needed services within the division, department, organization, and/or community. Who else within the organization is providing community reentry, aquatic therapy, or daylong services for career parents with special needs children? The analysis requires the manager to take a close look at census data and projections and services already in place in the geographic region. A manager is familiar with accreditation standards, reimbursement criteria, and legislation that impacts service parameters. Through this process, the manager becomes aware of internal and external audience perceptions, support, and educational needs. Also, trends likely to influence clientele, the profession, and health and human services are identified. From this investigation, the manager becomes aware of forces impacting the department service niche and influences within and outside of managerial control to which the department should be responsive. After a thorough marketing analysis, a manager is better able to capitalize on opportunities and to adjust planning strategies to manage competition, service excess or gaps, and market saturation.

## Marketing Goals and Objectives

Setting marketing goals and objectives provides direction for the department's marketing efforts. These goals and objectives are written for each selected target market after completing the assessments of the environment and target audiences. They guide the design of a marketing plan that is crafted to each target audience's needs. These statements relate to two types of intention. Image goals (NTRS, 1994) describe how service segments might perceive the department in the future. Action goals, on the other hand, present measurable department outcomes. Image goals relate to the changing and evolving nature of services that will attract and retain specific markets. Action goals describe quality indicators that position the department. Goal statements are broad general outcome statements that emphasize what the department will do. Objectives or outcome measures are written for each goal statement and lead toward identification of marketing strategies and action plans with each service segment or target market. An example for an internal audience with specific target segments is presented in Figure 12.1. Image, action goals, and objectives are also listed.

# Therapeutic Recreation Marketing Goals and Objectives

As with specific consumer goals and objectives, priorities are set. Prioritizing goals and objectives helps the manager plan appropriate budget allocations and resource distribution. After establishing marketing goals and objectives, the manager prepares or revises department mission and vision statements. The mission statement describes the current status of the department, and the vision statement projects future services and target markets. These statements are tools the manager uses to balance resources with demands. As described by Crompton (1983), a number of alternatives are available to the manager at any given time. Changes in one particular service affect a number of target audiences. With prioritized goals and objectives, the manager is able to anticipate the impact on present and future plans as adjustments are made to better address various service segments. Dynamic mission and vision statements help the department maintain its market position.

## Step 2: *Plan*

During this step the manager designs services to meet the marketing goals of each target market. Tools used during this stage are expressed in marketing terms as the marketing *Ps:* product, price, place, and promotion. O'Sullivan (1991b) suggests the nature of parks and recreation like other service industries must also consider several additional *Ps* such as physical evidence, people, policies and procedures, public image, and political impact. The manager contemplates each of these variables as planning decisions are made. This helps the department present the right services to the right market segment. As a result of this step service offerings are presented to each target population to accomplish its specific marketing goals and objectives.

## Product

The first *P,* product, is the service line a therapeutic recreation department offers. What unmet needs exist or will exist? For every service there are three levels or dimensions. The core or primary benefit is the fundamental or priority goal of intervention such as improved functioning or understanding of therapeutic recreation services. The second dimension O'Sullivan (1991a) refers to is the tangible aspects of service. Features such as service title, location and explanation of services, and perception of quality define this dimension. A third dimension pertains to the supplemental or additional services that complement the primary services. In therapeutic recreation settings this dimension might include assistance with transportation and the promotional packages available from the professional organizations used during "therapeutic recreation week." Traditional service lines in hospitals and community therapeutic recreation follow departmental lines (e.g., nursing, ancillary, support services). Service marketing uses integrated marketing techniques. As a consequence, services are being marketed along customized population-related segments and themes. The intent is to maintain relationships over time by providing services like referral planning and outreach programs.

A manager considers all of the services offered to each market segment by the department as decisions are made about adding new services, revising current programs,

---

**Figure 12.1 Marketing Goals and Objectives for an Internal Audience**

**Target Market: Agency Professionals**
1. Physicians
2. Administrators

**Goals:**
1. Image: To become the primary conduit for resource and referral planning.
2. Action: To increase the number of referrals and requests for transitional planning and assistance.
3. Objectives: After reviewing materials on therapeutic recreation and life satisfaction, physicians will identify the role assumed by therapeutic recreation in community reentry.
4. Objectives: After reviewing materials on therapeutic recreation efficacy, administrators will initiate contacts with therapeutic recreation staff to plan services for clients to gain skills necessary to community placements and leisure experiences.

and/or terminating existing services. As Crompton (1983) indicates, each service can be targeted to existing or new markets. Crompton (1983) and O'Sullivan (1991a) recommend that managers use a grid or cells to analyze options as they decide where marketing resources will be committed. Several options are available to use in building marketing strategies around present or new target groups or in reducing and redistributing resources to modified services. Crompton (1983) outlines each strategy available to managers:

1. Market penetration strategies attempt to achieve greater clientele support with current services and target markets. By increasing participation, revenues go up, clients achieve their outcomes more quickly, physicians make new referrals, and caregivers provide more transportation.

2. Market development strategies attempt to acquire new target audiences for present division or department programs. For example, recreation therapists have incorporated family members and buddies into leisure education programs and referral services. Alternative reimbursement sources (e.g., aquatic therapy and adventure-challenge participation) are also recruited to offset service expenses.

3. Reformulation and extension strategies attempt to modify and improve existing services for current audiences or to attract new target groups. The addition of new computer games may serve to breathe new life into a service. Taking services into clients' homes facilitates inclusive programming. Adding incentives recruits volunteers, and mailing additional information brochures alerts health and human service professionals to results of efficacy research.

4. Replacement strategies intend to increase satisfaction and perceptions of quality by current target groups either by replacing existing services with improved programs or by extending the services offered. For example, wellness programs have transitioned from a focus on physical health to total well-being. Therapists have incorporated occupational and physical therapists into community-reintegration trips to adjust to clients' decreasing lengths of stay and compensate for reduced client contact time. Summer day camps have become daylong services to accommodate career families.

5. Diversification strategies involve the introduction of new services to attract new clientele. This may involve a redefinition of the department mission. This could entail hiring new personnel, merging with other departments, and/or becoming accepted as a vital service in a new unit or geographic area. A department may decentralize so staff become integral members of outreach teams and/or recreation community centers.

6. Selected and general demarketing strategies involve deploying fewer resources to services in order to reconfigure the service or eliminate the service entirely. This occurs when services become too costly or the target markets are not realizing desired benefits. For example, in hospital settings first-line managers may reduce one-on-one contacts in particular care areas. In the community, however, service location is moved to accommodate target audiences from several different locales. Efforts to increase awareness about therapeutic recreation may also be shifted from primary caregivers to family members and support groups.

Decisions about service and target market priorities are affected by several factors most notably cost and revenue predictions. The manager considers financial investments required for the prepared services and strategies in light of the expected benefits. Manager's decisions are influenced by volume trends, profitability, and qualitative assessments (Van Doren, Durney, and Darby, 1993). An analysis of volume trends involves a reconsideration of target market descriptors and service dimensions and projecting market share changes or gains over the short and long term (e.g., one to three years). For example, managers might ascertain whether service levels for specific clientele will result in five percent or ten percent volume gains over the next three years or whether shifts in services rendered (e.g., inpatient to outpatient or adult- to youth-focused services) impact volume relative to other department service lines. Current and desired level of financial performance is assessed during this process.

Managers explore such variables as profitability or contribution margin of services, payer mix of clients in each service setting, and factors predicted to change (e.g., method of payment, cost of service components). Downward trends in some service reimbursements also require managers to consider specific cost reduction targets for service line components. As noted by Winslow (1992), managers consider both direct and indirect costs of services and generally target audiences that are most crucial to the department. Last, a manager compares quality improvements and service development, redesign, and/or termination with volume trends and profitability. A manager might question: What are the benefits to be derived from current and projected service lines with various market segments? Managers establish the role of their division or department in the provision of service lines by carefully reviewing assessment data and contemplating the evolving nature of the department's mission within the larger health and human service community. These preliminary financial considerations prepare the manager to make decisions about price, the second *P* of the marketing mix.

# Price

Price, according to O'Sullivan (1991a), affects each of the other primary marketing mix variables (product, place, and promotion). What is the financial goal of the department, and how does each particular service line and target market relate to the goal? Developing a pricing strategy requires a knowledge of the department's or organization's mission, funding options, and target market "opportunity costs." Opportunity costs relate to target market characteristics such as time and travel distance and service dimensions such as quality perceptions and supplemental benefits. Potential clientele must perceive that service benefits outweigh their personal costs. The nature of an organization's financial base is evident in its mission. For-profit businesses require service lines that produce revenues greater than service costs. Nonprofit agencies, however, market service lines so that fiscal year records report equity in financial expenditure and income. Relationship of the therapeutic recreation department budget to the overall budget influences pricing of service lines (e.g., leisure education) and service components (e.g., assessment). To illustrate, services within one unit may or may not need to generate profit monies if the difference can be reflected in the larger organization budget. Funding options, a third variable affecting pricing strategy, require the manager to have knowledge of reimbursement figures and protocols, payer standards, regulatory criteria, department and organization policy, and billing procedures.

## *Pricing Variables*

Prior to setting a price, a manager identifies direct and indirect service payments and the opportunity costs. In health and human services, these factors include consideration of related demands placed on clients such as payments to other caregivers and time already devoted to transportation to and from services. The direct price is the amount the user is charged. Market price relates to service use and may involve transportation, supply fees, equipment fees (e.g., sport chairs, card holders) and maintenance or membership fees. O'Sullivan (1991a) identifies three types of opportunity costs: time, association, and effort.

Time considerations involve actual service time and time associated with accessing the service. Managers also assess the timing of their services in relation to other obligations such as scheduled therapy times and special education class calendars. Another timing consideration is the desired service outcome. Therapeutic recreators design interventions to affect change which varies with each client and target audience. One service may capture desired audiences if offered in briefer time increments over ex-

tended time periods while another retains market volume when provided in longer time frames of shorter duration. Time of day, season, and time of contact are also marketing influences. Marketing services early in the morning is difficult because audiences such as persons with physical disabilities require time to complete activities of daily living (ADL) prior to any other activity. Yet marketing to agency and community professionals at that time might gain support through breakfast meetings. Winter months inhibit service access in some geographic areas while summer services are curtailed during the heat of summer time in others. Client contact time is briefer in health and human services. Further, the amount of time available determines how a first-line manager markets service lines and/or service components. To illustrate, referral planning and redistribution of services promotes a focus on inpatient assessments and outpatient leisure skill development in clinical settings and use of computerized community leisure directories through community therapeutic recreation services.

Association refers to perceptions of relationships with service provision. What is the value associated with therapeutic recreation when compared to other services (e.g., occupational and physical therapy), service locations, and service components? Caregivers might perceive the value of an experiential modality such as aquatics or horticulture to be greater than an intervention such as values clarification or assertiveness training due to the association of the intervention with tangible rather than intangible service features. Likewise, a service offered at a clinical or program site might be perceived as having more value than one offered in an outreach mode. Benefits associated with occupational therapy and physical therapy are perceived to have different merits when aligned with therapeutic recreation, which appears to be less intrusive. Therapeutic recreation departments operating autonomously are perceived differently from services provided through, for example, physical medicine or special services. Managers assess association as they anticipate service provision to target audiences because this affects who is attracted to the service and how it is packaged.

A third type of opportunity cost is effort. In therapeutic recreation, consideration of effort is crucial because the effort needed to access and participate in opportunities can mitigate inherent experiential values. The effort of caregivers influences consumer participation opportunities. The effort put forth prior to, during, and following the actual experience is also weighed by clients, caregivers, and professionals. An overall effort to provide on-site rather then outpatient or community outings is minimal, yet experiences in the "home" community may be more relevant and attractive to clients and caregivers. The effort needed to develop and adapt alternative skills influences client program preferences. The extent of effort consumers must put forth to continue to benefit from a service affects retention rates (e.g., rural driving distances curtail outpatient contacts and summertime intervention services). In some instances, therefore, regardless of direct price amounts, services remain unattractive because the effort to use the service outweighs perceived benefits. The opposite may also be true. Regardless of direct price (within reason) and the amount of effort necessary to access the service, the benefit is perceived as significant. This might be the case with arthritic swim programs.

The host agency or therapeutic recreation department mission translates into pricing objectives. For-profit units will have generation of revenue in excess of costs as their objective while not-for-profit units desire to operate in a cost recovery mode taking into consideration a percentage of charitable care and bad debt clients. A host agency may identify profit centers and services that are built into a per diem rate. A challenge course may be considered a profit center of the host agency or therapeutic recreation department. Assessment costs may be built into the room rate or the bed rate. Therefore, within the agency or department, service prices may be established to generate surplus revenue, (surplus maximization) or to recover the full cost of operation (cost recovery).

In therapeutic recreation the pricing objective is influenced by funding options. Funding alternatives relate to the payer mix for each service line and the relationship of the therapeutic recreation department budget to the host agency budget. The nature of the setting often determines the payer mix, the clientele make up, and the types of services provided (e.g., outpatient, ancillary services, assessments, leisure education). Consequently, reimbursement for services rendered may be for those considered necessary for specific diagnoses (e.g., head and back trauma). When therapeutic recreation is considered in this manner, reimbursement comes through daily or per diem charges and by direct billing to consumers with various insurance companies reimbursing according to preset rates. Where consumers have selected to participate and/or their diagnoses preclude insurance reimbursement, payment for services rendered may be adjusted to amount of time services are rendered or prorated according to a percentage of the total program fee (individual portion of group rate). The mission of the host agency or therapeutic recreation department may determine whether or not the pricing objective is to recover the full cost per client per service or to allow select services to make marginal contributions to the cost recovery of all services rendered by each service unit. Therapeutic recreation managers may garner funds through donations, grants, and contributions in order to assist with client costs (e.g., camp scholarships) and to cover indirect services such as research when their operating policies allow for this type of fund-raising. Pricing objectives for the unit, therefore, may include intents to raise external funds to offset program enhancement and service extensions.

## Place

The place or setting influences program operation and consumer's perception of the product or services rendered. Specific places vary with regard to target markets (Winslow, 1992). One marketing publication (NTRS, 1994) notes when clients want services yet cannot access them, a serious marketing problem exists. Kuramoto (1993) indicates services have been canceled because of inconvenient locations or failure to employ strategic market planning in placing programs at particular sites. Ultimately, consumers weigh tangible benefits of location against opportunity costs. Mahoney (1994) lists four factors to consider as place of service is determined: positive reputation, welcoming facility, convenient access, and safe location. Negative perceptions attributable to each of these factors become barriers. The location of professional offices and service centers reflects and influences the perceptions of various target audiences about the value of therapeutic recreation services.

The trend to place services in relevant cost-effective environments has resulted in a service shift from inpatient to outpatient and centralized to decentralized offerings. Marketing services "closer to home" promotes functional well-being. In this respect, therapeutic recreation managers must assess the importance of client contact time and the relevance of intervention outcomes to real-life circumstances. The likelihood is that both will be enhanced when services are brought into the consumers' living areas. Additionally, target audiences such as caregivers, reimbursement agents, colleagues in related professions, and administrators have firsthand opportunities to observe the benefits of interdisciplinary problem resolution. The experiential benefits of therapeutic recreation are most evident in naturalistic environments. Managers assess service offering locations in terms of accessibility, convenience, and opportunities to each target audience. The quality of the service environment directly affects users and those who interact with users. The support of this latter group is essential to retention of consumers.

## Promotion

Promotion is one element of marketing and is a form of communication. What is the desired image of therapeutic recreation within the host agency and community? The intent of promotion is to inform consumers of services offered, then to convince them to participate and/or support participation of a specific target audience. The greatest challenge is to ensure that persons for whom services are intended receive information in a timely manner. Four basic types of promotional tools have been identified (NTRS, 1994): advertising, personal contact, incentives, and publicity. Kuramoto (1993) suggests that choices of promotional tools are tied to cost factors; those achieving high levels of exposure are more costly (e.g., TV promotionals are more costly than newspaper ads). The costs and tools selected by a therapeutic recreation manager will be affected by the degree of responsibility assumed by the department. Where marketing is a host agency responsibility, a therapeutic recreation manager's role may be to identify target markets and to generate ideas leaving actual promotional production and dissemination costs to the marketing department. When responsibility falls to the therapeutic recreation department, management and staff may jointly promote all services, and/or individual services are marketed by staff assigned to the particular service.

A first-line manager's responsibility is to use promotional tools to develop an image that places the unit in a desirable market position. Each target audience uniquely relates to promotional media, and each service is suited to particular promotional tools. Each type of promotional tool is presented with illustrations of the target audience and service lines provided.

## Advertising

Advertising is a paid form of nonpersonal communication. Information is shared through radio, television, and printed media such as brochures, posters, and catalogs. Vendors use catalogs as do therapists when sharing information on adapted resources. For-profit agencies use TV ads to market private mental health services to adults. Public leisure service departments use public service announcements (PSAs) to inform community clientele about special services. A manager may also prepare and distribute a brochure on therapeutic recreation department services to other colleagues in the setting and professional community.

## Personal Contact and Word of Mouth

Personal contact and word of mouth remain significant communication tools. Quality service may be the factor that separates competitors. Good service results in positive comments, retention, and referrals. Former clients, support groups, advisory committees, letters from significant community members, and support from key figures, represent personal contacts. For example, Special Olympics Inc. and United Way have benefited from promotionals by popular athletes and well-known public figures. Former clients effectively communicate the benefit of therapeutic recreation services to other health and human service professionals. Managers who choose to sit on advisory boards and become active in professional associations also serve as advocates. Participants are key marketers because they transfer information in a timely, convincing, and personal manner by word of mouth. The market position of a department may well be a reflection of clientele satisfaction or dissatisfaction.

## Incentives

Incentives or sales promotions have financial value and are offered to consumers in exchange for their participation. For example, therapeutic recreators encourage family members to participate at no cost so clients benefit from family member awareness of their skills and needs. Buddies are used in some cases to facilitate barrier-free participation. Dealers also loan equipment to departments so clients may consider future purchases. Although not always philosophically desirable, group or special rates permit access that might not otherwise happen. A therapeutic recreation manager who invites professionals to benefit from a challenge course experience is exchanging information on the efficacy of this intervention for potential future referrals. Incentives also promote volunteerism and are used to promote consumer participation in wellness programs. In these situations a manager uses incentives to activate and change consumer behavior.

## Publicity

A fourth type of promotional tool, publicity, is used to inform target groups about the department. Publicity is not directly sponsored or funded by the unit but results from the efforts of others. Publicity results when departments receive national professional awards, and their names appear in print or on recognition awards. A professional who represents his or her department is publicizing the unit. It is publicity when vendors refer to a department that has purchased their products. Helmet safety programs, road races to benefit a particular diagnostic group, and tournaments to raise funds for accessible trails are examples of ways to attract the attention of local news media. Open houses, tours, and in-services also publicize services without incurring major costs. Awareness in a variety of target groups encourages exchange of in-kind services and creates networking opportunities.

According to Mahoney (1994), a well-conceived promotional campaign incorporates a mix of each promotional type to attain three goals: recruitment, retention, and reputation. Systematic promotions result in quality service distribution, referrals, and enhancement of department evaluation. The effectiveness of each tool is determined through formative and summative evaluations. Frequent changes of promotional tools are not necessarily essential because once a tool has been successful, it is likely to be continually effective (NTRS, 1994).

## The Service *Ps*

The traditional marketing *Ps*—product, price, place and promotion—evolved with the manufacturing of tangible products. Because leisure and therapeutic recreation involve exchange of long-term relationships for quality experiences rather than the one-time purchase of a tangible good, O'Sullivan (1991b) suggests that strategic market planning also includes several additional *Ps* such as physical evidence, people, policies and procedures, public image, and political impact. These factors are important to the therapeutic recreation manager because they become evident as therapeutic interventions occur, and they impact the evaluation of therapeutic recreation services by consumers. These marketing variables are planning factors for which first-line managers have primary responsibility.

## Physical Evidence

O'Sullivan (1991a) notes that the physical evidence surrounding or inherent to the experience is critical since the outcomes of participation are not always tangible. In therapeutic recreation physical evidence involves the area where the intervention occurs, tokens received from participation, and documented outcomes of the exchange. Managers must consider how to make the experience more attractive. For example, contact in an activity area would be perceived by a consumer as more pleasing than contact in a home or at hospital bedside. Retention is strengthened with feedback reporting progress that may not be visually apparent. Colleagues perceive the presence of the work environment to reflect the significance of their colleagues' work. External target audiences also gain impressions from the ambiance of the delivery setting. These impressions influence whether consumers chose to return and advocate on behalf of therapeutic recreation.

## People

A helping relationship is a key element in the therapeutic recreation process. Additionally, caregivers and family are integral to the process. Where experiences occur in groups, interactions with others influence service delivery. Thus, therapeutic experiences are impacted by people. As staff are hired and trained, managers assess their (staff) potential to enter into helping relationships. Caregiver and family perceptions of illness and disability directly influence whether consumers gain access to services and how effectively therapeutic outcomes are integrated into a consumer's lifestyle. The presence of consumers in groups adds to and/or detracts from the therapeutic nature of experiences. In some instances, for example, families and consumers make program selections that accommodate their feelings about others in the groups. Managers therefore assess service format and placing and distribution of services as they plan participant mix and target marketing strategies.

Another "people" element the manager must consider is the ability of various target audiences to comprehend information about therapeutic recreation. Bright (1994) suggests that the extent to which the audience understands the message is influenced by their frame of reference, ex-

perience, and education levels. Consumers of health and human services listen and respond because change is desired, yet they may not be motivated to take the necessary action. They may have had little previous exposure to therapeutic recreation services. Consumers and caregivers tend to rely on hearing what sounds most promising or is most relevant. Consequently, managers plan to use multiple promotional tools to ensure message retention. Also, managers rely on the expertise and trustworthiness of staff as credible information sources to whom target audiences will relate and listen.

## Policies and Procedures

Policies and procedures impact marketing. Internal and external regulations influence product, pricing, place, and promotion. Managers are aware of a number of factors that determine which services will be reimbursed, what conditions affect the service delivery setting, and how information about therapeutic recreation is shared with target audiences. Safety, risk, and infection control processes guide content selection and therapists' interactions. Managers examine operating documents with the intent of encouraging participation by various target audiences. The challenge becomes respecting the rights and confidentiality of various clientele.

## Public Image

Positioning in the marketplace is affected by *image*. Target audiences have perceptions about therapeutic recreation compared with related health and human service professionals. Since image is intangible, managers attempt to create concrete symbols to portray quality and service impacts. The slogan "TR riffic" used by the Therapeutic Recreation Division of the Cincinnati Recreation Commission connotes invaluable service results. Happy face buttons or stickers imply positive experiences. The quality of promotional materials and supplemental benefits such as refreshments creates a service image. Managers must also consider image as they hire staff. Whether consumers choose to return or not depends heavily on the image they retain after service completion.

## Political Impact

Political impact results from formal sponsorship of legislation as well as informal connections. Several illustrations follow. Legislative advocacy is a primary function of professional organizations such as the American Therapeutic Recreation Association (ATRA) and National Therapeutic Recreation Society (NTRS). Consumer groups (e.g., United Cerebral Palsy Association) can also become politically involved as they lobby for barrier-free experiences. Clients and caregivers who attend Individual Education

Plan (IEP) meetings and sit with the treatment team are using political power to gain service options. Therapeutic recreation has benefited from the political nature of social issues (e.g., accessibility) and vested interest groups (e.g., senior citizens). Managers must apprise themselves of political agendas of target audiences such as elected officials, insurance companies, corporate healthcare, and potential philanthropic groups. Each of these groups may have special interests or contacts that can lead to funding decisions, directions and alternatives. Coalitions of various health and human service professionals and organizations serve as conduits to legislative sponsorship and political recognition. Politics affects decisions managers make about service packaging, prices, promotionals, and distribution. Politically astute managers realize the linkages between financial resources and department well-being.

## Relationship Marketing

The intent of relationship marketing is to keep the client in the system. This is accomplished through integrated strategic market planning. Planning to meet the needs of the consumer is the central feature of integrated marketing, yet to meet the needs of the client, a number of other audiences are targeted. Access to services is simplified. Consistent follow-up and advocacy occur. A variety of promotional strategies are planned to accommodate each target market. Because of the unique needs of each audience serviced, planning to maintain a positive image can be challenging (Thorn, 1984). An action plan is written for each target audience in order to achieve its goals and objectives. According to Thorn (1994), at least four distinct markets require action plans: consumers, referral sources, third-party payees, and the professional community. An outline for a marketing plan with a client market is presented in Figure 12.2 (page 182).

The department manager orchestrates relationship marketing strategies as resources, staff, and services are coordinated. The staff and manager plan together to create a consumer-oriented service. Barber (1989) suggests a consumer-oriented service is characterized by a well-conceived department mission, availability of department resources to conveniently address consumer needs, and a staff who are client conscious or client friendly. The staff and manager focus on continuous improvements, and, as they are made, better plans evolve from direct service. Planning emphasizes process and performance outcomes. Delene (1992) indicates that relationship marketing is individually intensive and demanding. Improving the human relations skills and communication abilities of all practitioners is a management goal.

Delene (1992) believes internal department marketing is central to successful relationship building and quality improvements. Therefore, managers build their department

image from the inside out through consistent staffing practices and development planning. Staff commitment and motivation are enhanced as they increasingly contribute to consumer-oriented services. Kuramoto (1993) believes effective target marketing requires the best possible working environment for staff. Further, Kuramoto (1993) describes marketing as a team effort that involves the manager and staff jointly setting the mission, defining specific marketing activities, and implementing the plan.

## Step 3: Implementation

Implementation involves putting the respective integrated marketing plans into play. This management process entails putting each plan into action in an appropriately timed sequence of events with full awareness of each action's impact on the target audience's perceptions of the department and its services. Once each audience has become aware of department services, the focus turns from "external" to "internal" marketing, or from recruitment to retention and reputation. A manager makes conscious decisions based on prioritized target market needs and the marketing costs of each action plan. Winslow (1992) notes that the potential costs of completing a comprehensive market plan may be beyond the parameters of a particular budget, so the most important strategies and those likely to succeed are implemented. Crompton (1983) encourages the design of both long- and short-term strategic marketing plans to allow for adjustment in department resources during periods of dynamic change.

### Implementation Tasks

Tasks undertaken during the implementation step involve: (1) prioritizing the department's most critical target markets, (2) selecting the most financially reasonable and practical marketing strategies, (3) preparing a time table to implement these strategies, (4) preparing the promotional materials, (5) implementing the action plans, and (6) formatively evaluating outcomes of the marketing plan.

The first step involves a reconsideration of identified target markets and their specific needs in view of the department's mission. Managers discern which target audience goals and objectives are crucial to the credibility and viability of department services. Consequently, several target groups may require continuous and simultaneous information about therapeutic recreation services. A manager then studies the marketing strategies proposed with each target audience to discern financial implications. Prudent financial decisions might involve using one strategy (e.g., brochure or PSA) to achieve the marketing goals of more than one target audience or to coordinate the timing of several strategies to recruit and retain consumers. For example, incentives distributed while clients begin and terminate services are likely to market services immediately

---

**Figure 12.2 Marketing Plan Outline**

**Target Market: Consumers**
   *Goal:* Increase awareness of therapeutic recreation efficacy.
   *Objective:* Increase number of client contacts in leisure education by articulating outcomes related to well-being.
   *Service:* Leisure education.
   *Strategy:* Market penetration and extension.
   *Price:* Cost recovery.
   *Funding options:* Per diem; fee for service.
   *Place:* Relevant or home community and/or technology simulation.
   *Promotion Advertising:* Department brochure describing demonstrated efficacy of services.
   *Personal contact:* Consumer advocates; consumer and/or peer support group; one-on-one client-therapist assessment interviews.
   *Incentive:* Speaker's bureau participation by manager; caregiver participation; leisure buddies; recognition program (i.e., client participation).
   *Publicity:* Therapeutic recreation week materials from ATRA/NTRS; buttons sponsored by arts and crafts vendor; wearing apparel sponsored by clothing company; outpatient tape; host agency sponsorship of community sporting event.
   *Physical evidence:* Division logo on paper and pencil leisure education games; staff T-shirt logo.
   *People:* CTRS credentialed staff; consumer groups formed with those having similar assessed preferences.
   *Policy/Procedures:* Transportation risk management policy; computerized directory referrals by "confidential" passwords.
   *Public Image:* Department slogan: "Quality well-being through quality services—enhancement through therapeutic recreation service."
   *Political Image:* Community referral network; help lines.

---

and also extend service awareness to potential recruits. Therefore, a marketing timetable denotes a systematic effort to implement strategies that maintain the position of the department in the "competitive" marketplace. Using computer software packages, a manager may design a timetable that depicts the prioritized target markets, marketing strategy, timetable, and staff responsible for each action. To illustrate the third step a timetable to increase consumer contacts is presented here for each of the primary markets identified by Thorn (1984). The goal is to increase consumer referrals through awareness of therapeutic recreation efficacy (see Table 12.1).

While responsibility to prepare and implement marketing action plans falls to the entire department, assignment to actually prepare particular promotional tools, implementation task four may be handled by the staff, manager, department personnel, and host agency public relations personnel. Desktop publishing and available software are used by staff and managers to prepare department promotional pieces. Preparation of significant pieces (e.g., annual report, special event banner) may be contracted out to a commercial firm with staff design of content and layout. Information on the preparation of promotional tools is available through commercial vendors and professional publications and workshops. A number of specific illustrations and design specifics are reported in programming texts (e.g.,

Carter, Browne, LeConey, and Nagle, 1991; Rossman, 1995); marketing publications, (e.g., NTRS, 1994; O'Sullivan, 1991a); and administration texts (e.g., Winslow and Halberg, 1992). Professional associations (e.g., ATRA and NTRS) make available promotional materials for therapeutic recreation week (e.g., a week in June identified annually to promote the professional mission).

A managerial approach used to implement action plans, step five, is to maintain an updated list of target market contacts with specifications unique to each contact so timely information is made available in the desired format to actual target markets and to those who are responsible for distribution (e.g., newspaper, agency public relations personnel). Even if the manager and staff prepare, distribute, and monitor promotional tools within the host agency, protocols may require prior authorization and site-specific distribution assignments. That is, a stamp of approval must be received before materials are placed in certain locations. Public departments also have protocols stating who is permitted to use what type of promotion and make which type of contacts. Consequently, for example, before a PSA is sent to various news media, department employees must secure agency permission.

Formative evaluation, step six, occurs as the manager monitors implementation of the action plans. The manager ascertains if the appropriate strategies are being used in

**Table 12.1   Timetable**

| Target Market | Priority | Strategy | Timetable | Staff Resp. |
|---|---|---|---|---|
| Client | 1 | Newsletter Fact Sheet | Time of Contact Follow-Up | All Staff |
| Third-Party Payees | 2 | Brochure | Ongoing | Manager |
| Referral Sources | 3 | Brochure | Time of Contact | Manager/Staff |
| Professional Community | 4 | Staff Development Speaker's Bureau | Ongoing | All Staff |

a timely manner to inform targeted markets of department services. Managers consider marketing costs, staffing assignments, effectiveness of various strategies, and target market response. One accountability tool used by managers is a media file. Actual copies of printed media and documented target market contacts resulting from particular marketing strategies are saved. Such files are also appropriate to use with exemplary marketing strategies gathered from other departments through professional contacts and resources.

## Community Relations

Nestor (1992) notes that establishing long-term relationships with major communicators in the community is as important as developing long-term client relationships. The intent is to partner with various media for the purpose of community-based image development. Media reaches vast audiences overnight. Community service projects with media also facilitate significant exposure with relatively few dollars invested by the department. A manager whose department becomes involved in the community is building networks that promote access and cost containment. Collaboration fosters resource sharing and distribution of services in the home community. The focus is shifted toward education and prevention from treatment. Public accountability is increased through image building activities such as service or educational programs, volunteerism, and charity services. Public relations and marketing promote community benefit programs responsive to client needs. Therefore, marriage with the media and other professional colleagues positions the department to serve its target markets efficiently.

## Advocacy

The urgency to assume a proactive role in service provision has been precipitated by not only healthcare reform issues but also the movement toward managed care, in-

creasing levels of consumer sophistication, concern for accountability and quality, and the constantly changing nature of health and human service delivery options. Managers assume advocacy positions as they champion the values of therapeutic recreation. Although service quality does foster consumer retention, future scenarios require that managers become actively involved in promoting the profession. Managers are individual advocates as they interpret the inherent values of therapeutic recreation services with consumers, caregivers, and support networks.

As professional advocates, managers articulate the merits of therapeutic recreation services with referral agents, third-party reimbursers, colleagues, and political agents. Managers disseminate results of research and efficacy studies, and they participate in evaluation projects to gather data used in analysis of therapeutic recreation benefits. Additionally, managers monitor legislative transactions and communicate with political decision makers the essence of their services. For example professional advocacy occurs as service descriptors are shared with colleagues from other health and human service disciplines. When professionals recruit new organization members and/or serve on professional committees, they are advocating for their professional future. Professional advocacy is also in evidence during interdisciplinary meetings when therapeutic recreators clarify the relationship of quality well-being to therapeutic recreation interventions.

## Managerial Roles

Managers are central figures in community relations programs and advocacy efforts. These are ongoing activities that occur as the target market plans are implemented. Managers coordinate staff efforts and serve as the link between department actions and marketing by the host agency. Their focus is on ensuring the availability of resources and information to staff and agency public relations personnel in efficient and effective ways. Additionally, managers oversee the collection of formative data to determine if quality services are enabling recruitment, retention, and referrals. Observations, interviews, surveys, and case studies are used to collect data relevant to each target market's objectives. Staff responsible for the market action plans also may assume responsibility to evaluate each marketing strategy.

Marketing, like programming, is cyclical; processes are ongoing. Formative information enables immediate change in marketing strategies, and strategies are then adjusted to coincide with changes in the programming cycle that affect each target market. Implementation timetables assure that information has a consistent and timely distribution so that clients remain aware of available services, and new markets are attracted to replace those that have been referred elsewhere.

## Step 4: Evaluation, Trends, Strategies, Issues

### Evaluation

Summative evaluation concludes the strategic market planning process. The intent is to identify how well the goals of each target market have been realized. In addition, the manager is concerned with where the department is in relation to where it wanted to be. A marketing audit identifies for image goals if the desired target audiences have been reached and for action goals if the right services have been distributed to the right people. From the feedback received, a manager reaffirms or redefines the department mission statement, goals and objectives, and marketing strategies for each target market. Evaluation also takes into consideration unforeseen opportunities or adverse system influences that have arisen and might require modification in the marketing plans.

During a marketing audit each of the *Ps* is reconsidered. Successful elements are retained while those that are less successful are modified and reshaped. Input is gained from each target market. As a result of this feedback, one target market or service may be substituted for another, profit centers may be created or cost recovery programs maximized; location may be made more convenient to minimize opportunity costs; types of promotional tools may be diversified further to better integrate marketing strategies; and changes in staffing, policies, and the work environment may be undertaken to improve intangible qualities of therapeutic interactions. Evaluation, therefore, is helpful in reconsidering each of the preceding planning steps and the decisions that have occurred as the marketing plan evolved. Results are reviewed in light of costs as well as goal attainment. Monies are devoted to action plans likely to be of the most benefit to the greatest number of crucial target markets. Managers annually review their marketing costs as department budgets are prepared for the coming

fiscal year. The amount of funds approved is likely to impact the extent to which the various target market action plans are implemented. The monies allotted have a direct influence on which services and target markets are expanded, contacted, changed, and how vigorously available resources are balanced to address the department's potential consumers.

### Trends

In addition to those mentioned in the opening chapter section, a number of trends will impact therapeutic recreation marketing. These trends will result in a variety of new marketing strategies being incorporated into market plans because the composition of target markets is likely to change. In the future, a number of aging cohort groups with unique service needs will exist. Also, a number of users will not be tied to family units or supportive caregiving groups. Diversity will also characterize the health and human service needs of target markets.

Technological advances will impact how practitioners promote their services. As computers become more user friendly, responsibility to prepare promotional tools will fall to first-line managers and direct-service personnel. A commonly articulated change is the continued focus on wellness and health promotion. The trend away from treatment and toward prevention will eventually be supported by readjusted third-party reimbursement strategies. The management of health and human services will continue to undergo dynamic change (e.g., mergers, consolidations, reorganizations, buy outs). And professionals operating within these environments will continue to experience redefined missions. The nature of their services will become increasingly specialized yet integrated along market segments and customized service lines.

### Strategies

A number of marketing strategies have evolved in the 1990s and will continue into the twenty-first century. Marketing strategies will increasingly rely on technological applications and home-based computer systems to bring information directly to the client through interactive healthcare information systems. Practitioners in one location will consult via telecommunications with managers and recreation therapists in regional locations. Therapeutic recreation research and efficacy will be promoted through computerized database systems easily accessible to consumers, referral agents, third-party payees, and the professional community.

O'Sullivan (1991a) uses the phrase "bundling of benefits" to describe the integration of service benefits into a marketing mix (integrated marketing) with a particular program. Holistic well-being marketing strategies will result from the continuing wellness focus. Practitioners will package a service line targeting various age cohort groups. Benefits peculiar to each target segment will be promoted through referral programming to maintain long-term relationships with clients. The "smart" customer of the 1990s is likely to become even smarter as a result of technological access to information. As this occurs, client concern for quality services supportive of life satisfaction through leisure well-being as one healthcare alternative will increase. Customized, convenient, and timely access to services will remain a marketing strategy. As services continue to become more community based and inclusive, marketing strategies will focus on the relevance and appropriateness of the "right" service within the client's "own" living environment. Marketing efforts will also link clinical and community therapeutic recreation services in order to retain clients in comprehensive service networks.

Strategic market planning will continue to remain a critical first-line manager task. Increasingly, target marketing is a conduit to alternative funding and the competitive edge. Managers will incorporate marketing concepts and strategies and communication and information technology know-how into staff training and development programs. Ultimately, the entire staffing process will focus on consumer-oriented practices.

## Ethical Issues

Health and human services are businesses that operate at the margin of the market economy. Ethical dilemmas arise as a result of this situation. Billing therapeutic recreation services under other professional areas (e.g., occupational therapy) may well be an outcome precipitated by market demands. Conversely, the provision of therapeutic recreation services for reimbursement without proven effectiveness of the intervention contributes to resource waste and fraudulent billing. Clients in health and human service systems may lack the information to compare systems. When marketing strategies are used that require target audiences to analyze service advantages, the client may be confused and, as a result, create imperfect images of the intent of therapeutic recreation. First-line therapeutic managers will continue to focus on client education and awareness through external marketing. With internal efforts the manager will develop customer friendly work environments that encourage staff morally to commit to the department mission. Marketing plans designed with consumer concern as the central focus will guide staff decisions while helping clients.

# Summary

A number of factors have contributed to the introduction of marketing strategies into therapeutic recreation. Competitive health and human service alternatives, dynamic change, cost containment, accountability, managed care, and the consumer's demand for quality effective and efficient services are elements that worked to bring about marketing strategies to ensure the development of exchange relationships. Strategic service marketing is vital to department well-being and survival.

The marketing process, like the therapeutic recreation process, involves the following four steps: assessment, planning, implementation, and evaluation. In the initial assessment step, target markets, department strengths and weaknesses, opportunities, and competition in the service market are identified. Target markets are characterized by five descriptors (service needs and interest, geographic location, sociodemographics, behavioral, and synchronographics) that are assessed to determine which audiences are likely to be attracted to therapeutic recreation services. The target markets of therapeutic recreation include agency professionals, support staff, committee and board members, caregivers, general public, insurers, managed care providers, policymakers, community health and human service agents, peer professionals, and resource providers. Managers assess the service environment to ascertain a likely niche, evaluate the effectiveness of present and past marketing processes, and predict the future trends likely to affect the department's marketing position. As a result of the assessment, a manager designs image (e.g., perception) and action (e.g., outcome) goals and objectives for each target market. These guide the design of strategic action plans with each target market.

During the planning step the marketing mix variables are studied and organized with each target market. The service marketing mix consists of product or service, price, place or location, promotional tools, physical evidence, people, policies and procedures, public image, and political impact. Managers consider each of these variables with each target market in order to select an appropriate marketing strategy. Several strategies are used by managers to market the right services to the right target market. These include penetration, development, reformation, extension, replacement, diversification, and demarketing. As managers plan which strategy to use with each target market, they consider the financial demands compared to target market benefits. This involves an assessment of direct and indirect expenses and opportunity costs prior to setting service prices. Opportunity costs are the time, association, and effort target markets invest in participation. Managers also consider the mission of their department and funding options as they determine service prices. Managers consider where they place services because location affects retention and recruitment. The trend is to place services closer to clients or in relevant communities.

Four types of promotional tools are used to inform potential target audiences about services: advertising, personal contact, incentives, and publicity. Each promotional tool is suited to particular audiences and service offerings. The manager chooses those that best position the department. The additional marketing *Ps* of physical evidence, people, policies and procedures, public image, and political impact are relatively intangible factors that affect the perceived outcomes of therapeutic recreation services. The manager works with staff to create a dynamic mission and strategic action plans suited to each target audience. Market planning, therefore, also includes staffing and resource planning.

The third step in the marketing process, implementation, involves putting each target audience's marketing plan into action. Managers develop timetables with goals and objectives that identify target markets, marketing priority, selected strategy, assigned staff, and an action time line. During implementation, managers become involved in community relations programs to increase client referral options and to promote department services. Advocacy is essential to professional well-being. Managers represent their departments as professional advocates in a number of work and collegial situations. As action plans are implemented, managers collect formative data so immediate changes can be made to ensure the unit's market position.

The concluding step in the marketing process is the evaluation of the respective plans. Results are studied in view of costs incurred and benefits accrued. Each of the marketing mix variables may be adjusted to address target market needs properly. The amount of monies allotted to marketing is likely to determine which markets and services become the focus of the department. A number of trends will likely affect future marketing efforts and managerial decisions: target market diversity, technology advancements, increasing wellness focus, and an ongoing change in management and health and human service delivery systems. A number of marketing strategies have evolved to address these trends. Strategies likely to continue into the twenty-first century include integrated marketing, interactive computerized health networks, service line or segmented marketing, customized service referrals, and networking of relevant services.

Managers assume key roles in the development of target market action plans and preparation of promotional tools. They also orchestrate the creation of customer-friendly service environments and oversee employees who are customer conscious. Their responsibilities place them in vulnerable positions as they attempt to meet individual consumer needs while operating on the edge of the business economy. Further, ethical practices related to billing, service descriptors, efficacy, and client autonomy are involved as marketing decisions occur. Managers contemplate their own values and staff beliefs as they balance resources to ensure that the department remains in the competitive market.

# Discussion Questions

1. What are the factors that have contributed to the necessity to market therapeutic recreation services? What are the five characteristics assessed with each target market?
3. Describe the seven *Ps* included in the marketing mix.
4. What is meant by opportunity costs?
5. Who are the target markets of therapeutic recreation practitioners?
6. What are the elements of a target market action plan?
7. What are the four types of promotional tools used in therapeutic recreation?
8. How do trends affect marketing in therapeutic recreation?
9. What ethical dilemmas does the manager face when marketing therapeutic recreation?

# References

Barber, E. H. (1989). Customer service: The competitive edge. *Journal of Park and Recreation Administration, 7:4,* 10–20.

Bright, A. D. (1994). Information campaigns that enlighten and influence the public. *Parks and Recreation, 29:8,* 48–54.

Carter, M. J., Browne, B., LeConey, S. P., and Nagle, C. J. (1991). *Designing therapeutic recreation programs in the community.* Reston, VA: American Alliance for Health, Physical Education, Recreation and Dance.

Chilingerian, J. A. (1992). New directions for hospital strategic management: The market for efficient care. *Health Care Management Review, 17:4,* 73–80.

Crompton, J. L. (1983). Formulating new directions with strategic marketing planning. *Parks and Recreation, 18:7,* 56–63, 66.

Delene, L. M. (1992). Relationship marketing and service quality. *Journal of American College Health, 40:6,* 265–269.

Kuramoto, A. M. (1993). Marketing university-based continuing education programs. *The Journal of Continuing Education in Nursing, 24:2,* 61–65.

Mahoney, D. F. (1994). Marketing healthcare programs to older adults: Strategies for success. *Geriatric Nursing, 15:1,* 10–15.

National Therapeutic Recreation Society (NTRS). (1994). *Promoting therapeutic recreation: A marketing guide.* Arlington, VA: National Recreation and Park Association.

Nestor, S. E. (1992). Marketing to consumers: Unleashing technologies to help the public choose health service options. *Topics in Health Care Financing, 18:3,* 28–37.

O'Sullivan, E. (1991a). *Marketing for parks, recreation, and leisure.* State College, PA: Venture Publishing, Inc.

O'Sullivan, E. (1991b). Marketing experiences: It's the how not the what. *Parks & Recreation, 26:12,* 40–42.

Rossman, J. R. (1995). *Recreation programming designing leisure experiences* (2nd ed.). Champaign, IL: Sagamore Publishing, Inc.

Thorn, B. E. (1984). Marketing therapeutic recreation services. *Therapeutic Recreation Journal, 18:4,* 42–47.

Van Doren, D. C., Durney, J. R., and Darby, C. M. (1993). Key decisions in marketing plan formulation for geriatric services. *Health Care Management Review, 18:3,* 7–19.

Winslow, R. (1992). Marketing therapeutic recreation services. In R. M. Winslow and K. J. Halberg (Eds.), *The management of therapeutic recreation services* (pp. 115–136). Arlington, VA: National Recreation and Park Association.

Winslow, R. M., and Halberg, K. J. (Eds.). (1992). *The management of therapeutic recreation services.* Arlington, VA: National Recreation and Park Association.

# Chapter 13

# Staffing

## Introduction

Staffing provides for the proper mix and skill level of personnel to deliver quality services. If the staff within a therapeutic recreation division or department lack skills, experience, or motivation, the unit operates ineffectively and inefficiently and, more important, consumer service quality is affected. Thus, competent personnel are essential. What does the first-line manager do to ensure that there is an adequate mix and number of personnel to transform the department's philosophy and goals from abstract to reality?

The responsibility of staffing may be dispersed throughout the entire agency. A first-line manager may work with the human resource division to design therapeutic recreation job descriptions, plan interviews, formulate specific screening tests, and select staff. In another scenario, the manager may oversee hiring that encompasses agency employment processing and documentation. In some instances (e.g., special recreation districts), the manager may oversee a personnel specialist who holds an administrative position and guides the manager in processing all personnel and volunteers. In each case, the manager is involved in personnel decisions. The intent of this chapter is to consider the essential elements of staffing.

Health and human services are undergoing major scrutiny as the demand to deliver quality services at contained costs escalates. First-line managers must consider the cost involved in all aspects of department functions. A major portion of the total budget is always personnel costs. Managers must also consider the cost of training and development, benefits, and retention. Therefore it is crucial to employ therapeutic recreation specialists who meet client needs while performing cost effectively.

As the twenty-first century approaches, the changing nature of the work culture becomes a staffing consideration. Connolly (1993) projects that many health and human service professions will reexamine their entry-level work force as the composition of workers and nature of services change. Futuristic planners view departments as components of a system with changes and interactions that will have domino effects throughout an agency or organization. The relationship of each employee to every other employee impacts service outcomes. Systems management approaches such as total quality management (TQM) rely on human resource investments and performance to maintain and improve client services. The ability to perform as a team member is a human resource consideration. Systems respond to their environments through change and transformation. Motivation to change, adapt, and grow as the work culture evolves are future employee qualities and selection considerations.

First-line managers are impacted by a number of legal regulations and professional standards designed to protect the employee and employer and to promote fairness in the work environment. Professional standards also encourage employees to maintain and upgrade their professional competence. Managers who elect to incorporate these criteria into job specifications develop privileging protocols. Responsibility then rests with the manager to tie performance criteria to therapeutic recreation practices. The first portion of this chapter, therefore, covers legal and professional regulations and standards.

The second portion of this chapter outlines recruiting processes and practices. An initial management task is to outline current and future staffing needs and to develop a plan to meet these needs. Available practitioner surveys suggest trends as well as immediate hiring needs. Managers develop job specifications keeping in mind legal and professional standards, present and future staffing needs, and the local environment. Selecting the appropriate media to use in recruitment is a management task that also takes into account internal and external sources and appropriateness of the technique to the personnel being recruited.

Once a pool of applicants becomes available, the manager's task is to determine the right mix and number of personnel to hire. That is the focus of the next segment of this chapter. A number of screening and assessment processes are available, and managers may elect to use a combination of methods. Common practice is to review resumes and/or portfolios, conduct interviews, and administer tests. Applicants are also required to submit application forms, background information, and job-related health data. The manager then synthesizes the information, makes a decision, and presents a compensation package to the successful candidate. During this step, as with each of the others, a number of issues may arise. Consensus on the appropriate mix of personnel may not be a singular decision. The last portion of this chapter addresses issues that arise throughout the staffing process.

# Legal and Professional Regulations and Standards

Commencing in 1935, a number of federal laws and court decisions have been implemented that affect employment practices. Amendments to original legislation, court interpretations, and executive orders contribute to ambiguity and inconsistency in practice. Yet, the responsibility lies with the first-line manager to comply with the intent of laws and legislation. In an attempt to ensure quality consumer services, professional credentialing bodies and societies have recommended minimal and expected educational experiences and credentials. Further, in a number of practice settings privileging practices to promote maintenance of staff competence are outlined. Noncompliance to laws exposes the manager to liability. Adherence to professional guidelines, however, facilitates the hiring of staff who are eligible to meet personnel criteria and who have been exposed to competencies believed essential to quality therapeutic recreation service delivery.

## *Legal Regulations*

1) The National Labor Relations Act (Wagner Act) of 1935, the Labor Management Relations Act (Taft-Hartley Act) of 1947, and state right-to-work laws govern relationships among employees who are union or nonunion members and the first-line manager who is responsible for conducting fair labor practices. First-line managers in clinical and community settings interact directly or indirectly with unions as they employ and supervise staff. A city park and recreation department or a hospital may be unionized and have union members within the agency. In either situation the manager needs to be familiar with union conditions and practices that govern collective bargaining. In some instances, first-line therapeutic recreation managers rely on union members to carry out supportive tasks critical to program delivery such as room setup or equipment maintenance. Therefore, the manager must plan to accommodate stipulated work practices and include monies to cover the deployment of essential support services in the budget.

2) The Equal Pay Act of 1963 prohibits pay discrimination on the basis of sex. This act eliminated a tradition of paying wages at a rate less than would be paid to the opposite sex when the same skill level, knowledge base, and tasks are performed. Entry-level employees or non-supervisory staff as well as first-line managers are covered by this law and its amendments (e.g., 3) 1972 Equal Employment Opportunity Act). Private as well as government institutions are required to comply. Thus, whether the department is part of a larger city or county government agency or a private hospital, first-line managers are required to have equitable pay scales.

4) The first-line manager is directly responsible for the enforcement of the fair employment provisions of the Civil Rights Act, Title VII of 1964. This law and its court interpretations ensure that discrimination in hiring, firing, wages, terms, conditions, and privileges of employment do not occur. The courts have decreed that an applicant is to be judged based on ability. Prerequisites for a position are to be job related; therefore, if cardiopulmonary resuscitation (CPR) and first aid are employment requirements, they are to be tied to client safety during service provision. When employees are subjected to testing, it must be job-related (e.g., civil service tests administered by public agencies). Differential compensation rates and employment conditions may exist if part of a seniority system or merit program, yet they must not be discriminatory.

5) The Civil Rights Act of 1991 restored provisions (e.g., hiring, firing, or promotion) lost through Supreme Court decisions following the enactment of the 1964 law. Supervisors must be aware of hiring and promotion practices, known as the "glass ceiling effect," (e.g., artificial barriers) that adversely impact protected classes, seniority systems, and persons whose age might be considered an

employment factor. First-line managers may adopt policies that prohibit employment of people who use or possess illegal drugs (Murrell, Dwyer, Murrell and Coleman, 1992). Racial or sexual harassment on the job is prohibited, and individuals may seek punitive damages in intentional discriminatory claims. If a first-line manager elects to require passage of the certified therapeutic recreation specialist (CTRS) and/or certified leisure professional (CLP) exam as a criterion of employment, the responsibility lies with the manager to relate successful completion of the test to the employee's job tasks. According to Murrell, Dwyer, Murrell, and Coleman (1992), the first-line manager must be able to establish that success on these exams is predictive of job performance. Murrell, Dwyer, Murrell, and Coleman (1992) also noted that evaluation systems during training and in employee performance reviews are to be job related and technically sound. Thus, the design of employee privileging programs and performance appraisal processes is based on the knowledge, skills, and abilities (KSAs) to perform as a therapeutic recreation specialist.

The Age Discrimination in Employment Act of 1967, amended in 1978, makes it illegal to discriminate against persons 40 years of age or older in employment selection, retention, promotion, and compensation. Employers affected are those with 20 or more employees and government agencies such as municipal leisure service departments. As suggested by Robbins (1995), the only exceptions are instances in which a first-line manager can demonstrate that advanced age may affect client safety and organizational efficiency.

The Equal Employment Opportunity Act of 1972 established the Equal Employment Opportunity Commission (EEOC) to enforce the 1964 and later the 1991 Civil Rights Act. This law expanded Title VII to include employers with 15 or more employees and state and local government employers. Consequently, many first-line therapeutic recreation managers are affected. The law further requires the preparation of an affirmative action plan. Affirmative action plans identify guidelines affecting position advertising, application forms, and recruitment practices. Advertisement is to be nondiscriminatory in nature and must not indicate a hiring preference. Applications are to be job specific. During interviews, for example, the first-line manager cannot inquire about arrest records unless driving is a job requirement and the questions focus only on driving performance as it relates to job outcomes.

An affirmative action officer is identified within each organization. This person oversees the preparation of the affirmative action plan and reviews advertising, recruiting, and selection documents and processes to ensure compliance. For example, the writing of policies on sexual harassment is the duty of the affirmative action officer. An EEOC statement is developed and used on written communications such as job position announcements and offi-

cial documents. Within an agency the first-line therapeutic recreation manager may be appointed as the department officer or liaison to the affirmative action office.

The Americans with Disabilities Act (ADA) of 1990 addresses discriminatory practices against persons with disabilities. Title I of this act presents employment criteria. A first-line manager must make reasonable accommodations to provide access for a qualified person to a position. This may include technology such as physical access at the site of employment and special hearing and/or reading equipment to do the job. Also, on- and off-site locations for training and development programs must be accessible.

The Family and Medical Leave Act of 1993 affects all public employers and private employers with 50 or more employees. When an employee has worked for an employer at least 12 months, the employer must provide eligible employees with up to 12 weeks of unpaid leave per 12 month period for child care, care of an immediate family member, and an employee's own serious health condition that precludes job performance. With this particular law the first-line manager's concern becomes establishing policies to ensure that the law is implemented fairly and making sure that service quality is retained during staff absences.

## Professional Standards

Laws and court decisions affect how first-line managers conduct staffing processes and what policies and procedures are developed to administer departments. Credentialing bodies and professional groups set standards that affect what managers include in job specifications. The minimal staff requirement delineated in professional standards of practice (ATRA, 1993; NTRS, 1995) for the therapeutic recreation specialists is state licensure and/or certification with the National Council for Therapeutic Recreation Certification (NCTRC). Additionally, the department plan of operation is to require periodic reviews that ensure minimum standards of practice are being met and continuing education and development to maintain competencies and certification are taking place. NCTRC (1995) defines the bachelor's degree with minimal credit hours in recreation, therapeutic recreation coursework, and supportive content courses. A culminating internship with a minimal number of clock hours and length of time under a CTRS is the eligibility criteria for the entry-level certification exam. Upon successful completion of the exam, certification extends for five years with annual renewal maintenance fees. Following the five-year period, accumulation of experience and/or educational hours or successful reexamination ensures recertification. The first-line manager may elect to include the requirement of state licensure, CTRS certification, or eligibility to sit for the CTRS exam as job specifications. If this course of action is taken, the manager must relate job KSAs, job responsibilities and dimensions reported in the NCTRC job analysis. (See Appendix B for full discussion of the national certification program administered by NCTRC.)

Professional practice documents refer to therapeutic recreation specialists that maintain their competency through experience and education while adhering to policies, procedures, and clinical privileges where appropriate (ATRA, 1993; NTRS, 1995). Where credentials specify minimal professional expectations, privileging identifies specific agency or department practice requirements. A privileging plan sets minimal employment criteria such as possession of the CTRS credential, CPR, first aid, and experience(s) in specific settings. These are considered provisional privileges. According to Hatfield (1991), when the probationary period is successfully completed, the new employee must display competence in specific department KSAs to gain full privileging rights and retain employment. Specific privileges are gained with higher or more specific levels of knowledge and training (e.g., assertiveness, stress management). Privileging is granted for a predetermined time period after which the employee must document the continuing competence essential to quality service delivery. A first-line manager in a clinical setting may include privileging criteria in job specifications. In a community setting, similar criteria may be listed without direct reference to privileging requirements. In both settings the use of professional credentials and specific privileging or performance criteria with the demonstration of ongoing competence requires that the manager continually ensure the relevance of job specifications to therapeutic recreation practice.

# Human Resource Planning

Proactive human resource planning requires the first-line manager to continually assess and reassess staffing needs. As managers probe ways not only to streamline but also to diversify consumer services, staffing patterns remain in flux to accommodate new and changing department goals. The manager assesses current human resources, considers future needs, and develops a plan to ensure that the right mix and number of personnel are in place to meet future goals. From review of updated personnel files and portfolios, the manager develops an inventory of staff KSAs including education, experience, training, languages spoken, credentials held and specialized skills (Robbins, 1995). From this inventory the manager discerns department talents and anticipates training and development needs.

Future needs are considered by comparing results of the inventory to the organization's goals and the department's objectives. What new or changing skills will therapeutic recreation specialists (TRSs) need in the future that they currently do not have and/or use? For instance, the decreasing length of stay in clinical settings and the increasing focus on inclusion in communities will continue to shape job specifications. TRSs will have to become adept at brief treatment, home-healthcare planning, wellness interventions, participatory management, and training recreators to incorporate individuals with disabilities into community services. What other dynamics will shape the future of health and human services and how will managers define future job tasks? After determining present capabilities and projecting future needs, the first-line manager estimates the types and levels of staff KSAs needed to address client services and continue to deliver safe quality services. The manager then outlines training and development needs and plans for hiring, retraining, and staff realignments.

## Job Descriptions

A manager develops job descriptions by clustering job tasks so work that accomplishes the objectives of the department is done. A job description describes what, how, and why a job is done. Descriptions are fluid; managers redevelop them to address the changing human resource needs of the unit. Job descriptions, as described by Robbins (1995), are formal documents considered fundamental to supervisory appraisals and need-for-training decisions. Additionally, job descriptions help staff learn their duties by clarifying the outcomes management expects. Edington and Griffith (1990) note that job descriptions also allow prospective employees to be self-selective as they consider alternative positions. For example, if they ascertain that their qualifications are not compatible with the description, they may decide not to apply. Collectively, job descriptions present a picture of the department's human resources to internal and external audiences (Grossman and Ray, 1989).

Job or position descriptions tend to be comprised of several parts (see Figure 13.1): position title and classification, superior and subordinate relationships, objective or job statement, general and specific responsibilities, duties to be performed, qualifications, and skills. The first-line manager works with the human resource division or specialist to design job descriptions that reflect professional criteria (e.g., CTRS and department privileging criteria or performance standards). O'Morrow (1995) describes the process organizations use to complete job evaluation studies in order to assign relative worth to job tasks so that each position is ranked or classified in relationship to every other organizational position. Results of these studies are also used to set salaries and ensure pay equity. Usually the job description lists a job class or position as well as unique qualifications which are sought.

## Figure 13.1 Job Description

Iowa Methodist Medical Center of the Central Iowa Health System
Des Moines, Iowa

**Employee Job Description**

Title _____Recreation Therapist_____ Job Code # _____0848_____
Exempt _Exempt Professional_____
Department Name & Number _____Recreation Therapy—#640_____

Prepared By _____ Approved By _____
                                                    Dept. Head        Vice President

Date Effective_____ Date Reviewed _____

*Primary Function and Relationships to Total Organization:*
The Recreation Therapist is responsible for promoting the development, maintenance, and expression of an appropriate leisure lifestyle plan as related to quality patient care.
*Reports To:*
Director of Recreation Therapy
*Supervises:*
Student affiliates, student nurses, and volunteers

*Job Functions*

1. Essential Functions and Frequency:
   a. Completes leisure assessment on patients and assists with establishment of realistic goals and objectives related to assessed patient needs. (Occasional to Frequent)
   b. Plans and conducts patient recreation programs, out trips, evening activities and facilitates team interrelationships. (Frequent)
   c. Evaluates patients' functional skills within the leisure lifestyle component, records observations, and reports findings at medical staff conferences. (Frequent)
   d. Organizes leisure resource information and provides leisure education related to community resource use. (Occasional)
   e. Provides input to the director regarding program development and participates in establishing and achieving departmental goals. (Occasional)
   f. Responds to physician, staff, and family member referrals for patient recreation needs throughout the medical center. (Occasional)

2. Other Functions:
   a. Compiles and records statistical data regarding patient participation in planned activities.
   b. Demonstrates knowledge regarding professional trends; attends professional meetings and seeks opportunities for professional growth.
   c. Demonstrates effective communication skills, both written and verbal, and maintains a positive working relationship with staff departmentally and throughout the medical center.
   d. Performs functions other than described above due to extenuating circumstances.

*Personal Specifications*

1. Qualifications/Experience:
   Completion of an internship in a clinical setting under supervision of a Certified Recreation Therapist.

***Figure continues on page 194***

**Figure 13.1 Continued**

2. Education:
   a. Must be certified at the Therapeutic Recreation Specialist level with National Council for Therapeutic Recreation Certification.
   b. Rehabilitation therapist must be willing to become certified as a communication assistant through training provided by the Head Trauma Team and the Speech and Hearing Department.
   c. Must be willing to obtain a chauffeur's license.
   d. Must have current CPR and First-Aid Certification or be willing to obtain both.

3. Mental/Cognitive Demands:
   a. Must have ability to coordinate aspects of a program toward a recognized goal and follow through with a plan. (Frequent)
   b. Must be able to interact well with various patients, staff members throughout the medical center, and the director. (Continuous)
   c. Demonstrate ability to express self well in written and verbal language. (Frequent)
   d. Demonstrate ability to function effectively during tense and emotional situations. (Occasional)

4. Physical Demands:
   a. Must pass a physical examination as required by the medical center. (Occasional)
   b. Must be able to handle patients in wheelchairs and do lifting as it pertains to various recreation activities. (Frequent)
   c. Must be able to move around the medical center as necessary. (Frequent)
   d. Typically moving about the center a minimum of five (5) hours of an eight-hour (8-hour) day. (Continuous)
   e. Lifting up to 50 pounds. (Occasionally)
   f. Lifting up to 25 pounds. (Frequently)

5. Working Conditions:
   a. Working varied hours, weekends, and holidays as necessary to meet patient needs. (Occasional)
   b. Must be able to cope with working in various temperatures (i.e., summer heat during planned outings). (Occasional)
   c. May be required to work in an environment where patient smoking is allowed. (Occasional)
   d. Involvement in patient care may result in unavoidable work-related injury or illness. (Occasional)
   e. Works with patients/families who may be verbally abusive or physically violent. (Occasional)

## *Job Specifications*

Job specifications detail job descriptions. The specific minimum acceptable KSAs needed to effectively perform a given job are identified. Robbins (1995) suggests the job specification is the standard against which applicants are compared. Since the description is used as a recruitment notice, information on application deadlines, procedures, and materials to submit are listed. Job specifications, however, may also include salary information, benefits, work conditions, employment date, and specific duties. In practice, subtle differences unique to each setting exist between job descriptions and job specifications (see Figure 13.2).

The first-line manager in smaller organizations may prepare job specifications and receive applications when positions open. In larger agencies the first-line therapeutic recreation manager may assist the human resource department or specialist in the preparation of job specifications. When this occurs, materials are submitted to the human resource department or specialist who screens applications and forwards to the manager only those applications that satisfy the preferred specifications.

When positions do open, the position may be reevaluated to determine the necessity of the position in the achievement of department objectives and agency goals. The evaluation study may result in salary adjustments and/or job reclassification. Consequently, positions are eliminated, temporarily not filled, and duties are reassigned with or without salary adjustments. If jobs are reclassified, the manager reexamines the effectiveness of the structure to achieve desired outcomes and determines the appropriate mix and number of needed staff.

## Recruiting Process

With completion of the inventory, job description, and job specification, the manager is ready to prepare a plan to recruit applicants who meet the department's human resource

## Figure 13.2 Job Specifications

Title: Recreation Service Area Coordinator—Therapeutic Recreation

*General Statement of Duties*
The Recreation Service Area Coordinator (Therapeutic Recreation) Supervises Division of Therapeutic Recreation with the operation and personnel management of all special population programs. This employee develops, organizes and implements programs designed to offer services to the Community in accordance with the policies of the Recreation Commission and the Division of which the service area is a part.

*Examples of Work Performed*
- Required to prepare and monitor the budget for all Therapeutic Recreation programs and services by gathering data and information and organizing it into a format to be interpreted by the District supervisor.
- Maintain records and accounts of attendance, inventories, financial charges and receipts and other matters requiring systematic recordkeeping.
- Supervises administrative (Therapeutic Recreation Community Center Director II), clerical, contract and part-time personnel (i.e., personnel evaluations, attendance control, training, motivation).
- Required to recruit, hire, train, and evaluate part-time and contract personnel.
- Required to evaluate service area programs for quantity and quality as they relate to the standards of practice for Therapeutic Recreation service.
- Maintain cooperative working relationships with public and private agencies serving the disabled (i.e., Special Olympics, United Cerebral Palsy, Stepping Stones Center for Developmental Disabilities, Board of Mental Retardation).
- Works with the service area advisory council on a regularly scheduled basis to identify recreational needs of the disabled.
- Assures that therapeutic recreation programs are offered for all disabilities, age ranges and skill levels.
- Assists District Supervisor in setting service area goals as they relate to the departmental goals established on an annual basis by the Cincinnati Recreation Commission.
- Maintains specialized equipment in proper and safe working condition.
- Identifies and reports maintenance needs in facilities where therapeutic recreation programs take place.
- Interprets Civil Service Rules, City Personnel Policies and Procedures, and Departmental Rules and Regulations for service area employees.
- Investigates and resolves all complaints and problems involving service area operations, program members or staff.
- Required to hold regular meetings with service area staff to discuss ongoing activities and keep them informed of changes that affect programs.
- Handles service area emergencies quickly and effectively (i.e., staff replacements, investigation of accidents and injuries, follow-up on safety measures).
- Required to develop and present training courses to service area personnel.
- Provides periodic training sessions for other Community Activities Division personnel on programming for special populations.
- Performs related duties, as required.

*Examples of Knowledge, Abilities, Skills and Personal Characteristics*
Knowledge of:
- Policies and Procedures of the Recreation Department.
- Emergency, safety procedures.
- Basic management techniques, goal setting.
- Principles of supervision.
- Basic accounting and bookkeeping fundamentals.
- Community resources, existing support agencies providing services for the disabled.
- Core program of the Therapeutic Division/Community Activities Division.
- Theory, practice and administration of Therapeutic Recreation Programming.
- Disabilities and the implications for Therapeutic Recreation service to disabled individuals.

*Figure continues on page 196*

**Figure 13.2 Continued**

- Therapeutic Recreation techniques such as assessment, activity analysis and activity adaptations.
- Accessibility guidelines and architectural barriers.
- Normalization principles.
- Physical and behavioral sciences.

Ability to:
- Establish work priorities.
- Determine area staff and equipment requirements.
- Monitor an assigned budget and determine work schedules of staff.
- Facilitate staff/volunteer/area advisory council meetings.
- Provide training where needed.
- Maintain a professional manner in stressful situations.
- Work as a team member with area staff, peers, support agencies, and community groups.
- Perform basic statistical functions.
- Plan appropriate programs for targeted populations.
- Mobilize human resources.
- Interview and assess abilities of job applicants.
- Facilitate problem solving at the area level.
- Assist area staff in designing programs for special populations.
- Review and assess the extent to which activities and services are meeting needs and interests of area's special populations.

*Required Education and/or Experience*
Graduation from college with a degree in recreation with an emphasis in Therapeutic Recreation and five (5) years of experience directing community recreation programs for special populations.

**or**

Graduation from college in a related field (i.e., special education, psychology, sociology, rehabilitation counseling) and six (6) years of experience directing community recreation programs for special populations.

**or**

Graduation from college with a Masters Degree in Recreation with an emphasis in Therapeutic Recreation and three (3) years of experience directing community recreation programs for special populations.

**or**

Graduation from college with a Masters Degree in a related field (i.e., special education, psychology, sociology, rehabilitation counseling) and four (4) years of experience directing community recreation programs for special populations.

*Note:* Community Recreation Programs for special populations are those having a target population of adults or children with physical, mental or emotional handicaps which are staged in a community center, playground, day camp, YMCA, etc. This does not include those programs at institutions such as hospitals, psychiatric or educational institutions.

*Note:* Candidates must be eligible for Certification by the National Council for Therapeutic Recreation Certification.

needs. Identification of resources available to make potential applicants aware of position openings is the first task. As these resources are identified, the manager considers employment variables such as salary, geographic location, culture of the organization, and local community (Edington and Griffith, 1990). To illustrate, as reported by O'Morrow (1995), a CTRS presently employed in the Northeast or Pacific regions might find the salary ranges and fringe benefits of the Great Lakes or Southeast less attractive. Consequently, advertisements in national professional publications targeting applicants in different regions might not be as effective as intraregional flyers, state, and regional conference announcements. Selection of recruitment sources considers marketing costs as well as those variables that affect whether applicants will be attracted to particular openings.

Recruitment resources rely on both internal and external audiences. Internal searches are preferred by some managers because they are more likely to have access to detailed candidate information and the opportunity may be viewed by their staff as a career advancement or professional development option. With organizational structures becoming flatter and creating limited career ladders in therapeutic recreation, external searches rather than lateral transfers are probable. Managers consider variables that attract candidates as well as the type of position or level of responsibility for which applicants are being recruited. For example, a first-line manager's position is more likely to appear in the American Therapeutic Recreation Association (ATRA) or the National Recreation and Park Association (NRPA) placement bulletins than in a local newspaper. Entry-level CTRS positions, however, are likely to be advertised in the local newspaper as well as national professional bulletins. Robbins (1995) suggests upper level positions that require more specialized skills, experiences, and training are more widely recruited.

Individuals likely to perform effectively are usually found through direct contacts, recommendations from current employees, and/or referrals from colleagues in other therapeutic recreation agencies. Establishing ties with colleges and universities by serving on advisory committees, guest lecturing, and providing field visit opportunities or internship supervision links managers with students seeking entry-level positions. Alumni are also a good referral source. Placing announcements in professional organization bulletins, newsletters, and journals allows a wide audience of experienced professionals contemplating position changes to be reached. Professional convention job marts can attract both new recruits and experienced applicants. Unsolicited "walk-ins" whether by letter, phone, fax, or in person are prospective applicants. Even if there are no openings at the time of contact, applications are kept on file in anticipation of future vacancies. Persons seeking to relocate from one region of the country to another use professional employment services and/or make direct contacts through professional association directories. College bulletin boards and career centers are also resources for persons relocating from one area of the country to another. Word of mouth through professional networks continues to be a widely used source of employment opportunities.

The time frame available to recruit influences the selection of recruiting media. In some instances, searches remain "open until filled." These job announcements are likely to read "open until filled with screening commencing on . . . date." Organization policies also specify recruiting time frames. For example, in public agencies the vacated position must be left open for two weeks before advertisements are posted. Once posted, applications are requested for a two-week period. The fiscal year and budget conditions result in recruiting delays (e.g., positions are filled after the new fiscal year commences). Funds allotted to recruitment also influence the length of time positions

are advertised and sources used to notify potential applicants of position openings.

## Screening and Selecting

Recruitment results in a pool of potential applicants. The size of the pool, the nature of the position, and the size of the organization and department influence the manager's role in screening and selection decisions. A number of preliminary reviews are introduced and search committees are formed to ensure comprehensive objective applicant assessments. The manager coordinates with human resource personnel to define screening criteria and to facilitate objective on-site selection procedures.

### Preliminary Screening

In the absence of a perfect method to select candidates, first-line managers tend to use a variety of screening methods to identify the most appropriate candidate. Traditional methods have included application forms, resumes and portfolios, written and performance-simulation tests, interviews, and background examinations. According to Robbins (1995), use of a number of selection devices is intended to reduce accept and reject errors. An accept error is the selection of a candidate who subsequently performs poorly on the job, while a reject error is rejecting a candidate who would later have been successful on the job. In either situation, the outcome is costly because direct service time is ultimately lost and recruiting and screening are time consuming and expensive. A correct decision is made when the applicant is predicted to be successful on the performance criteria used to evaluate therapeutic recreation specialists. Robbins (1995) notes that a correct decision also occurs when applicants are predicted to be unsuccessful and would not meet expectations if hired. Thus, the first-line manager chooses those screening methods that are most likely to predict which applicants will be successful if hired.

Screening methods must be valid, reliable, and in compliance with legal and legislative directives. Valid methods demonstrate a relationship between the screening tool and job performance. For example, experience with documentation and assessments is a valid screening method to use in Commission on Accreditation of Rehabilitation Facilities (CARF) and Joint Commission on Accreditation of Healthcare Organizations (JCAHO) accredited settings where staff must complete these tasks. Likewise, skill proficiency in the use of wheelchairs and mobility aides is a valid screening method employed by community special recreation associations. Reliable screening tools yield consistent results. In other words, the characteristics being measured are considered to remain stable over time. Eubanks (1991) suggests the use of structured interviews to identify whether candidates' values and beliefs are compatible with organizational processes. If a consensus is not reached about the candidate's "organizational fit" after interviews by a number of different staff, the degree of reliability of the interview as a screening tool in this instance would be questioned. As screening methods are selected, Spencer (1994) suggests the manager also consider factors such as cost, time, ease of administration, interpretation of results, and staff capability to administer and use the selection methods and results.

The first screening step is to determine who is minimally qualified to perform the duties required in a particular position. It may neither be cost nor time effective to interview and test each applicant, so the manager uses application forms, resumes or portfolios, and/or background information to establish which candidates possess minimally desired qualifications. Weighing or rating systems are designed to assess information presented by applicants. Established criteria reflect job relatedness. For example, experience with aging adults with strokes would be weighted higher than would experience with well elderly when the manager is hiring for a rehabilitation unit whereas the opposite would be true if the position were in a community senior center. An applicant who possesses the CTRS and CLP credentials might be given higher ratings than the applicant who has yet to be declared eligible to sit for either exam if the manager chooses to tie the job responsibilities tested by each exam to the respective job tasks of the open position. To comply with legal directives, Grossman and Ray (1989) note it is the manager's responsibility to use and design methods that gather information related to *bona fide* position qualifications and to establish who is minimally expected to perform successfully.

## Application Forms

Application forms are one of the more traditional screening tools. The form should have sufficient questions to gain a picture of the applicant's potential but not be too lengthy as to discourage application completion. When the parent organization requires information irrelevant to the therapeutic recreation department, length may become an issue; conversely, the organization form may be so brief that the first-line therapeutic recreation manager must use a supplementary form. The form may be as brief as to require only name, address, phone, and emergency contacts or be as detailed as to require comprehensive profiles on education, experience, references, and KSAs related to particular therapeutic recreation positions. Grossman and Ray (1989) caution the manager to avoid questions that might be perceived as discriminatory (e.g., date of birth, sex, age, religion, maiden name, number of children, nationality, handicap, credit rating) as the application is designed.

## Resumes and Portfolios

Resumes and portfolios provide detailed information on applicants' qualifications. Resumes may precede, accompany or follow application submission. Managers may review unsolicited resumes then send an application to those who appear qualified. This practice serves as an initial screening and cost savings as the processing of each application might involve review by a human resource specialist to ensure compliance with EEOC. Another scenario finds job descriptions written so that potential applicants request an application then submit the completed application form with a resume, portfolio materials, reference sources, and actual reference letters. When this procedure is followed, the intent is twofold: (1) to determine if the applicant is truly interested in the position as demonstrated by actual follow-through, and (2) to ascertain the applicant's ability to follow procedures. When resumes accompany applications, the human resource specialist and manager compare documents to determine if gaps need clarification or explanations require more detail and to assess how thoroughly the documents have been prepared and submitted. This also permits simultaneous review for EEOC and therapeutic recreation expectations by those most qualified to conduct the assessments. A third scenario finds submission of a resume and/or portfolio materials upon managerial request following preliminary screening of application forms. This approach, as with the first, conserves time because the manager only reviews documents of applicants who have met minimal qualifications.

Managers study resumes and portfolio materials such as work samples, goal statements, and personal philosophies to determine depth and scope of qualifications in relationship to human resource needs and the professional practices of the department. These sources are considered to ascertain qualities and characteristics related to job performance such as organization, accuracy, neatness, completeness, professional presence, and thoroughness. Qualities such as adaptability, professionalism, and ability to function as a team member are judged by studying the number of reported continuing education units (CEUs) and professional development activities and evidence presented about collaborative activities. Resumes and portfolios are tools used to predict the likelihood of job success.

## Background Data

Background data are a third category of preliminary screening information. Application forms, resumes, portfolios, and contacts managers make as potential applicants are referred serve as primary sources of background information. Verification of application information is a fact-finding process. Job tasks completed in former positions are indicators of future job performance. The reliability of the applicant's information is ascertained at this stage.

Caution is advised, however, with information garnered from reference checks. Professional colleagues can confirm the applicant's commitment to therapeutic recreation but may not be able to report the applicant's individual work style and behaviors. In weighing the validity of information gained from personal references, the manager considers the length and nature of the applicant's relationship with the informant. It is an ethical responsibility to gain first written permission from the applicant and then secure reference information from the present employer. Even with permission, disclosure of information about the applicant's intent violates confidentiality and could impact future career options. Background investigations help the manager clarify past practices and future directions. Insight into why job changes have occurred or what needs the applicant might have from the community or geographic region where the anticipated job is located are gained from these searches.

Managers may have the opportunity to involve staff in preliminary and subsequent screening activities. In smaller agencies the therapeutic recreation manager and full- and part-time employees are more likely to carry out the entire selection process. If materials are mailed directly to a human resource department or personnel specialist, preliminary screening is conducted at this level with or without input from the manager and therapeutic recreation staff. Those who meet minimal qualifications such as the possession of a bachelor's degree, CTRS or CLP credential, and specific population and setting experience make up the *applicant pool*. The weighing or rating system prepared with human resource support is then used by the manager and/or staff to identify *top* candidates from the pool to participate in on-site screening. Several candidates may come simultaneously for comprehensive assessments, or each candidate may be invited beginning with the candidate who has received the highest reviews. When this procedure is followed, and the top candidate does not accept the invitation, the candidate with the next highest evaluation in the applicant pool is brought on site. This process continues until either the position is filled or the process terminated, and the search is reopened under new guidelines.

## On-Site Screening

On-site screening consists primarily of individual and/or group interviews, and performance simulation tests. In some instances, health tests are necessary to satisfy insurance benefit criteria contained in the compensation package. In public agencies such as municipal leisure service departments, employees are required to take civil service tests. Test questions are developed from site-specific job specifications and existing professional standards such as the NCTRC exam content outline (NCTRC, 1995). Tests are administered periodically through the human resource department. Therapeutic recreation managers serve as con-

tent experts for a personnel specialist who ensures compliance with legal mandates, test validity, and reliability standards. Applicants are ranked by score results. Agency-wide policies then determine who is selected for on-site interviews.

### Performance Tests

Performance tests require candidates to demonstrate work-related skills such as computer assessments, incident reporting, and writing client treatment or activity plans. Staff request that candidates use client data to complete desired forms. Candidates also may be asked to participate in role-playing situations like those that occur as services are delivered (e.g., assisting caregivers and clients with community leisure resource awareness or leisure family planning). First-line managers may have their staff and colleagues from other units and the community critique candidate performance according to the preset weighing or rating systems.

### Interviews

Interviews, like application forms, are a universal screening criteria. The interview process is planned. Significance of the position, number of candidates, and the time devoted to interviewing procedures will affect the interview approach. Regardless of the approach used, each interviewee should have, as nearly as possible, the same interview experience. A uniform rating procedure is used by all interviewers to document responses to each question or category of questions. Edington and Griffith (1990) suggest that interview questions determine if the candidate (1) has the KSAs to perform the expected duties, (2) would fit with others in the department, (3) displays the demeanor and other behaviors consistent with the organization's policies, and (4) has the qualifications reported on preliminary screening documents. The interview brings the candidate into the work environment and community culture. These factors can influence career decisions. Consequently, managers plan for the interviewee to become acquainted with features of the entire system.

A direct or pattern approach to the interview involves each candidate responding to the same set of questions. Following completion of all interviews, raters compare interviewee responses to each question. Edington and Griffith (1990) note this approach is reliable and minimizes interviewer bias. Open-ended questions are used in nondirect interviews. This approach may lead to a more comprehensive awareness of the candidates' qualities but is time consuming and not as reliable as pattern interviews. A third approach, group interviews, involves several candidates appearing before interviewers sequentially or simultaneously. This does create a degree of interviewee discomfort, but it enables the manager to discern responsiveness to "team-like" situations.

Planning an interview, therefore, involves preparation of questions and arranging for the on-site visit. Robbins (1995) suggests that interview questions should provide insight into the candidate's education, work experience, abilities, and motivation. As interview questions are developed, certain considerations should be kept in mind:

- Prepare open-ended questions rather than "yes" or "no" response items.
- Develop inquiries that begin with how or why which tend to result in more explicative responses.
- Avoid questions that lead to telegraphic responses (e.g., Would you agree that you have qualities supportive of teamwork?).
- Avoid bipolar questions that require respondents to choose from two alternatives (e.g., Do you prefer working with clients individually or in group sessions?).
- Develop questions that clarify background data rather than repeat factual information presented on applications, resumes, and portfolios.
- Encourage the interviewee to elaborate on areas where there appear to be gaps in information (e.g., You appear to have experiences in . . . interventions. How will you gain experience in . . . interventions used with this particular clientele?).

Examples of specific questions that exemplify the suggested question preparation criteria and that might be used to gain insight into the education, work experience, abilities, and motivations of applicants are presented here:

- How did your education prepare you for this position?
- What are some reasons why you selected recreation therapy as a major?
- What have you done in previous positions to demonstrate teamwork, discharge planning, leisure education?
- What are some outcomes of service delivery you have focused on in previous positions and what were the experiences selected to meet these goals?
- What were objectives in the performance appraisal process or professional development plans in previous positions and why or why not were they achieved?
- How and why is therapeutic recreation significant to the health, functional well-being, and quality of life of persons with disabilities?
- What specific therapeutic recreation skills will you bring to direct client supervision?
- What abilities acquired through previous work experience will help you perform successfully in this position?

- What are your plans for self-development during the coming year?
- Choose a song, poem, novel, video, movie, or person that reflects your character and explain why.
- Where do you see yourself, careerwise, in three years?
- Why should I hire you?

When the manager involves staff in interviews, each question should be asked by the same interviewer and in the same sequence with each applicant. The rating or weighing of responses occurs as quickly as possible after the interview and is done independently. Note taking during the interview is kept to a minimum. Interviewers complete their notes, rate responses to each question, and then collectively study results of analyzed ratings. Managers prepare their staff for interviews by coaching them on how to apply the rating criteria, when and what to document, and how to observe interviewee statements made during and immediately following the interview.

Another preparation step is to set up a schedule for the on-site visit. When managers interview one candidate at a time, the concern is to sequence the visit so that all staff and organization personnel who need to meet the candidate have an opportunity to do so. The manager must also make certain that the candidate has enough time to explore community concerns (e.g., housing, recreational opportunities). When all or most candidates are to be scheduled over several days or in one time frame, the manager ensures consistency with each candidate's schedule and plans staffing schedules to minimize service interruptions. Confidentiality becomes an issue when group interviews are scheduled. The manager plans for this through scheduling and discussion with candidates prior to the on-site visit.

The first-line manager sets the tone of the interview through opening comments and introductions. The intent is to relax the applicant and to establish rapport. Additionally, the manager identifies what topics are to be discussed, how long the interview will take, and how the questioning will proceed. A brief orientation to the agency, therapeutic recreation service, and the position follows. Opening questions relate back to already presented background information so that the interviewee feels confident to respond to further questioning. The manager uses probes, repetition, and paraphrasing to gain insight into how the applicant's KSAs relate to the job specifications. Silence also encourages response. The manager concludes the interview by asking the interviewee if there are any details about the position, organization, or community that require clarification. Additionally, the manager identifies the next step in the hiring process (e.g., when a decision will be made, how the notification will occur, and what follow-up steps might be required of the candidate).

The manager and staff are alert to remarks made after concluding the interview when applicants relax and present true impressions. During and following the interview, observation of gestures, mannerisms, and nonverbal cues may provide the manager with valuable clues about the applicant's "fit." Documentation of verbal and nonverbal responses and behaviors establishes if the candidate is qualified and likely to perform successfully in the position if hired. Grossman and Ray (1989) suggest one of the best predictors of future work patterns is past performance. Consequently, throughout the interview and review of applicant materials, the manager assesses relatedness of previous work characteristics to demands of the position to be filled.

## Selecting

Selection and rejection are the final steps in the screening process. This may be difficult since each candidate brings unique qualities to the position. When qualifications of several candidates appear equal, the ability to fit into the department and meet future human resource needs are deciding factors. Although the first-line manager is responsible for the hiring decision, it is wise to work through staff and upper level management to gain consensus and support. This is especially true if the new employee will be working with other organization employees and representing the department at agency events.

Notice to the selected candidate precedes rejection notification to unsuccessful candidates. In the case that a selected candidate rejects the offer, the door remains open to offer the position to the next most qualified candidate. A reasonable deadline is allowed for acceptance or rejection so that the manager is able to contact the next candidate without alerting him or her that he or she is not the first choice. Individuals who are seriously considered but not hired are possible candidates for future positions. If applicants are unlikely to be considered again, a personal letter explaining why their qualifications did not satisfy the job specifications is a professional courtesy. Documentation from all candidate screening is retained in the event questions about hiring and rejection decisions arise in the future.

Compensation is negotiated and finalized with selection of a successful candidate. Job specifications usually identify a starting salary range commensurate with the applicant's qualifications. Additionally, a benefits package includes insurance, retirement, leave of absence, vacations, holidays, professional development incentives and other fringe benefits. A therapeutic recreation manager usually makes the decision about the exact amount of the starting salary while human resources presents the organization's alternative benefits packages. Whether or not the candidate elects to accept the offer may be deter-

mined by his or her perception of the total package and factors outside the actual offer (e.g., geographic location, community resources). Consequently, the manager is aware that extraneous factors may determine whether or not a candidate accepts or rejects a particular offer.

The likelihood exists that the top-rated candidates may decline the offers. When this occurs, Grossman and Ray (1989) advise that it is better to reinstitute the recruitment and selection process than to employ a therapeutic recreator who will be a liability to the department. It is also possible that those involved in making selection recommendations to the manager may not agree or come to a consensus on the preferred candidate. The manager's challenge is to create a work environment supportive of each new employee. Team building strategies can be used to dissipate differing opinions. Also, reference to objective performance criteria in job specifications validates management decisions.

# Probationary Periods

Organizations use probationary periods to confirm that a proper mix or match has been made. These periods vary from several weeks to a few months. This variation is due to the size of the organization and the position level. Usually the larger the organization and the more responsible the position the longer the period. During this period suitability of the new employee to the position and the position to the new employee is determined. Is the employee likely to perform successfully as a continuing member of the department? To predict the likelihood of success managers incorporate personnel training, development, and evaluation processes into this orientation period. A new employee is introduced to position duties, trained in site-specific practices, and evaluated on service outcomes. Compatibility between the manager and employee is ascertained as the new employee is coached in the design of an individual development plan and becomes familiar with the department privileging and/or performance expectations. Managers use the new employee's development objectives and performance criteria from position specifications to evaluate progress toward performing the job tasks of the newly acquired position.

A candidate who does not perform successfully or appears unlikely to be able to develop the KSAs in the job specification is not selected for the position. If the manager documents behaviors or performance that do not satisfy expectations, the candidate is released prior to or at the end of the probationary period. A candidate may voluntarily elect not to remain as an employee and terminate the probationary experience. The intent of the probationary period is to enhance the probability of making a correct decision rather than either an accept or reject error.

# Staffing Issues

Several issues affect recruiting and screening processes. What the manager may say and do during candidate selection is governed by a number of laws, court decisions, and executive orders that affect the staffing process. Managers must ensure job relatedness of questions and statements. In therapeutic or caring relationships personal qualities and subjective characteristics such as empathy and active listening skills are perceived as essential yet may not be listed as specific job tasks. Consequently, asking a candidate a direct question about his or her abilities to be empathetic might be perceived by the candidate as inappropriate. Therefore, the manager develops simulation or role-playing scenarios to assess these types of communication skills to ensure the screening activities remain job related.

Another issue is the job relatedness of credentials such as the CTRS and CLP. Is a person with these credentials likely to be more successful than the individual without the credentials? Although the competencies covered by the exams have been tied to job responsibilities, research has yet to link the competencies with indicators of quality in service outcomes. The same analogy holds true for experience. Do two years of experience with developmentally delayed persons prepare a candidate to complete the therapeutic recreation process in behavioral medicine? Further, persons who have experienced injuries or have experience with family members with disabilities may seek employment in therapeutic recreation. Interview questions on medical background and family history are illegal. Are these experiences relevant to the ability to perform as a therapeutic recreator?

While experiencing continuous change, health and human services are also undergoing major scrutiny. Quality services are expected within contained costs. Are today's staff KSAs relevant to future delivery approaches? Predicting successful performance is, therefore, an issue of the present and the future. The manager's dilemma is to recruit staff capable of performing the job tasks and adapting to future human resource needs. What combination of screening methods is predictive of present and future job success? While it is desirable to plan for future human resource needs, the task is formidable.

Recruiting is costly and time consuming. Which source attracts the most qualified pool of applicants in a timely manner? Word of mouth through professional networks is a common referral practice. Each candidate undergoes a similar screening process, but the politics of acknowledging a referral contributes to manager discomfort when the desire is to maintain professional relationships and access to future candidates. Employee's friends and contacts are potential applicant pools. The manager's task is to ensure that the screening process remains bias free. Training em-ployees to complete objective ratings reinforces the importance of fairness in staffing decisions.

When a manager works with human resource departments or specialists to screen applicants, the manager is the content or field expert while the specialist is the process or technical expert. The relationship a manager has with the department or specialist affects the degree of input managers have as each screening step is undertaken. When mutual respect and confidence exist, the therapeutic recreation manager is likely to be involved from the onset. Thus when the applicant pool is complete, desired therapeutic recreation KSAs are evident in each candidate's materials. Although cumbersome and sometimes time consuming, operating without assistance and clearance from specialists and EEOC personnel can place hiring decisions in jeopardy.

Assurance of the proper mix and number of competent staff rests with the first-line manager. The probationary period is a critical supervisory period, and experiences or patterns are valid predictors of future performance. Thus, behaviors and performance during this period are not to be overlooked or excused as "new employee" errors. Managers and employees take this probationary period more seriously when identifying staff training needs in a personal development plan is a goal. In public agencies probationary employees can be dismissed without adhering to the traditional termination steps. Therefore, it is actually easier to let a probationary employee go than to terminate an employee after successful completion of the probationary period. The tendency of many is to presume the selection process is final when an offer is accepted. Yet, in reality, the selection is finalized with demonstration of the KSAs expected of a successful therapeutic recreation specialist during the probationary period.

# Summary

Every first-line manager will be involved in staffing decisions. The nature of this involvement depends on whether the parent organization has a human resource department or specialist. In small organizations therapeutic recreation managers conduct recruiting and screening with consultation from a personnel specialist. In large organizations, however, the human resource department oversees and guides hiring practices. A manager is the content specialist while the personnel specialist gives technical and legal assistance. A therapeutic recreation manager, therefore, needs to not only be aware of the qualifications and performance expectations of therapeutic recreation specialists' positions but also those standards and practices that impact how recruiting and screening are conducted. Ultimately, the first-line manager is responsible for selecting persons who are likely to perform successfully on the job. This chapter covered material on the standards that affect recruiting and screening and the methods and sources a manager uses to ensure an appropriate mix of human resources to deliver safe quality services.

A number of laws, court decisions, and executive orders have been enacted that influence recruiting and screening processes and decisions. These include the National Labor Relations Act, Labor-Management Relations Act, Equal Pay Act, Civil Rights Act (Title VII), Age Discrimination in Employment Act, Equal Employment Opportunity Act, Americans with Disabilities Act, and the Family and Medical Leave Act. Professional standards of practice and credentialing bodies recommend qualifications that therapeutic recreation managers may choose to include in job specifications. The issue for the manager becomes establishing the job-relatedness of the credentials (i.e., CTRS, CLP) and the recommended experience and educational standards (i.e., ATRA, 1993; NTRS, 1995). Privileging protocols use these criteria as entry-level expectations with site specific standards added to ensure competency maintenance.

The manager plans for present and future human resource needs which change with the evolving directions of health and human services. As the manager develops job descriptions, an inventory of present staff KSAs and training and development needs is completed. This permits the manager to select candidates that have talents and capabilities to adapt to future transitions. Job evaluation studies also help the manager to develop job specifications.

As a recruiting plan is developed, the manager considers those variables such as salary, organization, and community culture that might influence one's decision to apply for a particular position. Recruiting materials are designed to target specific audiences. Job specification content is used to develop recruiting announcements. Word of mouth and personal referrals tend to be effective methods of recruitment. Other sources include colleges and universities, professional job bulletins and conferences, professional contacts and networks, and various public news media.

Because no singular screening method has been found to result in selection of the "right" candidate, a number of methods or tools tend to be used during the selection process: application forms, resumes and portfolios, background checks, tests, and interviews. The first three are used to form applicant pools. Tests and interviews are costly and time consuming. Usually the finalists are asked to complete performance simulations and interviews with staff and management. Final selections occur after probationary periods of varying lengths are completed. Screening methods must be valid, reliable, job-related, and objective. Weighing and rating systems are developed to factor each screening tool into the final decision.

The probationary period is the final opportunity to assess compatibility and the proper staff mix. During this period the manager supervises training, development, and evaluation processes so that the final decision is correct and not an accept or reject error.

Issues arise throughout the staffing process. The manager's challenge is to ensure the best staff mix. Any decisions made must be tied to job relatedness. When CTRS or a bachelor's degree in therapeutic recreation are listed as job specifications, the manager documents the relationship between service quality and outcomes and the competencies represented by these criteria. This chapter also considered how a manager adjusts for the possible bias introduced when colleagues refer potential applicants or friends of current employees apply.

# Discussion Questions

1. Identify and summarize the laws and professional standards of practice impacting staffing processes and decisions.
2. What are the primary steps in human resource planning?
3. Describe the contents of job descriptions and job specifications. What is the relationship between the two?
4. What are primary recruiting methods and what factors does the manager consider as they are used?
5. What are the primary screening techniques and how is each used in relationship to each of the others?
6. What are predictors of a "proper" fit and how does a manager factor these into a final decision?
7. Summarize the issues a manager faces as staffing processes and decisions are carried out.

# References

American Therapeutic Recreation Association (ATRA). (1993). *Standards for the practice of therapeutic recreation and self-assessment guide.* Hattiesburg, MS: Author.

Connolly, P. (1993). Balancing changing healthcare needs with the shortage of quality healthcare professionals: Implications for therapeutic recreation. *Loss, Grief & Care, 6:4,* 15–22.

Edington, C. R., and Griffith, C. A. (1990). *The recreation and leisure service delivery system.* Dubuque, IA: Wm. C. Brown Publishers.

Eubanks, P. (1991). Hospitals probe candidates' values for organizational "fit." *Hospitals, 65:20,* 36, 38.

Grossman, A. H., and Ray, M. B. (1989). Recruiting and selecting professional personnel. In A. H. Grossman (Ed.), *Personnel management in recreation and leisure services* (pp. 91–116). Reston, VA: American Alliance for Health, Physical Education, Recreation, and Dance.

Hatfield, R. (1991). Credentialing and privileging in therapeutic recreation: Practical professional necessities. In B. Riley (Ed.), *Quality management applications for therapeutic recreation* (pp. 163–172). Hattiesburg, MA: American Therapeutic Recreation Association.

Murrell, D. S., Dwyer, W. O., Murrell, P. A., and Coleman, L. K. (1992). The civil rights act and parks and recreation. *Parks and Recreation, 27:11,* 58, 61–62.

National Council for Therapeutic Recreation Certification (NCTRC). (1995). *Candidate handbook.* Thiells, NY: Author.

National Therapeutic Recreation Society (NTRS). (1995). *Standards of practice for therapeutic recreation services and annotated bibliography.* Arlington, VA: Author.

O'Morrow, G. S. (1995). *Therapeutic recreation practitioner analysis, 1994.* Arlington, VA: National Therapeutic Recreation Society.

Robbins, S. P. (1995). *Supervision today.* Englewood Cliffs, NJ: Prentice Hall.

Spencer, A. (1994). The right choice. *Nursing Times, 90:5,* 59–61.

# Part 4

# Human Service Management

# Chapter 14

# Effective Communication

## Introduction

People communicate even when they do not speak. The hallmark of an effective manager is effective communication which is a complex process that requires skills on individual, group, and organizational levels. Managers participate in formal and informal communication, and the size of the organization influences the quality and formality of the communication. As a change agent, the manager's role is facilitative and integrative. Through communication the manager shares information and accesses resources so that others perform effectively to deliver quality services. The intent of this chapter is to explore communication from an individual perspective as a supervisor or at the group level and within the organization.

What is successful communication? Is it overcoming resistance to change, gaining staff cooperation, negotiating higher salaries, and handling criticism? The first section of this chapter explores personal and interpersonal communication skills. As noted by Austin (1997), one must have basic interpersonal communication skills to perform as an effective helper. People communicate using a number of methods, yet even during personal interactions, barriers arise. The first portion of this chapter reviews strategies and techniques that foster effective interpersonal communication.

The authors consider the relationship of effective communication as part of managerial roles and functions in the second portion of this chapter. Supervisory-subordinate relationships emanate from the "authority" position of the manager. Yet paradigm shifts in management to participatory styles affect communication between first-line managers and employees. Managers seldom see the end of a change event because they are busy and their work is fragmented. Information is transmitted orally and through a variety of media to accomplish goals of the department and organization. In addition to personal skills, managers use processes like delegation, negotiation, and collaboration to accomplish results.

In the concluding section of this chapter, communication within the organizational structure and as a professional representative of the organization and profession are explored. Within organizations formal and informal patterns of communication exist (Robbins, 1995). Protocols structure interactions. Barriers exist. Strategies that enhance organizational interactions also contribute to effective interpersonal and managerial communications that ensure employees have the information necessary to maintain and improve service quality. Therapeutic recreation managers represent their departments and organizations professionally. Interactions with associates, colleagues, clients, and caregivers leave an impression.

## Personal and Interpersonal Communication

The business of helping is a human enterprise that uses day-to-day communication skills. According to Austin (1997), the higher one's level of personal communication, the higher the potential to function effectively as a helping professional. The manager who does not communicate properly will have an ineffective department. Managers and therapists communicate formally and informally through a number of media. The intent of this communication is to share ideas, thoughts, or emotions with each other so the meaning of the content is understood by both. Liebler, Levine, and Rothman (1992) identify four pieces to the communication process: initiation, transmission, reception, and feedback. The sender begins interaction by transmitting the message formally or informally to a receiver. A receiver acts upon the message from a particular frame of reference through feedback. This feedback, according to Liebler, Levine, and Rothman (1992), acknowledges the information in the form of acceptance, nonacceptance, modification, or suppression. The effectiveness of communication is influenced overall by assumptions, perceptions, feelings, past experiences, present surroundings, and interpretations of the sender and receiver as well as the context in which the communication occurs. Understanding the ideas of others is essential to delivery of quality health and human services.

## Communication Avenues and Influences

In formal communication each party is aware of the avenues used, while in informal communication one or the other party is unaware of the avenues being used or that a message even exists. This latter form of communication is referred to as the grapevine or the political context of communication. As listed by Robbins (1995), formal communication takes place through verbal and nonverbal communication, behavior, written documents, and technology (e.g., electronic mail).

### Formal Communication

#### Verbal Communication

Verbal communication is perceived as a quick way to transmit information and as a way to build trust and support. In contrast to other avenues, the spoken word conveys a personal caring. Day-to-day managerial interactions rely heavily on the spoken word. A verbal exchange is comprised of voice, message, response content, and methods used to transmit and receive information. Emotions are expressed orally. Tone, word choice, use of silence, accents and intonation, speed of delivery, clarity, and articulation are verbal exchange factors. Genetics and culture affect these qualities. Additionally, as noted by Liebler, Levine, and Rothman (1992), professional preparation trains managers and therapists to deliver information in a certain fashion.

Word meanings vary with the setting in which they are used. For example, boardroom and hallway conversa-

tions have different connotations. Content is also affected by the positions held by the receiver and sender. Familiarity with each other, the setting, and content information influence how well messages are understood. Methods used to transmit and receive information influence the meaning and understanding of messages. Talking on the phone or via teleconference is distant and not necessarily as revealing as face-to-face exchanges. Listening in a crowded hallway versus a private office introduces different distortions. Moreover, one's ability to listen and attend is influenced by communication methods. Listening as a message is transmitted by phone demands less attentiveness than listening during face-to-face interactions.

#### Nonverbal Communication

Nonverbal communication accompanies oral communication and is present in body language, posture, distance, eye contact, and body movements. Interaction is initiated through nonverbal avenues such as eye contact or gestures then continued through oral exchanges. Phone conversations are dependent on oral exchanges; however, silence and intonation convey unspoken thoughts. Talking at an intimate distance, 18 inches or less, is less formal, usually, than discussion during public distances, 12 or more feet. Folded arms and legs crossed away from the speaker suggest nonreceptivity while open posture toward the speaker implies acceptance. Likewise, eye contact and hand gestures connote degrees of attending and active listening. A soft-spoken voice creates a different meaning from a loud voice. Robbins (1995) indicates that oral communication carries a nonverbal message which is likely to have the greatest impact on the meaning and understanding of transactions. How something is said is as significant as what is said.

Dress is another nonverbal communication form. Unwritten and written rules govern professional attire. Written rules specify colors for specific therapies or days when staff shirts are to be worn, location and type of professional identification, and appropriateness of accessories or apparel regarding safety issues or organizational protocols. For example, if practitioners were to wear sandals or jewelry, consumer interactions might be affected, and if the manager were to wear casual rather than formal attire on board meeting day, the impression left might be less than the desired *professional image*. Impressions are created by attire and personal identification—the impact of a briefcase, business card, and lapel name pin. These impressions reflect feelings or beliefs about the department and therapeutic recreation as a profession. Social norms and work culture determine dress protocols and standards. To illustrate, if Fridays are viewed as "casual attire" days, how are clients and staff distinguished during Friday night socials? Therapists promoted to managers consider the unwritten dress codes that influence how other professionals respond to the authority of the new position. As a result "meeting room" rather than "functional activity" attire is more frequently worn.

## Conscious and Unconscious Behaviors

Conscious and unconscious behaviors affect oral communication. During conscious exchanges the speaker is aware of the content, direction, and intent of the interaction. Unconscious motives and behaviors such as desires, fears, mind set, and beliefs are "hidden," yet they affect behavior. Word selection and use do the same. For example, to say "finish the report" as opposed to saying "please finish the report by the end of the workday" projects two very different attitudes.

## Written Documents

As noted by Robbins (1995), written documents are official, have long-term implications, and present complex information. Written documentation is as simple as a memo and as sophisticated as an annual report. The message may be as personal or informal as "Enjoy your birthday off" or as formal as the action plan following a performance review. Writing commits thoughts and feelings to record; a paper trail is created that later can become "permanent binding statements" to which a manager is legally committed. Although writing tends to reduce ambiguities, the reader may have a different understanding of the written material from the writer. Telephone messages or e-mail are examples of communication in which what is written may be as significant to the message as what is not written. Understanding written communication is affected by factors such as the type and quality of handwriting or printed word, word choice, composition level and complexity, volume, organization, and presentation of the material. To illustrate, a bound laser-printed report is received differently from a stapled dot-matrix-printed document.

## Technology

Technology has added new methods and forms of communication to therapeutic recreation management and personal interactions. Through computers, cellular phones, videoconferencing and networking, personal communiqués are transmitted more quickly over longer distances, and access to others is easier. Since several people receive one message simultaneously, the volume and number of interpersonal exchanges are increased. These forms of communication rely on the manager's ability to use and access equipment. Consequently, they are not available to the same extent at all work sites. Another concern lies with the translation of the message to written word: Is the meaning lost? Or, are there thoughts that are not articulated?

## Informal Communication

Informal communication occurs through informal networks or the grapevine (i.e., gossip or the rumor mill). It is not uncommon for the person accountable for change to be the last one to become aware of desired actions or the impact of actions on others. Rumors begin for a number of reasons: words have different meanings or are interpreted differently, time lapses occur between senders and receivers, mediums are distorted, messages are incomplete, and anxiety creates ambiguity. Less time is available on a daily basis to communicate increasing amounts of information. Further, the personal context of a message is easily lost in an informal transmission.

One reacts differently to informal networks and grapevines and these personal reactions affect how one responds personally and professionally to messages circulated in this manner. The grapevine does, however, act as a feedback loop to help judge accuracy and appropriateness of messages. To illustrate, if the message through the grapevine was that one appears to dominate conversations, one has the opportunity to assess interactions and adjust verbal and nonverbal contributions accordingly.

## Communication Barriers

A number of conscious and unconscious barriers contributes to the meaning of exchanges being confused or misinterpreted. These interferences can originate with the sender, receiver, methods of communication, and the message itself. Robbins (1995) suggests that barriers to effective communication result from word usage, poor listening or attending, limited feedback, perceptual differences, role or status differentials, use of inappropriate communication methods, and variances between the sender and receiver with regard to honesty, emotions, and orientation:

1. **Word usage.** There is a tendency to believe that the words and terms used to send messages have the same meaning for the receiver. Yet, the use of language is not uniform (Robbins, 1995). Age, education, culture, and role or status tend to influence language use. Witness the various meanings the words play and leisure have for a child, adult, and a professional therapeutic recreator. Likewise, qualitative words used to describe size, amounts, and range have unique meanings to each of these groups.

2. **Listening or attending.** Listening and attending are distorted by one's mind set, perceptual defenses, sensory overloads, and thinking about the receiver or response one anticipates. Robbins (1995) also suggests that a person tends to listen for agreement and disagreement rather than for meaning. Listening involves attending, interpreting, and remembering. Consequently, environmental distractions, inability

to focus on the moment at hand, and/or the sender's behavior contribute to *inactive* listening. The friend who wears a color one dislikes, the loud radio on a colleague's desk, and the desire to be elsewhere at the moment are examples of situations that cause nonlistening.

3. **Feedback.** Feedback is essential information given by the receiver to the sender that helps the sender judge effectiveness of the transmitted message. Feedback reveals how behavior appears to others or affects others' feelings. Without feedback or reliable evaluative feedback, one does not know if the message has been received as intended (Robbins, 1995). There are several legitimate reasons for the absence of feedback: (1) receivers may choose not to respond; (2) responses may not be forthcoming as the respondent fears the consequence of giving feedback; and (3) the time to respond may not permit adequate responses.

4. **Perceptual differences.** Perceptual differences between senders and receivers interfere with interpretation, transmission, and understanding of meanings. Assumptions, attitudes, past experiences, expectations, cultural perspectives, educational and philosophical orientations, and family and caregiver values influence how one interprets and responds. Thus, senders and receivers view a situation from their unique perspective. To illustrate, consider the differing viewpoints held by the public and those in health and human services toward disabilities that are visually apparent and those that are "hidden."

5. **Role or status differentials.** One engages in behaviors that typify the roles one plays (e.g., child, mother, father, employee, employer). Roles have certain expectations. For example, mothers nurture, children respect parents, employees and employers are loyal. These role expectations create differentials and a frame of reference from which communication is interpreted. Those in professional roles use technical terms or *jargon* that is not necessarily understood by other professionals. At any given time, one assumes multiple roles that may interfere with another. For instance, the desire to be home with the family after a program has ended contributes to the recording of brief notes on client outcomes.

6. **Selection of communication methods.** According to Robbins (1995), communication methods vary in the richness of information transmitted. Oral, one-to-one contact is more direct, complete, and personal than e-mail or phone contact. Complex, ambiguous messages are better committed to writing; however, time and resources may preclude accurate reporting. Out of frustration a request is committed to writing when a verbal reminder would bring about the desired change, or one might say "thank you" when a letter in a personnel file was justified. The nature of the message also influences selection of the communication method. However, these are not always matched and issues arise as a consequence of the incongruity between content and process.

7. **Sender and receiver variances.** A number of factors contribute to the inability to be honest and open regarding communication. One may desire to avoid confrontation that causes someone to become upset or resistive. One may say what others want to hear to gain their support or a political advantage. One may temporarily withhold communication in order to allow for time to gather additional information or to calm tempers. Increased tension and creation of additional communication barriers is a consequence of not being open and timely with communication. Openness and honesty are compromised by extreme emotions such as frustration and anger or excitement and happiness. As noted by Robbins (1995), one is likely to disregard rational thinking processes when these emotions are present. Time, place, situational set, and people in the environment influence emotional response and how messages are received and sent. The nature of the therapeutic recreation work environment is supportive to open communication, yet the practitioner may need to repeat the information in a formal meeting so that the consumer grasps the significance of the recommended intervention.

Senders and receivers are preoccupied with their respective orientations. Each is concerned with achieving his or her own objectives or sending and receiving messages that leave others with positive impressions. One becomes insensitive to the needs of others when one promotes the self. Communication is most effective when the sender anticipates how the receiver will respond and what the meaning of the message will be for the receiver.

## Effective Communication Techniques

Effective communication results when the sender and receiver interpret the intended meaning of the message similarly and respond accordingly. Although some communication blocks such as word usage and perceptual differences are less pliable, techniques such as feedback and active listening are improved with practice. Objective analysis also improves communication. As reported by Liebler, Levine, and Rothman (1992), objectivity involves observing, attending, responding to requests, and checking information. A skilled observer separates personal interpretations and perceptions from the reality of an event. Awareness of self permits one to understand a message as intended in its original meaning. A person who attends listens actively and focuses on what is said rather than what the response is likely to be. An active listener responds to the true, conscious and unconscious, meaning of a message. Further, communiqués are presented with differing agendas. Objective listeners sort through the layers to discover the real meanings of the exchanges. Finally, by requesting feedback, a listener checks for accuracy of the interpretation. Clarification, paraphrasing, and summarizing are techniques used to check information.

The personal characteristics of therapeutic helpers are believed to be effective in promoting communication (Liebler, Levine, and Rothman, 1992). Qualities such as genuineness, empathy, caring, humor, congruence, respect, and trust enhance communication processes. Effective helpers and communicators display compatibility between what is known, how it is expressed, and the actions that are taken. They are true to their own feelings and accept the feelings of others; thus, information is shared openly. Respect and a mutual commitment are evident, and the significance, uniqueness, and contributions of each are affirmed.

## Feedback

Misunderstandings occur without feedback. Feedback is a way of giving help. Without feedback, one is unaware of how one's communication, verbal or nonverbal, affects others or one's behavior appears to others. Feedback is confirming or correcting. With either, one may choose or not choose to change or improve oneself and the quality of one's services. As suggested by Denton (1987), several techniques improve the effectiveness of feedback:

- Specific rather than general statements are more accurate and lead to action (e.g., "Your reports will be read by colleagues when better organized" rather than "Your paperwork is sloppy").
- Action rather than inaction statements motivate change (e.g., "Is there a way that you could improve report writing?" rather than "There does not seem to be a way to improve the situation").
- Descriptive rather than evaluative statements help clarify meaning (e.g., "When you do not document your observations the team is unaware . . ." rather than "Your documentation does not reflect client outcomes").
- Feedback that presents options is more likely to be received than input that does not permit choices (e.g., "Could you chart daily or work with a co-therapist?" rather than "Entries are required each session").
- Feedback is given immediately or within a reasonable amount of time after the incident. During a time lapse, emotions build and more information is "stored up" than one is capable of accurately sending or receiving.

## Active Listening

Active listeners receive and understand the whole message. Several factors cause people not to be active listeners. These include judging or speculating on the speaker's motive, planning responses while spoken too, interrupting the speaker with information that finishes the thought, and sensory overload. Additionally, as noted by Denton (1987), past experiences create a set of expectations that may either help one to understand the new ideas or cause one to mold the information to the present situation. Physical health or medical condition may discourage active listening as well. To improve active listening, one should become aware of these blocks and distortions.

The active listener understands the communication from the speaker's point of view. Robbins (1995) notes that this is accomplished by listening with intensity, empathy, acceptance, and a willingness to assume responsibility for completeness. Concentration permits the active listener to place each new piece of information into the context of preceding information. Empathetic listeners step into the "shoes" of the speaker suspending personal thoughts and feelings. Active listeners withhold judgment on the content until the speaker finishes. Further, Robbins (1995) suggests that active listeners take actions necessary to receive the intended meaning of the communication (e.g., shut a door, ask the speaker to restate the message).

Knippen and Green (1994) describe four techniques used by effective active listeners: restatement, summarization, responding to nonverbal cues, and responding to feelings. Active listeners restate or repeat messages by paraphrasing in their own words what the speaker has said (e.g., "What I hear you saying is that you prefer briefer more frequent meetings"). Summarizing occurs when the important points of the speaker are listed at the conclusion of the conversation as occurs during assessment interviews. The active listener often acknowledges and verbalizes nonverbal cues by stating the effect of nonverbal messages (e.g., "I hear you saying you don't mind adjusting your schedule yet your slow response time indicates otherwise"). Responding to feelings permits verbalization about perceptions and unexpressed feelings (e.g., an astute manager aware of staff concern about client progress might state "I see the lack of client progress and motivation are contributing to your frustrations").

A number of specific active listening strategies can be used to enhance communication effectiveness during conversations. They are summarized here:

1. Metzger (1982) suggests the judicious use of silence. When questions are asked at the beginning of conversations, allow silence to motivate response.
2. Open-ended questions allow the respondent to truly present the type of information perceived as important (Metzger, 1982).

3. Emotional filters cause misinterpretation when one feels strongly about a subject. Metzger (1982) suggests a third party or resource person be asked to join a conversation to facilitate objectivity.

4. Metzger (1982) notes most people listen for facts to the exclusion of feelings and the speaker's point of view. Paying attention to the way the speaker delivers the message clues the respondent into the speaker's true meaning. Impressions are checked by asking questions after the speaker concludes.

5. As noted by Robbins (1995), eye contact with a speaker focuses the respondent's attention, reduces the likelihood of being distracted, and encourages the speaker.

6. According to Denton (1987), a number of nonverbal techniques or *back channels* indicate interest. An active listener uses affirmative head nods, facial gestures, and attending actions such as "uh-huh" to denote interest.

7. When time is limited, rather than interrupting the conversation, the stage is set to continue at another time (e.g., "Excuse me, I apologize for disrupting your thoughts, could we plan to complete this conversation when time permits both of us to concentrate . . .") (Robbins, 1995).

8. A conversation is viewed as a "whole" rather than as separate pieces. Questions are asked that ensure understanding of the entire puzzle (e.g., "You have shared several ideas . . . are we looking at the need to restructure program offerings?").

9. Confront biases that prohibit accurate evaluation of the message source. As illustrated by Robbins (1995) appearance, speaker credibility, and personal mannerisms cause one to draw premature conclusions about the speaker.

10. Statements that begin with "I" clarify, show ownership of conversations, receipt of messages, and reflect feelings (e.g., "I understand the need for additional time to complete . . .") (Denton, 1987).

11. Robbins (1995) recommends thinking before acting. What outcomes are expected? The message should be organized, and a method of delivery chosen that is congruent with desired outcomes and the receiver's needs and resources (e.g., e-mail is quick yet not always available and does not permit "rich" exchanges).

12. Language choice is critical. Jargon and professional terms facilitate meaning for those who understand but cause confusion for those unfamiliar with the terms (Robbins, 1995).

13. Actions give meanings to words. When words and actions are congruent, they act as motivators and credibility and trust develop. Relationships are strained when actions do not back up words.

According to Robbins (1995) conversation may have at least six messages:

- what the speaker means to say,
- what the speaker actually says,
- what the listener hears,
- what the listener thinks he or she hears,
- what the listener says, and
- what the speaker thinks the listener said.

Facilitation skills, especially the ability to communicate warmth and be an active listener, are essential to helping and leading (Carter, Van Andel, and Robb, 1995). Assertiveness training, values clarification exercises, and role playing are methods to cultivate awareness of personal communication processes. A first-line manager's personal communication skills become evident during supervisory-subordinate relationships.

# Managerial Communication

The typical workday of a first-line therapeutic recreation manager consists of numerous meetings, informal interactions, one-on-one supervisory conversations, personal contacts with clients and caregivers, and colleague contact via phone, fax, and e-mail. Instead of following a detailed schedule, supervisors find they spend the day reacting to people and situations. Robbins (1995) notes that the majority of time on a particular workday is spent communicating. Effective managers learn to separate important from insignificant messages and to manage their time so that disruptions do not prevent them from achieving department goals.

The power invested in a managerial position gives the first-line manager the authority to act through employees to achieve unit and organizational outcomes. Through processes such as delegation, negotiation, and collaboration, the work of practitioners, volunteers, and seasonal employees is facilitated. Supervisory interactions do result in criticism, complaints, and confrontation which can be managed in order to gain support for accomplishing work initiatives. The effectiveness of supervisor-employee exchanges determines the efficiency with which the unit operates to achieve its goals.

## *Social Context of Managerial Communication*

A manager's communication is embedded in the social context or culture of the employing organization. Consequently, exchanges are judged within an organizational climate. Formal avenues of communication and the grapevine are channels of information exchange. For example, protocol may dictate how and when upper level decisions on benefit packages or new services are to be communicated by the supervisor, while the grapevine simultaneously generates rumors speculating withholding and service adjustments. Managers are challenged to respond to organization protocols and meet the information needs of department employees. As suggested by Grossman (1989), prior to supervisor-employee exchanges, the manager should consider the social context of each communiqué as follows:

- Who will be affected by the information and will action be required?
- What parts of the information are critical to employees' actions (e.g., Do they need all of the pieces or facts?)?
- Do protocols require certain avenues or timing of the exchanges?
- Is the idea clear and how should it be interpreted for staff?
- Is the information accurate and does the message contain the "why" of the desired action or change?
- Is a feedback mechanism built into the exchange?
- Is the anticipated response one that can be tolerated?
- Is the expectation congruent with the employee's job specifications and professional development goals?

## Delegation

To accomplish the work of the department the manager delegates responsibility to employees to make decisions and take actions toward accomplishing unit goals. Delegation shifts "power" from the first-line manager to an employee. First-line managers may hesitate to relinquish a portion of their "authority" for a number of reasons (e.g., I can do the job better, time is of the essence, staff are inexperienced, work loads will become imbalanced). Consequently, they may underdelegate. *Overdelegation* occurs when the first-line manager relinquishes inordinate amounts of authority. A number of reasons such as dislike for certain paperwork tasks, feelings of being overworked, awareness that certain employees appear to be interested in specific tasks, and the manager's own inexperience in a management position contribute to overdelegation. Hansten and Washburn (1992) recommend consideration of the following four factors to determine when and what to delegate:

1. **The task.** Certain tasks remain the responsibility of first-line managers (e.g., personnel and fiscal matters, and policy-related actions). Staff carry out direct service interactions such as initially responding to client and caregiver inquiries and soliciting programmatic input.
2. **The employee.** Employee job specifications, privileging protocols, and plans of operation identify who

has specific knowledge, skills, and abilities (KSAs) and is to perform certain responsibilities. For instance, asking a volunteer rather than a department employee to dispense medications on an outing would be inappropriate and outside the purview of a volunteer's job duties.
3. **The message and the medium.** Written communication is used with significant messages such as documentation of client outcomes, while phone contact or a hallway conversation is appropriate to gain an update on a coming special event.
4. **The feedback.** Evaluation during and after task completion ensures accountability and proper employee recognition. Feedback gives the manager a status report while acknowledging the employee's contribution to department goals. Thus, when tasks are assigned, time and resources are also planned to gain input.

Employees are empowered through participation in decisions that direct, coordinate, and control their work. Delegation is the primary means a supervisor has to empower employees. A first-line manager accepts and expects mistakes within this process, but he or she institutes feedback controls so that the costs of errors do not exceed the learning that occurs (Robbins, 1995). Redesigning job specifications is another process used to delegate. This occurs as positions are vacated, when mergers occur, and through restructuring. Job specifications are rewritten during retreats and with design of professional development plans. As outlined by Robbins (1995), effective delegation is mutual: The task is clearly delineated; the employee has the authority and resources to accomplish the task; the employee has the competence and has agreed to accept the responsibility; other employees are informed of the delegation; and the employee is expected to respond to problems that arise as the task is carried out.

## Negotiation

Managers communicate through negotiation. Effective negotiation sets up a win-win work environment. An effective negotiator recognizes the needs and objectives of others while expressing in a professional manner points of view that facilitate achievement of unit goals. Negotiation skills are used during performance reviews, employee coaching, conflict resolution, and planning quality improvement programs. Official negotiations occur with collective bargaining and contract agreements. On a daily basis, the first-line manager negotiates for meeting times, program space or areas, employee benefits, and client contact time. Each of these encounters involves distribution of resources among work units to accomplish outcomes. The quality of manager-employee relationships and relationships with other organizational units is impacted by the manager's ability to look for solutions to promote positive outcomes among all parties.

Viewing an issue as one to be resolved jointly enhances the probability of a win-win situation. When a win-lose situation is created, those who lose become resentful while those who win may use power inappropriately; either condition is counterproductive to long-term working relations among people and organizational units. A problem-solving approach creates win-win situations (e.g., mutually define the problem, look for alternatives, select and implement the most feasible option, and evaluate and plan for follow-up). Robbins (1995) suggests the following guidelines as issues are negotiated:

- Consider the needs, interests, and strategies of all those affected by the situation.
- Consider the significance of the issue to the operation of the department and the needs of the unit's constituents (e.g., how critical is the pay raise or van access to employee morale or client programming?).
- Think small and positive. When initial overtures reflect reconciliation and agreement, others are also more likely to result in *give-and-take*.
- Issues are depersonalized so that perceptions do not distort communication. Real issues are identified so feelings and misinformation don't become "fog" factors.
- Negotiating is a continuous process of informing and monitoring outcomes. Professionals agree to disagree professionally. Avenues to ensure continuous exchanges are established (e.g., weekly briefings).
- When third parties mediate, confidentiality of information is cautiously regarded.

## Collaboration

Collaboration is the outcome of win-win situations (Robbins, 1995). Robbins (1995) characterizes collaboration as involving open discussions, active listening, understanding and identifying differences, and deliberating over all possible solutions. Team building and networking are collaborative. These efforts have become more critical in health and human services as a result of reduced resources, briefer intervention periods, increased accountability demands and attention to measuring outcomes, and the ongoing impact of change on service quality and improvements.

Managers empower staff by creating collaborative environments in which staff have the support and resources to react and change events. This occurs through communication that fosters feelings of trust, risk taking, openness, equity, and opportunity finding. According to Stevens and Campion (1994), several features define collaborative communication. These are listed here:

- Communication is behavior or event focused rather than "personal."
- Messages are specific rather than general, descriptive rather than evaluative, and they make comparisons to objective standards rather than subjective standards.
- Congruence is evident among what collaborators do and say.
- A manager's messages validate staff feelings and decisions (e.g., they do not convey superiority or rigidity of position).
- Encounters are conjunctive, allowing everyone an opportunity to speak and be perceived as competent.
- Each party takes responsibility and is held accountable for its ideas and actions.
- Techniques that avoid conformity to majority opinions such as brainstorming, nominal group techniques, and simulations facilitate change and empowerment.
- Discussions are scheduled when facts are fresh. Investigation and documentation prior to exchange save time and aggravation.
- Personal biases are confronted in order to dissipate strong feelings that could distort communication.

Successful collaboration is dependent upon cohesion and dedication to a service mission that reflects common values. Managers create linkages among their staff that promote cooperation, respect, and integration of individual talents so that collective achievement of goals enables unit change.

## Criticism, Complaints, and Confrontation

Although the desire is to create win-win situations (see Strategies for Conflict Resolutions in Chapter 11), managerial exchanges and actions do result in criticism, complaints, and confrontation. These occur for a number of reasons, but primarily because no one is perfect all the time. Further, these outcomes need not always be perceived as negative because they are valuable self-assessment tools. The manager's challenge is to identify underlying issues or needs and redirect energies toward effective encounters. Managers also separate the significant from the insignificant to identify those requiring responses.

This profession is naturally more vulnerable to criticism, complaints, and confrontation because one is on the "front lines" working with those who have health and well-being needs. Fear, frustration, and anxiety contribute to complaints, criticism, and confrontations. According to Deering (1993), practitioners make critical decisions in high-stress situations that do not always bring the desired success or help. A first-line therapeutic recreation manager is in the middle of the communication loop between upper level managers who have the resources or authority and staff who use these resources to achieve organizational goals. This position requires interpreting communiqués from two viewpoints which may or may not be congruent. A therapeutic recreation manager, therefore, is the potential recipient of criticism, complaints, and confrontation for a number of reasons and from a variety of sources.

A first-line manager must model ways to give and receive criticism, complaints, and confrontation in order to promote constructive outcomes. Complaints arise for a number of reasons. As Davidhizar (1991) notes, complaints may be an attempt to meet information needs, express discomfort, and gain control, or as the result of an effort to seek clarity in confusing situations. Criticism is caused by a negative evaluation of personal actions and is usually considered unpleasant (Davidhizar and Wysong, 1992). Confrontation results from discrepancies between performance and expectation. According to several authors (Davidhizar, 1991; Davidhizar and Wysong, 1992; Deering, 1993), the manager may elect to receive and respond in a number of ways to promote positive outcomes from criticism, complaints, and confrontational situations. The following list highlights some of these ways:

- Confidentiality promotes an atmosphere conducive to disclosing feelings (Davidhizar, 1991).
- Active listening enables the manager to listen to the verbal and nonverbal message and respond to the *whole.* A response like "I agree with you as do other staff" may be enough to enable the manager and staff member to cope with the situation.
- Credibility of the involved parties can be maintained by investigating, determining the real problem, and deliberating alternatives.
- To avoid escalation of the problem and embarrassment to those involved, consideration is given to the timing and location of intervention (Deering, 1993). When intervention does occur, the problem behavior and the desired behavior are identified so that the employee is able to regain control and feel positive about self and work.
- When employees participate in actions that affect their responsibilities, job satisfaction tends to increase and negative input decreases. Employee confidence and cooperation is gained by explaining *why* and *what for.*
- Responses are presented in a manner of "kind firmness" and expectations are stated concretely with specific examples of acceptable and unacceptable responses.
- Even when formal grievances have been filed, the manager should respond with consistency and respect. Responses are nonthreatening and "save face"

for the manager and employee. A request for feedback or an apology help the manager gain additional evaluative information and handle feelings of inadequacy that may have been projected onto staff.
- Therapeutic recreation managers work in stressful environments. Humor is a constructive mechanism that promotes communication. Davidhizar and Wysong (1992) suggest that an appropriately timed laugh creates avenues to exchange perceptions and interpretations with others while helping take the error more lightly.
- Practitioners tend to respond to fair challenges. The key to change is moving from small points of consensus toward overall agreement. The competent manager agrees with valid complaints, criticism, and confrontation and sets the expectations so that each change or accomplishment is acknowledged and rewarded. Sometimes public reward is all that is needed to gain positive momentum.

A prudent manager accepts complaints, criticism, and confrontation as an inevitable part of first-line supervisory duties. By modeling constructive ways to receive and respond to these situations, the first-line manager helps staff gain insight into their own behaviors. Professional actions can correct the erring, consider personal communication styles, and initiate change so that problem behaviors are changed into constructive relations.

Through delegation, negotiation, and collaboration the manager guides staff to carry out department goals. A positive response to criticism, complaints, and confrontations facilitates the risk taking necessary to change and improve. The first-line manager assumes a key role in organizational communication that usually implies a position somewhere between upward and downward channels.

# Organizational and Professional Communication

To achieve organizational goals effective communication is essential. Formal communications are sanctioned and occur through meetings, memos, executive sessions, and individual management-staff supervisory sessions. Informal communication takes place through the grapevine and may or may not promote the goals of the organization. Organizational communication patterns have become more complex in health and human services. Factors like professional specialization, decentralization of service centers, use of cross-disciplinary teams, corporate mergers, and reductions in the number of mid-managers present challenges to the transmission of messages in a timely manner to appropriate personnel.

The first-line manager is a central figure who represents therapeutic recreation within the organization and to public and professional audiences external to the organization. Employees expect the manager to be informed and are quick to realize when their supervisor is "mouthing" organizational policy or has been bypassed in the communication chain. First-line managers direct and/or redirect formal communications from upper level management. In their positions, first-line therapeutic recreation managers inform and educate department staff, organization employees, clients, caregivers, and colleagues about the mission of unit services and scope of professional practice. Through research, evaluation, presentations, and publication of written materials, the therapeutic recreation manager conveys the essence of the profession at the work site, within the community, and to the profession at large. This advocacy role is evident in management meetings, at communitywide special events, and during professional leadership functions.

## Organizational Communication

Formal communication within an organization is directional and supportive of organizational goals. Usually, a hierarchy of roles guides the direction of communication (e.g., a first-line manager normally does not walk into the chief executive officer's office unannounced to request additional storage space). Formal verbal communication occurs at management meetings; board, committee, and team meetings; staff training and development sessions and meetings; and in strategic planning sessions, budget hearings, and public forums. Nonverbal formal communication is written or transmitted through goal statements, manuals, executive orders or directives, employee direct mailings, paycheck inserts, flyers, e-mail, bulletin boards, and training session handouts. As identified by Liebler, Levine, and Rothman (1992), informal communication is not necessarily directional and may circumvent formal channels. Gossip and rumors are not always accurate but they result from situations important to the employee (Robbins, 1995). Rumors persist until expectations causing the uncertainties are fulfilled and anxieties reduced. Managers use the grapevine as a barometer and feedback mechanism to judge success of formal communication and identify relevant employee concerns.

### Blocks to Organizational Communication

As with personal and interpersonal communication, a number of factors block or distort organizational communication. Liebler, Levine, and Rothman (1992) note that the grapevine and a number of other factors associated with groups of people working together day-to-day in a structured environment influence communication. These factors are presented here:

- **Language.** Jargon or technical terms used by the practitioner may be unfamiliar to upper level administrators or colleagues from other health and human service professions.
- **Unconscious motives.** Staff have thoughts or feelings based on real and/or perceived events that interfere with their ability to view the current events and communications from an objective perspective (e.g., previous budget cuts affect willingness to risk change and innovation).
- **Status and position.** Real and perceived differences in rank, title, and physical location of divisions or departments inhibit exchanges and interactions.
- **Organization size and structure.** The larger the organization the greater the number of contacts or channels through which messages are transmitted. Within self-governing teams and participatory management roles, the diversity of responsibilities assumed by managers and staff contribute to increasing numbers of employees becoming part of communication networks.
- **Logistical factors.** Support factors such as space, availability of technology and computers, skill and resources of available administrative assistants, work schedules, location of direct services in relation to management, and time permitted for clerical work affect the nature of face-to-face interactions, written communication, and feedback.
- **Work culture and environment.** Rapid client turn around or dramatic increases in the number of clients with diverse, multiple needs and severe deficits creates staff frustration that inhibits communication. When the intensity of the work varies with seasonal changes or client turnover, communication becomes labored and distorted as a result of staff stress and pressure.
- **Employee composition.** Each age group brings unique features to the work environment. Values, beliefs, experiences, and expectations vary when there are employees from various age cohorts working together.

### Improving Organizational Communication

Centrality of the manager's role to the flow of communication requires that conscious actions be taken to develop linkages throughout the organization. Several strategies used to facilitate organizational networking are listed here:

- The manager gains the confidence of others by remaining impartial and consistent, responding promptly to requests, and representing the interests of department employees to other management levels and throughout the organization.
- Accurate information is transmitted between levels. If communication bypasses levels or goes through informal channels, it is acknowledged.
- Individual efforts and the work of the department are recognized publicly and before upper management levels.
- The manager impresses upon the staff that ineffective communication can mean wasted time and resources. Staff also are made aware that communication is subject to organizational controls as are other organizational functions (e.g., fund-raising, marketing). This helps employees understand why compliance with protocols and proper use of communication tools enhance the *image* of the department.
- The manager creates multiple avenues through which messages are transmitted so that the meanings benefit from the impact of repetition.

Organizational communication is also enhanced by careful planning and analysis of formal and informal exchanges. Planning and evaluating the transmission of written documents and documentation improves the effectiveness of message sending and receiving. When forms are used properly and reports completed in a timely manner, others view the department positively. All persons associated with a situation are informed of the outcomes (e.g., minutes of staff meetings sent to upper level management garner support and awareness). The appearance of official documents leaves an impression that influences responsiveness. Committing agendas and problem alternatives to writing, for example, allows others to prepare for exchanges. The first-line manager solicits input on the relevancy of communication methods to determine their appropriateness to various audiences. For example, paycheck inserts and e-mail may elicit more input than bulletin boards and flyers.

Verbal exchanges are also planned. Location of verbal exchanges are contemplated. Confidential material is discussed in private as is any topic that might arouse emotional responses. Discussion between staff and management regarding resource allocations occurs on *neutral territory.* Verbal exchanges are planned to occur after all facts are carefully analyzed for accuracy. Positions of communicators in the conversation are planned (e.g., space between speakers or height of speaker-respondents is arranged). Discussion is focused by controls such as time, *Robert's Rules of Order,* or third-party facilitation. The intent of conversations is stated at the outset, and summarization brings closure at the conclusion. Talking with constituents prior to structured meetings clarifies and gathers information and permits the manager to gain insight into the situation. Formally acknowledging hallway communications also helps informal communications become barometers for needed formal communiqués. Conducting communication audits to request input on how information and ideas are shared and what the satisfaction level is with these patterns helps organizations plan proper uses of formal verbal and nonverbal communication processes.

## Professional Communication

The manner in which communication is shared within and outside the organization leaves an impression about therapeutic recreation. Through a number of media such as in-services, presentations, reports, research, articles, and voluntary contributions, the first-line manager is a role model for staff, a representative for the organization, and an advocate of the profession. As a role model, the first-line manager shares professional resources, publications, contacts, standards, and protocols with staff. Likewise, staff present information from off-site professional meetings to unit colleagues during in-services. Managers encourage their staff to present agency-wide in-services on therapeutic recreation. As noted by Austin (1997), first-line managers interact with staff during clinical supervision to ensure that their performance promotes department accountability which will be considered in more depth in Chapter 20.

First-line managers represent their departments and the organization as they network and collaborate in the agency, community, and profession. Their poise, appearance, mannerisms, promptness, and timeliness are qualities reflective of personal professional standards of excellence. The manager's written and oral accuracy, follow-through, receptivity, and quality of delivered materials, project an *image.* Real and perceived impressions of the manager affect others' thoughts and feelings about the manager, organization, and profession.

Managers are also judged by the "company they keep." Power associated with positions and roles is communicated through associations. Responsiveness to a manager occurs in a political context. Judgments affect what and how others share information. Before a manager communicates externally, organizational protocol requires that proper internal personnel have been informed and that information to be disseminated has received clearance. Professionals ensure that the positions and roles of others are respected, and, in return, they expect the same of colleagues.

When a therapeutic recreation manager disseminates publications, research findings, and results of service evaluations, information representative of the profession is being conveyed to clients, caregivers, and colleagues. Through professional writings and presentations and community service projects, therapeutic recreation is promoted as a viable health and human service. The advocacy role is evident in one-on-one interactions and during professional conferences. This advocacy role is carried out in a number of ways such as program tours, advisory board meetings, support group facilitation, resource sharing, volunteerism, cosponsorships, and student intern training.

Professional communication is unique because of the distance communication travels and the impact it makes on audiences wider than those within the organization. E-mail, telephones, formal letters, committee reports, and conference calls are impersonal and do not permit the message to project feelings or subjective interpretations. Each professional reads and hears the message from his or her own perspective. Because this frame of reference is unique, the sender and receiver ascribe different meanings to the message. Therefore, to ensure congruence the first-line manager carefully constructs the message, seeks review prior to transmission, and solicits feedback from the receiver(s) to gauge accuracy of understandings. A correspondence file permits revisiting previous communications to verify information transmitted. Additionally, the manager devotes certain daily time periods to prioritized communications. Brief notes are made summarizing appointments, calls, and contacts. Busy work times (e.g., Monday mornings or budget hearings) are avoided. A resource file is maintained to ensure ongoing communication and networking.

Organizational and professional communication are multidirectional and multifaceted. The first-line manager is often the person between and through whom organizational messages are transmitted. Communicating the right message at the right time to the right person is a major responsibility of management. Internal and external professional exchanges leave long-lasting impressions and are primary tools through which the professional and profession mature. How, what, and when messages are conveyed influence perceptions others have of therapeutic recreation.

## Summary

This chapter began by identifying the components of interpersonal communication and the nature of formal and informal communication processes. The interchange between formal written and verbal exchanges is influenced by the nonverbal manner in which messages are conveyed. Successful communicators exhibit congruency in the manner messages are shared and received. Also, effective communicators consider the barriers that occur and result in real or perceived differences in message content and interpretation. Personal characteristics of "effective helpers" promote effective communication. Feedback and active

listening are two tools that enhance communication when used properly.

Interpersonal communication skills are employed during managerial exchanges. A first-line manager's day-to-day transactions are brief yet focused so that employees have the support and resources to perform department tasks. As a clinical supervisor, the first-line manager ensures that those within the unit and those that support unit activities, have timely, factual, accurate information. Through delegation, negotiation, and collaborative processes, the manager communicates so that win-win situations accomplish unit and organizational goals. When criticism, complaints, and confrontation do arise, the manager separates the significant from the not so critical in order to discern real needs and action steps. With humor the stress created in problem situations can be dissipated.

Organizational and professional communications extend the first-line manager's network beyond the division or department. These exchanges inform and educate others about therapeutic recreation while advocating for the contributions made by professionals. Although barriers exist within the organization and public domain, the professional is able to analyze situations so that the appropriate image is projected and clients, caregivers, and colleagues have accurate impressions of the nature of the profession.

## Discussion Questions

1. Identify the avenues of formal and informal communication and describe how each affects message transmission.
2. How is the manager's role as a change agent affected by formal and informal communication avenues?
3. Explain the critical roles of active listening and feedback in overcoming communication barriers.
4. What steps can be taken to improve message sending, transmission, receiving, and feedback?
5. Summarize the nature of managers' daily communications incorporating a discussion of the social context of communication.
6. What steps can a manager take to improve the processes of delegation, negotiation, and collaboration?
7. How are criticism, complaints, and confrontation managed so win-win situations result?
8. Identify organizational blocks to communication.
9. How does a manager enhance organizational communication?
10. What practices contribute to effective professional communication?
11. Summarize the relationships between effective communication and successful management.

# References

Austin, D. R. (1997). *Therapeutic recreation processes and techniques* (3rd ed.). Champaign, IL: Sagamore Publishing, Inc.

Carter, M. J., Van Andel, G. E., and Robb, G. M. (1995). *Therapeutic recreation: A practical approach* (2nd ed.). Prospect Heights, IL: Waveland Press, Inc.

Davidhizar, R. (1991). The employee who complains: Understanding and responding to staff complaints. *Hospital Topics, 69:4,* 16–19.

Davidhizar, R., and Wysong, P. R. (1992). Positive and negative criticism: Strategies for professional growth. *Critical Care Nurse, 12:6,* 94–99.

Deering, C. G. (1993). Giving and taking criticism. *American Journal of Nursing, 93:12,* 56–62.

Denton, P. L. (1987). *Psychiatric occupational therapy: A workbook of practical skills.* Boston, MA: Little, Brown and Company.

Grossman, A. H. (1989). The two-way streets of communication, authority, and responsibility: Aspects of delegation. In A. H. Grossman (Ed.), *Personnel management in recreation and leisure services* (pp. 153–164). Reston, VA: American Alliance for Health, Physical Education, Recreation, and Dance.

Hansten, R., and Washburn, M. (1992). How to plan what to delegate. *American Journal of Nursing, 92:4,* 71–72.

Knippen, J. T., and Green, T. B. (1994). How the manager can use active listening. *Public Personnel Management, 23:2,* 357–359.

Liebler, J. G., Levine, R. E., and Rothman, J. (1992). *Management principles for health professionals* (2nd ed.). Gaithersburg, MD: Aspen Publishers, Inc.

Metzger, N. (1982). *The healthcare supervisor's handbook* (2nd ed.). Rockville, MD: Aspen Systems Corporation.

Robbins, S. P. (1995). *Supervision today.* Englewood Cliffs, NJ: Prentice Hall.

Stevens, M. J., and Campion, M. A. (1994). The knowledge, skill, and ability requirements for teamwork: Implications for human resource management. *Journal of Management, 20:2,* 503–530.

# *Chapter 15*
# Motivation

## Introduction

A first-line manager creates a work environment in which an employee is motivated to want to work. Motivation is the stimulant to need fulfillment. A therapeutic recreation manager's challenge is to create a work environment that encourages or empowers staff to carry out mutually developed division or department goals. Productivity and accountability result when practitioners are "turned on" to their job tasks. To motivate effectively, a manager must be in tune to each practitioner's personal needs and the interchange between the work environment and employee needs and abilities. The intent of this chapter is to explore the relationships among employee motivation, department outcomes, and the manager's responsibility to create a productive work environment.

What is motivation? Motivation is a degree of readiness or the desire or willingness within an individual to pursue a goal. As suggested by Robbins (1995), motivation is conditioned by the ability of the action taken to satisfy a need. First-line managers choose how to motivate their employees. The challenge is to create an environment where staff become self-motivated as a result of meeting their personnel needs. The manager seeks to create an environment in the department that enhances each practitioner's willingness to work.

Each staff member is unique. What is significant to one person is not necessarily important to another. Likewise, what motivates a practitioner at one particular time may not be something that fulfills a personal need in the future. The first section of this chapter identifies causes of individual differences and needs that are fulfilled through work.

A number of theories explain motivation. The principles derived from these theories are universal. Their application in a particular situation, according to Edginton and Griffith (1990), will determine the success or failure of the first-line manager to empower staff. A manager's perception of human nature and individual differences affects his or her management philosophy. The second section of this chapter reviews the theories that help explain a manager's choice of motivational strategies.

Successful managers blend individual employee needs with department expectations. The extent to which harmony prevails determines performance outcomes. A positive supportive environment is created by effective application of motivational concepts. While remaining aware of personal needs, the first-line manager seeks to expand the zone of acceptance within staff or department goals. This chapter's third section presents strategies a manager uses to create a supportive environment that promotes staff performances.

Employees are significant organizational assets. Their needs change within the dynamic work environment. Therapeutic recreation practitioners of the future are likely to be more demanding, mobile, and to have a different value perspective about work than current staff. A first-line manager will experience challenges unique to a diverse work force. The closing section of this chapter highlights a few of the issues likely to influence choices managers make as they balance practitioner needs with the changing work environment.

# Individual Need Fulfillment

A number of factors contribute to individual differences: age, education, upbringing, experience, value systems, expectations, feedback, perceptions, goals, and learned behaviors. Robbins (1995) suggests that five particular personality characteristics are relevant to understanding varied practitioner motivation and behavior. The first, locus of control, describes a person's belief about being the master of his or her fate. Persons with an internal locus of control perceive they are responsible for their own actions and, as a consequence, are less likely to blame the outcomes of their actions on luck or chance. Need fulfillment is their assumed responsibility. Staff members who attribute actions and their outcomes to someone other than themselves display an external locus of control. Persons with this focus are likely not to assume responsibility for their actions and attribute consequences to factors over which they have little control. Persons with an internal locus of control are inclined to satisfy their needs through inherent work values, while those with an external locus of control are more apt to gain work satisfaction through rewards such as paychecks.

A second factor that tends to affect individual perceptions about work is employee perceptions of power. Some employees perceive power to be inherent in their positions. Others perceive that power results from achievement of outcomes. In the former situation, a staff member is more prepared to be accepting of department protocol. An employee motivated by the end product is more apt to "bend the rules" to achieve department outcomes.

Self-esteem, a third factor, is a personality trait that influences one's degree of self-acceptance. According to Robbins (1995), persons with high self-esteem believe they have the ability to perform while those with low self-esteem are more susceptible to external influences and are motivated by the expectations and external reinforcement of others.

A successful employee adapts to the work environment and is capable of adjusting to changes in the workplace. Liebler, Levine, and Rothman (1992) suggest that a practitioner who fits into the department and values the role of a therapeutic recreation specialist is more easily motivated. Robbins (1995) refers to this fourth characteristic as the ability to "go with the flow" or to be self-monitoring. Self-monitoring personalities are more likely to discern situations that require change and flexibility. Persons who are low self-monitors, however, tend to be rigid and to show their "true colors" when their course of action is disrupted. Someone who self-monitors is more capable of performing in diverse work roles and with team members having various expectations.

A final characteristic to differentiate staff is the ability to assume risk. Robbins (1995) indicates that some people are more willing to act with less information than others. Those with high levels of confidence tend to make more rapid decisions because they believe in their ability to operate with the resources available. Thus, a risk taker is more willing to try a new technique or to initiate a new service than is an employee who dislikes risk taking. Risk taking facilitates change. The manager's challenge is to decide the degree of *risk* that is necessary to support staff as they adapt to the changing work environment.

## *Individual Needs and Work*

Accepting and understanding individual uniquenesses help the manager plan alternative motivational strategies for staff. Efforts to hire, train, and develop the "right" staff are likely to have negligible impacts on performance and "organizational fit" if managers are unsuccessful in matching motivational strategies with staff needs. Staff and volunteers are motivated to work in leisure and therapeutic recreation for a variety of reasons. The desire to help others, contribute to health and well-being, improve the system, and give back time and support to the community are needs met through volunteerism and paid positions. According to Edginton and Griffith (1990), financial reward, status, recognition, relationships, and growth are work incentives. For some, money is a major motivator; for others, only the amount of money necessary to ensure relative comfort is essential. Status associated with certain employment settings (e.g., clinical or community) or work groups (e.g., teams or committees) varies. Persons who perceive associational status differences are, therefore, likely to act accordingly to satisfy their needs.

Recognition in therapeutic recreation practices often does not come directly from the clients who most benefit from practitioner's work. Caregivers, colleagues, significant others, and siblings tend to recognize outcomes of intervention. Also, the type of recognition received is not always what a practitioner desires to hear. For example, clients and caregivers tend to perceive that therapeutic experiences are "fun" but that intervention can cause discomfort at times. Incentives to perform may emanate from peer recognition and rewards external to the work setting such as professional recognition. Professional associations recognize outstanding professionals and departments during annual meetings. The source of recognition influences worker behavior.

Employees are motivated by personal needs and group interactions. Relationships formed with colleagues on treatment teams or staff in the department motivate work behaviors. Likewise, interactions between staff and support groups, advisory committees, and/or parents stimulate staff initiatives. Summer staff and volunteers return, in part, because their relations with staff have been enjoyable.

Edginton and Griffith (1990) report that staff are more likely to remain in a position when they experience a sense of growth. Growth experiences are unique to each individual. For some, the opportunity to apply new interventions constitutes growth while for other practitioners, a change of clientele or setting is enough to stimulate the interest in learning and acquiring skills.

The first-line manager aware of individual differences also accepts the significance of personal needs as motivators in the work environment. No single work incentive addresses the complexity of human behavior. Motivation comes from within the staff member and department. Employees perform because they desire to do so. Employee behavior impacts others and, as a consequence, contributes to other's harmony with department protocols and directions.

# Motivational Approaches

The goal of a first-line manager is to accomplish department goals while giving practitioners the opportunity to meet their needs. A number of theories have attempted to interpret alternative approaches for motivating employees. These theories change with time and tend to reflect the psychosocial views prevalent during particular time periods. A brief review of these views reveals shifting explanations for employee motivation.

## *Maslow's Hierarchy of Needs*

According to a number of authors (Liebler, Levine, and Rothman, 1992; Murphy, Niepoth, Jamieson, and Williams, 1991), one of the most elementary yet influential understandings of motivation was presented in 1943 by Abraham Maslow. Maslow's hierarchy of needs theory suggests the key to motivation is to determine where along the developmental continuum (i.e., physiological, safety, social, esteem, self-actualization) an employee is functioning and focus motivational efforts at this level. For example, money is essential to satisfy physiological needs; an adequate paycheck becomes a desirable goal when securing a position. Employees pursue goals to satisfy their needs. The need to fulfill one's potential is at the highest level of the continuum. Consequently, employees strive for growth through professional training, job advancement or sharing, and employment with different agencies. Needs from each of the five levels are important at different times. No need is ever fully met yet a substantially satisfied need (i.e., comfortable income) no longer motivates one's actions.

## *Herzberg's Two-Factor Theory*

Frederick Herzberg's concept of motivators parallels Maslow's concept of higher level needs (i.e., esteem, status, self-fulfillment) and, as noted by Murphy, Niepoth, Jamieson, and Williams (1991), was built on experiments conducted in the work environment. According to Herzberg, when most practitioners' lower level needs have been met, the manager creates work environments in which higher level needs such as status and recognition can be achieved. The needs that motivate staff to achieve in the work environment are satisfiers. Practitioners expect adequate wages, good working conditions, and quality supervision. Activities (referred to as "hygiene") directed toward meeting these needs contribute to dissatisfaction in the work environment when absent. Liebler, Levine, and Rothman (1992) report that motivators provide satisfaction from the job itself and are found in opportunities for advancement and promotion, greater responsibility, challenge and growth. The manager's task is to create a challenging work environment through such activities as job enrichment and professional development opportunities. Robbins (1995) suggests that the manager who eliminates factors that contribute to job dissatisfaction while creating a comfortable work setting is not necessarily motivating staff toward the intrinsic rewards of "working." Satisfied workers are not necessarily motivated workers. Manager's motivate by expanding jobs vertically and by encouraging practitioners to learn new things and reach for new goals.

## *Argyris Maturity-Immaturity Continuum*

First postulated in the late 1950s, the Argyris maturity-immaturity continuum is also based on a behaviorist perspective and is grounded on a continuum approach. Individuals vary in their level of maturity along a relative continuum from total immaturity to total maturity. Grossman (1989) suggests that when managers recognize practitioners' relative level of maturity they create within the work environment a climate to meet individual needs based on respective maturity levels. Edginton and Griffith (1990) propose that immature employees tend to be more dependent, lack self-awareness and view outcomes from a short-term perspective. Mature employees operate independently, exercise self-control, and view operations from a long-term perspective. The manager's challenge is to view each employee from his or her respective maturity level and to create a work environment that recognizes each employee's uniqueness. To motivate employees, managers acknowledge staff differences yet are fair and consistent. Argyris advocated for job enlargement. As noted by Grossman (1989), this means that the manager gives employees a greater number and variety of tasks so that they are motivated by higher level needs such as responsibility and control.

## McClelland's Achievement Theory

Some practitioners strive for personal achievement through seeing their work through to successful completion. Robbins (1995) suggests that the drive to succeed, rather than rewards of success, compels these individuals. McClelland describes this drive for personal achievement as a higher level need similar to Maslow's esteem and self-actualization higher order needs. An employee operating with this motif is intrinsically motivated, displays a high degree of self-control, and desires to perform more efficiently. High achievers avoid risky tasks or those that might succeed or fail if outcomes were left to chance (e.g., intervention like high elements of an adventure-challenge course). The manager's task becomes assigning responsibilities of moderate risk while delegating enough authority so the employee is self-regulating and receives appropriate recognition. Grossman (1989) submits that these employees prefer work environments in which social interaction facilitates performance feedback—a need similar to Maslow's social needs. A manager operating under this premise incorporates into the work environment social recognition (e.g., employee of the month) and opportunities to see moderately challenging tasks from start to successful completion (e.g., redesign of department assessment tools).

## McGregor's Theory X and Theory Y

Coincidental with Herzberg's and Argyris' theories, McGregor presented Theory X and Theory Y to explain two types of management. McGregor observed from studying traditional organizational structures that some workers dislike their work, avoid responsibility, lack initiative, and prefer strong direction (i.e., Theory X). Motivation is derived from satisfaction of lower level needs (salaries and fringe benefits). This approach has been labeled the "carrot-and-stick" management style. A manager who operates according to Theory X leads with an authoritative hand or bribes employees to perform using extrinsic motivators such as financial reward. This theory assumes the lowest levels of need satisfaction like Maslow's and Argyris' motivate behaviors.

McGregor proposed an alternative theory, Theory Y, based on higher levels of need satisfaction. Motivators create opportunities for self-control, self-direction, and self-esteem building. The assumptions undergirding this theory view human behavior positively and hold that work is as natural as play. McGregor believes people seek self-control under the right conditions, learn to accept respon-

sibility, commit themselves to meaningful tasks or department goals, and seek quality in personal and professional tasks. As summarized in Murphy, Niepoth, Jamieson, and Williams (1991), an interrelationship exists between satisfaction of personal and professional needs. As an employee's personal needs are met, work performance is apt to reflect this achievement positively. The manager is challenged to create an environment in which Maslow's higher order needs are achieved. Grossman (1989) states that managers must arrange department conditions to ensure that employees achieve their personal goals by controlling their work efforts as they achieve the unit's goals. (Effective management of self-regulating teams represents the tenets of Theory Y).

## Vroom's Expectancy Theory

In the mid-1960s a number of theories purported that behavior is not merely motivated by need satisfaction alone; employees' perceptions and expectations of the work environment influence outcomes of work behaviors. Expectancy theory suggests that an employee must expect that his or her behavior will lead to satisfaction or a desired outcome. Robbins (1995) outlines the relationship among three primary tenets of the theory: effort-performance, performance-rewards, and rewards-personal goals. An employee is motivated when effort leads to positive performance appraisal and proper recognition which satisfy the employee's personal goals. Motivation decreases when probability of goal attainment is low and/or value attributed to the reward is low.

Vroom's theory suggests the manager should be aware of the unique needs and values of his or her staff. Each staff member places different value on work motivators such as security, financial reward, and recognition. Likewise, the needs fulfilled by work vary. Some therapeutic recreation specialists need praise from a supervisor while others need collegial recognition; some need "to give or help" while others need to be a part of a "medical team." Also evident from this theory is the significance of a manager's explanation of the reward structure and performance expectations. First-line managers must clearly articulate the relationship between performance and departmental goals and the significance of the department's award structure to each member's individual goals.

## Equity Theory

Similar to the expectancy theory, equity theory describes the relationship between individual effort and reward and employees' perceptions of the effort and reward received by others. Equity exists when an employee subjectively determines that the ratio of his or her input to reward or outcomes is comparable to that of other employees. When an imbalance exists, the tension that is created causes the employee to be motivated to reduce the inequity and to achieve fairness.

Employee input includes a number of factors such as effort, experience, education, and competence. Reward is also broadly defined to include salary level, fringe benefits, recognition, working conditions, and department rewards. Tension is created when, for example, two employees of the same age and years of accumulated work experience are rewarded differently. Robbins (1995) indicates this theory helps to explain why employees reduce their work efforts when they perceive they are not rewarded fairly. Some employees may even resign when they perceive their relative condition compared to others in the department seems inequitable.

## Ouchi's Theory Z

William Ouchi described a contemporary motivational approach that focuses on increasing productivity through participatory management. As described by Liebler, Levine, and Rothman (1992), the Theory Z approach recognizes quality outcomes and participatory decision making found in present-day healthcare and human resource initiatives and management models. Murphy, Niepoth, Jamieson, and Williams (1991) suggest this approach supports both Theory X and Theory Y because employees and managers alike participate in making decisions that effect department outcomes.

A holistic perspective permeates management. Each staff member's efforts are significant to the department and work of the team. Quality circles work on solving job-related quality problems such as client scheduling and/or transportation. As a result of feeling a sense of commitment from the department, employees tend to plan a life-long career with the unit. Relationships forged by group efforts support each employee's individual needs and job satisfaction.

To summarize this section, each theory offers alternatives to managing motivating environments. Traditional theories tend to limit motivation to behaviors that satisfy needs. Fundamental differences in these theories relate to descriptors of lower and higher level needs to be satisfied through work. More recent theories attribute motivation to broader concepts of need satisfaction. These theories suggest employee behaviors tend to be affected by perceptions and judgments of relationships among a number of factors including how employees compare and relate to one another. Systematic management practices derived from the most recent theories acknowledge the influence of the total work environment on the achievement of personal needs and on the inherent relationship between satisfaction of personal needs and department goals.

# The Manager, Work Culture, and Motivation

Grossman (1989) contrasts motivation to a coin. Each has two sides. On one side, the manager must develop and use himself or herself to motivate practitioners. Employees also must satisfy their needs in the work environment and/or through alternative experiences. A manager's challenge is, therefore, twofold: (1) to hone personal professional qualities and practices to engage staff and volunteers in experiences that result in fulfillment and (2) to create a work environment supportive of personal satisfaction and development and achievement of department goals. A manager is aware of human characteristics and qualities that contribute to positive supportive relationships. Additionally, a sensitive manager is aware of work environment factors that enhance the well-being and productivity of staff and volunteers. As a result, actions are taken to orchestrate a mutually beneficial work experience. Liebler, Levine and Rothman (1992) indicate that high-level performance is consistently achieved when managers focus on ability, support, and effort. In this section, motivation is considered from the manager's and department's perspective. Managerial guidelines drawn from the theories, study of manager behaviors, and organizational climate are presented. The section closes with a summary of strategies to encourage high-level performance.

## Qualities and Practices of the First-Line Manager

How does a manager make staff and volunteers want to work? A conscious planned effort is essential. A first-line manager's behaviors and practices create a presence and an environment in which staff and volunteers are comfortable working toward personal and professional goal achievement. Managers frequently "dress in front of the mirror" to reflect on qualities and actions that influence other's behaviors. Several authors (Edginton and Griffith, 1990; Grossman, 1989; Murphy, Niepoth, Jamieson, and Williams, 1991) suggest that a manager must develop certain human characteristics in order to create an environment where people want to work and are self-motivated. Some of these critical managerial characteristics are listed here:

- knowledge of self, especially strengths and weaknesses, and what does and does not motivate personal actions and managerial behaviors;
- knowledge of staff and volunteers and their personal and professional needs and goals;
- a sense of sincerity and responsibility to meet the needs of others and commit to their well-being;

- willingness to change and respond to dynamic and constantly fluid work expectations and socio-economic-political variations;
- self-respect, integrity, acceptance and respect of others (e.g., unconditional positive regard);
- active listening, feedback, and commitment to authentic, open, trustworthy communication;
- a patience and tolerance for growth in oneself and others;
- the ability to discipline oneself to accomplish immediate and long-range outcomes; and
- the ability to accurately self-assess and separate personal from professional judgments.

## Work Culture and Motivation

A number of variables within the work climate directly influence motivational levels of managers, staff, and volunteers. First-line managers have the opportunity to affect change in some of these variables while other variables remain outside their realm of influence. With an awareness of these variables, managers are open to opportunities that promote achievement of staff and department goals.

One variable over which a first-line manager has minimal influence is the complexity of the department and/or relationship of the unit to the organization. Communication flows through more channels in larger organizations. Structure of the department and its relationship to other units and/or the organization also is a function of size. Formal policies and procedures codify behavior in larger complex work environments. Edginton and Griffith (1990) note that specialization in larger organizations adds to complexity. Where size and complexity are factors, managers hope to structure unit tasks so that practitioners perceive trust, openness and support within the department for their needs.

A variable over which the manager does have some influence is the climate within the department. Within the department a manager structures the physical environment to support interpersonal relationships and a collective commitment to the mission. Amenities like access to a mail drop, coffee pot, fax machine, and comfortable office space boost morale. Grossman (1989) suggests that managers structure opportunities to communicate personal and career goals at the department level. The degree of control a first-line manager has within the unit is relational to organizational variables. Consequently, the climate set at the macro level permeates managerial actions within the service unit. Individual work units are only as healthy as the overall work environment.

A number of administrative processes like personnel selection, reward structures, financial management, and supervisory communications affect department environments. Competent personnel can be expected to perform if given necessary support, resources, and appropriate recognition. Conversely, marginally qualified persons are not as likely to perceive their jobs in a positive manner regardless of the quality of work environment and reward system. Achievement is promoted by properly rewarding performance. Motivation results when staff value the reward and the reward is commensurate with their efforts. The degree of financial solvency within the division, department, and organization contributes to worker security and morale. For example, uncertainties about pay raises or fringe adjustments create discomfort and lead to job dissatisfaction. Supervisory communications affect the work environment and, therefore, influence practitioner motivation. Tools and avenues used to transmit information stimulate positive employee interactions and/or discourage open exchanges among department employees. Further, the leadership style a first-line manager uses affects department communication (see Chapters 4 and 20). Examples are set as the manager communicates during formal meetings and informal supervisory conversations. Thus, communication explicitly and implicitly motivates (see Chapter 14).

Work culture broadly describes the atmosphere and nature of a job setting. A number of factors over which the first-line manager has varying degrees of control and influence contribute to the work climate. For instance, the size, complexity, and structure of a department and organization directly affect job comfort and performance. Satisfaction is enhanced with the presence of amenities and open interactions. The manner in which a manager transacts duties also sets a certain tone and sends specific messages. A positive work environment finds manager and staff equally committed to the achievement of personal goals and the department mission.

## Guidelines to Build a Positive Motivational Atmosphere

A successful manager blends individual needs with department goals. As Murphy, Niepoth, Jamieson, and Williams (1991) point out, a motivational manager makes available appropriate resources and support for satisfaction of employee needs. If the work environment creates a spirit of camaraderie, staff and volunteers feel empowered to communicate with candor and openness. Grossman (1989) indicates the manager's ability to release staff capacities is influenced greatly when a motivational environment exists. There are many actions a manager can take to promote worker desire to achieve personal and departmental goals. A number of authors (Edginton and Griffith, 1991; Grossman, 1989; Murphy, Niepoth, Jamieson, and Williams, 1991; Robbins, 1995; Young, 1992) present guidelines managers should consider as they organize the work setting to promote worker satisfaction and performance. The following list highlights these guidelines:

- become familiar with employee needs in order to relate these to department goals;
- communicate candidly so that each staff member and volunteer feels significant to department outcomes;
- increase practitioner ability to achieve personal and professional goals through training and development;
- introduce challenges so that expectancy is increased, performance is improved and workers experience a higher level of job satisfaction;
- encourage commitment to the course of action by involving staff and volunteers in decision-making processes so that commitment to the course of action results;
- promote team initiatives and building processes because unity results in productive units;
- structure the work environment so that practitioners have the freedom to accomplish clearly delineated tasks and then reinforce productivity with positive feedback;
- encourage cooperation and respect for each person's unique contributions by individualized reinforcement, praise, and recognition;
- epitomize ethical behaviors such as being consistent, objective, equitable, and reliable;
- maintain a healthy lifestyle on and off the job;
- match practitioner preferences, knowledge, skill, and abilities with work tasks;
- guide practitioner actions and review progress by setting up observable, measurable goals and planned formal and informal sessions;
- link rewards with performance and seek ways to increase the visibility of the reward (opportunities to link monetary rewards with performance should not be overlooked); and
- continuously evaluate the work environment to ensure motivational strategies are in place. If performance problems become apparent, participatory efforts should openly address environmental deficiencies causing worker dilemmas.

Managerial actions that promote motivational environments are interrelated. Also, when one element like individualized recognition, is in place, another is likely to be positively impacted (e.g., performance reviews). The autonomy of the therapeutic recreation department may determine the manager's relative control over motivational strategies. A number of these guidelines appear to have evolved from previous theories (i.e., expectancy, equity, and Theory Z). Management views tend to promote work environments that facilitate satisfaction of higher level needs (e.g., self-esteem, self-fulfillment) through staff and volunteer involvement in day-to-day decisions and planning. This stimulates cohesiveness and unity between personal and unit goals.

## High-Level Performance

Effective managers motivate staff and volunteers by providing adequate human and technical resources and support. When competent people have the necessary support, they will exert the work effort needed to achieve high-level performance. Liebler, Levine, and Rothman (1992) indicate that continued education is essential to maintain and enhance staff in health and human service agencies. Support is necessary so that staff abilities and competence are fully utilized. This support includes not only equipment and safe areas for intervention but also proper guidance and supervision. Department goals must be attainable and the first-line manager must work together with upper level management to secure required resources. When competent staff have proper support, they are likely to put forth the effort to do their jobs well. Therefore, first-line managers should focus their actions on ensuring competent staff, adequate support, and worker effort. As presented by Liebler, Levine and Rothman (1992), the strategies managers use to enhance each of these areas are summarized here:

1. Strategies to promote staff competence and ability:
   - delineate desired knowledge, skills, and abilities in job descriptions and specifications;
   - communicate achievable staff performance goals;
   - communicate formally and informally with upper level management particular staffing capabilities and trends;
   - create a positive department image so that people desire to work in it; and
   - remain informed on relevant employment trends in therapeutic recreation and communicate this to upper level management.
2. Strategies to garner department support and resources:
   - provide constructive feedback;
   - maintain only necessary policies and protocols;
   - meet routinely with staff to assess resource needs;
   - pursue acquisition of the best possible resources; and
   - create a socially dynamic and fluid work environment.
3. Strategies that encourage staff effort:
   - set performance objectives and standards for evaluating results;
   - provide rewards and reinforcement commensurate with achievement of performance expectations;
   - communicate with upper level management performance accomplishments of the department;
   - maintain a degree of presence and visibility in the unit and within the organization; and
   - remain a confident, enthusiastic role model.

These strategies summarize effective human resource management helpful to the first-line manager where limited control of work environment variables is evident. The success a therapeutic recreation manager experiences is in the interactions between the first-line manager and upper level management.

One of the more specific functions of a first-line manager is the job design process. Robbins (1995) reports that one of the more important factors influencing employee motivational levels is the job structure. Through the job design process, managers enrich employees' jobs and increase their motivation to achieve high-level performance. According to Robbins (1995), every job has five key characteristics, and, when each is present to a high degree, the job is potentially motivating. Needs of the employee determine the motivational effects of each characteristic reported by Robbins (1995):

1. the degree of skill variety (routine or multifaceted),
2. degree of task identity (whole or partial completion),
3. degree of significance (minimal to substantial impact on others),
4. degree of autonomy (discretion to determine intervention), and
5. degree of feedback (source of information about effectiveness of therapeutic recreation services).

Although each staff member's needs will determine the motivational influence of each of the five job characteristics, the manager's actions contribute to the motivational potential of a particular job. Robbins (1995) outlines five steps first-line managers may take to accomplish job enrichment:

1. increase skill variety and task identity by combining responsibilities;
2. create natural task units so an employee conducts the whole job (e.g., assessment through client evaluation);
3. increase skill autonomy and feedback by helping staff establish professional relationships with consumers;
4. increase autonomy by delegating unit tasks like risk management to staff; and
5. provide timely relevant feedback to open communication channels (this is as effective as prescheduled performance reviews).

Designing motivating jobs requires the manager to contemplate the inherent motivational features of each position. To do this, a manager projects the level of productivity each employee is expected to achieve. In these projections, the manager considers how each employee's needs will be fulfilled and how each employee's achievements relate to department goals. Job design is foundational to department motivation and high-level performance.

# Future Motivational Challenges

A number of management trends, healthcare initiatives, and social demographics create challenges in the work environment. Health and human service work settings will experience increasing rates of change, accountability, and quality concerns with a reduced work force and resource base. Cultivating a work environment supportive of staff needs will become increasingly challenging. Traditional motivators like promotional opportunities, blanket healthcare coverage, and wage increases will become less significant in the employee recognition process. Human resource management will focus on high-level performance through conscious efforts to match personal and professional growth needs to achieve measurable outcomes.

Participatory management, accountability, and quality monitoring are trends impacting employee motivational strategies. Self-regulating teams, supervisor-employee design of development plans, and management-staff operational planning exemplify participatory functions likely to influence practitioner motivation. Managers empower staff to become intimately involved in these activities to encourage self-efficacy and department advocacy and growth. Decision-making opportunities promote perceptions of value, worth, and control—qualities necessary for one's self-fulfillment.

A focus on accountability requires each practitioner to assume responsibility. Accountability is known through feedback. Positive feedback affirms responsible actions and fosters motivation. First-line managers transfer to practitioners an increased degree of authority to ensure responsible use of limited departmental resources and client contact time. Managers help staff through the time-consuming "paper trails" so that practitioners are made acutely aware of the results of their interventions. Formal and informal acknowledgments reward contributions.

Continuous quality improvement processes focus on individual staff efforts, garnering necessary support, and maintaining competent professionals—the three variables of high-level performance. Managers guide staff in their self-assessments and team building. Increasingly, first-line managers will advocate for necessary resources and devote their time to staff enhancement, change, and growth. Managers will possess training and financial management skills and will create a work environment of expectancy and self-direction.

Health and human service professionals are experiencing decreased direct client contact, blending of professional roles, and relocation of services. These trends either motivate or demotivate. Managers will facilitate personnel transformations, assist during periods of role ambiguity, and train staff as referral and transition specialists. Without adequate managerial support, employees are likely to perceive job insecurities, feelings of incompetence, and professional abandonment.

Managers face the challenge of helping staff realize their contributions to the whole intervention or program process regardless of service setting. Therapeutic recreators will apply the therapeutic recreation process across disciplines and settings. Managers will also help their staff and volunteers advocate for the significant role therapeutic recreation assumes in the quality of life and well-being. Additionally, a work culture will cultivate flexibility and adaptability so that helping skills are applied not only at one work site but also in several delivery settings. Feedback from delivery networks will help staff realize that the therapeutic recreation process is carried out even when settings change and jobs are not titled "therapeutic recreation specialist."

Just as the work setting and way work is managed are changing so is the nature of the work force. The work force will be more diverse, more technologically and scientifically astute, and individually value laden. These characteristics will influence who, when, how, and why services are offered. Traditional students (e.g., chronological age 18–21) comprise a smaller percentage of campus student bodies. Persons reentering the work force, changing careers, and/or seeking to complete entry-level credentialing criteria will continue to change the makeup of the classroom and work force. Flex time, job sharing, permanent part-time positions, and as-needed basis positions are factors contributing to a diversified work force that will provide therapeutic interventions. Employees will be technology literate and capable of using the latest innovations in management and delivery of therapeutic recreation services.

Why will careers in therapeutic recreation be attractive? A shifting value system will orient inward toward individualized commitments and inherent worth of personal services rather than commitment to "company" outcomes and department recognition. As Robbins (1995) notes, employees will place their allegiance with the profession rather than a particular work site. Future employees will tend to be as sensitive to job design as to money. As with volunteers, "what's in it for me" will become the double-edged sword of management.

To motivate, managers will focus on intangibles as well as tangibles in the work setting. Factors like autonomy, variety, group cohesiveness, peer recognition, personal development options, and self-determined work schedules will become commonplace in the work environment. Amenities like e-mail and access to alternative program resources through telecommunications will accompany the coffee pot and company wellness program as standard employment benefits. Staff and volunteers will more readily achieve high performance in a work culture supportive of flexibility, professional growth, and self-management. The manager's challenge becomes communicating options through strategies like delegation, negotiation, and active listening. Traditional management preparation tends to focus on day-to-day tasks like budgeting, marketing, and supervision. Future processes will emphasize concepts found in clinical supervision, self-efficacy, and human resource development.

# Summary

Motivation is an inherent feature of management. The future will see an increased focus on the first-line manager's ability to motivate staff and volunteers. This is due in large part to the changing nature of the work environment, work force, and health and human services dynamics. As traditional motivators like money and advancements become less available, the manager's ability to manipulate areas that influence the work environment become more critical to effective department operations. The intent of this chapter was to present options managers introduce into the work environment to empower staff so that work outcomes are mutually beneficial to staff and department goals.

The initial section of this chapter dealt with a motivation prerequisite—the fulfillment of individual needs. A number of factors (i.e., locus of control, perceptions about power, self-esteem, employee fit, risk taking) contribute to individual differences. When a manager recognizes these uniquenesses, it is easier to match individual need satisfiers with performance outcomes. The work environment or work culture is shaped by the manager. The support and resources of the environment add or detract from relationships formed in the work environment. Thus, the manager blends the work culture with uniquenesses of employees to accomplish personal goals and department outcomes.

A number of theories have explained motivation. Each purports concepts applicable to manager-practitioner motivational variables. One of the more elementary but significant theories is Maslow's hierarchy of needs. Several behaviorists, Herzberg, Argyris, and McClelland, employed the concept of need satisfaction along a continuum from lower to higher order needs to describe the significance of need satisfaction to personal development and achievement in the work setting. McGregor's now infamous Theory X and Theory Y also applied similar concepts to explain the difference between workers who require a carrot-and-stick approach and those who are motivated by self-growth opportunities. Theories proposed since the 1960s (e.g., expectancy, equity) suggest that behavior alone does not motivate action. Workers are also motivated by perceptions of others and comparisons between their efforts and rewards and that of other employees. The more recent Theory Z contends that participatory management strategies enhance workplace motivation.

From these theories and management writings, a number of motivational guidelines are drawn. Specific managerial qualities and practices trigger motivation. These characteristics are summarized because they are key to facilitating employee self-motivation. A second source of motivational factors is the work culture. The work culture is impacted by complexity, structure, administrative processes, and communication processes. First-line managers have varying degrees of control over these motivators and demotivators. A motivational atmosphere is positive and supports realization of staff and department goals. Specific guidelines are listed for creating positive work settings. All managers desire high-level performance, but the manager who properly addresses employee competence, provision of department resources, and effort is likely to facilitate outcomes reflective of high productivity.

A closing section addressed challenges therapeutic recreation managers may anticipate in the future. Management trends, healthcare initiatives, and social demographics are causing dynamic work settings, work forces, and adjustments to the way therapeutic recreation is practiced. In the future, managers will focus on tangibles and intangibles to create motivating workplaces. Further, tradition-

ally assumed motivators like financial reward will be supplemented by creative job design and management of the social fabric of one's work cultures. Managers will need to craft flexible, dynamic open networks where interpersonal and professional development focus on achievement of personal and departmental goals.

# Discussion Questions

1. What are the primary factors that explain individual differences in the workplace? Explain how each influences motivation.
2. What are the key theoretical concepts that have influenced management of employee motivation? Summarize points of each that will influence futuristic management styles.
3. What specific manager characteristics affect motivation?
4. What work culture variables influence employee motivation?
5. How is a positive motivational atmosphere created in the workplace?
6. What are the three key elements that motivate high-level performance and how do they interrelate?
7. What is the manager's role as it relates to futuristic job design?
8. How will managers motivate in the year 2000 and beyond?

# References

Edginton, C. R., and Griffith C. A. (1990). *The recreation and leisure service delivery system.* Dubuque, IA: Wm. C. Brown Publishers.

Grossman, A. H. (1989). Developing and implementing motivational strategies. In A. H. Grossman (Ed.), *Personnel management in recreation and leisure services* (pp. 133–151). Reston, VA: American Alliance for Health, Physical Education, Recreation and Dance.

Liebler, J. G., Levine, R. E., and Rothman, J. (1992). *Management principles for health professionals* (2nd ed.). Gaithersburg, MD: Aspen Publishers, Inc.

Murphy, J. F., Niepoth, E. W., Jamieson, L. M., and Williams, J. G. (1991). *Leisure systems: Critical concepts and applications.* Champaign, IL: Sagamore Publishing Inc.

Robbins, S. P. (1995). *Supervision today.* Englewood Cliffs, NJ: Prentice Hall.

Young, B. (1992). Motivating your part-time staff and volunteers. *Parks and Recreation, 27:9,* 92–95.

# Chapter 16

# Performance Appraisal

## Introduction

One of the more challenging tasks experienced as a first-line manager is performance evaluation and review of subordinates which is both a personal and a professional responsibility. This overlap occurs on the job as the manager communicates and motivates employees; yet it is most evident as the manager attempts to evaluate deficiencies and recognize accomplishments. Each employee brings to a position personal characteristics and behavioral traits with professional knowledge, skills, and abilities (KSAs). To attain division or department goals, a manager capitalizes on each employee's resources to benefit the client, employee, and organization. This means helping employees to appraise and continue to improve their performance.

Quality management approaches, health and human service reforms, accountability demands, cost containment efforts, and the focus on service outcomes necessitate competent therapeutic recreation professionals whether their roles are full time, part time, seasonal, or volunteer. Along with the ever increasing rate of change, these concerns require the manager to ensure that staff remain competent and able to adapt to future job expectations. Thus, performance reviews are integral to human resource management decisions related to staffing, training and development, and planning future personnel needs. Also, as noted by Sullivan (1994), a manager may be held liable if an employee fails to practice competently. For the manager the challenge is to shift the focus from documentation of personal attributes and behaviors to assessing the profes-

sional partnership between the manager and individual and/or team so that human resources within the system are properly used to achieve department outcomes. A manager completes a number of tasks in preparing and completing performance reviews.

The development of a personnel evaluation and review system involves structuring formal and informal reviews and communicating on a continuous basis. The manager prepares and implements these processes after considering a number of factors including professional and legal directives, the nature of employees' positions, the organizational context in which reviews and evaluations occur, and strategies that enhance manager-employee participation in appraisals. In the first section of this chapter, the authors introduce a number of variables the manager recognizes and prepares for as systems are designed. In the second section, the development and implementation of appraisal forms and processes is studied. Constructive continuous feedback is generated with proper design of evaluative tools and interview methods. A number of human and system elements, however, may enter into the process and reduce validity, reliability, and objectivity of the process. The first-line manager implements several strategies to compensate for these compounding factors.

A third section outlines the steps and alternatives that follow actual appraisals. After the manager and employee have reviewed the information collected and have completed a formal appraisal, an action plan is designed. Managers use outcomes to facilitate staff potential and to plan training and supportive resource development. Results are also considered in promotions, reassignments, maintenance of privileging status, monetary adjustments, and terminations. Evaluation of others is inevitable. If done well and on a continuous basis, outcomes are motivational, encouraging stronger working relationships among the employee, team, and manager. Conversely, if results are used improperly, fairness is jeopardized and service quality is placed at risk.

# Planning Personnel Evaluation Systems

Personnel evaluation is a vital component of human resource management. Persons who possess the desired KSAs are hired. Then they are oriented and trained to perform their jobs so that department goals are achieved and, finally, they are evaluated to ensure that the mix of personnel and resources remain optimal. According to Halachmi (1993), evaluation is a joint effort by the first-line manager and the therapeutic recreation specialist to find out what needs to be done to achieve desired client outcomes, what and how the therapeutic recreation specialist can contribute, and what the first-line manager must do to create a work environment that helps staff contribute to department outcomes. A personnel evaluation system must be congruent with the protocols of the organization and uphold the tenets of the profession. Like other human resource functions, evaluation systems must be free of bias and job related.

Performance appraisals and reviews operate under several assumptions which undergird design considerations. The following list highlights assumptions drawn from the literature (Ghorpade and Chen, 1995; Robbins, 1995; Sullivan, 1994):

1. Each employee brings unique KSAs to a position and differs in how able and motivated he or she is to apply these KSAs to the duties.
2. Each employee's performance quality influences the degree to which the department is able to achieve its goals. Therefore, appraisal is needed to determine if the department is getting its rightful due.
3. Evaluation is an integral part of development and provides for assessing each employee's potential to gain from training and development opportunities.
4. Through ongoing formal and informal supervisory communication and feedback, evaluations and reviews encourage continuous quality improvement.
5. Job performance which includes one's ability to be a team player is a part of each therapeutic recreation specialist's contributions to the department and team thus, peer reviews confirm validity of the process.

6. Formal appraisal is essential to legally defend the organization against claims of inadequate service outcomes.

Evaluation is a serious activity with consequences for both the employee and the manager. The primary intent of evaluation is to foster an employee's growth and development within the department so that organizational goals are continuously achieved. Appraisal outcomes are also weighed in a number of other management decisions and actions:

1. Evaluation is necessary to determine the effectiveness of human resource efforts such as training and development.
2. Evaluation is a form of systems or managerial analysis that enables decisions to be made about relationships, organizational structure, and resources as they relate to personnel performance.
3. Documentation resulting from evaluation and reviews is used to support references and administrative decisions on personnel status and reward.
4. Feedback and development from evaluation results help staff remediate and improve in order to prevent adverse personnel actions and to enable the manager to help each employee realize his or her full potential.
5. As suggested by Dwyer and Cripe (1984), evaluation judges adequacy or appropriateness of placement with part-time and seasonal employees. Does the employee possess the necessary KSAs to return next summer? Would the employee benefit from reassignment of part-time work hours to another shift or sequence of days or hours?
6. Evaluation and performance appraisals are a form of quality improvement; therefore, as recommended by Ghorpade and Chen (1995), causes of variation are identified and improvement strategies are planned in the same manner that other deficiencies are noted and resolved.
7. McGee reports (1992) that appraisals and reviews lead to opportunities for improved communication between the first-line manager and employees throughout the year and are a form of participatory management that motivate employees to provide input into the department strategic plan.

This list presents the complexity of management decisions emanating from performance appraisals. As suggested by Ghorpade and Chen (1995), it is becoming progressively more difficult to retain the qualities desired in the system such as validity, reliability, objectivity, job relatedness and importance to job success. The onus of responsibility lies with the first-line manager to ensure these measurement qualities.

## Organizational Considerations

The organization in which the therapeutic recreation program is housed greatly influences the manager's role in performance reviews. Rarely does the first-line manager have complete discretion in personnel evaluations (Robbins, 1995). It is not uncommon for an organization to use or recommend the use of standardized forms and/or review processes during formal evaluations. In some instances an abbreviated or generic form is provided, and the manager assumes the responsibility to identify individual employee job factors and quality indicators to be included during actual evaluation sessions. Managers develop job specifications and select staff according to organizational policies and protocols. Within any organization, personnel carry out the tasks delineated in their respective job specifications according to operational codes. Managers cognizant of these organizational factors incorporate assessment of organizational expectations into the evaluation.

Politics and the working environment or culture within the organization also impinge upon worker performance and are considered as systems are designed. Results of evaluations have implications for relationships among employees, employees and managers, and managers and upper level administration and they are important in salary, promotion, and retention actions. A manager's budget requests to upper level administration include personnel justifications. Employees' perceptions of their manager rest upon how well the manager has fostered their potential and has supported their resource needs. While working together to improve client well-being, each employee anticipates a return for his or her contribution to the client's satisfaction. Therefore, there is an ever-present reality that employees, the manager, and upper level administrators are influenced by the political consequences of actions directly or indirectly tied to performance evaluations.

A number of precipitating factors have contributed to the manager's role as a department facilitator. Decreases in funding and staffing levels, increases in accountability measures, shorter length of stays, and reduced length of program sessions have fostered collaboration and teamwork. Clients gain from collective expertise and resource access. Berryman (1989) suggests that employees benefit from participatory management practices because the environment is nonthreatening, and they are more likely to be motivated to apply their KSAs, to change, and to improve their performance. Collaboration, networking and teamwork rely on each employee to contribute to the team and to be a good *team player*. These qualities are often better assessed by those who share in these strategies than by the first-line manager (Robbins, 1995). Thus, peer reviews and group evaluations, if included in the performance appraisal process, encourage autonomy of working groups, reinforce cooperation, and increase the validity of the process (Robbins, 1995).

## Professional and Legal Considerations

The manager's responsibility to ensure compliance with professional practice standards in the workplace has contributed to closer scrutiny of the tie between organizational and departmental personnel evaluations and professional training and credentials. A manager is aware that *qualified* therapeutic recreation specialists and leisure professionals with similar credentials (i.e., certified therapeutic recreation specialist [CTRS], certified leisure professional [CLP]) have varying practice styles based on training and experience (Sullivan, 1994). Also, part-time and seasonal employees with credentials in other health and human service professions may be qualified to practice in specific positions such as day camp leaders, aquatic supervisors, and adventure-challenge specialists where their expertise is applicable and contributes to improved client functioning. Managers design evaluation systems to recognize differences while noting acceptable practice modalities. Where staff hold credentials outside the professional purview of therapeutic recreation managers, appraisal systems incorporate performance indicators that assess contribution to departmental outcomes but do not require the manager to judge the competence of the staff member as, for example, a special education teacher, nurse, or relaxation therapist. The manager's challenge is to create performance systems that determine if competent professionals are able to apply their KSAs clinically or functionally in practice. Standards of practice (ATRA, 1993; NTRS, 1995) define service scope and depth and describe the types of services to be delivered by competent professionals. In essence, these are *worker-oriented* jobs because they present what content experts see as essential to successful therapeutic recreation practice. Inclusion of evaluative criteria that recognize these practices enhances the validity of appraisals (Dwyer and Cripe, 1984).

Lawsuits arise when managers say or do something that employees believe affects them adversely. Usually associated with organizational appraisal forms and processes are personnel policies and handbooks. These documents are increasingly recognized by the courts as binding unilateral contracts (Robbins, 1995). Consequently, if the manager inadvertently does not follow or follows improperly these guidelines, the organization may be held accountable. Managerial position training during orientation incorporates discussion of staffing and particularly those practices that, when not adhered to, could result in legal action. A human resource department, personnel specialist, or an attorney who specializes in employer-employee relations is usually a primary resource in interpreting legal connotations of personnel policies.

Equal employment opportunity laws require that all staffing practices be free of bias and job related. Evaluation criteria, review methods, instrumentation, and documentation must be designed to ensure objectivity, validity, reliability, and job relatedness. A good manager is astutely aware that a number of factors contribute to the employee's perceptions, beliefs, and interpretations of supervisory actions. Rondeau (1992) has noted the following as primary influences on the employee-manager relationship:

- employee's experience and length of service,
- employee's and employer's motivational states,
- capability of the manager to communicate information,
- employee's receptivity to constructive criticism,
- manager's knowledge of the employee's performance,
- manager's ability to control significant sanctions and rewards, and
- degree of trust each has in the other's motives.

The manager's task is to ensure that the employee does not believe or perceive decisions, actions, and communication to be the result of personal bias, prejudices, or idiosyncrasies. To avoid this, the manager should include employees in the evaluation of the performance system and the appraisal of supervisory staff, including the manager. Additionally, connections between the reward system and job retention and/or termination should be clearly articulated. Managers must encourage personnel to view appraisal as one element having significance equal to any other in the continuous process of improving service outcomes.

## Quality Management Considerations

Since performance appraisals are intended to stimulate individual staff growth and development, aid employees to realize their potential, and measure their contributions to the department's outcomes, each performance appraisal is unique. As the manager assesses the situation, reviewing and collecting available documents and using recommended evaluation techniques can add to the credibility of the implemented processes. Colleagues from other units within the organization or other agencies have access to tools and may be willing to share resources. Agencies also tend to distribute supportive materials with personnel appraisal forms, and instruments are available through conference presentations and professional reading. Likewise, texts on evaluation and personnel management may include sample documents and recommended guidelines to follow as personnel evaluation systems are designed. A number of strategies are recommended for developing performance systems so that they are congruent with quality management principles and the unique features of a particular work environment:

1. Ghorpade and Chen (1995) suggest that evaluation considers two types of behavior—task performance and quality improvement. Organizations invest resources to attain goals and to preserve the viability of the organization. In turn, workers complete tasks relevant to goal attainment and which promote teamwork and system improvement.

2. Personnel evaluation is an ongoing process with informal and formal reviews. A personnel file is maintained on each employee and the manager continually documents specific incidents (Robbins, 1995). Generally, the longer the manager has been familiar with the employee, whether full or part time, the more accurate the performance assessment (Dwyer and Cripe, 1984).

3. Training leads to more accurate rating and evaluation of employee and system factors. Employee evaluations are tempered by the knowledge that the behaviors and/or outcomes the rating is based on are influenced by factors within the organization and department over which the employee has no control or responsibility.

4. Information is collected from multiple perspectives or raters including the person being assessed. Multiple raters increase reliability as illustrated with sports competition when the judges drop the highest and lowest scores (Robbins, 1995). Additionally persons in other positions and units are often in better positions to identify system factors than the therapeutic recreation manager who, for example, may not have firsthand observation of teams on which staff sit.

5. Evaluation considers employee potential and barriers to potential improvement and growth. Feedback is less confrontational when the emphasis is placed on improvement rather than blame for specific problems. Assessment of potential allows the employee to project future career options and growth targets.

6. Evaluation focuses on behavior since behavior is observable, inherently job related, and relatively more controllable by the worker (Ghorpade and Chen, 1995). Raters are, therefore, more likely to observe behavioral indicators than traits like initiative or intuition which are desirable but are more likely to be appraised from the rater's viewpoint or bias.

7. Absolute, or noncomparative, and relative, or comparative, standards are combined in the design of personnel evaluation systems. Absolute standards direct employees toward quality output without concern about a competitive position with their peers; however, absolute standards tend to be biased by inflationary pressures as, for example, high rankings (Robbins, 1995). Relative standards inhibit teamwork and minimize actual variability among employees yet facilitate individual awareness of behaviors perceived significant within the team or department. Using both absolute and relative standards enables the manager to present information relative to other

personnel in the organization as each unit manager may use different rating forms and assign values to rankings differently.

A number of factors can distort the evaluation process. To illustrate, managers may hesitate to categorize their employees or assign ratings to behaviors because evaluations have negative connotations rather than being viewed as development tools and quality indicators (Edington and Griffith, 1990). Managers may think that evaluations tend to cause staff to become unmotivated or that staff have difficulty accepting criticism. Further, the employee may not have control over certain circumstances like length of stay or client registration in particular community-based programs which results in the employee being concerned about achieving client outcomes and performing his or her job as expected. According to Rondeau (1992), four out of five employees entering into formal appraisals feel they are performing at an above-average level and, as a consequence, may receive information they do not want to hear and may want to discount. This situation creates managerial discomfort and may prevent first-line managers from providing unflattering feedback. The strategies mentioned earlier help the manager plan personnel evaluations so factors that distort the process are taken into consideration.

# Designing and Implementing Personnel Evaluations

By assessing the environment in which personnel evaluations are to occur, the manager becomes aware of resources, guidelines, and constraints that will affect the design and implementation of evaluations. The next step is to determine the performance standards, communicate these expectations, and gather information or data to use in making judgments on performance. During orientation and probationary periods, the manager and employee review position specifications and discuss the evaluation process. In these discussions the distinction among setting performance objectives for development plans, reviewing development plans, and completing formal performance appraisals is clarified. The relationship of each activity to the reward system is also explained. The time frame for setting objectives varies with the time necessary to measure accomplishment of the behaviors described in each objective. Development sessions follow measurement of individual development plan objectives and serve the purpose of revising development plans based on the assessment of objective outcomes. The usual pattern of activity involves holding a yearly session dedicated to performance appraisal that incorporates information from earlier objective and development sessions.

A number of reward systems exist in organizations; the most predominant is financial. Usually salary adjustments occur after the probationary period and at regular intervals thereafter, none of which are necessarily congruent with or contingent upon the time frame of objective setting or development plan discussions. Most organizations combine feedback sessions on salary adjustments with appraisal sessions (Rondeau, 1992). Shortly after being hired, therefore, the manager and employee define performance expectations and the context in which personnel evaluations and reviews occur and are linked to the organization's reward system.

## *Determine Performance Standards*

The initial task in setting expectations is to translate job specifications into performance criteria and to relate these to employee performance objectives. As Robbins (1995) states, the three most popular sets of criteria used in personnel appraisal are job outcomes, behaviors, and traits. Outcome evaluations focus on the end result or product such as delivery of a special event or the client's ability to participate successfully in a leisure decision-making process following completion of a leisure education session. When employees work together as teams or in staffing a particular program, it is difficult to identify outcomes attributable to one person. In these situations, it is not unusual to appraise individual behaviors like responsiveness, thoroughness, accuracy, and respect for client confidentiality. The link between traits and job outcomes is weaker than the criteria in the other two areas, yet organizations tend to incorporate trait measurements into the appraisal process (Robbins, 1995). Because traits like dependability and cooperativeness refer to potential predictors of performance (rather than performance itself), they are often included on rating forms and in the manager's written descriptions of employees' interpersonal skills.

The manager reviews each employee's job description and specifications to identify outcomes, behaviors, and traits. Simultaneously, the manager identifies statements that require translation into outcomes, behaviors, or traits. For example, statements like "maintains proper documentation" or "leads group sessions" require identification of tasks, whether they be outcomes, behaviors, or traits observed when the task was successfully undertaken. However, a task like "files weekly session reports" is phrased as an outcome statement and would require no further interpretation.

As the job roles and responsibilities are clearly identified, consideration is given to how performance criteria integrate into quality controls and improvement plans of the department and organization. Individual development plans reflect each employee's contribution to the unit outcomes. To illustrate, one criterion might read, "Participates in department operations demonstrating professional behavior, supporting unit goals, and maintaining an accounting of resource use." Rewritten as a quality control measure, the statement would be broken into several components:

- the employee contributes to writing unit goals that improve operations;
- the employee exhibits ethical, safe behaviors that comply with standards of practice and protocol; and
- the employee recommends cost-effective ways to deliver therapeutic recreation services with available resources.

A lengthy list of criteria identifies performances expected of persons with the KSAs in each position. Organization personnel policies and performance appraisal handbooks may outline generic areas to be appraised. For example, all employees are to meet standards in the areas of resource management and organization, quality of service and role accountability, interpersonal skills and teamwork, and knowledge and skills of their profession. A second example might list the following areas: professional development, ability to supervise, program development, budgetary and communication skills, and work performance as a practitioner. Generally, generic forms also allow for the projection of improvement areas and reporting of recognized contributions.

The challenge for the manager is to integrate into the generic form and/or process each position's performance expectations and to interpret the relationships of each position's expectations within departmental or organizational criteria. This would apply also to seasonal and part-time employees who might not have formal objective setting or development plan sessions but would be expected to meet operational standards and carry out protocols. For these employees the link between performance expectations and financial reward is viewed from a different perspective than that of a full-time practitioner; the opportunity to retain part-time hours or to return the following summer might be as significant as salary adjustment.

## Determine Format for Performance Review

After the manager and employee have determined the criteria that either stand alone or become integrated into existing forms and processes, the format for collection of data is either designed or reviewed (if in place with generic forms and processes). Information is gathered using absolute or relative standards, objectives, and eclectic measurements represented by total quality measurement (TQM) approaches. The first three methods tend to evaluate individual performance; the last focuses on measurement of system variables impacting individual employees.

Absolute methods do not compare employee performances to one another. Formats include essays, critical-incidents, checklists, graphic rating scales, and behaviorally anchored rating scales (BARS) (Robbins, 1995). The essay or free-form narrative is a descriptive response format that enables the manager to elaborate on the quality of the employee's performances in each performance category or for each criterion. Commonly, this subjective format is used with more objective rating scales. Essay results may reflect the manager's writing ability rather than the employee's performance. The critical-incident approach permits the manager to observe employee performances in specific situations over time. The longer the manager is familiar with the employee and the more incidents that are documented, the more accurate the evaluations tend to be. This documentation type permits the manager to explain why performance is effective or ineffective and which outcomes, behaviors, or traits require improvement. Checklists allow the manager to note whether performance has (yes) or has not (no) occurred (e.g., "Does the employee maintain progress notes on each client?" or "Is the weekly petty cash report accurate?"). Checklists tend to reduce critical criteria to absolutes; however, adding narrative comments to each question offsets this disadvantage.

Graphic rating scales are among the oldest and most popular appraisal formats according to Robbins (1995). Each performance criterion is rated on a Likert scale along a continuum that best describes the employee's behavior. The format is appropriate with objective criteria such as quality of service, job skills, and knowledge. The scales are popular because the items are standardized, the data are easily compiled, and they are less time consuming than, for example, essay and critical-incident formats (Robbins, 1995). Table 16.1 presents an illustration of generic criteria presented in a graphic rating scale format.

A frequently used format, BARS combines major elements of the critical-incident and graphic rating scale methods (Robbins, 1995). Managers rate employees along a scored continuum according to actual behaviors performed on the job. Each job responsibility or dimension is defined as having varying performance levels using observable, measurable behaviors. The process of developing the instrument is valuable because it clarifies to both manager and employee the quality of performance expected. To illustrate, one of the National Council for Therapeutic Recreation Certification (NCTRC) job responsibilities, selection of programs and activities to meet client needs, is presented in the BARS format in Table 16.2 (page 240).

The second category of formats uses relative standards. Relative standards compare one employee's performance with other employee evaluations. Ranking systems use a standard distribution curve or a comparison of individual

## Table 16.1  Graphic Rating Scale Format

| Criterion | Performance Ratings | | | | |
| --- | --- | --- | --- | --- | --- |
| | 5 | 4 | 3 | 2 | 1 |
| Resource Management | Uses time productively and maintains supplies and equipment at highest level | Uses time wisely; reports problems with equipment and supplies | Usually uses time wisely; does acceptable job in maintaining equipment; only rarely wastes supplies | Occasionally misuses time and equipment in unproductive effort | Often misuses time, equipment and supplies; does not report problems |
| Quality of Service, Role Accountability | Produces well-organized work and maintains all documentation | Produces high quality work and usually keeps updated documentation | Work is acceptable with some corrections and documentation sometimes falls behind | Fair quality of work with errors and corrections needed in documentation | Work and documentation have errors and require correction routinely |
| Interpersonal Skills, Teamwork | Always co-operates and contributes to group effort | Willing to help and support work of others | Helps others and usually contributes to group effort | Frequently has difficulty working with others and contributing to group initiative | Cannot comfortably contribute as group member |
| Therapeutic Recreation Specialist Skills, Knowledge | Exhibits KSAs required of position; exceptionally executes job | Exhibits KSAs; seldom requests manager assistance | Completes routine tasks; seeks help with some tasks | Seeks assistance with client-related duties and supportive roles | Usually seeks help from others with client and supportive duties |

employees to obtain a ranked list (Houston, 1995). The effectiveness of this method varies with department size and would be inappropriate with smaller units. The manager using a group ranking places employees in classification categories described by the normal distribution curve (e.g., top one-third or two-thirds). For individual ranking, the manager lists employees in order from highest to lowest performance. As Robbins (1995) points out, the major disadvantage of ranking systems is that a mediocre employee may score high because he or she is "the best of the worst" while an outstanding employee is rated poorly because he or she is evaluated against others who are also performing as expected.

Management by objectives, the third format, uses the individual development plan objectives or performance objectives prepared with each employee as the focus of results or outcome evaluations. The time frame for accomplishment of each objective becomes the guide to scheduling appraisal sessions. When objectives are matched with

criteria derived from job specifications, they provide a fairly accurate assessment of overall employee performance (Robbins, 1995).

TQM approaches promote evaluation of factors in the system that contribute to service quality rather than quality of individual differences among employees. One of the formats to evolve with TQM was the quality circle. Self-regulation is characteristic of systems management where focus is on human resource development and growth. Peer reviews and teams are evident in clinical therapeutic practice while networking and "advisory" committees are community-based therapeutic practices. A manager's task in either setting is to "partner" with the team or employee and colleagues because peers know when performance standards are met and expected outcomes achieved (Sullivan, 1994). A dilemma arises when measuring group effectiveness and each staff member's contribution to the team or staff which are both essential to department outcomes. One alternative is to consider group

**Table 16.2  Behaviorally Anchored Rating Scale**

| CTRS Criterion | Rating |
|---|---|
| Could be expected to select services that enable each client to achieve program/treatment plan objectives | 5 |
| Could be expected to recommend services enabling client achievement of program/treatment plan objectives with occasional supervisory guidance | 4 |
| Could be expected to identify alternative services appropriate to client objectives for staff review and program determination | 3 |
| Could be expected to seek approval for recommended services to achieve objectives from staff and manager | 2 |
| Could be expected to seek assistance from staff and manager for identifying appropriate alternatives to achieve client objectives | 1 |

effectiveness for evaluation and reward while individual evaluations are done by peer work groups. Validity is enhanced with this approach, and ongoing competency assessment and program improvement are promoted.

## Performance Review Errors

A combination of formats is commonly used to gather information. The literature confirms that results-centered (management by objectives) behavioral systems (BARS) and TQM approaches that combine outcome with behavioral appraisals tend to be the most job related and fair. In preparation for gathering information, the manager reviews existing forms and formats and attends supportive training sessions. Training allows practice with the tools and opportunities to give feedback or to coach employees on their performances. These sessions also alert managers to the types of errors likely to occur as information is gathered. Introduction of personal bias or imposition of subjective judgment into personnel evaluations reduces the legitimacy of the results. Through training, a manager becomes aware of these errors and how to avoid them.

A first-line manager has a value system that acts as a standard against which judgments are made (Robbins, 1995). Consequently, ratings may be high or low according to perceptions of the value of a particular criterion. For example, if the manager places a great deal of importance on teamwork and values resource management to a lesser degree, employee ratings would be weighted differently than if the opposite were true. A positive leniency error underestimates performance which reduces the ability to discriminate among employees' performances. By using multiple raters and combining relative with absolute standards, this tendency is minimized.

When considering performance over a long period of time, there is a tendency to give more weight to what happened last week than to the performance of two months ago. This is referred to as the recency error. There also is a tendency known as the halo effect to rate all factors high or low as a result of remembering the most notable performances during the whole evaluation period. Accuracy of ratings is increased by continually gathering information and involving peers, clients, and colleagues in the evaluation process.

A manager may evaluate based on qualities like organization and timeliness that the manager possesses so that an employee with similar behaviors is assessed differently from the employee who does not display these characteristics. This is a similarity error. When a manager does not like the exhibited behavior, the horns effect is present. Use of BARS tends to compensate when this form of personal bias is introduced. The use of objectives and quality circles or similar participatory evaluations also balances these rating errors.

It is possible regardless of who is being evaluated or what format and criteria are being used that the pattern remains the same: The manager tends to rate everyone in the middle rather than discriminate "outstanding" from "unacceptable." Consequently, performances appear more homogeneous than they really are, the error of central tendency (Robbins, 1995). Using multiple raters and combining formats (e.g., essay with critical incident) helps to improve accuracy and reduce uniform ratings.

One issue that has become more apparent is the tendency to inflate ratings. There has been a tendency to evaluate with less rigor and to reduce the consequences of unsatisfactory performances (Robbins, 1995). Fear of retribution, concern for equality, and a prevailing philosophy that promotes "freedom to make decisions" discourage managers from issuing "average" or "needs further development" ratings. A focus on quality improvement and the contributory role of each employee to the department outcomes encourages managers and employees to move beyond mediocrity.

## *Gathering Performance Information*

As managers supervise, they may choose to note performances informally, record anecdotal notes, and document observations and discussions with employees using department and organization personnel forms or guidelines. Additionally, most organizations require formal reviews and appraisals at least once or perhaps twice each year. During new employee orientation or probationary periods, the manager and employee review informal and formal processes and forms and plan the time for the formal biannual or annual appraisal to coincide with the unit and organization time requirements (e.g., anniversary date of employment or fiscal year dates). Common practice has the manager completing a performance appraisal form then conducting an interview with the employee to discuss and consider or reconsider the assigned ratings. At the conclusion of the appraisal discussion, the document is signed by the employee and manager and placed in an official personnel file.

Formal reviews serve important functions; information from informal observations and supervisory communications is organized and processed. As Berryman (1989) notes, the intent of sessions is to motivate staff to improve performance and to engage in professional development activities. Formal appraisals encourage practitioners to examine their own contribution to the organization in relationship to their KSAs and job specifications (Robbins, 1995). Each participant is presented with the opportunity to explore ideas, interests, and meanings so that each is more aware of the other's *modus operandi*.

Preparation for the formal appraisal is critical. The exact location and time of a meeting must be arranged to avoid interruptions and to allow adequate time. It is better to meet earlier in the work week than later because it allows time for follow-up before the weekend. An agenda with objectives is mutually prepared. Employees review their job specifications, development plans or performance goals, and may elect to present self-appraisals. This approach helps to shift the manager's role from that of judge and jury to that of a counselor (Rondeau, 1992). In combination with peer and client evaluations, self-appraisals both facilitate collaborative activity and enhance the practitioner's self-respect because these appraisals present the most complete picture of one's performance. Additionally, Rondeau (1992) points out that when the manager

incorporates all of these pieces of information into the review, there is a greater probability that the appraised employee will be more accepting of the manager's message. The following is a list of questions that might be helpful to both the manager and employee as they prepare for the interview (Eggert, 1993):

- How has performance compared to objectives?
- What has been achieved?
- Where could there be improvement?
- In what situations is performance best?
- How consistent has performance been?
- Are the KSAs present or appropriate to job specifications?
- What training and development targets should be set?
- What resources and support are necessary to achieve performance objectives and unit outcomes?
- What specifically can the manager do to increase the likelihood of the therapeutic recreation specialist (TRS) achieving personal performance objectives as well as unit outcomes?
- How does current performance relate to career aspirations?
- How do the manager and employee see the department changing in the next few months (years)?

Before beginning the session it is important for each participant to be at ease. Each will be less able to understand messages or participate willingly in identifying change strategies if "nerves" prevail (Rondeau, 1992). A problem-solving approach rather than a "tell-and-listen" approach facilitates mutual consideration of performance. Several specific strategies for actually conducting the appraisal session and creating a "partnership environment" are highlighted here:

- clearly state the objectives and agree upon confidential content;
- encourage discussion of present and past performance as well as what has been gained or learned;
- initiate conversation with positive feedback and specific examples rather than fat phrases (e.g., "You were late in completing three client assessments last month" rather than "You are always late");
- move into areas of improvement with feedback consistent with previous informal and formal communications;
- set specific goals and time tables so that each participant knows what has been done well, what requires improvement, what the plans are to improve, and what performances are expected in the future; and

- specify a follow-up plan to examine progress and obstacles to goal achievement with identified review dates during the coming six months or year.

If generic organization forms are used, the manager and employee review performance within each category interpreting how the employee's performance did or did not meet the standards and why specific ratings were assigned. Each job task on the position specification is also reviewed. Through the exchange it may be discovered that position descriptions require rewriting. Time is also devoted to assessing each employee objective. This helps the manager and employee acknowledge achievement and validate performance. Designating a finish time is useful because the tendency is to continue discussions beyond comfortable active listening limits. Before closure, the manager's feedback is checked via paraphrasing or rephrasing as with routine therapeutic intervention sessions. Action steps to be taken by the manager and employee are committed to writing to ensure follow-up and affirm session outcomes.

The manager's effectiveness as a manager is likely to be judged by the employee's perception of fairness, meeting efficiency, and the relation of the outcomes to the employee's job. It is critical that both the style and substance of feedback are properly managed (Rondeau, 1992). If the style is incongruent with the substance, the utility of the message is diminished. To illustrate, when the employee demonstrates performances that do not meet criteria, the manager's role becomes that of a teacher who outlines corrective actions with clear performance measures and time frames. Conversely, when the employee is a high performer and demonstrates potential for growth, the manager assumes the role of a problem solver or mentor, and joint resolution and direction are planned. Thus, the manager tailors feedback to the characteristics of each employee as well as toward the department's and organization's processes and objectives (Rondeau, 1992). Actual documents considered and comments recorded during the appraisal session are placed in the employee's personnel file and, if appropriate or required, shared with the human resources department or personnel specialist.

# Managing Outcomes and Follow-Up

The purpose of appraisal is to effect change in the performance of others. Yet, the outcomes of personnel evaluations are factored into a number of management functions and decisions that affect the employee and manager. Immediate tasks resulting from completed appraisals are to design an employee action plan and process information to use with quality controls and improvements. In addition, evaluation outcomes are used to take personnel actions like promotions or terminations, to plan training and development programs, to adjust system operations or department management, and to reward performances.

## *Designing an Action Plan*

According to Eggert (1993), a follow-up plan identifies measurable outcomes, time or dates by which goals will be achieved, roles of employee and manager, and the resources necessary to realize the employee's potential and to enhance service quality. Committing this information to paper encourages goal-oriented behaviors and focus on service improvements. Also, the establishment of more frequent time periods for discussion of progress (e.g., every few months as opposed to once a year) increases work-related communication among staff and management (McGee, 1992). This acts to discourage the buildup of frustration by providing opportunities to express concerns about such things as resource limitations or appropriateness of client placements. This plan is prepared as a stand-alone document; however, statements from the document are integrated into quality improvement plans, development plans, training inventories, and staff performance objectives. Thus, both the employee and manager are planning for the measurement and reward of future performance. The format of the plan might resemble a client's discharge plan or transition plan with a listing of objectives, target dates to review accomplishments, required resources, and progress notations. With this form of ongoing communication incorporated into routine supervisory sessions, fear created by once-a-year reviews is minimized and energies are refocused toward personal success and department or organization improvements.

The action plan is a tool used to improve quality. The plan identifies steps an employee might take to gain the KSAs necessary to deliver services in compliance with job specifications and professional standards of practice. Team effectiveness might be improved by changes in staffing assignments or other work processes that encourage interdepartmental communication and coordination. To illustrate, an objective on an employee's action plan might be to improve documentation or to incorporate assessment results into referral plans so that the team is more accurate in projecting length of stay. With seasonal or part-time staff, action plans help managers judge appropriateness of staff assignments. For example, teachers who have experience with special needs students are often hired in summer day camps. A job responsibility is to lead a variety of therapeutic recreation activities. A first-line manager may discover after a month of the program that day campers are repeating the same activities weekly. Together the manager and summer employee plan to add diversity to the offerings and base these offerings on client objectives for the summer. If a second review a month later were to also note no new or additional services, the manager might recommend additional training prior to authorization for hiring the employee the following summer. Time is an essential quality control factor. An employee's action plan may require improvements in completion time of work tasks like individual assessments or preplanning for large group activities like outings or family events. The completion of these tasks in a timely manner is essential if subsequent services dependent upon these initial actions are to be expedited efficiently. The action plan commits the manager and employee to ongoing communication and problem solving. The focus becomes what can be done better rather than what is being done incorrectly.

## Personnel Actions Following Performance Reviews

Evaluation outcomes are used in personnel decisions. If outcomes of formal reviews are positive, the manager reinforces the behavior with incentives through the reward system and the development plan. If the manager determines that performance does not satisfy expectations, corrective action is incorporated in the follow-up document. Depending on the degree of variance from the standard, disciplinary action can be initiated. This action may lead to employee termination or separation from the unit. Generally the types of variances that require the manager's attention include attendance, on-the-job behaviors (e.g., carelessness, insubordination), deviation in protocol or practice that impacts services delivered, safety and risk incidents, client-management errors, and dishonesty and/or misuse of resources.

Performance appraisals measure employee actions against expectations. Some variance is anticipated in all performance; therefore, it is critical that the first-line manager determine an acceptable range of variation (Robbins, 1995). In some instances, the slightest deviation (e.g., noncompliance with safety policies) is extremely critical while in others there appears to be a greater degree of tolerance (e.g., misuse of craft supplies or outing funds). The manager's role is to help the employee adjust performance to acceptable levels, revise the standards, or both. In the first instance, a manager may, for example, remind the employee of transportation safety rules; while in the second, the manager may determine that since storage space is limited, the employee needs to dispose of partially used containers rather than attempt to reorganize the storage area. The manager might work with staff to secure additional and/or better organized storage areas.

## Corrective Actions and Controls

The type of corrective action included in the follow-up plan is actually the last alternative or correctional control that is intended to prevent any further problems. To illustrate, a follow-up goal regarding safety might have the employee conducting a presafety and a postsafety inspection with each outing so, with repetition, the employee commits to practice and memory safety protocols. Preventive control anticipates and prevents unacceptable performance. Thus, including examples of proper procedures (e.g., safety drills or discussion about financial impacts of inappropriate resource usage) in new employee orientation is preventive control. A first-line manager's daily tasks entail the third form of control, concurrent control. With firsthand observation, the manager identifies or anticipates behaviors that could become problems. The difficulty is that first-line managers are not necessarily available to observe direct service provision if responsibilities take them to meetings or service areas other than where practitioners are interacting with clients. When the manager does observe ineffective performance attributable to the employee rather than to standards, a *memo for the record* is placed in the employee's personnel file after the issue is discussed with the employee. This documentation is used, if necessary, during the formal review and/or in support of disciplinary action.

Effective controls increase the likelihood that staff will attempt to meet expectations according to Robbins (1995). As previously mentioned, since a first-line manager cannot control everything that happens in a department, controls like training, regulations, and performance appraisals cover the key indicators that contribute to quality outcomes. In previous illustrations, generic evaluation forms stated what the organization, division, or department considered to be key performance indicators. Employee development plan objectives or performance goals may challenge or stretch an employee's KSAs, or privileging criteria may motivate staff to attend continuing education unit (CEU) programs, but these criteria are reasonable and within reach. If the manager and employee discern through performance discussions, that particular goals have been set too high, follow-up action is taken to reset the goal or to allow more time to achieve the desired results.

According to Edington and Griffith (1990), the perceptions of the employee and the therapeutic recreation manager influence how the staff member views follow-up and corrective actions. An employee may resist because he or she perceives he or she is being "checked up on." Work performance may be adversely affected because the employee feels "mistreated." Coaching, team support, quality work groups, and self-assessments are techniques to close the gap between performance and expectations. These methods encourage employees to operate independently and to make decisions that control their work activities.

## Disciplinary Actions

When variance is significant and the manager determines the deviation is directly attributable to employee action or inaction and not the standard, a verbal warning may accompany the written follow-up plan. This warning serves as the first notice of action taken to enforce department and organizational rules. A verbal warning informs the staff member that, if the action is not corrected (e.g., compliance with safety protocols), subsequent disciplinary action is likely. The warning states the specific policies that are violated and details subsequent steps in the discipline process. When the first-line manager pursues a course of disciplinary action, a personnel specialist or human resource department employee advises the manager of due process requirements and proper legal procedures. Normal sequence of events is to issue a verbal warning followed by one or two written notices, suspension, demotion, pay cut, reassignment, and dismissal (Robbins, 1995). The challenge for the manager is to help the employee to separate disciplinary action from the action identified on the follow-up plan. To illustrate, the follow-up plan might have the employee attend an in-service on transportation safety and management of client behaviors in vehicles with other staff members to ensure all outing safety regulations are followed. At the follow-up conference with the manager, the employee would report on the effectiveness of these two controls in achieving the specific follow-up objective on safety.

Like corrective action, perceptions of management and staff influence whether disciplinary action is transmitted and received in a nonthreatening way and results in cooperative behavior. A manager determines whether the employee has the ability and the influence to correct performance (Robbins, 1995). Were there uncertainties, unexpected events, or inadequacies over which the employee had no control that influenced outcomes? Or, does the manager view the employee as having the potential to perform as expected? The follow-up plan is a form of preventive correction because it guides the manager and employee to take steps that deter the reoccurrence of problem behaviors. A follow-up plan also may help both parties realize that the situation is not workable. As a consequence, the employee may choose to "separate," or seek reassignment, within the organization or corporation. A manager may encourage an employee to seek employment elsewhere if the follow-up plan confirms that an employee's abilities are not adequate.

## *Performance Outcomes, Rewards, Training and Development, and System Changes*

Performance outcomes that are considered in employee rewards are more likely to be repeated. Also, motivation to continue to perform as desired is encouraged if the reward is contingent on performance. Thus, rewards are a form of management control. The desirable scenario is to reward employees for the attainment of specific development plan or performance goal accomplishments. Yet the timing of a formal annual or biannual reward may not coincide with individual employee goal achievement. To compensate for this difference managers have instituted recognition systems like "employee of the week" (or month), newsletter features, yearly service awards, and increased opportunities to attend off-site meetings and professional development seminars. These formal signs of recognition are accompanied by informal "thank yous" and letters placed in personnel files. As opportunities for promotion and position upgrades decrease with *flattening career ladders,* the value of such recognition systems is becoming more significant.

Evaluation outcomes help managers and staff plan needed training and development programs. Follow-up action may suggest in-service programs that cover certain regulations and personnel policies or incorporate similar content in seasonal orientations. The effectiveness of training and development sessions is judged by how well staff perform on the job. Evaluation outcomes also provide managers and staff with information needed to take steps that correct system dysfunction. As mentioned earlier, standards are reconsidered. Managers often rethink the methods they use to give feedback and conduct their daily interactions with staff. A manager might discover that staff complete tasks in a certain fashion because "this is the way we've always done it," and no one has offered alternative strategies. Involving multiple performance ratings and raters is likely to reveal system inadequacies and to gain consensus for major department change.

With the discussion that has surrounded performance appraisal systems, it is amazing they continue as a form of management control. Yet without feedback, either positive or negative, behavior is unlikely to change. The work force of the future will expect to have more say about what they do and how they do it. When the manager incorporates employees in targeting performance expectations, a partnership is formed that is no longer contaminated by the prospects of reward and discipline but instead is driven by support and an ongoing search for quality (Halachmi, 1993).

# Summary

This chapter began by establishing that evaluation is concerned with gathering information to determine if employees have achieved work expectations and performance goals and have contributed to department service outcomes. Rarely does the first-line therapeutic recreation manager have sole responsibility for designing, implementing, and conducting performance follow-up. Through a human resource department or personnel specialist, the manager acquires and perhaps gives input into forms and processes used agency-wide. The primary role of the manager to gather information, give feedback, and determine the support needed by each employee to perform as expected and to maximize his or her potential was discussed.

The authors cited evaluation literature and research that suggest a number of steps a manager can take to ensure instruments and processes satisfy standards of objectivity, reliability, validity, and administrative practicality. Outcomes, behaviors, and traits identified by the manager and incorporated into the agency form or used to design individual review forms were discussed. Format for information collection may include essay, critical-incident, BARS, graphic rating scales, rankings, and management by objectives (MBOs). More recent systems management uses quality control methods that incorporate self, peer, and results-centered approaches because they are more job related and fair.

The manager may use several techniques to compensate for potential rater errors (e.g., leniency, recency, similarity, central tendency, inflation, and the halo and horns effects). Informal collection of information is ongoing. Formal reviews usually occur once or twice a year which allow the manager to share informal observations and encourage the employee to continue to improve and achieve. A manager's feedback is tailored to the employee, department, and organization needs and processes.

A follow-up action plan jointly prepared and routinely discussed emphasizes continued improvement, quality control, and employee potential. Objectives and target dates encourage ongoing employee-manager communication.

The plan is also a correction control tool as it helps the employee perform as expected so that problems do not escalate. The plan also aids the manager in correcting inappropriate operational standards and performance criteria. In essence, the follow-up plan prescribes what the employee and manager must do together to avoid disciplinary action.

Performance outcomes are weighed in a number of management decisions including planning and evaluation of training and development sessions, reward and recognition processes, department management changes, and adjustments within the organization. The manager's challenge is to create a supportive environment that focuses energy and resources on those areas of employee performance which contribute to quality outcomes and ongoing service improvements.

# Discussion Questions

1. Describe the professional and legal factors a manager considers as personnel evaluation systems are designed.
2. Describe several steps a manager takes to design evaluations that are congruent with individual staff needs as well as unique system features.
3. Identify and explain the three types of performance criteria.
4. Explain and give the advantages and disadvantages of each method used to rate information gathered on performance criteria.
5. What are the appraisal errors commonly made by managers and what control features are introduced to reduce these tendencies?
6. What techniques are used during formal appraisals to create a problem-solving approach to performance issues?
7. What is a follow-up action plan and how does it relate to corrective and disciplinary actions?
8. Summarize the variables affecting the manager's role in performance appraisals and evaluations. Discuss how the outcomes of performance reviews impact other management functions.

# References

American Therapeutic Recreation Association (ATRA). (1993). *Standards for the practice of therapeutic recreation and self-assessment guide.* Hattiesburg, MS: Author.

Berryman, D. L. (1989). Evaluating professional personnel. In A. H. Grossman (Ed.), *Personnel management in recreation and leisure services* (pp. 207–237). Reston, VA: American Alliance for Health, Physical Education, Recreation, and Dance.

Dwyer, W. D., and Cripe, R. (1984). Evaluating seasonal employees. *Parks and Recreation, 19:10,* 56–58.

Edington, C. R., and Griffith, C. A. (1990). *The recreation and leisure service delivery system.* Dubuque, IA: Wm. C. Brown Publishers.

Eggert, M. A. (1993). In praise of appraisal. *Nursing Times, 89:9,* 28, 30.

Ghorpade, J., and Chen, M. M. (1995). Creating quality-driven performance appraisal systems. *Academy of Management Executive, 9:1,* 32–38.

Halachmi, A. (1993). From performance appraisal to performance targeting. *Public Personnel Management, 22:2,* 323–344.

Houston, R. (1995). Integrating CQI into performance appraisals. *Nursing Management, 26:3,* 48A–48C.

McGee, K. G. (1992). Making performance appraisals a positive experience. *Nursing Management, 23:8,* 36–37.

National Therapeutic Recreation Society (NTRS). (1995). *Standards of practice for therapeutic recreation services and annotated bibliography.* Arlington, VA: Author.

Robbins, S. P. (1995). *Supervision today.* Englewood Cliffs, NJ: Prentice Hall.

Rondeau, K. V. (1992). Constructive performance appraisal feedback for healthcare employees. *Hospital Topics, 70:2,* 27–33.

Sullivan, C. A. (1994). Competency assessment and performance improvement for healthcare providers. *Journal of Healthcare Quality, 16:4,* 14–19, 38.

# Chapter 17

# Staff Training and Development

## Introduction

According to Sandwith (1993), the triple threat in most health and human service organizations is simultaneous demands for continuous quality improvement (CQI), cost savings and reductions, and the rapid rate of change and innovation. For managers this translates into a need to maintain and upgrade therapeutic recreation specialists' knowledge and skills. Managers must provide responsive training programs that address staff needs accurately, quickly, and cost effectively.

Through the 1990s and beyond, training and development will be integral parts of most jobs. The goals of continuous improvement, high quality, cost-effectiveness, worker efficiency, and adaptation to change require that managers and staff be in a constant state of learning and development. Additionally, as reported by Metzger (1982), research has shown that properly trained employees have less absenteeism and turnover. Another trend contributing to the growing interest in employee training and education programs is the use of systems management approaches like total quality management (TQM). TQM philosophy values the role that employees play in the success of health and human service agencies. Each system component, such as the employees, contributes to organizational outcomes. At the core of "service" organizations is employee knowledge and skill. As the health and human service dollar becomes more scarce, formalized programs to update and maintain staff competence and efficiency become imperative.

Training refers to learning experiences that result in a relatively permanent change in an individual that improves his or her ability to perform on the job. As described by Robbins (1995), this change occurs in the practitioner's knowledge, skills, attitudes, and/or behavior. Development addresses the personal and professional nature of a career and is concerned with more conceptual understanding of why and how skills or behaviors relate to the broader context of an organization and profession (Arnold and McClure, 1989). Staff development is the broader concept that includes training and is intended to prepare practitioners for continuous growth beyond day-to-day job demands (Carter, Browne, LeConey, and Nagle, 1991).

Sandwith (1993) notes that managers engage in a broader range of activities than was once thought and use skills associated with leadership such as facilitation, coaching, problem solving and negotiating. Management in therapeutic recreation encompasses competencies from several domains: conceptual or creative, leadership, interpersonal, administrative, and technical. Training and development programs address the needs of managers and practitioners in each of these areas.

The first section of this chapter considers professional standards that support training and development. Various types of training and development are also presented. Personnel needs assessments in each competency area are described in the second section. With this information a comprehensive training and development program is designed. The third section of this chapter addresses the learning styles and principles of adult learning that influence the methods used to present material and the types of training and development programs included in a comprehensive staff training and development program. Implementation of training and development programs—section four—involves the manager in a number of tasks, the result of which is delivery of relevant and useful options. The final section considers evaluation of training and development programs. Evaluation helps to justify training expenditures. The manager conducts evaluations to ascertain if staff enhancement has occurred and if outcomes are relevant to organizational and client needs. Specific evaluation strategies are introduced in the fifth section of this chapter. This chapter concludes with an overview of trends and issues in therapeutic recreation training and development.

Throughout this chapter, the role of a first-line manager in training and development is considered because responsibility for knowledge of department personnel competencies lies with the first-line manager. The manager is also aware of the problems to be resolved and decisions to be made as personnel adapt to change within the organization and profession. Further, managers oversee the budget. Changes in productivity and outcomes are reflected in the budget, and a manager's task is to relate the cost of training and development to changes in worker productivity and outcomes. Formalized training and development programs address the needs of all personnel (seasonal, part-time, interns, volunteers, on call [PRN], and full-time employees) as each contributes to the department's accomplishment of service goals and outcomes. Thus, managers monitor comprehensive programs that meet their needs and the needs of those who carry out the unit's mission.

# Composition of Training and Development Programs

Professional standards documents (ATRA, 1993; NTRS, 1990, 1995) identify staff training and development guidelines. These are cited as either stand-alone criteria or as criteria in a plan of operation. Continuing education, training, and professional development are intended to ensure that staff remain current and abreast of knowledge and skills so that they function as competent employees and professionals. The manager assures that staff are competent to deliver quality client services. This is accomplished with the preparation of individual development plans, written annually, that conform to the department's plan governing staff development (ATRA, 1993).

A written plan of operation includes policies that promote training and development and procedures for periodic assessment of therapeutic recreation staff educational needs (ATRA, 1993). Also, as an element of CQI, staff are to participate in periodic evaluation of the department's professional development plan and make recommendations

for improvement (ATRA, 1993). A professional development plan supports a wide range of opportunities for continuing education and training. This plan identifies policies that establish minimum staff participation, and guidelines for practitioners' individual development plans (ATRA, 1993; NTRS, 1990). The ultimate outcome of properly planned and executed staff training and development programs is client and caregiver satisfaction with staff performance.

Literature sources (Carter, Browne, LeConey, and Nagle, 1991; Grossman, 1989) and professional standards (NTRS, 1990) suggest that a number of types of formal training are incorporated in a comprehensive staff training and development program. An orientation program, the first type, is a systematic training aimed at introducing new employees to the department. This orientation generally introduces staff to several different components of the organization such as:

1. the vision, mission, goals, objectives, and services;
2. the policies, procedures, manuals, and plan of operation;
3. the areas, facilities, resources, and work stations;
4. the protocols and standards of practice;
5. the clientele and coworkers; and
6. the performance expectations and privileges associated with each position.

Orientation programs are distinct from and/or included in the probation period. Formal orientation usually occurs for a briefer period commencing with initial processing. Probationary periods extend from a few weeks to months in length after which the employee gains full privileges and is held accountable for the duties of a particular position.

Pledge (1993) indicates that an in-service training program is based on service needs of clients, staff, and supervisors. The goal of this second type of staff training and development is to enable practitioners to fulfill the expectations of their positions with the highest degree of competence possible and to maintain performance at that level as long as the position is held. According to Grossman (1989), keeping staff at peak performance and up-to-date requires that opportunities be provided to review previous knowledge and skills (e.g., documentation) and to acquire new information and developments (e.g., computerized assessments). Organized in-service training programs occur through regularly scheduled staff meetings; agency-sponsored workshops and seminars; and the use of outside consultants, media, and technology (NTRS, 1990).

Professional development programs, a third type of staff training and development, are becoming increasingly more important. As managers and staff must meet the changing health and human service needs of clients within a dynamic environment, development training addresses both department needs and practitioner needs. Each job is viewed as an activity unto itself and as it contributes to the department and the profession (Arnold and McClure, 1989). The intent is to improve an employee's promotional opportunities within the department while creating opportunities for professional advancement. Development training reflects the variety of knowledge, skills, and abilities (KSAs) in each of the five competency domains (conceptual, leadership, interpersonal, administrative, and technical) found as practitioners consider career options.

Managers facilitate development training by knowing goals, performance records, and expectations of professional positions. Managers "coach" practitioners as individual development plans are written to include desired training and continuing education. Further, first-line managers help staff access specialized conferences, institutes, and meetings through use of time off, travel support, and direct service coverage. In return, staff are expected to present in-services reporting benefits of their development experiences that are applicable in their current positions (NTRS, 1990).

Technological advancements and development and the constantly increasing rate of change have an impact on what staff and first-line managers do. Retraining, a fourth type of training and development, has emerged to accommodate practitioner needs to remain abreast of changing work environments and demands. Evidence of the rapid rate of change in the clinical setting is the more frequent publishing of the Joint Commission on Accreditation of Healthcare Organization's (JCAHO) standards and the decreasing length of client stays. In the community, practitioners respond to legal directives like the Americans with Disabilities Act (ADA) and the fairly recent acute health needs of persons returning to their homes from clinical settings. As a result of impacts such as these, managers are faced with new and changing roles that must be affected immediately if standards are to be met and costs recovered. Although retraining needs are felt by all, the responsibility lies with the manager to remain abreast of career trends and support access to continuing education and professional development. The intent of these experiences is to ensure staff gain the KSAs necessary to stay productive and marketable while delivering quality services efficiently. Retraining occurs through position exchanges, long-distance learning, computerized self-paced programs, acquisition of credentials in other professional areas, return to school, and conventional in-service programs.

# Training and Development Assessments

The first step in an effective training and development program is to determine the needs of the department. Pledge

(1993) reports that this process is generally not standardized and usually combines reactive responses to external requirements (e.g., JCAHO and ADA) with internal suggestions from staff. This approach does not necessarily ensure that energies are also being focused on department and client needs. A comprehensive needs assessment focuses on the resources and expertise necessary to provide services to clients while continuing to incorporate staff perceptions of client needs and professional growth issues (Pledge, 1993). A comprehensive needs assessment gathers relevant data from the department, identifies alternative training resources and performance expectations, and ultimately creates a department-wide atmosphere supportive of training and development programs.

As the therapeutic recreation manager plans and conducts needs assessments, several factors are considered. According to Arnold and McClure (1989), needs assessments are conducted under conditions that are as close as possible to normal working conditions. Perceptions can be inaccurate if ratings are completed when work loads are high. Input is gathered from all persons affected by change. For example, if client confidentiality policies are revised, all employees including volunteer, part-time, and seasonal personnel attend training sessions. Assessments focus on issues raised rather than who raised the issues. Managers ensure staff that confidentiality of information sources is maintained. Assessments consider needs of each practitioner level within the department while also taking into account emerging day-to-day direct service needs. The first-line manager is the link between upper level management goals and operational needs of staff. Responsibility falls on the manager to balance these perspectives.

Several types of assessments are designed to determine staff and department needs. Primary types of assessments include interviewing, questionnaires, observations, group surveys, and participatory meetings. In health and human service settings managers have also employed focus groups, case conferences, and individual staff development plans to ascertain needs and provide continuing education opportunities (Denning and Verschelden, 1993; Kaplan and Breslin, 1989; Pledge, 1993). These approaches tend to be more integrative because they recognize the relationship between client needs and staff performance which is an integral element in department CQI plans.

To determine the needs of a particular position a traditional form of needs assessment is a job or task analysis. This analysis determines what is to be performed; how often or frequently the task is performed; how important or significant the task is to services provided; and how difficult it is to develop the KSAs to perform the task. Job descriptions, performance appraisal criteria, professional certification plans (NCTRC, 1997), and licensure requirements are resources of expected therapeutic recreation specialist job responsibilities. Task analyses prepared from review of such documents are used to compare staff performance with competencies expected of professionals in similar positions. Discrepancies become the focus of individual development plans. Each plan identifies specific performance outcomes to alleviate deficits found in actual job behaviors. The manager uses data from staff development plans and department assessments to prepare training and development goals. These goals identify information to be acquired by practitioners and the challenges they will face as newly acquired knowledge and skills are put into practice.

Because managers are responsible for the performance of their staff, it becomes their responsibility to ensure that employees are properly trained. The role assumed by the first-line manager depends on a number of the following factors identified during the assessment process: the size of the department; funds available for training; the manager's and employees' training skills; and access to resources through professional associations, the department, and in the community. Robbins (1995) indicates that the larger the department or agency, the more likely there will be a separate training department or specialist with support resources to conduct specialized training. With available funding, experts are brought into the agency, technology is purchased so distance learning and teleconferences are possible, and staff are reimbursed for participation in professional training sessions and conferences. Supervisors' training and clinical supervision skills vary. Some have developed particular expertise through training and experience and are comfortable planning and conducting educational sessions. Likewise, staff with special experience are also able to develop and present programs. The scope and depth of available personnel resources affect the therapeutic recreation manager's training and development roles.

Training and development resources are found within the agency, local community, and through professional contacts and networks. Affiliation with state and national professional organizations is a conduit to training and development expertise and materials. Other therapeutic recreation, health, and human service personnel in the agency and community bring expertise to bear on issues of common concern. Community and professional contacts, in essence, validate the findings of assessments. Additionally, they provide resources to help managers and staff remain abreast of global professional issues. Attendance and participation in agency, community, and professional activities is, therefore, one avenue to access training and development resources while also remaining aware of management trends.

# Design of Training and Development Programs

Training and development programs are ultimately judged on how well they meet the agency's, department's, and practitioner's goals. Through the needs assessment process the manager identifies the training and development goals and challenges staff will face as they attempt to apply newly acquired knowledge and skills. The manager prioritizes training and development goals from the needs assessment. Objective statements are then written to delineate specific employee behavioral changes. Objectives in each employee's development plan guide the manager as department priorities are set. Likewise, the manager reassesses agency goals to ensure the department's plan will prepare staff to contribute to the achievement of agency outcomes.

One of the challenges considered as objectives are developed is time. Objectives guide manager's decisions about content. The time available for the practitioner to become familiar with the content and to practice newly acquired skills is influenced by impending accreditation visits or health and safety inspections among other things. Therefore, as objective statements are written, the manager takes into consideration the time it will take for employees to demonstrate performance changes.

Available training time and the nature of the content also influence the type of training and development provided (i.e., orientation, in-service, professional development, retraining). For example, for staff and management to keep abreast of the impact of legislative reform on client services, a professional development program provides information over a period of time as legislative actions are taken. Retraining is appropriate when access to new intervention modalities such as adventure-challenge courses or horticulture therapy becomes available through community networking because acquisition and skill practice need only a brief time period. In-service sessions are appropriate when updating of existing knowledge and skills is required; thus, if staff have experience with computerized functional assessments, the introduction of the functional independent measure (FIM) on the computer would take a relatively short time. Arnold and McClure (1989) suggest new information acquired during an in-service is easier to learn in shorter rather than longer time blocks, while continuous practice is necessary to the acquisition of new skills. Orientation programs are usually longer in length as skill practice is required in order to assure performance. Orientation sessions introduce new seasonal staff or employees to department procedures and protocols prior to actual on-the-job performance. It is desirable to keep the time lag between acquisition of new information and its application as short as possible; thus, orientation precedes the new program cycle or the retraining occurs immediately prior to use of the new intervention with clients. Managers also consider time when they assess the system-wide impact of anticipated staff changes. When the introduction of new interventions or revised evaluation instruments affects personnel in other units, additional time and training is scheduled.

The manner in which adults learn and change behaviors also influences training time and content. Managers and employees have different levels of skill, interest, experience, and motivation. Consequently, adults learn and change behavior differently and at different rates. Entry-level behaviors and motivation to learn more or new information are not uniform among personnel. Managers employ several techniques to accommodate different learning and behavior change styles and rates. To increase motivation, learning experiences are linked to employee development plan objectives. Performance is enhanced when staff "know what's in it for them," and interest is maintained when expected outcomes are known prior to the training and development experience. Each training and development session should have identified outcomes with objectives that delineate each skill to be acquired as outcomes are achieved. This whole-part-whole method is an effective adult teaching strategy.

Motivation to change is related to the manager's support for change and the practitioner's perceived need to change. The greater the discrepancy between employees' performances and desired outcomes, the more frequent and immediate is the need for the manager's feedback, reward, and/or reinforcement. As suggested by Robbins (1995), this also increases the likelihood that the new behaviors will be repeated. A completed job analysis identifies the frequency with which knowledge and skills are practiced. When skills are more significant and more frequently used, employee interest is maintained by providing a commensurate amount of training time and practice. Practice builds confidence and is self-motivating because it rewards or reinforces demonstrated abilities. Thus, during training and development experiences, trainees practice job-related tasks. The rate at which practitioners acquire knowledge and skills tends to decrease as objectives are achieved. Also, learning plateau's are unique to each trainee and, as a consequence, learning occurs at different rates. Managers encourage staff to assess their performance at periodic intervals rather than at uniform times (i.e., every six months or once a year) to accommodate varying rates of behavioral change.

Learning styles also vary among practitioners. Ismeurt, Ismeurt and Miller (1992) describe two types of learning styles in their research. Field-dependent learners tend to prefer discussion, guided discovery, and demonstration methods while field-independent adults tend to prefer observation, experimentation, and interaction with others to acquire new information and skills (Ismeurt, Ismeurt, and

Miller, 1992). Field-dependent trainees tend to be influenced by feedback while field-independent trainees tend to be self-motivated and to respond better to situations that permit active participation and leadership. Therefore, as the manager designs the content and plans for the practice of newly acquired staff knowledge and skills, adult learning styles are considered.

Training objectives guide the selection of content and methods used to present the information. Each type of content (i.e., conceptual, leadership, interpersonal, administrative, technical) lends itself to particular instructional methods. For example, when the training outcome is from the leadership or technical domain (conducting debriefing following adventure-challenge course participation), psychomotor or performance skills is the learning focus. Role-playing, simulation, and demonstration methods are effective instructional strategies when outcomes are action oriented. If a conceptual or interpersonal outcome such as strategic planning or communicating effectively are training outcomes, the cognitive domain is the content focus. Lecture, discussion, reading, and viewing tapes are effective training methods with cognitive information. When content involves leadership, interpersonal, and administrative competencies, learning involves socioemotional skills as well as skills from the psychomotor and cognitive domains. Multidimensional behavioral changes are supported by methods such as job rotation and sharing, internships, coaching, case study analysis, supervisory conferences, profiling, portfolio development, and professional conferences and workshops. The manager first analyzes each objective to determine the content needed to enable trainees to achieve specified outcomes. Next, the methodology appropriate to present the content is determined. Selected methods must also be compatible with adult learning styles and the type of training and development provided.

Prior to implementation of a comprehensive training and development program, therapeutic recreation managers plan how to evaluate the outcomes of the program (i.e., summative evaluation) and each training and development opportunity presented (i.e., formative evaluation). Training objectives tied to CQI plans and staff development plans become indicators of outcome achievement. Habel (1994) notes that an outcome-based service focus requires evaluation to demonstrate the difference training and development makes in job performance and ability to adapt to future professional challenges.

Training and development effectiveness is judged by how well staff performance addresses agency, department, and personal and professional goals. Thus, evaluation assumes a three-dimensional perspective. Upper level managers are generally concerned with whether employees work efficiently to meet agency goals. First-line managers, however, focus on the quality of client services. Arnold and McClure (1989) suggest employees measure training and development by how much they can apply to their immediate responsibilities and future obligations. Similar to needs assessments, a number of methods are available to validate learning and its impact on service outcomes. According to Habel (1994), primary evaluation approaches are verbal and written feedback, demonstration, and observation of job performance following introduction of new knowledge and skills. The manager's task is to identify an approach and to design tools appropriate to each evaluation audience. Ultimately, the manager must prepare an evaluation plan that projects how achievement of objectives will be measured and reported to document the effects of training and development on job performance and service outcomes (Habel, 1994).

# Implementation of Training and Development Programs

When preparing to conduct or facilitate participation in training and development programs, the first-line manager undertakes several tasks to ensure that the delivery is relevant and useful:

- inform staff about the opportunities;
- arrange for staff attendance or access;
- prepare the delivery methods and setting;
- ensure that offerings are related to staff development plan goals;
- plan for applicability of programs to the job or professional growth of each trainee; and
- project follow-up and continued training and development needs.

While training and development programs are in progress, the manager monitors change through formative evaluations with upper level management, trainees, service recipients, and anyone affected by therapeutic recreation services. Formative or process evaluations involve the manager in staff discussions, work site observations, portfolio reviews, performance appraisal documentation, financial reporting, and CQI or service quality monitoring.

## *Informing Staff*

Informing staff about training and development opportunities is essential for several reasons. If behavioral change is expected, staff must know about and be motivated to attend programs to gain access to knowledge and skills. Acquisition of continuing professional development points to maintain certification requires systematic planning to accumulate the required number of points in the defined time period. When participation occurs during work time, impact on programming and direct client services is considered. Additionally, the manager plans for the equitable

distribution of time and financial resources among personnel. One information method is a training and development calendar (see Figure 17.1). This calendar identifies on-site programs for a period of time such as a month, or fiscal or calendar year. This helps managers plan for service continuity, and staff select opportunities that best relate to their particular needs. Also, the calendar becomes an educational tool that apprises colleagues of common issues and networking opportunities. Other methods used to announce training and development opportunities include flyers, electronic mail systems, table tents, bulletin board displays, and department circulars. A technique used to inform personnel of off-site professional workshops and conferences is association mailings of training and development calendars.

## *Facilitating Access*

Managers facilitate access to training and development when they circulate information and arrange program coverage. Lead time is required to submit financial requests and to plan adequate service supervision when off-site programs are attended. On-site arrangements for teleconference hookups or media rentals are made through a training specialist or human resource personnel. With brief lunch or after-program in-services, circulating a sign-up sheet permits employees to rearrange personal schedules and managers to have the proper amount of training materials. When opportunity permits, staff who conduct in-services for other agency employees gain personal satisfaction and recognition while promoting awareness of therapeutic recreation services to others agency-wide. Department membership in professional organizations and the opportunity to attend a national conference are staff motivators. Managers conscious of these employment perks budget accordingly.

## *Preparing Delivery Methods*

Training and development programs are conducted in ways that help trainees remember and use information and skills. The environment in which programs take place and the resources used during programs are arranged or planned to support trainee goals. As previously noted, presentation methods recognize the nature of the content and learning needs of practitioners. When the training environment resembles the work setting, trainees transfer more quickly the newly acquired information and skills. Further, when training and development experiences closely align with work tasks, transfer is facilitated. Presentation methods such as case studies, simulations, gaming, and role playing enable practice of therapeutic recreation situations. Learning results more readily from seeing rather than being told. Visual media such as interactive tapes, films, transparencies, computer graphics, and teleconferences are accessed

**Figure 17.1 Training and Development Calendar**

MONTH:    June, 19___

Educational Services
Iowa Health System
Des Moines, Iowa

Woodland Center
1313 High, Ground Floor

Preregistration is required on all classes. To register, call #6398.
For detailed information on these classes, consult your "Educational Services Catalog."

| MONDAY | TUESDAY | WEDNESDAY | THURSDAY | FRIDAY |
|---|---|---|---|---|
| | | | (1) | (2) |
| (5) New Employee Orientation 8-4:30; IMMC-Hill Aud | (6) | (7) | (8) | (9) Q2/Care 8:30-4; Woodland Center #3 |
| (12) | (13) Q2/Care 4-9 p.m; ILH-Conf Room A/B | (14) | (15) | (16) |
| (19) New Employee Orientation 8-4:30; ILH-Conf Room A/B | (20) | (21) | (22) Q2/Care 8:30-4; Woodland Center #3 | (23) |
| (26) | (27) Supervisors' Forum 1:30-2:30 pm; IHL-Conf | (28) Supervisors' Forum 8:30-9:30; IMMV-Hill Aud repeated 1:30-2:30; IMMC-Hill Aud | (29) | (30) |

253

through purchase, rental, and collegial networks. Nontraditional devices such as equipment used in therapy sessions and during recreation experiences motivate participation by appealing to the primary senses and the desire to "learn by doing."

## *Relating Training and Development to Staff Needs*

A manager helps to ensure the relatedness of training and development programs to staff needs by including staff in program design and implementation. Staff participate in needs assessment processes and the preparation of the department's annual training and development plan. Also, along with the manager, staff develop goals for each program. This fosters interest and enthusiasm which motivates staff to learn, remember, and use acquired information and skills (Arnold and McClure, 1989). Managers also encourage staff to link their individual development plan goals to those for each training and development program. Each learning opportunity is then linked to the goals of the department's annual plan. When staff conduct programs, they are more likely to relate training content and outcomes to their particular situational needs.

## *Applicability of Training and Development*

Another technique to motivate change and growth is to relate learning outcomes to practice and professional development. This is accomplished by including in the programs situational sets found in therapeutic recreation practice. When staff conduct programs or attend programs presented by other therapeutic recreators, they benefit from "ownership" of the experience and relating to "common" professional issues. Attendance at professional meetings also exposes staff to analogous situations. Evaluations that require respondents to identify how session knowledge and skills will be applied to practice also helps trainees realize how they are expected to improve or change performance as a result of attendance.

## *Projecting Follow-Up*

A final management task prior to implementing training and development programs is to project what follow-up is necessary after staff participation. Dramatic change in the work environment requires additional practice, managerial feedback and support, and recognition of achieved training and development goals. Follow-up occurs when staff return to the work site to present materials and resources acquired at off-site meetings to those in the department who did not attend. Follow-up also involves planned observations and reviews of tapes to critique practices and compare "before" with "after" performances. The use of written checklists to confirm completed job tasks is a follow-up strategy and self-correcting tool to incorporate into personnel appraisal processes. Follow-up needs are projected in order to prepare the resources and continued training and development opportunities that ensure use of newly acquired abilities and to overcome challenges to the introduction of new behaviors in the work setting.

## *Implementing Training and Development Programs*

While training and development is in progress, the manager oversees program delivery, facilitates application of knowledge and skills, and conducts formative evaluations. Specific tasks include managing site logistics, collecting and analyzing evaluation information, monitoring application of learned skills, documenting and verifying continuing education credits, tracking financial and travel reimbursements, and ensuring continuity of department programs and services. Through postevent follow-up, managers observe how newly acquired knowledge and skills relate to department services and professional practice. A primary concern for the manager is the match between individual development goals, department annual development goals, and the outcomes of each particular training and development experience. When incongruencies are observed, the task becomes reconciling available opportunities with annual staff and department development plans. Locating and offering different opportunities and/or revising staff and department plans are options. Change has a domino effect. As change resulting from training and development is monitored, performance expectations and development plans are updated to ensure that indicators of quality improvement are continually achieved.

Implemented training and development programs vary with the needs of the staff, situation, department, and agency. The needs of volunteer, intern, seasonal, and part-time employees are more diverse than full-time staff. As a consequence, orientations and in-services cover broader topics, but they are less in depth. With full-time staff, development and retraining are focused and in depth while emphasizing the knowledge and skills necessary to update, enhance, and/or revitalize performance.

Situational needs also influence program implementation. Resources and interventions are unique to each setting. Professionals who relocate may find it necessary to attend orientations or in-services to become familiar with protocols peculiar to new positions. Implementation is also affected by relationships and timing of department and agency programs. The therapeutic recreation manager monitors the timing and content of department and agency programs to encourage maximum staff involvement and support and to avoid duplicating efforts.

## Implementing Orientation Programs

Managers involve staff in conducting orientations with, for example, summer or seasonal employees or new full-time employees. Content acquaints personnel to the mission and direction of the department and agency operational policies. Topics presented by managers and staff include but are not limited to the following:

- agency mission, goals, and structure;
- department clientele, services, and operating protocols;
- areas, facilities, resources, and use procedures;
- risk management, infection control, and quality and safety plans;
- employee benefits, forms, policies, and performance expectations;
- work rules and standards;
- privileging procedures and professional opportunities;
- personnel introductions; and
- credentialing requirements and opportunities.

## Implementing In-Service Programs

In-services are generally implemented on site in brief time periods (e.g., over the lunch hour or during "nonprogram" time). Employees and resource people within and external to the agency present information helpful to current job performance. Some general, yet not all-inclusive, in-service topics are:

- marketing and promotion,
- referral and transition planning,
- managing safety and risk,
- use of software resources and technology,
- interdisciplinary and teamwork strategies,
- managing assistive devices,
- volunteer management,
- caregiver training and support,
- application of specific interventions (i.e., brief treatment), and
- adapting programs and resources.

## Implementing Development Programs

Development opportunities like attendance at local workshops or out-of-state professional conferences (see Figure 17.2, page 256) are widely recognized as effective motivators and employment perks (Carter, Browne, LeConey, and Nagle, 1991). Implementation of development in-service and retraining sessions are guided by professional standards (Riley and Connolly, 1996) and emerging trends that affect staff career plans. Development addresses systematic issues such as the following:

- legislation and legal directives,
- advocacy,
- technological and scientific discoveries,
- ethics and professionalism,
- innovative interventions,
- philosophical paradigms,
- research and efficacy,
- health and human service reforms, and
- changing demographics and clientele needs.

## Implementing Retraining Programs

First-line managers and staff may be unaware of the impact of change. The need to retrain, therefore, becomes a viable retraining program to implement. Attitudinal and behavioral change occurs over time and through novel approaches like job sharing or exchanges. Self-monitoring of continuing education units (CEUs) through readings, tapes, and videos permits access to newly developed resources. Clinical supervision of interns is a form of retraining because students tend to bring recently acquired resources to placement locations. When orientation, in-service, and development sessions expose trainees to updated therapeutic recreation practices, retraining occurs. Implementation of retraining is critical during transitions like mergers and restructuring or reorganizing. Training is provided by persons already in similar positions from within the agency or agencies with similar cultures. Retraining sessions are implemented over extended time periods or through intermittent briefings.

Managers monitor the selection of content and the implementation of training and development programs to assure immediate staff performance and long-term growth and professional development. Monitoring also ensures compatibility between agency and department efforts and the appropriate balance among orientation, in-service, development, and retraining programs. Collection of formative data enables immediate adjustments to staff, department, and agency development plans. As systems analysts, managers measure immediate outcomes and monitor quality indicators to project future plans and directions.

# Evaluation of Training and Development Programs

How are the results of training and development programs measured? What indicators verify adaptation to the domino effect of change? Reorganizing staffing patterns, implementing cost-effective delivery systems, and improving quality within a framework of declining resources mandate that management and staff respond to change. Training and development are the tools that enable change to take place; evaluation determines the effectiveness of training and development. The complexity of change and each

---

**Figure 17.2 Development Programs**

**Managing Diversity**

DATE:             March 30, 19__

TIME:             8:30 a.m.–12:00 p.m.

PLACE:            Educational Services, Classroom #3

INTENDED
AUDIENCE:         Managers and Supervisors of Central Iowa Health System (CIHS)

PURPOSE:          To discuss the multicultural work force of the future, exploring the differences of managing this
                  work force, and how to use coaching techniques.

OBJECTIVES:       At the completion of this program, the participant should be able to:

                  1. Identify six (6) basic diverse work groups at CIHS.
                  2. Examine three (3) steps in understanding and managing these diverse work groups.
                  3. Discuss the changing attitudes and values in today's work environment and the impact
                     on patient care.

FACULTY:          Educational Services

REGISTER:         Call 241-6898

MCE–3.5

This program has been approved for four (4) contact hours/0.4 CEUs by an Iowa Approved Provider #31, Educational Services, Iowa Health System.

Used by permission of Iowa Methodist Medical Center of Central Iowa Health System, Des Moines, IA.

---

person's responsiveness to change result in a variety of content and methods being used to accomplish training and development goals. Systematic evaluation strategies are, therefore, needed to validate achievement of planned outcomes.

Evaluation has several benefits. For instance, evaluative measures determine if programs are producing the results for which they were intended, thereby justifying the time and money budgeted. The feedback provided enables the manager to improve offerings. A comprehensive evaluation plan is prepared during the design phase to assess each training and development program. Jeska (1994) reports that managers determine the focus of evaluation plans by considering cost, volume, and significance of each program. The higher or more crucial each of these variables is to the trainees and service quality indicators, the more intense the evaluation effort. Orientation and retraining sessions typically focus on new staff or new procedures and are more costly, time consuming, and significant to service outcomes than are in-service or development programs. As a result, data collection is more carefully

planned and carried out with the former than with the latter types of programs.

Training and development evaluations have tended to focus on trainee opinions of programs and perceptions of what trainees have learned. Robbins (1995) notes these forms of evaluation are unduly influenced by the difficulty of the learning experience, its entertainment value, and the personality of the instructor. According to Jeska (1994), a comprehensive objective evaluation plan measures four facets: employee reactions, learning, transfer of new knowledge and skills to job performance, and results or impact on service outcomes. Additionally, Sims (1993) suggests that evaluation of each training and development session has five goals which influence the manager's selection of evaluation audiences and determination of the evaluation schedule:

1. to determine how well or what the trainee does during each session;
2. to determine if objectives of individual, department, and agency development plans are achieved;

256

3. to determine whether trainee effectiveness is improved (e.g., is there an impact on consumer services?);
4. to ascertain if the session was efficient or if alternative types of training and development might achieve the same objectives; and
5. to ascertain relevance of content and methods to training and development objectives (e.g., were topics related to job and career goals and were appropriate methods used to deliver content?).

To obtain maximum benefit from a program, trainees must like the opportunity. Employee reactions are usually evaluated by conducting interviews or administering questionnaires immediately following the program. The intent, according to Sims (1993), is to determine if trainees liked the program, if they felt the instruction was helpful, and if they learned from the presented materials. Typical questions may include:

- How well were trainees' personal objectives met?
- How well were the identified program objectives met?
- How effective was the instructor in delivering the content?
- Were the environment and instructional aids conducive to learning?

Learning evaluations, the second form of evaluation, determine if the trainee is able to demonstrate understanding of presented content. Skill demonstrations, cognitive tests, role playing, and case study analyses determine how well trainees acquire KSAs from each of the five competence domains. Test performance may neither reflect what is actually learned nor the ability to apply the KSAs to work or career goals; however, when used at the conclusion of a program, tests are reliable, easy to administer, and objective in their assessment of the trainee's grasp of presented content.

Transfer of KSAs toward improving job performance and/or agency effectiveness is one of the most critical outcomes of training and development (Sims, 1993). Information is of little value unless behavior or performance changes. The main question becomes, "Does the trainee assimilate learning within the practice setting?" This form of evaluation occurs at defined intervals after participation in training and development. The amount of time to incorporate new information into behavioral patterns varies with the difficulty level of the competencies. For example, soon after an in-service on new petty cash (e.g., administrative competency) or equipment use (e.g., technical competency) procedures, the therapeutic recreation manager observes and/or interviews staff to confirm use of the new procedures. Self-assessments and peer reviews evaluating outcomes of work delegation (e.g., interpersonal competency), time management (e.g., leadership competency), or strategic planning (e.g., conceptual competency) sessions occur on several occasions over extended periods of time because of the complexity of behavioral change. Listed here are some questions to assess the transfer of KSAs to job improvement:

- Compared to two months ago, has the supervisor delegated work assignments more effectively?
- Do recorded work activities of this month reflect improved time management as compared to the calendar kept prior to the in-service last month?
- Have practitioners revised their individual development plans since the implementation last month of the department's new mission and plan of operation?

The fourth component of comprehensive evaluation is the result or impact of training and development on service outcomes. The purpose of training and development is to increase or improve effectiveness through achievement of department goals. In health and human service agencies the primary evaluative question is "Did training and development result in enhanced client well-being?" In therapeutic recreation the manager might ask, "Was service maintained or improved through cost reductions, enhanced use of personnel or physical resources, and the application of specific interventions?" Impact evaluations are accomplished through cost-benefit analyses, audits, trends reports, and follow-up client and caregiver questionnaires or surveys. Results of this form of evaluation are directly correlated to department goals. A manager reconciles impact outcomes with staff and agency development goals, and adjustments occur when goals are not reached or incongruencies are evident among development plans.

The evaluation plan is based on the department's training and development needs and goals and the objectives of each particular program. A manager prepares instruments and identifies techniques to collect data in each of the four areas—reaction, learning, performance, and impact—for each training and development opportunity provided. The task is to match each form of evaluation with the type of training used to reach identified outcomes. As shown in Table 17.1 (page 258), performance and impact evaluations are appropriate to development and retraining sessions, while reaction and learning evaluations are administered with orientation and in-service sessions. With each training and development program one or more evaluation audiences (e.g., staff, managers, clients, caregivers, administrators) respond to or are the subject of assessing outcomes. After an in-service, managers interview staff to ascertain if they learned how to conduct client assessments differently. However, after a retraining session, both managers and staff participate in peer reviews on adapting to agency-wide changes. A comprehensive evaluation plan depicts the department's assessed needs, the programs designed and

**Table 17.1  Training and Development Evaluation Plan**

| Domain | Goal/Need | Program | Evaluation Type | Audience |
|---|---|---|---|---|
| Conceptual | Adapt to change | Retraining | Impact | Manager & staff |
| Leadership | Build teams | Development | Performance | Staff & clients |
| Interpersonal | Manage conflict | Development | Performance | Staff & colleagues |
| Administrative | Design development goals | Orientation | Reaction | Staff & administrators |
| Technical | Conduct assessments | In-service | Learning | Staff |

implemented to meet these needs, and the forms of evaluation used to collect the data to determine the benefits of training and development (see Table 17.1). An evaluation plan, therefore, interrelates the assessment, design, implementation, and evaluation steps of comprehensive planning.

Managers revise, replace, or retain programs based on evaluation outcomes. These decisions relate training and development outcomes to performance and service delivery effectiveness. Compatibility among the department's, agency's, and staff's development goals and evaluation results is assessed. The manager determines which behaviors and performances have changed, the longevity of the changes, and the relationship of the changes to service outcomes. Goals in each of the plans are rewritten and training and development opportunities are reconsidered if incongruencies exist. For example, the orientation content or schedule might be revised while in-service sessions are replaced by more relevant or current topics on medication side effects and accessible transportation alternatives.

Professional conventions provide staff and managers with development and retraining opportunities. Attendance decisions are usually based on location of the meetings, funds available, and a rotation schedule that enables staff participation on an alternating basis. Yet, if staff performance warrants updating, managers make funding decisions based on revised attendance schedules. The therapeutic recreation manager uses evaluation results to make immediate adjustments in development goals and to plan for long-term development that will impact future department services.

## Training and Development Trends and Issues

Society is undergoing very rapid change in a number of ways including the manner in which the practice of thera-

peutic recreation is conducted. Dynamic work and social environments require that professionals continually update knowledge and skills in order to adjust to the needs of clients and the profession. Health and human service organizations are a portion of the growing service industry where "people skills" are fundamental to quality of services delivered. It is evident that therapeutic recreators rely on communication skills more and more to maintain and improve client well-being. Further, information is acquired and communicated more rapidly with the computer and other electronic and technological resources. The increasing significance of information as a commodity is evidenced in network information systems and through emerging forms of electronic leisure. The pace of change intensifies with information exchange.

Each therapist will continue to need knowledge and skills about how to process and access information via technology. Increasing amounts of information will be communicated in the practice setting to consumers, caregivers, and colleagues. As demands for accountability, continuous improvement, cost reductions, and service redistributions magnify, the time to communicate becomes less while the necessity to communicate the value of therapeutic recreation becomes greater. Consumer well-being is the central focus of intervention. The challenge is to synthesize vast amounts of information so that the intent of professional practice is properly communicated while consumer well-being is maintained and enhanced.

Therapeutic recreation specialists will continue to need to develop communication skills, and management will have to evolve to meet changing social philosophies. Competency in communication skills such as conflict resolution, negotiation, individual and group facilitation, public speaking, problem solving, and empathetic listening are fundamental to service delivery approaches that emphasize participatory management and interactive leadership. As the information age brings people closer together,

1. Orientation
2. In service
3. Professional development

4.

communication with others whose backgrounds, experience, and education are more unique and varied increases. Consequently, communication is an avenue to cultural awareness and skill building. Advocacy depends on effective communication. The intent of therapeutic recreation is communicated through research, evaluation, and efficacy studies. Thus, competence in all forms of communication is necessary and continues to be a training and development need.

Training and development provides opportunities to study ethical dilemmas. To illustrate, "doing the right thing" receives mixed signals in the workplace, profession, and society. Therapists increasingly experience dilemmas in situations that involve service marketing and competition, financial reimbursement, consumer confidentiality and self-determination, and collegial interactions (e.g., teamwork and networking). Training and development teach the facilitation skills necessary to resolve situational and professional practice dilemmas and to communicate the beliefs and ethical standards of therapeutic recreation.

How does one cope with change? The interpersonal aspect of therapeutic recreation contributes to the need to adjust to the changing perspectives of clients, caregivers, and management. Therapeutic recreators, like other members of health and human service teams and networks, require support as the work environment becomes more people and information intensive. Support can be found in time and stress management sessions and self-help books that represent an attempt to adapt personally to changing professional interactions and pressures. Training and development offers avenues to adapt to changes that would otherwise contribute to "professional burnout."

## Summary

The intent of this chapter was twofold: to introduce the tasks in preparation and delivery of staff training and development programs and to explore the roles and responsibilities of first-line managers in staff training and development. The need for such training and development has evolved out of the rapid rate of change in society and the workplace. Professional practice standards include guidelines pertaining to annual department development plans and personnel training and development goals. A therapeutic recreation manager is the intermediary between the development goals of the agency, department, and staff and is expected to know the competence of employees and outcomes of each position. Consequently, the manager is held responsible for achieving agency and department goals through staff activities. A comprehensive training and development program is integral to continuous quality improvement and delivery of relevant services.

Four types of staff training and development are orientation, in-service, professional development, and retraining. Training goals are established through assessments, and a plan is developed to address specific objectives. These objectives guide the selection of training content and methods. A number of adult learner characteristics are taken into consideration as the first-line manager designs each program. Also considered are the compatibility of methods to each competency domain (e.g., conceptual, leadership, interpersonal, administrative, and technical) in which behavior is learned. Managers facilitate access to training and development opportunities and conduct sessions in which the content and methods appropriate to each type of training and development are presented.

The manager also designs an evaluation plan that collects formative and summative data to ascertain if newly acquired practices result in client-related benefits. A comprehensive evaluation plan assesses four types of trainee outcomes: reaction, learning, performance, and impact. The type of evaluation chosen is compatible with the training offered. Where higher levels of resources are invested, evaluation efforts are more intense.

Viable training and development topics continue to be adaptation to change and the use of technology to access information and apply newfound knowledge and skills to practice. A number of training and development topics emanate from the aspect of therapeutic recreation that deals with different people day in and day out. The challenge is to validate the linkage between training and development, professional practices, and client services.

## Discussion Questions

1. Describe the purpose of orientation, in-service, development, and retraining programs.
2. Outline the criteria on training and development presented in professional standards documents.
3. What considerations are involved in developing and conducting needs assessments including job analyses?
4. What factors and challenges are considered as training and development programs are designed?
5. Explain how adult learner and behavior characteristics impact implementation of training and development programs.
6. Explain how the manager selects and uses each type of evaluation. What are the goals of training and development evaluations?
7. Generate responses to the following statement: In the future training and development in therapeutic recreation will likely focus on—and will be delivered through—media.

# References

American Therapeutic Recreation Association (ATRA). (1993). *Standards for the practice of therapeutic recreation and self-assessment guide.* Hattiesburg, MS: Author.

Arnold, W. E., and McClure, L. (1989). *Communication training and development.* New York, NY: HarperCollins Publishers.

Carter, M. J., Browne, B., LeConey, S. P., and Nagle, C. (1991). *Designing therapeutic recreation programs in the community.* Reston, VA: American Alliance for Health, Physical Education, Recreation and Dance.

Denning, J. D., and Verschelden, C. (1993). Using the focus group in assessing training needs: Empowering child welfare workers. *Child Welfare, 72:6,* 569–579.

Grossman, A. H. (1989). *Personnel management in recreation and leisure services* (2nd ed.). Reston, VA: American Alliance for Health, Physical Education, Recreation and Dance.

Habel, M. (1994). Planning an agency-wide in-service. *Journal of Nursing Staff Development, 10*(3), 133–136.

Ismeurt, J., Ismeurt, R., and Miller, B. K. (1992). Field-dependence/independence: Considerations in staff development. *The Journal of Continuing Education in Nursing, 23:1,* 38–41.

Jeska, S. B. (1994). Evaluation: An important aspect of staff development service. *Journal of Nursing Care Quality, 8:4,* 55–65.

Kaplan, G., and Breslin, L. (1989). Education and training on a shoestring: The clinical case conference as a staff development tool. *Administration and Policy in Mental Health, 17:1,* 47–49.

Metzger, N. (1982). *The healthcare supervisor's handbook* (2nd ed.). Rockville, MD: Aspen Systems Corporation.

National Council for Therapeutic Recreation Certification (NCTRC). (1997). *Updated NCTRC exam content outline* (Supplement to the NCTRC Candidate Bulletin). Thiells, NY: Author.

National Therapeutic Recreation Society (NTRS). (1995). *Standards of practice for therapeutic recreation services and annotated bibliography.* Arlington, VA: Author.

National Therapeutic Recreation Society (NTRS). (1990). *Guidelines for the administration of therapeutic recreation services.* Alexandria, VA: Author.

Pledge, D. S. (1993). Staff development needs in a community mental health center. *Administration and Policy in Mental Health, 20:3,* 175–182.

Riley, B., and Connolly, P. (1996). *The 1996 job analysis: A simulation.* Paper presented at the 1996 American Therapeutic Recreation Association, San Francisco, CA.

Robbins, S. P. (1995). *Supervision today.* Englewood Cliffs, NJ: Prentice Hall.

Sandwith, P. (1993). A hierarchy of management training requirements: The competency domain model. *Public Personnel Management, 22:1,* 43–62.

Sims, R. R. (1993). Evaluating public sector training programs. *Public Personnel Management, 22:4,* 591–615.

# Chapter 18

# Volunteer Management

## Introduction

Management of volunteers is an integral component of personnel management. The significance of volunteers to practice is noted by the inclusion of governing standards in professional practice documents (NRPA, 1990). The intent of this chapter is to present information on each phase of volunteer management in therapeutic recreation. Material is organized according to those areas a manager needs to cover when designing a volunteer program which may be the sole responsibility of the therapeutic recreation manager or shared with those responsible for the agency-wide volunteer and staff development program when agency-wide recruitment, placement, supervision, and evaluation of volunteers are involved. Issues and dilemmas that arise as staff, clients, and volunteers interface are introduced. Illustrations are drawn from actual agency and department materials.

## Volunteers

### Volunteer Planning

Volunteer preparation begins with the organization of program staff and resources to ensure recruitment and selection of mutually compatible volunteers. After this has been completed, a cadre of volunteers is chosen to extend, enhance, and expand programs, services, and resources. Organization involves:

1. assessment of the department strategic plan;
2. identification of standards and practices impacting volunteer management;
3. delineation of relevant management policies and protocols;
4. determination of staff, consumer, and volunteer roles and responsibilities; and
5. design of job descriptions and management documents.

With completion of organization tasks a department is ready to recruit volunteers. Recruitment alerts potential volunteers to the needs and benefits of giving of their time and resources. Recruitment entails developing a marketing plan to:

1. identify target volunteer audiences;
2. coordinate internal (agency, division, or department) and external (community) promotions;
3. disseminate information about the department, clientele, and services; and
4. evaluate the effectiveness of the marketing plan to ensure the retention of a volunteer pool.

Volunteer recruitment is an ongoing process. Selection is ongoing and/or periodic (i.e., coincides with program start-up or staff development cycles). Volunteer selection involves:

1. application and credential review and verification,
2. candidate screening and interviewing, and
3. candidate disposition and documentation.

Results of planning for volunteer management include a structure, policies, and job descriptions to organize volunteer operations and relationships of volunteers, staff and clients; a marketing plan and promotional materials to use in recruitment and retention; and strategies and processes to use in initial screening and review of potential volunteers. The nature of this planning is influenced by the agency's mission and the therapeutic recreation department's role in achieving that mission. To illustrate, when the department is in a primary care hospital where length of stay averages less than two weeks, volunteers provide hospital-wide support with assistance during recreational outings and pet therapy sessions. When the department is an autonomous entity as in a transitional living center or special recreation district, volunteers support staff in all phases of service delivery and are trained specifically to meet client needs during therapeutic intervention.

## Volunteer Organization

Assessment of the department's mission and strategic plan are undertaken to determine the attitude toward volunteers and the roles and relationships of volunteers within the agency to the department. The vision, mission, and goals guide the manager's planning (Carter, Van Andel, and Robb, 1995). Study of organizational charts also shows the relationship of volunteers within the agency to each department. When volunteers are identified in these documents, their functions are essential to service outcomes, and resources are devoted to volunteer management.

Review of these documents also reveals whether volunteer management is centralized or decentralized. In centralized management settings such as veterans affairs hospitals, one unit is responsible for hospital-wide volunteer coordination. This centrality is noted by identification of an autonomous unit that has parity with other hospital-wide units (e.g., marketing, finance, research). In decentralized management, each department such as therapeutic recreation or Region I (e.g., geographic unit) is responsible for volunteer coordination in its particular unit. To illustrate, when volunteer management is centralized, one or more persons manage volunteer operations of the entire hospital. In decentralized settings, staff in each unit such as aquatics, community integration, and pet therapy oversee direct service responsibilities and manage the volunteers assigned to their areas.

A number of publications include volunteer management guidelines. Professional organizations (NRPA, 1990) incorporate statements in standards of practice on administration of therapeutic recreation services. Literary sources (Tedrick and Henderson, 1989) report practices in health and human services. Accreditation statements (NRPA, 1992) reference volunteers in personnel management standards. All recommend that procedures similar to management of permanent staff be instituted with volunteers. These sources also present samples of tools such as job descriptions and evaluation forms.

Specific volunteer management directives are found in state laws, city ordinances, risk management plans, insurance, and workman's compensation regulations which outline limits of direct volunteer service roles, legal precautions, and compensation related to health and medical needs. The essence of these directives is reflected in job descriptions, contracts, and department policies.

Volunteer management practices are governed by general and specific policies emanating from the agency and department. General practices are found in placement procedures, contracts, orientation and training materials, job descriptions, supervisory and evaluation plans, productivity measures, risk management plans, safety policies, infection control plans, and personnel codes on workman's compensation.

Specific policies cover legal and risk concerns and client and staff functions and interactions. Legal and risk documents identify specific volunteer roles on outings, when transporting, in emergencies, and when documenting or reporting client information. Treatment protocols specify client-volunteer interactions. To illustrate, volunteers may not be permitted to transfer patients without a qualified therapist present, or during a community outing a volunteer may not be permitted to refer to an agency by name if the reference would violate client confidentiality.

Generally allowable roles are defined by agency and department policy documents. The manager assesses unit needs to determine desired volunteer skills, expertise, and roles. Roles and responsibilities usually fall within three categories: direct service, supportive services, or administrative services. Direct service roles involve provision of services, programs and resources to clients. When a volunteer assists a client during Special Olympics or on a challenge course, it is direct service. Volunteers who accompany staff on outings or during group sessions to complement and supplement staff skills provide supportive service. Administrative roles enable service delivery but do not directly involve clients as when volunteers repair equipment, secure alternative funds, or write computer programs.

Volunteer roles are intended to extend, enhance and expand current staff capabilities and consumer services. A number of factors influence volunteer roles. These factors include:

- number of staff available, their competence and interests;
- staff to consumer ratio;
- consumer abilities and preferences;
- length and nature of interventions;
- safety, risk, and emergency practices;

- available work stations, space, and resources; and
- policies governing consumer interactions.

The manager develops an inventory listing volunteer needs. From this list, job descriptions are generated. These are developed for each direct, supportive, and administrative role. Each description presents information in several categories:

- agency and department information, position title, work sites;
- purpose or objective of job;
- performance expectations;
- job requirements (e.g., duration, hours, days, orientation, training);
- qualifications (e.g., job-related education, training, competence, credentials, experience, membership dues, insurance, equipment, dress, medical tests and treatments, legal screening, transportation);
- authority and supervision (e.g., limits to authority, relationships with staff, consumers, other volunteers, and job supervisor, and evaluation, separation, and recognition procedures);
- comments (e.g., in-kind benefits, unusual job site demands, medical coverage, emergency protocols, disclaimers); and
- date of job description preparation, revision, approval.

As with descriptions for permanent positions, these descriptions are updated periodically and used as recruiting tools. Because they define expectations, they are foundational to supervisory and evaluation plans. Contracts are written after the review of job descriptions and unit policies.

Contracts detail the relationship between each volunteer and the placement site. Therefore they usually consist of two parts: one portion outlines the volunteer's commitment while the second describes the placement's responsibilities. Volunteer contracts outline minimal practice standards and performance expectations. Consequently, along with job descriptions they are used to formulate volunteer supervisory plans and evaluations. Signed contracts are placed in volunteer personnel files.

A direct service contract might include:

The volunteer agrees to:
1. become familiar with department policies and procedures;
2. work a certain number of hours at a particular site in the position of _____;
3. report to work according to the schedule and maintain a record of hours worked by clocking in and out;
4. provide 24-hour notice of nonattendance and notification of one week in advance of a leave of absence;
5. attend orientation and training sessions and undertake continuous educational development;
6. accept right of the manager to dismiss a volunteer for poor performance and attendance;
7. exercise caution when acting on behalf of the department to protect the confidentiality of the unit and its clientele;
8. abide by department rules specifically related to health, risk, safety, and emergencies; and
9. accept supervisory actions and functions as a team member contributing to professional working relationships among staff, clientele, and volunteers.

The unit agrees to:
1. train volunteers to a level permitting them to commence and continue work confidently and competently;
2. provide work conditions equal to paid staff;
3. conduct routine evaluations and provide references upon request;
4. offer promotions, new assignments and/or more responsible jobs upon mutual agreement and with commensurate training;
5. keep volunteers informed of activities and policies;
6. recognize volunteer service;
7. include volunteers in program planning where possible; and
8. provide benefits as appropriate (e.g., parking, proper identification tags, meals, access to medical library, fee waivers for cardiopulmonary resuscitation [CPR] classes, first-aid classes).

Sometimes more than one person from a service organization donates time in supportive or administrative volunteer roles to a department. In this situation a manager prepares a standard form letter that describes group responsibilities and serves as a contract between the department and service organization. For example, the letter details volunteer roles of the group for a one-time project such as a birthday party on the pediatric unit or spring cleanup of the challenge course area.

## Volunteer Recruitment

Designing a marketing plan to recruit volunteers begins by determining the roles to be played by volunteers in reaching the department mission. What are potential roles of volunteers as services are provided in achieving unit goals? And as volunteers provide these services, what benefits do they receive? Volunteering is an exchange; the department provides growth, challenge, and experiences while volunteers give time, expertise, and resources. The design of a marketing plan begins with generating responses to questions like:

- What does the unit offer volunteers in exchange for what is desired from them?
- What motivates volunteerism?
- What rewards are volunteers seeking?
- What type of service commitment is desired?

Not all volunteers desire the same benefits or have the same motives, and each experience uniquely impacts each volunteer. Consequently, the manager identifies target volunteer audiences to maximize each volunteer's "product life cycle." Promotional effectiveness is more likely when the manager is aware of the type of service commitment and benefits anticipated by each target audience.

Several target volunteer audiences are likely to have an interest. Among these are older adults, students of medicine and health-related professions, caregivers, youth, court-assigned volunteers, and former consumers. Each of these audiences brings a particular perspective and expectation to the volunteer experience. To recruit these groups a first-line manager determines how to use their skills while offering an experience that both suits their personal needs and achieves the unit's goals.

Older adults gain a sense of belonging, recognition, companionship, and opportunities to remain a part of the social mainstream as they share their personal expertise plus encounters they may have had with healthcare settings. Students in medicine and health-related professions desire to receive evaluated work experience, explore career possibilities, and receive professional training. When a caregiver volunteers, focus may be on a member of his or her family or other persons with illnesses or disabilities served by the same agency (e.g., extended care facility). Caregiver needs encompass a desire to support a cause, to make system changes, alleviate boredom, compensate for losses, and process grief. For a caregiver, volunteering can be a form of leisure and self-help.

Youth volunteers bring novelty, energy, unconditional positive regard, acceptance, and a desire to help and to have fun to their experiences. Some desire to explore career options while others gain a sense of social responsibility desired by their parents or legal authorities. If volunteers are assigned by the courts, their primary objective may be to avoid institutional detainment, but authorities recognize the rehabilitative potential of volunteerism. Court-assigned volunteers also have a need to contribute to change, use their skills, and be a part of a group with socially acceptable leisure outlets. Former consumers have a vested interest and are influential recruiters (e.g., adult wheelchair athletes promote youth leagues). Their needs stem from a desire to give back to those who have enhanced their well-being and to advocate for constituent group needs (e.g., accessibility).

Person-to-person contacts and support from satisfied volunteers are the most effective recruiting tools. Managers select and coordinate the use of internal and external promotional resources suited to each target audience. Several details are considered as the medium is selected. Each message presents an "opportunity" through particular roles and unique experiences. Volunteers respond to familiar situations and those with known credibility. To illustrate, potential volunteers are more responsive to a call from the "hospital" coordinator of volunteer services than the less familiar department manager. Since people usually do not respond immediately to a call for volunteers, managers select media outlets that will keep their story continuously in full view.

To facilitate coordination of recruiting efforts a matrix is designed that identifies the media and contacts used with each target audience (see Table 18.1). This matrix is intended to ensure that each audience receives the proper amount of information in a timely manner. The matrix presents several target organizations as potential volunteer sources. Social service clubs and corporations periodically contribute both money and group efforts. These communal efforts create individual awareness and collective advocacy. Likewise when educational institutions and professional organizations donate expertise, they, too, are advocating for persons with disabilities.

Information dissemination results as the manager and therapeutic recreation specialists communicate with clients, caregivers, colleagues (doctors, nurses, social workers, other therapists), residents, and organizations. This communication is usually ongoing but can intensify at times which coincide with seasonal program cycles. When contacts are made, documentation on the matrix helps to determine if and when the audience should again be contacted. Although few volunteers drop in, a method should be in place to record both the nature of each inquiry and the source of information about the opportunity. Initial information to share with all audience types includes benefits of the opportunity, the length, frequency, clientele, location, educational and experiential requirements (e.g., certifications), training expectations, application and placement dates and deadlines, screening tests or procedures (e.g., references, police), and incentives.

Marketing outcomes are evaluated by identifying the number of new and retained volunteers. Marketing also educates others to client referral needs such as access to other hospital or community resources. Consequently, evaluation encompasses situations such as phone inquires, mail requests, newspaper clippings, observed television and radio releases, invitations to make presentations, and

## Table 18.1  Volunteer Recruitment Matrix

| Target Audience | Benefit | Media/Contacts | Record* |
|---|---|---|---|
| Older Adults | Recognition, companionship | RSVP, church group, radio, newspaper, displays, talks | |
| Students | Work experience, career choice | TV, classroom, career fairs | |
| Caregivers | Compensation, support | Open house, cable TV, support groups | |
| Youth | Social responsibility, careers | TV, service club, high-school counselor | |
| Court Assignment | Rehabilitation | Social workers, voluntary action center, flyers | |
| Former Client | Advocacy | Personal contact, incentives | |
| Social Service Agencies | Community welfare | Referral agencies, PSAs, human interest stories | |
| Corporations | Public relations | Gift brochures, chamber of commerce, posters | |
| Educational Institutions | Education | PTA(O), displays, bumper stickers | |
| Professional Organizations | Advocacy | Annual conventions, letter writing, publications | |

*Record name of contact person, address, response, type of media used and dates of use.

expanded client reentry opportunities. One approach is to allow space on the initial volunteer application for identification of where or how the volunteer became familiar with the opportunity.

Documentation of marketing costs is part of evaluating the benefits of a volunteer program. Figures on media and dissemination expenses are included in administrative budgets or individual program budgets. The manager compares the cost of gaining and retaining volunteers to worker year equivalents (e.g., 2,080 hours equal one worker year) or service extensions. Ultimately, evaluation determines if the form of marketing used was suitable to each target audience. Managers consider whether the right story has been told to a sufficient number of the right people. Marketing continues as volunteers are trained, supervised, and recognized. When satisfied volunteers are retained, the recruiting of new qualified volunteers is made easier.

## Volunteer Selection

Selection of qualified volunteers commences with application and credential review and verification. This review affirms the match between a volunteer's skills, priorities, and expectations and the department's goals and needs. During the recruitment process potential volunteers are given job descriptions and materials that delineate respective roles, needs, and expectations. They then complete applications that require presentation of personal information plus any credentials related to their job competence and qualifications.

When volunteer services are managed agency-wide, the application form may or may not present specific options (e.g., therapeutic recreation, hospice, special events). When decentralized, each unit solicits and processes applications. Generally, applicants present information in several areas:

- personal and business address, phone, emergency contacts, and procedures;
- employment and volunteer experiences with addresses and references;
- credentials, specialized training and skills, and educational preparation;
- commitment, time, duration, reason for seeking the opportunity, and source of information about the opportunity;
- previous experiences related to therapeutic recreation (e.g., setting, clientele, intervention); and
- job-related insurance, medical checkups, legal records.

A preliminary review validates accuracy of presented information, ascertains appropriateness of a volunteer to available positions, recommends further screening to specific agency and department interviews, and determines whether or not to refer the volunteer to other placements. A volunteer may appear to have compatible needs and goals yet lack proper training or experience, or the desired opportunity is not available at the time of application. Managers inform volunteers of such assessments and request that they return after training or at a later date.

During the selection process, managers involve staff associated with placements. This contact facilitates volunteer supervision and evaluation as staff carry out these tasks. Staff also have information about volunteers from previous contacts and are responsible for recruiting volunteers to their programs. This enables staff and managers to consider the merits of volunteer placements from both the management and programmatic perspective. Volunteer needs emanate from a sincere desire to be therapeutic helpers or to be "community do-gooders." Managers and staff balance these attitudes during the selection process.

Preliminary reviews result in one of the following actions:

1. information confirmation and referral of a volunteer to appropriate manager or staff member for interview and screening placement;
2. referral to another volunteer opportunity within the agency or community;
3. recommendation that further training or credentials be acquired with application at a more compatible time; or
4. nonselection because the applicant's skills and the department's needs and expectations are incompatible.

After successful reviews, candidates are screened and interviewed. These processes are used to match the volunteer with placement options, to identify training needs, and to orient the volunteer to the organization. The nature of each volunteer job influences the screening and interviewing processes. When applicants are being assessed for supportive roles (e.g., computer processing) rather than direct consumer services (e.g., community reentry buddies), the process is briefer because fewer consumer-related skills are evaluated. If the intent is to create a registry or list of potential volunteers, screening is also less detailed and time consuming.

Screening is done with individuals or groups by phone or in person. A manager informs applicants of the agency's and department's intent, operating parameters, and needs. Specifically, the volunteer is apprised of time commitments, work schedule, healthcare and childcare options, employee processing procedures, incidentals (e.g., parking, out-of-pocket expenses, insurance coverage), and client protocols. In turn, the volunteer clarifies and explains how his or her qualifications relate to the position. Screening may result in referral or application withdrawal because time commitments may be incompatible or education and training may not be appropriately balanced. If there does appear to be a match, formal on-site interviews are planned.

The interview continues the orientation process while confirming if a match between the volunteer and department is likely. Individual or group interviews are conducted by the manager and therapeutic recreation staff. Interviews for administrative or support positions are conducted by the manager while staff are likely to be included when applicants interview for direct service positions. Initial interviews help management and staff to determine if volunteers and staff are compatible and if volunteers are likely to contribute to consumer health, well-being, and leisure functioning. During initial interviews consideration is given to:

- program goals and client descriptors;
- agency and department structure and volunteer positions, roles, and responsibilities;

- relationships and communication among management, staff, and volunteers;
- commitment requirements (e.g., time, resources);
- ethics and practice protocols;
- training and supervisory requirements; and
- volunteer selection, placement, evaluation, recognition, and separation procedures.

An interview begins with the verification and clarification of information in application forms and credentials. Noting the way with which these documents were presented as well as any professional manner displayed during the interview are an indication of the volunteer's perception of the significance of the position. After clarifying application information, an interviewee responds to specific questions about each opportunity. Through the interview management and staff become aware of how the applicant's personal and professional competencies and character will or will not enhance program and client outcomes. Therefore attributes of effective helpers like empathy, unconditional positive regard, interviewing skills and any previous exposure to persons with disabilities are areas of investigation. Questions that might lead to interpreting personal-professional philosophies and practices include:

- What do you anticipate will be the outcomes of this experience?
- How have you become aware of this opportunity?
- What do you perceive to be the benefit of therapeutic recreation with our clients?
- What do you believe to be essential qualities of effective helpers?
- Describe your previous roles and interactions with healthcare systems and clients.
- Why do you recreate?
- What are your personal career goals?
- Interpret your assets and liabilities as related to the particular job.

Presentation of situations helps determine how a volunteer might respond to emergencies and to routine behaviors exhibited by various consumers. Also the volunteer becomes aware of the types of behaviors, needs, and situations that he or she is likely to encounter. Types of questions that illustrate possible scenarios include:

- What would you do if you and members of our staff were intervening when a consumer becomes resistive or combative?
- How would you respond on an outing if a consumer becomes disoriented and confused?
- How would you react to a consumer who uses inappropriate language to describe your character?

Direct questioning about the interviewee's health is inappropriate unless it is related to performance expectations (e.g., assisting with patient transfers). If the interviewee indicates need for job accommodations, the manager is obligated to discern what can be done to effect necessary changes (e.g., assign the volunteer to a unit where consumer's do not require physical assistance). Volunteer placements can be made contingent on outcomes of job-related physical examinations.

During the interview process, time is permitted for the interviewee to ask questions and to observe activities at various work stations. Managers seek permission to check references, to conduct a police record check, and to contact former supervisors and employers. At the conclusion of the interview, the manager summarizes factors that either confirm or negate a match, referral, training needs and/or trial placement.

With acceptance, rejection, or referral written notification is sent to the volunteer and placed in permanent volunteer records. Acceptance letters are accompanied by contracts that inform volunteers of their assignments, workdays and hours, length of commitment, client and program protocols, training, supervision, and recognition processes. Rejection letters to volunteers present other options, suggest needed training, encourage application at a later date, recommend trial placements, and/or cite reasons for incompatibility.

## Volunteer Training and Supervision

Successful completion of volunteer planning results in a cadre of volunteers who appear to be compatible with the agency and department. The next phase of volunteer management involves placing volunteers, providing education and training on their roles, and supervising their performance. Specifically placement involves:

1. orientation to the agency and department,
2. introduction to specific jobs, and
3. trial and final placement.

After probationary periods volunteers begin their jobs. Preparation to perform day-to-day tasks is acquired during in-service training and professional updating occurs through continuing education. Training and education of volunteers involve:

1. designing training and education materials,
2. providing job-related training and education,
3. facilitating access to continuing professional development, and
4. monitoring and facilitating staff and volunteer infusion.

Managers supervise staff and volunteers as they work together to provide consumer services. Managers communicate and interact while documenting volunteer performance and maintaining records. Supervision involves:

1. communication with volunteers and staff,
2. documentation in personnel and department records, and
3. retention and promotion or termination and separation.

Adequate training and supervision enables effective volunteer performance and efficient volunteer management. Training and supervision, like planning, are influenced by the agency mission and relationship of the therapeutic recreation department to agency goals. Consequently, managers either assist the agency-wide volunteer manager or assume total responsibility for these functions in their unit.

## Volunteer Placement

Orientation introduces volunteers to the working environment and to expectations. The goal of orientation is to ensure basic awareness and compliance with policies and codes while acquainting volunteers with department mission, resources, and personnel. Orientation periods extend over a period of time to avoid information overload. Consumers and caregivers are involved as volunteers are made aware of the unique focus of the department. Orientation topics and activities include:

- history and mission of department;
- volunteer roles in the department;
- organizational structure, management team, and staffing protocols;
- financial and promotional protocols;
- personnel policies relating to insurance, liability, consumers' rights, parking, personal identification, reimbursement, emergency, safety and infection controls, disaster plan, health codes, ethical conduct, and personal recordkeeping (e.g., time cards);
- management, staff, volunteer introductions, responsibilities, and interrelationships;
- volunteer "boundaries" and performance criteria;
- identification and location of agency-wide service units and resources; and
- medical, health, and legal clearances and reporting of test results.

Introduction to specific work assignments and job responsibilities occurs either as the volunteer is oriented to the agency or as a department orientation is conducted. This orientation takes place at the conclusion of the agency ori-

entation or at a subsequent time period. Orientation activities attempt to instill confidence in the volunteer through a thorough understanding of assigned roles and tasks. Orientations are conducted by staff and managers and as a consequence staff-volunteer relationships are developed and staff learn to manage volunteers. Orientation to specific job responsibilities includes:

- introductions to staff, volunteers, and associated personnel in the unit including their roles, the chain of command, and the process for communicating among professionals, consumers, and caregivers (e.g., specifically things that can and cannot be said);
- identification of supervisory procedures, evaluation documents, and promotion and separation processes;
- location of space for personal items, what to do when reporting to work, specific identification tags, and parking assignments;
- review of job description, recordkeeping procedures, how to perform tasks, and location of people and resources;
- specific consumer and caregiver information, staffing and volunteer protocols, intervention protocols, and client management;
- managing consumer emergencies and unexpected work absences; and
- review of operation plan, internal and external accreditations, and professional standards of practice.

When orientations are completed, staff and volunteers have had opportunities to develop "teamwork" behaviors, and each accurately interprets the other's roles and responsibilities. Volunteers have experienced a sampling of tasks, and trial placements can occur as volunteers circulate through each work opportunity.

Trial placements encourage volunteers to explore where their skills and interests are best utilized while staff judge their suitability to program operation. For instance, trial rotations at each work site might determine that the *best fit* is with group experiences rather than during one-on-one sessions. Trial placements are also important because they help the manager identify types of in-service training and continuing education needed by volunteers. The scope of the program and a volunteer's skills influence the number and length of trial placements. Written documentation records placement activities including decisions made about final assignments, referrals, and recommendations.

Final assignments are made during—or following—trial placements by the manager and staff taking into consideration volunteer preferences. Assignments are made in writing and include workdays and hours, length and location of commitment, in-service training requirements, supervisory procedures, and client-related protocols (e.g., confidentiality, public disclosure, record access). If a contract is required, both the manager and volunteer sign the document a copy of which is placed in the volunteer's permanent file.

## Volunteer Training and Education

Training begins with orientation and continues as long as necessary to ensure the volunteer remains updated. Education refers to those opportunities which enhance the volunteer's comprehension of practice (e.g., professional development experiences). Training and education experiences are intended to develop job-related skills, expand practice knowledge, facilitate volunteer-staff partnerships, and provide opportunities that might lead to promotion. Managers prepare and organize in-service and educational materials. Volunteer job descriptions and department goals guide the manager in this task. Volunteer manuals are developed which serve as training and education resources (Appendix C is an example of a volunteer manual). A content outline for a manual reflects the volunteer management process and the unique features of a particular department (see Figure 18.1).

In addition to the manual, a manager organizes staff and resource people, including caregivers, to present in-services on topics such as communicating with a recently traumatized patient or lifestyle monitoring in cardiac rehabilitation. Managers also develop resource files and libraries to support volunteer training and education.

Job-related training and education sessions are scheduled with orientation sessions and during probationary or trial periods. Also, managers plan intermittent sessions to coincide with natural program breaks and client routines. To illustrate, shortly after volunteers begin their trial placements, managers can conduct volunteer-staff training to review compliance with protocol, to monitor staff-volunteer working relationships, and to require monthly in-services to update staff and volunteers on new equipment or resources.

Managers facilitate access to continuing professional development opportunities through other resources such as service organizations (e.g., Red Cross) and professional associations (e.g., American Therapeutic Recreation Association [ATRA] and National Therapeutic Recreation Society [NTRS]). Volunteer contracts require acquisition and retention of credentials (e.g., first aid). Managers also elect to send volunteers to educational sessions as incentives or for promotional opportunities (e.g., state or regional ATRA or NTRS training). Consultants and educational sessions are brought into a facility via satellite or media networks. Each training and education session is evaluated to ensure that volunteers perceive experiences to be applicable to their respective assignments and to the goals of the department.

Managers oversee volunteer-staff-client interactions. Staff vary in their degree of exposure to volunteer supervision. As a consequence, managers facilitate communication links and encourage the proper balance between authority and delegation of responsibility. Appropriate volunteer-client interactions are monitored. With staff, managers instill respect for volunteer roles so that volunteers are "not taken for granted" while they guide volunteers to ensure they do not "overstep boundaries" by assuming professional roles for which they are not qualified. Staff and volunteer roles are combined so that consumer goals are the focus of service.

## Volunteer Supervision

Supervision is an ongoing process that involves communicating and documenting volunteer performance for the purpose of retention, promotion, or termination. When successful, supervision enables volunteers to perform skillfully with enthusiasm and motivation. Volunteer retention diminishes with inadequate supervision and limited personal contact. Managers guide volunteers, create good

---

### Figure 18.1 Content Outline of a Volunteer Manual

**Department Background**
- Vision, mission, goals
- Service description
- Consumer needs
- Volunteer opportunities

**Volunteer Program**
- Organization and structure
- Volunteer jobs and contracts
- Staff-volunteer communication and protocols
- Volunteer screening, selection, placement processes
- Orientation content and procedures

- In-service content and procedures
- Professional development opportunities
- Evaluation tools and procedures
- Retention, promotion, recognition standards

**Department Information**
- Policies, standards of practice
- Ethical practices
- Therapeutic Recreation process and interventions
- CQI and risk management practices
- Records and documentation

working climates, encourage interest, and maximize volunteer effectiveness through communication.

Feedback is ongoing, positive, corrective, and supportive. Routine one-on-one conferences are supplemented with phone contact, observation, informal discussion, and brief written "thank yous." Communication clarifies expectations, recognizes quality performance, monitors performance, and ensures safety. Constructive criticism promotes understanding (e.g., identifying a subtle client cue such as a change in body temperature that signals a need for professional staff attention). In order to have the most impact, feedback focuses on *how* rather than *why* and is given just prior to the time when the skill is to be used again.

Motivation is a key element in volunteer supervision. A manager balances volunteer needs with department goals so that the volunteer achieves his or her needs through assigned roles. "What's In It For Me" (WI/FM) aptly describes this task. Volunteers are empowered through job enhancement, relationships with staff and clients, and confirmation that their roles contribute to department goals. Volunteers are motivated by their perception of contributing to the well-being of others or "helping" someone improve his or her health. This volunteer role can also be significant because the volunteer may be adjusting to the unexpected presence of an illness in his or her own family.

Documentation is essential to volunteer management. Formative and summative supervisory evaluations are recorded in volunteer files or data banks. Information is used in planning, budgeting, quality control and improvement, risk management, job promotion, termination, and recognition. Quantitative data are collected using computer programs to generate statistics on number of volunteer hours, equivalent dollar value of volunteer hours, "prototype volunteers," and ratio of volunteers to clients. Managers document volunteer roles and responses in incident and accident reports necessary for liability and risk management. Routine supervisory sessions permit documentation of volunteer compliance with job assignments while casual observations permit documentation of skill development needs or quality of performance. Routine documentation occurs periodically during volunteer service (e.g., formative evaluation) and when volunteers complete their assignments (e.g., summative evaluation).

Volunteers outgrow their assignments, develop new interests, feel unneeded, burn out, experience change in their time commitments, develop improper attitudes, and/ or become dissatisfied. Managers observe and record behaviors to determine if volunteers have reached *plateaus* and would benefit from promotion or reassignment. A promotion results when a volunteer assists with another consumer or in another program area, and/or leads while staff provide support. Such an experience might lead to retention as the volunteer perceives his or her talents are better utilized. Administrative or supportive assignments

may seem to be monotonous due to the repetitive nature of a particular task. In this situation a manager promotes retention by reassigning the volunteer to direct service tasks or places the volunteer on call until his or her talents can be better utilized.

Performance reviews conducted during supervisory meetings compare volunteer performance with job descriptions and contract specifications. Termination or separation results when expectations are not met. Volunteers experience changes in their personal commitments that prevent them from fulfilling their intended obligations. In this situation the volunteer may choose to separate from the department by submitting a brief written request to relinquish the position. During sessions, managers may observe a *sympathetic* rather than *empathetic* relationship that compromises the consumer's goals. Managers might overhear conversations that compromise the consumer's integrity or confidentiality. In the later situations, after due process, volunteers are assigned to positions without consumer contact, or they are terminated. Following formative and summative supervisory meetings, managers document their actions (e.g., retention, promotion, or termination) in permanent files or data banks. These data are used to evaluate the operation of the volunteer program, recognize volunteer contributions, and prepare future references or recommendations.

## *Volunteer Evaluation and Recognition*

As managers formally and informally guide volunteers during supervisory interactions, the evaluation process commences. Volunteer program evaluation is one aspect of a comprehensive evaluation process. Comprehensive evaluation plans address personnel, programs, resources, clients, and management. Several tasks are involved in design and implementation of a comprehensive evaluation program:

1. design evaluation plan;
2. collect data, analyze results, and implement outcomes; and
3. maintain records and financial data.

Data from supervisory sessions and evaluation reviews guide the manager's decisions concerning recognition. Informal and formal recognition enhances volunteer retention and staff support of volunteer efforts. Additionally, public recognition promotes therapeutic recreation. Thus, managers oversee informal volunteer and staff recognition and formal and public volunteer and staff recognition.

### Evaluation Plan

A comprehensive evaluation plan is an element of professional practice standards (ATRA, 1993) and is a recommended programming practice (Rossman, 1995). Use of volunteers is impacted by or influences each element of comprehensive evaluations—consumers, programs, resources, personnel, and management. Evaluation plans are developed by responding to several questions:

- What will be evaluated?
- When will evaluation occur?
- How will data be collected and analyzed?
- Who will administer and who will respond to the measurements?
- How will the results be used and disseminated?

What to evaluate is determined by department goals, and professional and regulatory criteria. Fundamental questions to raise about the volunteer program include:

- What should the volunteer have done, was it done, why or why not?
- Did the volunteer's support improve client services or embellish service offerings?
- Were the volunteer's efforts successfully meshed with staff competence to create supportive relationships and an effective team?
- Was each phase of the volunteer process (e.g., planning, training, supervision, evaluation, recognition) successful, why or why not?

Quantitative data are helpful during continuous quality improvement (CQI) planning. Examples of outcome measures that might be useful to quality improvement include length of service, turnover rate, total amounts of individual and group volunteer time, number of volunteers with demographic variables, dollar value equivalents of hours contributed, costs per consumer or per program, expenditure per volunteer, and staff time per volunteer. Each of these factors provides information helpful to extension or enhancement of services.

The nature and length of a volunteer job influences the *when* or frequency and formality of evaluation. When volunteer assignments are in direct service rather than administration or supportive areas, more frequent formal evaluations are likely. Direct service volunteers are governed by practice standards that mandate research and evaluation. Also, the consequence of error in direct service provision is more critical to client well-being than in nonconsumer contact functions. When volunteer commitments are short term, evaluations also are less detailed. The evaluation plan identifies approximate times of formal and informal reviews so that both formative and summative information are made available to the manager as needed for day-to-day decisions and future improvements.

A number of data collection tools and methods are available. Selection is influenced by several qualities:

- validity (Does the instrument measure what it should?),
- reliability or dependability (Does the instrument have the same results with repeated use?),
- usability (Are resources available to administer evaluations, do staff have support for analysis, and is the evaluation method economical?),
- meaningfulness (Are significant features of the volunteer program assessed in an objective manner?),
- timeliness (Is the instrument used in a reasonable length of time and are the results readily available?),
- operational (Is information unique and does it contribute to action, and is the maximum amount of information gained through minimum effort?), and
- understandability (Are directions clear, are results readily interpretable?).

The intent of evaluation influences the type of tool or method selected. Managers may use questionnaires, interviews, observations, checklists, case studies, audits, self-appraisals, consumer ratings, cost-effectiveness studies, critical incidents, and a variety of participatory techniques (e.g., focus groups, quality circles, advisory groups, and staff-volunteer councils). Decisions made using data from a number of methods add objectivity to actions taken following evaluations. To illustrate, a triangulated evaluation approach might be used if the purpose is to determine appropriateness of a volunteer's placement and his or her ability to perform assigned tasks. Data are collected from three sources: the manager uses a checklist formulated from the job description and supervisory observations, the volunteer completes a self-appraisal, and the consumer gives input on a satisfaction scale.

The *who* are those impacted by the volunteer program. Thus evaluation audiences include volunteers, staff, consumers, caregivers, managers, committee or board members, colleagues, and peers. Each audience evaluates its respective roles with respect to each of the other audiences. To illustrate:

- staff respond to questionnaires noting volunteer compliance with job descriptions;
- volunteers complete surveys on training and supervisory effectiveness of staff and managers;
- consumers report their satisfaction with programs and personnel during exit interviews; and
- managers gain reactions of volunteers and staff to operational efficiencies during quality circles.

Managers determine who is most directly affected by the evaluation concern or purpose and then design the evaluation plan so all audiences are involved appropriately. Additionally, managers either administer or oversee information collection or delegate the responsibility to appropriate personnel.

The last step in designing an evaluation plan is to determine how the results will be used and disseminated to improve program quality. Managers determine how each aspect (e.g., consumers, program, resources, personnel, and management) may be improved. Also, the manager decides how each evaluation audience is to be informed and incorporated into follow-up as the evaluation results are used. The three options managers have are to maintain the status quo, to reassign or revise, and to terminate or discontinue. When results support achievement of performance indicators in the plan of operation, no change is necessary. When managers determine, for instance, that volunteer-staff relationships have not contributed to improved consumer functioning, reassignments or termination are plausible considerations. Evaluation information is considered confidential and disseminated with discretion. Results are placed in appropriate files and are included in reports to administrators, and governing boards.

## Collect Data, Analyze Results, and Implement Outcomes

Data are collected using the tools or methods selected or prepared by the department manager or agency-wide volunteer coordinator. Formative evaluation is done as volunteers complete their assigned tasks; summative evaluation occurs at the conclusion of particular duties. Forms incorporate more than one evaluation aspect (e.g., program evaluations include volunteer functions), or each major component may have individualized evaluations (e.g., personnel, programs, resources, clientele, management).

Analysis of formative data leads to immediate adjustments such as additional in-services on ethics in the workplace, or recreation therapist's contributions to consumer health and well-being; reassignment of volunteers to another unit or a different consumer; referral of a volunteer to supportive or administrative services; or recommendation of a promotion to another job. Analysis of summative data allows the manager to make judgments about future actions in order to improve services. Minimal change may be required or revisions and discontinuation may require major adjustments. Revisions that might result include additions to the orientation and training schedule such as more hands-on experiences with clients; modifications in the supervisory process such as additional self-assessments; alterations in contracts to better clarify job parameters; and/or redesign of evaluation tools to incorporate caregivers' comments.

Termination or discontinuation is the third summative evaluation outcome. Volunteers can be fired. Documentation corroborates contract violations and unmet job expectations. Termination results from noncompliance with consumer protocol, staff directives, ethical and professional standards, and operational policies. This action is appropriate regardless of the length of the intended commitment (e.g., after an outing or one event a volunteer is released if his or her actions placed the consumer in an at-risk position). When supervisory communiqués are ineffective over an extended time, volunteers are relieved of their duties. To illustrate, volunteers may tend to talk among themselves rather than focus on the consumer's needs, and although this is not detrimental to the consumer's health, over time such actions detract from consumer skill acquisition and program quality.

## Maintain Records and Financial Data

Managers maintain records on each program aspect. A number of computer programs are available which permit data manipulation so that productivity measures and impact figures can be generated to use in both annual and monthly trends reports. Records facilitate preparation of cost-effectiveness data and strategic plans. Volunteers use records for income tax statements and educational and employment applications. Managers use records to support supervisory feedback and recognition programs.

Volunteer records document work outcomes and performance-related activities. Permanent reports and records include job descriptions, contracts, supervisory plans, training results, performance appraisals, recommendations, referrals, promotions, terminations, recognitions, service data, staff evaluations, risk management, and CQI information.

As suggested by Henderson (1988), relative worth of a volunteer to the agency is determined by cost-effectiveness analysis. Figures show output per dollar spent on each volunteer and are similar to productivity measures. Managers use statistics to show costs per volunteer, per consumer, per program, and per volunteer service hour. The intent of presenting this information in annual and monthly reports is to show the value of added service that contributes to reduced healthcare costs and increased consumer and staff effectiveness. Managers use 2,080 hours, or one worker year, and the salary ranges of equivalent professional positions to generate dollar value amounts contributed through volunteer service hours. Financial reports are shared with current supporters and prospective external funding sources to promote the department and to solicit future resources.

## Informal Volunteer and Staff Recognition

Recognition energizes the work environment by supporting and motivating staff and volunteers. Since it promotes the worth of volunteers and therapeutic recreation to the agency and community, recognition is also a form of public relations. Recognition and praise counter feelings of insecurity and inadequacy. And when consumers are unable to express appreciation, acknowledgment from staff is imperative.

Intrinsic recognition tied to performance motivates behavior. Therefore, informal recognition associated with task completion tends to enhance retention and recruitment. Since volunteers value peer recognition and acknowledgment of their competence so, a "thank you," a handshake, or a "stickie" note can heighten motivation. Informal meetings among volunteers, staff, and management facilitate recognition and feedback. During supervisory sessions the suggestion of an additional assignment or promotion to another work area rewards quality and encourages service continuation.

### Formal and Public Volunteer and Staff Recognition

Formal awards are based on performance criteria. Specific goals or service levels each with commensurate forms of recognition identify volunteer service hours, financial contributions, innovative programming, and resource acquisition. A comprehensive recognition program acknowledges quality as well as quantity so traits such as dependability and promptness as well as extraordinary hours of service are rewarded. To foster support for the program and to design meaningful equitable criteria, managers solicit volunteer and staff assistance to select tangible rewards and plan public ceremonies. Family members and caregivers are frequently willing to participate in recognition events.

Managers use documented work hours, projects completed, funds raised, number of newly recruited volunteers, innovative programming ideas, and suggestions resulting in time-saving service improvements as achievement indicators. The chosen form of recognition must be perceived as valuable by the recipient. For example, a senior citizen who works on the pediatric unit would enjoy a luncheon, while a news clipping in the local newspaper would be more relevant in recognizing a service club. The nature of the contribution being recognized influences the nature of the tangible reward. Thus, if documented service hours is the chosen criterion, the value of the reward increases as the hours escalate (e.g., pins are given for 500 hours while plaques are presented for 1,000 hours). When ideas result in service improvement (e.g., adapting equipment) the contributions warrant a write-up in the agency newsletter.

Managers recognize staff for their support of the volunteer program. Staff train, supervise, and recognize volunteers. Such tasks consume additional time and effort worthy of recognition. *Team efforts* are the result of staff facilitating cohesiveness among consumers, volunteers, and colleagues. Managers incorporate recognition of such contributions into job performance standards on volunteer supervision, documentation of supervisory experiences, released time for special training in volunteer management,

letters of commendation in personnel files, and public acknowledgment before agency administrators, volunteers, consumers, and caregivers. Informal staff recognition (e.g., interoffice phone call) creates a cooperative work environment and garners support of management.

## *Related Considerations*

A number of trends and issues affect volunteerism. Levels of volunteerism have been on the decline. Volunteerism is a component of service learning in high schools and colleges. As social inclusion continues, volunteer buddies, aides, escorts, and pals become more integral to accessing relevant experiences. Also, with healthcare focusing on community and caregiver intervention, volunteerism becomes an essential element of the support network in home healthcare, outpatient, and transitional services.

A number of issues arise from these economic, social, and healthcare trends. Youth under age 18 seek out volunteer opportunities as alternatives to inaccessible paying positions and as service learning projects. Identification of placements appropriate to the youth and clients is a manager's dilemma. For example, youth unaware of secondary outcomes of a disability like head injuries or strokes become uncomfortable with inappropriate client behaviors or statements yet are bored if assigned supportive tasks.

Quality control and cost containment evident in the healthcare industry along with social inclusion necessitate intensive volunteer training and higher levels of competence to assist during consumer transitions. Staff train volunteers as advocates, companions, and aides. This is time consuming since the process is ongoing and individualized to each consumer's needs. Managers, therefore, institute staff development programs to train entry-level staff as trainers so they "coach" volunteers to monitor individual client progress. The importance of devoting time to volunteer training is further complicated by a decline in number of available volunteers, reduced amount of consumer contact time with professional healthcare providers, and implementation of quality control standards.

The use of consumers as volunteers presents several issues. Consumers perceive that through volunteering they may secure a permanent position yet may not have the physical or emotional tolerance to work full time. Problems arise when former consumers perceive that they are capable of helping recently traumatized patients while still adapting to their own changed lifestyles. Adult athletes who sponsor and train youth wheelchair athletes are effective role models as are formalized support groups where consumers and caregivers in various stages of recovery mentor one another.

Volunteer supervision has become more complicated due to the increasing number of standards, regulations, laws, and work demands. Staff may not perceive the necessity of volunteer accountability so managers monitor records pertaining to safety and risk issues as well as financial and personnel outcomes. Firing a volunteer and holding staff accountable for volunteer-consumer interactions require time and attention to protocols and standards of practice. Staff may perceive that volunteers are available to be used in tasks they would prefer not to undertake and/or that volunteers are available to carry staff overloads. Managers articulate expectations while carefully discriminating between professional and volunteer roles and the importance of each task to operation of the department.

# Summary

The intent of this chapter was to provide an overview of volunteer management. Major tasks in this process were briefly presented. Planning encompasses the paperwork steps prior to actual operation of a volunteer program. Is a volunteer program an element of the strategic plan and department mission, and are resources available to support the program? Professional standards, agency needs, and regulatory criteria guide design of volunteer policies, job descriptions, and contracts. Recruitment and selection of the right volunteer for the right job are fundamental. Target audiences such as older adults, students, caregivers, youth, court-assigned volunteers, and consumers each bring to the volunteer experience certain needs and anticipated outcomes that are matched with department goals.

Training and education begin with volunteer placements. Usually an orientation period introduces volunteers to the overall agency and department operation and its significance to services and outcomes. Orientation in therapeutic recreation includes responsibilities of volunteers within the unit and information about the focus and intent of the department within the setting. In-services prepare volunteers to complete daily assignments properly while educational sessions expose them to professional practices and issues. Supervision ensures compliance and performance of job expectations and a partnership among staff, volunteers, and management that benefits consumers.

Through informal and formal supervisory contacts, managers make decisions about volunteer retention, promotion, reassignment, and termination. Evaluative data affirm compliance with contractual expectations and contributions to service quality. Collected information is used to recognize volunteers and staff and to inform agency publics of the value of their efforts to program enrichment and improvement. Statistics used in cost-effectiveness ratios quantify the value of volunteers. Productivity measures incorporate cost of volunteer operation per client, per program, and per hour as performance is assessed. Trends report document value of volunteer hours per worker year (e.g., 2,080 hours times hourly rate of a comparable position times number of volunteers equals dollar value of volunteers to department). Issues arise with volunteer management. Age and maturity of volunteers, amount of time devoted to training, presence of client volunteers, relationships among staff, volunteers, and consumers, and accountability measures are management considerations.

# Discussion Questions

1. Identify and explain the outcomes of each phase—organization, recruitment, and selection—of department preparation of a volunteer program.
2. Explain the essential orientation topics to be covered as volunteer placements are made.
3. What types of resources are needed in volunteer education and training programs?
4. Feedback and motivation are integral to volunteer supervision. Explain the manager's role with each.
5. What types or forms of documentation and evaluation should managers retain with volunteer programs?
6. What is the significance of recognition in volunteer management?
7. Explore how healthcare trends impact use of volunteers in therapeutic recreation.
8. Examine the pros and cons of client placement in volunteer roles.
9. Discuss the relationship of volunteer contributions to cost analysis and accountability (e.g., how should volunteer management costs and benefits be reflected in the budget)?

# Selected Resources

Council of Better Business Bureaus, Inc. (1994). *The responsibilities of a charity's volunteer board* (Publication No. 25–015, E250594). Arlington, VA: Author.

Henderson, K. (1990). The market value of volunteers. *Parks and Recreation, 25*:6, 60–62, 84–86.

Independent Sector. (1994). *Giving and volunteering in the United States* (CAT# P100). Washington, DC: Author.

Loughton, J. (1993). The fundamentals of cultivation and solicitation. *Parks and Recreation, 28:12,* 38–43.

Markwood, S. R. (1994). Volunteers in local government: Partners in service. *Public Management, 76:4,* 26–31.

Pomerance, G. (1994). The care and feeding of volunteers. *Parks and Recreation, 29*(11), 54–55.

Scott, J. T. (1996). Volunteers: How to get them, how to keep them, how to treat them (and why). . . . *Parks and Recreation, 31:11,* 50–53.

Tedrick, T., Davis, W. W., and Coutant, G. J. (1984). Effective management of a volunteer corp. *Parks and Recreation, 19:2,* 55–59.

Weston, R., Owen, M., McGuire, F., Backman, K., and Allen, J. (1993). The intergenerational entrepreneurship demonstration project: An innovative approach to intergenerational mentoring. *Journal of Physical Education, Recreation and Dance, 64:8,* 48–50.

# References

American Therapeutic Recreation Association (ATRA). (1993). *Standards for the practice of therapeutic recreation, self-assessment guide.* Hattiesburg, MS: Author.

Carter, M. J., Van Andel, G. E., and Robb, G. M. (1995). *Therapeutic recreation: A practical approach* (2nd ed.). Prospect Heights, IL: Waveland Press, Inc.

Henderson, K. (1988). Are volunteers worth their weight in gold? *Parks and Recreation, 23:11,* 40–43.

National Recreation and Park Association (NRPA). (1992). *Standards and evaluative criteria for baccalaureate programs in recreation, park resources and leisure services.* Arlington, VA: Author.

National Recreation and Park Association (NRPA). (1990). *Guidelines for the administration of therapeutic recreation services.* Alexandria, VA: Author.

Rossman, J. R. (1995). *Recreation programming, designing leisure experiences* (2nd ed.). Champaign, IL: Sagamore Publishing, Inc.

Tedrick, T., and Henderson, K. (1989). *Volunteers in leisure.* Reston, VA: American Alliance for Health, Physical Education, Recreation and Dance.

# Chapter 19
# Intern Management

## Introduction

For purposes of this publication, the authors have chosen to define the internship and fieldwork experiences as follows: an internship is a structured career-related full-time work experience (e.g., 32 hours or more per week) of one or more quarters or semesters in duration (e.g., 10–16 weeks) for which the student receives academic credit and which occurs following the completion of the majority of major coursework during the junior and senior years in an upper division institution. A fieldwork or practicum experience may precede the internship experience or be the title assigned to experiential learning in the two-year or lower division institution. This experience or series of experiences is usually less than full time (e.g., 32 hours per week), may be completed as major coursework is taken, may or may not be graded independently of coursework, and serves as a prerequisite to the culminating internship.

Internships and fieldwork require agency preparation and devotion of staff time, resources, and expertise. Watson (1992) notes that cost-benefit analyses suggest that costs are rarely fully recovered. Why then would a manager consider having interns? According to Feldman and Weitz (1990), college students are benefited by the intern experience in several ways: professional interests and values are affirmed, the transition from the academic setting to the work environment is made easier, and the opportunity to secure employment is enhanced. Further, managers have the opportunity to observe potential employees prior to writing recommendations, links to academic settings create avenues of information and resource exchange, and the department serves as a professional development site.

Tasks undertaken, documents developed, management policies and responsibilities, and issues faced prior to, during, and following student placements are similar to volunteer management activities. Four major types of activities are undertaken by the manager: preplacement preparation, orientation, supervision and training, and evaluation and termination. Preplacement planning encompasses tasks necessary to establish a relationship with university programs including the delineation of department, student, and academic responsibilities; the incorporation of internship policies and procedures into department documents; the dedication of personnel and resources to support student experiences; and the preparation of documents and agreements used in student selection and training. Orientation commences with initial student contact and recruitment and continues as the student becomes familiar with the agency, department, staff, and potential learning experiences.

While students assume increasing degrees of responsibility and autonomy, managers both provide supervision and conduct training to enhance the intern's ability to respond to the new demands. Formal written evaluations take place at midterm and termination periods with intermittent weekly or biweekly reports submitted through the manager to the academic supervisor. Throughout the placement, the manager mentors, advises, models, and challenges the student to acquire and demonstrate ethical behaviors. Performance is guided by personnel standards, professional practice standards, on-site protocols, and the student's personal professional philosophy. During the placement, and as the experience terminates, issues may arise that require resolution. To illustrate, the intern may observe differing management styles between the academic and site supervisors. As the student internship ends, managers address transitions to be made by staff, students, clients, and caregivers.

This chapter is organized according to the primary steps completed in preparation, orientation, supervision and training, and evaluation and termination of interns. The focus is on the for-credit undergraduate experience. Graduate students may, however, enroll in such a course to gain additional experience or satisfy credentialing criteria. Watson (1992) notes that those students who are closely supervised and receive academic credit tend to be more reliable and motivated, and the agency is legally protected from accusations of unfair labor practices. Campbell and Kovar (1994) suggest that successful internships provide the proper balance of academic and agency guidance and independence so students mature professionally.

# Preplacement Planning

Preplacement planning tasks organize the department to support internships, formalize relationships with academic institutions, and secure a pool of internship applicants. Internship preparation, therefore, involves a number of the following management tasks:

1. delineate specific internship goals and objectives;
2. establish policies and procedures;
3. prepare staff and resources to support interns;
4. develop training materials;
5. delineate department, academic, and intern responsibilities;
7. negotiate affiliation agreement;
8. develop selection procedures;
9. design application and screening process;
10. disseminate information and recruit potential interns; and
11. select and interview intern candidates.

With the completion of these steps, interns are under contract, academic institutions have committed to fulfill specific contractual obligations, and the manager and staff are prepared to involve interns in daily department operations.

## *Department Preparation*

An initial management task is to delineate within the department mission the nature of an internship program. The scope and outcomes of structured internships are articulated in goals and objectives that appear in agency operating documents, marketing materials, and internship manuals. Collectively, these statements present the internship

focus and substantiate contributions of the department to internship training. These documents establish the parameters for the management of the internship program. Subsequent management tasks are guided by these directives. Figure 19.1 notes the therapeutic recreation internship goals of a community-based special interest group.

Existing department policies and procedures are studied to determine whether the manager will work with existing statements or develop new statements to define pertinent intern protocols. Intern policies and procedures are prepared and placed in internship manuals, affiliation agreements, recruiting materials, department policy manuals, and informative brochures presented to interested students and faculty. Statements are developed to describe personal and professional expectations and the resources that will be made available to students during the internship. Figure 19.2 illustrates information for the student from an internship policy and procedures manual.

The manager involves department staff in internship preparation to encourage their commitment to internship training. Student policies and procedures are incorporated into staff training in anticipation of student arrival. Sessions devoted to intern management prepare practitioners for transitions they will undergo as student interns assume increasing degrees of autonomy and responsibility. Simulations and role-playing during staff training help staff visualize the significance of their roles, anticipate areas in which students might require assistance, and gain familiarity with procedures and forms used during the internship. The manager prepares staff guidelines that are shared with staff and placed in internship documents.

The value placed on internship training by the manager is reflected in the access to resources provided to the student during the internship. In order for the student intern to complete assignments and communicate with the department and academic supervisors, access to office space, computers, fax, e-mail, telephone, duplication services, and supplies is necessary. Access to professional and medical libraries on site or through practitioners also helps the student make connections between theory and practice. Visits and observations with area practitioners and settings permit the student to become aware of relationships, issues, and practice similarities and differences. Opportunities to network through professional meetings and seminars heighten student awareness of the significance of professional membership and continuing professional development.

Training materials including an internship manual and recruiting packages are prepared to guide the student as the internship is completed. Contents and materials are similar to volunteer materials and are guided by professional standards (NTRS, 1997). A manual contains materials used in planning, orienting, training, supervising, and evaluating students. Items from the manual are used to recruit

**Figure 19.1 Goals of Student Internship Program**

The following are the therapeutic recreation staff goals for students involved in the internship program:

1. Provide students with the opportunity to practice skills learned in the classroom.
2. Promote the expansion of knowledge gained in the academic setting.
3. Facilitate the student's refinement of interpersonal skills and development of work attitudes.
4. Provide feedback for on-the-job performance with the purpose of guiding the student towards improved effectiveness.
5. Encourage the development of self-evaluation and problem-solving skills.
6. Provide role models for clinical therapeutic recreation treatment.
7. Serve as a transition from the role of student to the role of Therapeutic Recreation Specialist.
8. Meet the fieldwork requirements of the NCTRC.
9. Prepare the student for an entry-level position in the field of therapeutic recreation.

Used by permission of The Rocky Mountain Multiple Sclerosis Center, Denver, CO.

**Figure 19.2 Student Intern Information and Guidelines**

1. **Meals** are available in the dining room. Students receive the same discount rate on meals as employees.
2. **Dress code** is casual and appropriate according to activities. Athletic shoes are permitted but must be white leather and clean. Exercise attire can only be worn for exercise or sport activities. No blue jeans are allowed. Keep in mind the hospital is a professional setting and you want to present yourself in a professional manner.
3. **Phone calls.** When answering the department phone identify the department and yourself. Department phones should mainly be used for business matters. Personal calls should be kept to a minimum and should not interfere with work responsibilities.
4. **Working hours**—minimum 40 hours per week, minimum 15 weeks. Schedule is determined by unit. Evenings and weekends may be involved.
5. **Breaks.** You are entitled to a 30-minute lunch or dinner. You are expected to be in the building during working hours. If you leave the building, let your supervisor know (and have approval). Your supervisor should be aware of your schedule.
6. **Documentation of hours.** You must document hours (time of arrival and departure) on your weekly schedule.
7. **Illness.** If you are ill and cannot report to work, notify your supervisor by 8:30 a.m. Any hours missed due to illness or other personal matters will have to be made up if they interfere with the number of hours needed for completion of internship.
8. **Holidays** are observed as follows: New Year's Day, Memorial Day, Independence Day, Labor Day, Thanksgiving Day (and the day after), and Christmas Day. You may be scheduled to work during a holiday weekend, but usually not on the day the holiday is actually observed.
9. **Educational materials.** Books, videos, etc., belonging to the Recreation Therapy Department or Medical Library are available to students but must be signed out and returned.
10. **Housing.** Students are responsible for living arrangements. The Student Coordinator can be contacted for possible resources.
11. **Parking.** Do not park in the visitor parking areas. Please refer to the parking memo.
12. **Smoking.** This hospital is a smoke-free hospital. No smoking is allowed within the hospital or on the hospital campus. An outdoor smoking area for patients is located on the West End.
13. **Name tags.** You will be provided with a name tag. You will be expected to wear this during working hours.

Used by permission of Recreation Therapy Department, Chelsea Community Hospital, Chelsea, MI.

students. Managers organize packets to send to academic institutions that invite applications and specify how to develop relationships between the department and academic program. Documents sent might include application forms, job descriptions, agreement forms, and housing contracts (see Appendix D). The contents likely to be found in a internship manual are listed in Figure 19.3.

## Department and Academic Relationships

The internship experience is a triad relationship among students, departments, and academic programs. Introductory materials help define the expectations of each entity in detail. These expectations are further defined in a memorandum of agreement (MOA) between agency and academic programs (see Appendix D) and in contracts between the student and the department. Professional standards (NCTRC, 1994; NTRS, 1997) also provide directives helpful in developing relational documents. The supervisor of the internship should be qualified as a certified therapeutic recreation specialist (CTRS) with at least two years of professional experience and should ensure a highly structured experience that encompasses the practice as defined by the National Council for Therapeutic Recreation Certification (NCTRC) job analysis, professional standards of practice (ATRA, 1993; NTRS, 1994) and other external regulatory agents (Commission on Accreditation of Rehabilitation Facilities [CARF], Joint Commission on Accreditation of Healthcare Organizations [JCAHO]). The length of the internship experience and the number of required hours ranges from 20 hours per week for 18 weeks to 40 hours for a ten to 16 week quarter or semester. A minimum of 360 clock hours to a maximum of 600 clock hours is recommended.

Students, departments, and academic programs enter into agreements after confirming each is able to satisfy the other's expectations. To illustrate, managers may wish to only accept students who have majors in therapeutic recreation, attend Council on Accreditation (COA) therapeutic recreation accredited programs, and/or are supervised by an educator who holds the CTRS credential. Academic institutions may desire placements with agencies where at least two CTRSs are employed or where exposure to a variety of client populations rather than one particular clientele is guaranteed. Agreements specify who is responsible for purchase of liability insurance and who completes specific supervisory tasks. MOAs are usually in effect for a definitive time period or until one party dissolves the relationship. As agreements require legal development and review, it is not unusual that three or more months of lead time is required to consummate a relationship.

## Intern Selection Procedures

Intern selection processes are similar to the procedures used to hire employees. Selection processes require resume submission, on-site or phone interviews, verification of academic coursework, and proof of liability and health insurance. More detailed procedures require:

- transcript and copies of certification documents;
- recommendation letters;
- prerequisite experience in similar setting and/or with similar clientele;
- specific coursework (e.g., clinical psychology);
- maintenance of a specific grade point average (GPA) in therapeutic recreation classes;
- completion of all therapeutic recreation classes;
- application form and self-assessment profile;
- philosophical statement and career goals; and
- selection after department interview and university approval.

---

## Figure 19.3 Content Outline of an Internship Manual

1. Agency Overview
   - Vision, mission, goals, objectives
   - Organization, operational information
   - Clientele and service scope

2. Department Service
   - Vision, mission, goals, objectives
   - Organization and staffing
   - Services, scope of care, standards

3. Internship Program
   - Affiliation policy and agreement

- Responsibilities of department, student, academic program
- Procedures for selection and placement
- Goals, objectives, prerequisite competencies
- Department policies, personal guidelines
- Job description
- Application procedures
- Schedule and weekly expectations
- Learning outcomes and assignments
- Supervisor profile
- Personnel and evaluation forms
- References and resource materials

Managers base selection decisions on a first-come, first-served basis; preference may be given to students from academic programs with presigned agreements. Selection may also be based on the quality of each applicant. Submission of materials by specified deadlines also determines who is given further consideration. Agency-wide preset starting dates (e.g., June 1, September 1, and January 15) can also be used by the manager to select students available at these rotation intervals.

After the selection criteria are determined, a process is developed to receive and evaluate application forms and supportive student documents. This process is affected by a number of variables: size of the department, presence of an agency-wide clinical coordinator, supervisory assignments from semester to semester, existence or nonexistence of an agency-wide intern program, and the number of on-site student rotations available per semester (e.g., aquatic, outpatient, substance abuse). These variables also influence who is involved in actual intern selection and how and when selection takes place. A formal rating system that collapses a large amount of subjective information into quantitative terms may be used to assess the quality of the prospective student's application, and/or the decision may be made by the manager with input from staff that are assigned to supervise interns. Selection criteria consider the "goodness of fit" between student and department.

A pool of applicants can be recruited by personal contacts, participation on academic advisory committees, class presentations, mailing of materials to campus career centers, and through professional contacts. During professional meetings department information is displayed and distributed. Managers who serve on boards or make presentations have captive audiences with whom to share internship opportunities. Mailings to persons on professional membership lists access students. Academic programs host job and internship fairs, and alumni and agency placement days. Agency video or media presentations are used in introductory and seminar classes to inform students of intern options.

Managers may elect to screen prospective applicants with interviews granted to a select number of students. Managers may require on-site interviews or use alternatives like teleconferences, videotaped or written responses to questions, and/or phone interviews. These experiences are similar to hiring staff and placing volunteers. Interview questions emphasize the student's career goals and specific needs that might be served by a particular internship.

Interviews determine the "goodness of fit." Students may discover in an interview that they are not interested in a particular type of setting, or managers may ascertain that the student's goals would be suited to placement with clientele other than those served by the department. Interview outcomes are reported to the student as well as to the academic advisor in writing so that appropriate corrective action and/or follow-up can be taken. When a student is accepted, managers request return of an acceptance letter within a definitive time period. This is then followed by mailing of orientation materials including an internship manual. This begins to prepare the student for the department orientation.

# Department Orientation

Volunteer and intern orientations are similar. The structure of the internship experience is planned during the orientation. Student supervision, work schedules, assignments, evaluations, and communication protocols are arranged, and responsibilities and department-academic expectations are clarified. At this time, a student-department contract is formalized with clearly stated objectives, due dates, and tasks. Primary orientation activities include:

1. introduction to agency and department,
2. identification of training needs and expectations,
3. review of supervisory and evaluation processes and procedures, and
4. student-department contract negotiation.

## *Introduction to Agency and Department*

Topics like those under volunteer training and supervision are incorporated into an intern orientation. When a site is a clinical training site for a number of disciplines, a general agency orientation may occur independently of the department orientation. Regardless, the orientation period ranges from a few days to a few weeks (i.e., one or two). Informal orientation continues as the manager meets routinely with the intern. An orientation checklist (see Figure 19.4, page 282), helps the student organize information and resources accumulated during the experience.

Contents of the internship manual are reviewed and used to familiarize the student with the agency and department, and to help the student become comfortable with the supervisor's management style. When objectives are outlined in the manual, students and supervisors review the evaluative criteria so that students can anticipate internship outcomes. Visits to other sites and discussions with peer professionals during the orientation help the student become familiar with healthcare and human services and the role of therapeutic recreation across disciplines. When several services comprise a department, students rotate among the areas prior to actual placement with particular services. Academic expectations, assignments and forms are considered. Decisions are made as to which forms and assignments will be required. Recommendations from these discussions help the student focus on particular NCTRC job tasks, professional practice standards, and personal goals and needs.

---

**Figure 19.4 Orientation Checklist**

**The Rocky Mountain Multiple Sclerosis (MS) Center
Adult Day Enrichment Program**

| To be completed by the end of Week #1 | Check Off | Intern Orientation Checklist |
|---|---|---|
| | _____ | Tour of Facility |
| | _____ | Parking |
| | _____ | Securing Building |
| | _____ | Keys |
| | _____ | Employee Manual |
| | _____ | Policy and Procedure Manual |
| | _____ | Client Charts |
| | _____ | Meet with Director |
| | _____ | Meet with Adult Day Enrichment Program Staff |
| | _____ | Review of Clients |
| | _____ | Staff Meeting Schedules |
| | _____ | Program Brochure/Multiple Sclerosis Community Resources Information |
| | _____ | Communication Procedures |
| | _____ | "Typical Day" |
| | _____ | Introduction to Participants |
| | _____ | Lunch |
| | _____ | Job Descriptions of Adult Day Enrichment Program Staff |
| | _____ | Participant Rights/Application Process |
| | _____ | Office Supplies |
| | _____ | Phone System/Answering/Staff Lines |
| | _____ | Library/Multiple Sclerosis Community Resources |
| | _____ | Master File |
| Week #2 | _____ | Documentation Requirements |
| | _____ | Orient to Multiple Sclerosis Center |
| | _____ | Transferring |
| | _____ | Swallowing Protocol |
| | _____ | Time Sheets |
| | _____ | Mileage Reimbursement |
| | _____ | Petty Cash |
| | _____ | Emergency Protocols |
| | _____ | Other Events out of Adult Day Enrichment Program |
| Week #3 | _____ | Multiple Sclerosis Video |
| Week #4 | _____ | Participant Advisory Council |
| Week #5 | _____ | Budget |

Used by permission of the Rocky Mountain Multiple Sclerosis Center, Denver, CO.

---

## *Identification of Training Needs and Expectations*

Managers expose students to the full range of division or department services and alternative placement assignments in order to acquaint the student with the day-to-day expectations and potential internship outcomes. This may entail brief time periods devoted to each service, clientele group, and staff role, or more extended rotations after which the student is either assigned to rotate among particular staff and service areas or the student selects a specific area where the majority of the experience will occur. During introductory rotations the manager identifies potential roles and contributions that are likely to be made by the intern. Simultaneously, the academic supervisor and student review assignments (e.g., assessment, documentation, program and treatment planning) to discern which are most compatible with the intern's anticipated goals. Together the manager, student, and academic supervisor determine specific training needs and outcomes beneficial to the department and intern.

A schedule of rotations, job tasks, and learning assignments is prepared. Student expectations are defined by goals and objectives that specify a sequence of tasks to be completed as the intern assumes increasing levels of responsibility and autonomy. Specific due dates, assignments, and projects compatible with job tasks are defined. These are often organized in weekly increments. Interns are required to organize increasingly more hours daily as they perform higher order job tasks with equally high levels of effectiveness and less direct supervision.

## *Review of Supervisory and Evaluation Process and Procedures*

Managers, interns, and academic supervisors review criteria and forms to be used during supervisory contacts and performance reviews as the sequence of intern events is planned. Midterm and final evaluation forms and project evaluation forms are found in department and academic internship manuals. Additionally, student-generated documents like journals, logs, and weekly reports are tools used to assess intern progress and growth toward anticipated personal and professional goals. The nature and procedures for using these indicators help the manager plan feedback and debriefing processes.

Department supervision is influenced by a number of variables. Distance between the academic program and placement site affects the frequency and nature of contact between supervisors. To illustrate, internships completed more than a few hundred miles from the academic program necessitate phone, fax and/or e-mail contacts rather than in person exchanges. Staff-intern assignments determine whether or not the manager devotes time to student supervision or the manager supports staff in their supervision of students. When the manager is the only department staff person, time permits two or three formal reviews at designated times with casual observations during routine service provision. If interns rotate among staff or services, several supervisors provide input to the manager. Size and location of the service influences how frequently managers are able to complete casual observations and make informal contacts with the intern (e.g., with outreach services or community-based services that cover extended geographic areas fewer contacts are likely as compared to services in one facility).

As the manager and student review performance criteria, they establish a mutually beneficial communication process. Success of intern management, like volunteer management, is somewhat dependent on how effective the manager is in motivating, interpreting, and clarifying. Managers help the student apply knowledge to practice and to realize the impact of personal behaviors on therapeutic relationships. They have the arduous task of helping the student assimilate the impact of the "self" on therapeutic outcomes. Each must feel comfortable in approaching the other, giving and receiving constructive criticism, resolv-

ing interpersonal and professional conflicts, and respecting the other's competence and professional integrity. Awareness of alternative management styles is a benefit of the internship experience.

## *Negotiate Student-Department Contract*

Throughout the orientation period, managers, students, and academic supervisors work together to clarify and delineate internship assignments and learning experiences. Once finalized, they are organized on a document signed by the manager and intern and submitted to the academic supervisor with initial weekly reports. As shown in Figure 19.5 (page 284) this document contains the intern's goals and objectives, due dates, projects, learning activities, and special notations. The contract also specifies the dates upon which interns are to submit reports to the manager and academic supervisors. It is desirable for the student first to submit materials to the manager and respond to feedback before sending reports to the academic supervisor. This allows the academic supervisor to benefit from the manager's input and perspectives. Contract items are renegotiated when the manager detects that an intern's progress and task completion justify alterations. Adjustments are reported to the academic supervisor in revised weekly reports.

# Supervision and Training

Throughout an internship, managers monitor and model professional competencies, personal skills, and performance desired of interns. Training is planned to enhance the intern's skills and to permit the intern to share expertise brought to the placement. Volunteer and intern supervision and training are similar and entail three major tasks:

1. communication with and observation of the intern,
2. documentation of intern activities and experiences, and
3. provision of training and education opportunities.

With supervision and training, the professional growth of the intern is promoted, and entry-level practice competencies are reinforced. Managers also ensure that the intern is operating within department policies while contributing to its outcomes.

## *Communication and Observation*

Formal communication processes are identified when the student and manager negotiate the contract. Projects and reports guide the nature and timing of a manager's observations. Thus, prior to the due date, managers plan conferences and observations to ensure interns have completed tasks and are reporting factual, accurate information according to protocol. A weekly time period dedicated to

## Figure 19.5  Student-Agency Contract

**Student-Agency Agreement Form**

This agency is accepting the following student as an internship student as defined by the below listed specifications:

Name of Student _____

Starting Date _____ Terminating Date _____

Type of Insurance Coverage Provided _____
Wages, stipend, housing, meals, or other compensation the student may receive:

_____

_____

The policies and procedures governing this internship are delineated in the student manual, division handbook, the identified agency documents, and Ashland University MOA.

Assignment Completion
  1.  Research/Evaluation Project/Presentation Dates

      Agency _____ Ashland _____
  2.  Portfolio Dates

      Agency _____ Ashland _____
  3.  Readings/Resource File Dates

      Agency _____ Ashland _____
  4.  Weekly Reports/Experience Form

      (Due to Ashland by)        1. _____        8. _____

                                 2. _____        9. _____

                                 3. _____       10. _____

                                 4. _____       11. _____

                                 5. _____       12. _____

                                 6. _____       13. _____

                                 7. _____       14. _____

  5.  Evaluations

      Midterm on-campus meeting date          _____

      Final on-campus meeting date            _____

      Supervisor midterm evaluation           _____

      Supervisor final evaluation             _____

      Student Ashland curriculum evaluation date   _____

Used by permission of Ashland University, Ashland, OH.

**Figure 19.5 Continued**

Student Internship Goals
　　List five to seven as agreed to by yourself and your supervisor(s):

1.

2.

3.

4.

5.

6.

7.

Agency Assignments/Requirements
　　List specific projects or assigned tasks as determined by yourself and your supervisor, including agency due dates.

_____

Agency                                      Representative

_____

Date                                        Title

_____

Student                                     Date

---

discussion and review of the preceding week's events helps track progress and alerts the manager to impending issues and challenges.

Informal observations and contact occur throughout an internship. Managers focus on the quality with which the intern performs duties delineated in the job description and the internship objectives. Midterm and/or final evaluation forms are useful as guides for debriefing sessions and recommending corrective actions. When the intern keeps a log or diary, the manager is able to gain additional insight into his or her personal needs and perceptions. The manager draws student attention to qualities and performances that enhance or detract from the department's mission and the student's ability to perform interventions through helping relationships.

Communication between the manager and academic supervisor occurs as the student is supervised. Preset phone calls permit three-way conversations, and correspondence by fax and e-mail expedite contacts. Managers who choose to send written comments with intern reports are creating avenues for three-way communication. Intern progress is reported and suggestions on curriculum needs and resources are shared. Academic supervisors, in turn, confirm student preparation experiences and prior clinical training. Each supervisor is made more aware of what facets of professional practice and personal development are perceived as significant.

## Documentation of Activities and Experiences

The managers guide the interns as documentation skills are acquired and practiced. They also assist the students in setting aside time to complete department and academic projects. And, managers help the interns process issues and concerns resulting from their daily experiences. The type and amount of previous clinical experience may influence the interns' ability to document internship occurrences. Managers direct students to subtle cues and clinical manifestations that corroborate clinical decisions. When managers review intern reports that are to be submitted to the academic program, they make recommendations that help the interns clarify their actions. Managers also help interns organize their time to accomplish required written experiences. Last, managers encourage interns to complete self-assessments and analyze their personal diaries to gain insight into real and perceived problems or successes. In each situation, the desire is to enhance the interns' ability to document the effectiveness of therapeutic recreation interventions and helping relationships.

Managers document intern activities in several ways. First, they review academic assignments and agency projects to provide informal feedback. Second, they use periodic formal evaluations like the midterm and final exam to present written critiques. Third, managers review interns' actual documentation on services as they cosign reports. And, finally, they retain personnel files on each intern in which they document performances similar to those kept with personnel performance plans. The information accumulated from these sources helps the manager judge intern progress and take corrective actions. For instance, managers may require additional training, recommend alternative placements, or encourage adjustment in time spent in the department or on assigned tasks.

## Provision of Training and Education Opportunities

As managers prepare for the arrival of interns, they organize department resources useful to the advancement of the intern's education. Through the orientation experience and follow-up supervision, the manager ascertains the nature of the intern's training needs as well as the resources brought to the department by the intern. Interns have a need to acquire knowledge and apply skills in day-to-day operations as well as to gain insight into current professional issues and agendas.

In-services conducted by staff make interns aware of policies and operating protocols. Attendance at area professional meetings helps students build networks and become aware of the professional scope of service. Intern led in-services bring new theories and resources to department staff. Intern completion of a project that is incorporated into ongoing services also is mutually beneficial because interns and staff gain resources and contacts as the project is developed, implemented, and evaluated. Visits to other departments and interviews with colleagues in the agency and community facilitate intern application of academic knowledge and awareness of professional expectations and issues.

# Evaluation and Termination

Formative and summative evaluations occur routinely during and at the termination of the internship experience. They involve each of the three parties' (e.g., student, manager, academic supervisor) assessments of each other's contributions and needs. As the internship nears completion, a number of factors are considered. The manager makes decisions on how transitions will occur so minimal service disruption results. The intern brings closure to a significant life phase and anticipates transition into the career world. Major challenges and issues arise. Evaluation and termination of an internship involves:

1. formative evaluations,
2. summative evaluations, and
3. termination tasks and issues.

## Formative Evaluations

Throughout the internship, students, managers, and academic supervisors evaluate interrelationships and processes to ensure growth and development of the intern. According to Lamb, Cochran, and Jackson (1991), focus of student evaluation is on knowledge and application of professional standards, competency, and personal functioning. Department evaluation considers the manager's effectiveness to supervise and communicate with the academic supervisor and intern, the adequacy of department resources to support the internship, and the managerial compatibility with the intern's needs and goals. The academic program is assessed by considering the adequacy of student preparation, management of the internship, intern supervision, and department relations. During the orientation, the procedures and criteria to assess each of these areas are mutually agreed upon.

As noted by Lamb, Cochran, and Jackson (1991), timely and early feedback enables the manager and intern to address anxiety issues, to identify areas of concern, and to articulate specific training recommendations. Formative evaluation commences with initial supervisory sessions and continues as the manager reviews reports, monitors performance, and submits comments to the academic supervisor. Assessments consider how well the student integrates into the department and is able to apply knowledge to practice. The intern's ability to work with other staff and to follow operating codes is closely monitored. Skill deficits are noted so remediation strategies are incorporated into the internship.

Formative evaluation tools are intern reports, midterm written evaluations, and contacts between the manager and academic supervisor. If the internship is planned around a sequence of increasingly more difficult or autonomous responsibilities, evaluation focuses on the student's competence and willingness to assume these tasks and obligations and perform effectively. Managers document performance adequacy and recommend training needs. If there is impairment in the intern's performance other than what can be corrected by training, the manager, intern, and academic supervisor agree on appropriate alternatives, which could include reassignment or immediate withdrawal from the placement.

## Summative Evaluations

Summative evaluation occurs near the completion of the internship period. Managers complete forms that critique the student's personal and professional competence, the academic preparation and supervision of the student, and interactions with the academic supervisor. Students assess the adequacy of their preparation and the department to support the internship as well as their interactions and compatibility with both supervisors. Academic supervisors consider appropriateness of the manager's supervision and the department's support, compatibility of practice with standards purported in academic experiences, and the student's ability to synthesize theory and practice.

At the completion of an internship, the student has been given the opportunity to demonstrate entry-level practice standards as defined by NCTRC, the American Therapeutic Recreation Association (ATRA) and the National Therapeutic Recreation Society (NTRS). Managers use the standards documents of these organizations as measurements of the intern's potential to perform successfully as an entry-level practitioner. The manager also considers how well the intern integrates professional standards into his or her repertoire of professional behaviors. Additionally, the manager assesses the degree to which the intern has been able to respond positively to feedback. Comparison of midterm with final ratings reveals whether corrective action and training have resulted in progress and behavior change.

Summative evaluation considers changes and growth in the intern's personal functioning. How well did the student respond to supervision, manage stress and time, and work with and for other staff? What was the intern's comfort level with clients of diverse lifestyles? What was the intern's responsiveness to unexpected client behaviors? Did performance anxiety interfere with helping relationships? Are there mannerisms or behaviors that discourage active team participation? A number of personal qualities are essential to effective practice. The internship is the first opportunity to ascertain how well personal attributes, values, and attitudes intertwine with professional roles. The internship connects the theoretical with the practical. Transition between the two is enhanced by discussion of the exchanges between personal and professional roles and qualities.

## Termination Tasks and Issues

The internship brings closure to academic preparation while serving as the transition step into a professional role. Managers transition back into responsibilities partially or completely assumed by the intern. As the student separates from consumer, staff, and department contacts, managers provide emotional support. Procedures are instituted to integrate the intern's project into department services.

Before the completion date nears, planning the next professional step has begun. Managers expose interns to future opportunities through various professional contacts and meetings. Managers coach the intern on job search strategies and interview techniques.

A number of issues surface as transitions are made. The intern reflects on interactions with consumers and supervisors and their readiness to assume professional challenges. As the intern terminates helping relationships, issues of confidentiality and client autonomy arise. Consumer dependency behaviors may trigger the student's desire to share personal information and maintain contact after the internship. Although absolute confidentiality may not be attainable, relative consumer and department confidentiality are necessary and supported as the manager communicates to the intern permissible forms of follow-up.

The internship experience may be the first opportunity to compare personal management styles. Did intern experiences reflect academic underpinnings? Were communiqués from the supervisors to the intern relevant? Was feedback useful and focused on the intern's needs? An unusual internship would be one void of conflict. The manager's task is to help the intern learn to disagree without resentment. The manager and academic supervisor each have expectations. Issues arise when they are not compatible or vary in their level of expectancy. Managers and academic supervisors help the intern gauge the degree of autonomy achieved during an internship and their readiness to undertake future professional challenges.

Evaluations help the academic and department supervisor prepare for future interns. Managers cognizant of intern's perceptions about department acceptance, degree of assistance, quality of learning opportunities, and accomplishment of internship goals are able to make adjustments before the next interns arrive. More important, if the intern reports feelings of token acceptance or difficulty in approaching personnel or accessing resources, managers take immediate action as the intern's judgments are likely to be apparent with other department staff. The manager and academic supervisor guide the intern to experiences that resolve present issues while fostering future life and career successes. Interns are directed to alternative employment settings or clientele groups or asked to reconsider their chosen career field. Readministration of self-assessments facilitates rethinking of life and career goals and directions.

# Summary

Contents of this chapter have been divided into four sections descriptive of the steps undertaken as managers design, implement, and evaluate internship programs. A major portion of the time devoted to intern management actually occurs during the initial step or preplacement planning. Division or department preparation involves determining the intent and nature of the intern program within the unit and preparing the staff and resources necessary to support student placements. This step is followed by, or occurs as, cooperative relationships between the department and academic setting are affected which may involve negotiating MOAs. With legal documents in place, intern selection commences. These procedures are similar to employment processes and serve as a first step in the student's transition from academics to the work world.

The second step, department orientation, introduces the intern to agency operations and/or department services. Supervision and training are actually begun during orientation periods. Managers detail their expectations and clarify student assignments and academic requirements. The feedback loop begins as the manager and intern negotiate a student contract that structures the intern's weekly activities.

During supervision and training, step three of intern management, managers guide student acquisition of job-related knowledge and skills and professional competence and functioning. Through ongoing communication and observations, managers discern progress so that increasing degrees of autonomy are given to the intern. Through documentation and personal contacts, managers share constructive criticism and corrective actions with interns and academic supervisors. Training facilitates increased exposure to application of academic knowledge and helps the intern become aware of current practices.

Finally, evaluation and transition prepare the intern to bring closure to the academic experience while moving into a new life stage. Evaluation processes begin during orientation and continue throughout the experience. Formative evaluation occurs as the manager reviews intern reports and projects routinely submitted to the academic supervisor. Summative evaluations generate information on the intern's knowledge and application of professional standards, entry-level competence, and personal functioning.

Issues arise during the internship. Managers encourage conflict resolution and development of problem-solving skills. Yet, interns experience real-world dilemmas such as client confidentiality, supervisor approachability, and relevancy of academic preparation to practice. Clinical experiences initiated early in the academic program permit the student to apply knowledge and skills to practice while acquiring professional skills supportive of transition into a career.

# Discussion Questions

1. What are the major tasks completed by a manager as the site is prepared to serve as a training site?
2. What activities occur during the orientation that are critical to the outcomes of the intern's entire experience?
3. Discuss the significance of supervisory feedback as it relates to the intern's training needs and the academic and department expectations.
4. Discuss techniques that the manager and academic supervisor use to support increasing degrees of intern work autonomy and progress toward the application of knowledge to practice.
5. What types of formative and summative evaluation tools are used to assess intern performance and how do these tools measure the critical outcomes of an internship experience?
6. Consider the issues that might arise as an intern prepares to bring closure to the internship experience. Discuss how they might impact the intern's professional and personal goals.

# References

American Therapeutic Recreation Association (ATRA). (1993). *Standards for the practice of therapeutic recreation, self-assessment guide.* Hattiesburg, MS: Author.

Campbell, K., and Kovar, S. K. (1994). Fitness/exercise science internships: How to ensure success. *Journal of Physical Education, Recreation and Dance, 65:2,* 69–72.

Feldman, D. C., and Weitz, B. A. (1990). Summer interns: Factors contributing to positive developmental experiences. *Journal of Vocational Behavior, 37:3,* 267–284.

Lamb, D. H., Cochran, D. J., and Jackson, V. R. (1991). Training and organizational issues associated with identifying and responding to intern impairment. *Professional Psychology: Research and Practice, 22:4,* 291–296.

National Council for Therapeutic Recreation Certification (NCTRC). (1994). *Field placement information sheet.* Thiells, NY: Author.

National Therapeutic Recreation Society (NTRS). (1997). *NTRS internship standards and guidelines for therapeutic recreation.* Alexandria, VA: National Recreation and Park Association.

National Therapeutic Recreation Society (NTRS). (1994). *Standards of practice for therapeutic recreation services and annotated bibliography.* Arlington, VA: National Recreation and Park Association.

Watson, K. W. (1992). An integration of values: Teaching the internship course in a liberal arts environment. *Communication Education, 41:4,* 429–439.

# Part 5

# Consumer Management

# Chapter 20

# Service Delivery Management

## Introduction

The therapeutic recreation manager is responsible for delivering quality service to the consumer. This service is based on one's knowledge and professional standards and, in some settings, regulatory standards. However, there are also other perceptions of quality that must be managed and achieved.

There are a variety of customers in varied settings and organizations (e.g., clinical and community-based leisure agencies, Joint Commission on Accreditation of Healthcare Organizations [JCAHO], Commission on Accreditation of Rehabilitation Facilities [CARF], Medicare) who define quality differently from the therapeutic recreation manager. If their definition of quality is not met, and their perception of quality is not achieved, they will think that quality service does not exist. Health and human service organizations cannot tolerate much variability in quality service. The room for error in quality has become narrow, and it affects in many instances financial outcomes and public outcry.

This chapter considers specific factors associated with improving the quality of service delivery provided by the practitioner within healthcare facilities and community-based leisure service agencies. Quality work gets done when practitioners are encouraged to develop their strengths and abilities. This approach addresses both the need to accomplish the task at hand and the need to make an investment in the practitioner so that future work activities can be accomplished more efficiently and effectively.

Initially considered is scheduling. Assigning, staffing, and scheduling are the ways in which goals of the therapeutic recreation department are converted into concrete acts.

The next consideration is the therapeutic recreation process, a systematic approach to meeting consumer and group needs through recreative and leisure experiences. While there exists a number of therapeutic recreation service models identified as the National Therapeutic Recreation Society (NTRS) leisurability model (NTRS, 1982) initially developed by Gunn and Peterson (1978), the helping model (Carter, Van Andel, and Robb, 1985), and the outcome model (Carter, Van Andel, and Robb, 1995) all contain some form of the following steps: assessment, planning, implementation, and evaluation. Although these steps are discussed in detail in other texts, the concern here is to summarize briefly the salient characteristics of the steps or process because all managers need to be acutely aware of the steps to meet consumer and group needs and the knowledge and abilities needed by the practitioner to carry out the process and assure quality. In addition, brief consideration is given to protocols. Protocols assist the therapeutic recreation process. They are procedures or courses of action to be taken in specific situations.

Another responsibility of the manager in association with the therapeutic recreation process is documentation. The manager has a responsibility to ensure proper documentation, its appropriateness and correctness. Documentation is also linked to risk management programs.

293

Last, consideration is given to monitoring and reviewing practitioner performance relative to program effectiveness in order to meet organizational goals including those of the division or department. Discussion of this responsibility is not focused on the traditional annual performance evaluation of the practitioner as was discussed in an earlier chapter, but rather on the day-to-day performance of the practitioner and the interaction that takes place between the practitioner and manager or supervisor to improve job performance. It is a joint process meant to encourage frequent and open discussions of job-related issues and problems.

# Scheduling

Scheduling is developing a plan for where and when personnel are to work within the parameters dictated by the organization. It is one of the manager's most frustrating and least fulfilling responsibilities. The therapeutic recreation manager is usually responsible for developing the schedule since he or she is aware of consumer needs as well as the expertise, limitations, and personal needs of the staff. The chief goal is balance. Therapeutic recreation managers, when possible, involve staff in decisions regarding the staffing plan and thereby obtain their commitment to the results. In this way, plans become more individualized, promoting staff satisfaction and productivity. However, assigning program activities and consumer cases by matching work to be done with the experience of the practitioner can lead to more effective and efficient service delivery. Heavy work loads may necessitate the setting of priorities among various program activities and cases. Regardless of the assignments given to a practitioner, assignments must be allotted reasonable time to produce results. In healthcare facilities this may be difficult given the length of stay as dictated by insurance.

In the community setting the scope of service, consumer disabilities, resources, educational or experiential levels of staff and their availability affect scheduling. Factors which complicate scheduling within varied healthcare facilities might be types of consumers, consumer expectations, fluctuations in admissions, length of hospitalization, referrals, physicians' orders, nursing procedures, and services provided by other departments. In schedule planning, consideration must also be given to demands of staff that are not related directly to consumer service. In-service programs, staff meetings, charting, attending conferences, and getting supplies and equipment together are all necessary, but they take time away from the consumer.

Therapeutic recreation practitioners are associated with organizations that use the traditional eight-hour workday as the basis for scheduling; however, it is not unusual for practitioners, regardless of setting, to work some evenings, weekends, and holidays. In fact, it's more the rule than the exception. The seven-day week was created to confound managers. At least this is true in a society in which five-day work weeks predominate.

Unfortunately there is no therapeutic recreation scheduling model to follow regardless of setting although one might want to consider various nursing scheduling models if the staff is large (e.g., block scheduling, cyclical scheduling, computerized scheduling [D. O'Morrow-Snyder, personal communication, May 16, 1995]). Seasonally "starting from scratch" for many community-based programs and when admitted to the healthcare facility or referred to it, the therapeutic recreation manager develops the schedule taking into consideration quality and staff skills. The major advantage of this approach is its flexibility. Since the process or admission and referral is begun from scratch, any changes in the procedure can be worked into the new schedule. The disadvantage of this might be that staff skills and quality are uneven and costly.

## Goals of Scheduling

Regardless of the problems associated with scheduling, goals of scheduling can be summarized as follows:

1. achievement of department objectives, especially those related to consumer service;
2. accurate match of department needs with staff and volunteer abilities and numbers;
3. maximum use of manpower;
4. equity of treatment to all employees (or equal treatment for all employees within a similar job classification) and volunteers;
5. optimization on use of professional expertise;
6. satisfaction of practitioners (both as to hours worked and as to perceived sense of scheduling equity) and volunteers; and
7. consideration of unique needs of staff and volunteers as well as consumers.

## Scheduling Problems

In addition to the schedule problems noted above, there are several more: management of full-time versus part-time employees; creation of policies that control abuse of sick time; legal and administrative constraints on scheduling; and irregular hour scheduling practices.

Because of rapid turnover and retrenchment to accommodate the cost of services today, many health and human service organizations combine full-time and part-time practitioners in a therapeutic recreation department. While part-time practitioners may be qualified, there are usually problems or disadvantages in hiring them. These problems may consist of inequity in salary and benefits wherein the part-timer may feel inequitably treated. Use of part-time practitioners may pose a threat to continuity of service. It is also thought that part-time employees lack the commitment to the organization and consumer that is found with the permanent employees. In addition, part-time employees are usually involved in in-service training or ongoing education programs. Last, full-time practitioners may be shown some form of favoritism regarding work time scheduling for example.

While there is no universal solution to these problems, the manager, in cooperation with higher management, may be able to develop a benefit package that would be equitable for both full-time and part-time practitioners. Equity may involve pay or benefits in compensation for preferential hours. Full-timers may be more understanding of some favoritism in hours extended to a part-timer if they know that they have some recompensing factor, such as vacation prorated at a higher level, a higher pay scale, or some other benefit that compensates and equalizes the situation.

Abuse of sick time is another factor that can ruin a well-planned schedule. Some practitioners perceive sick time as time that is owed to them. They use sick days whether or not they are ill. Such practices can be curtailed by good personnel policies concerning chronic absences. Some organizations give back a proportion of unused sick days as extra days off. Other organizations allow the accrual of unlimited sick leave.

In devising schedules the therapeutic recreation manager needs to be aware of laws concerning work time. As noted in Chapter 13, there are federal, state, and even local laws and regulations which deal with wages and hours that must be followed. In most health and human service organizations the organization's personnel policies or personnel officer can inform the manager of the work hours for his or her department. If employees are unionized, it is important that the manager review any labor contracts for their impact on his or her staffing and scheduling.

In some settings, the ten-hour or other irregular hour shift (flextime) has come into popularity. One advantage of such a practice is that it often gives the employee three rather than two days off at a time. On the other hand, scheduling problems develop unless adequate full-time staff or part-time employees are used. The present trend is away from irregular staffing because it usually costs the organization more money.

These scheduling matters are not the only concerns of the therapeutic recreation manager. Other matters associated with the manager's role in scheduling may or may not include verifying to the fiscal office services provided to consumers for billing purposes or collecting fees; monitoring supplies and equipment used; approving department staff payroll; monitoring personnel schedules (e.g., sick time, volunteers); and monitoring productivity (e.g., cost of program A relative to program B or effectiveness rela-

tive to efficiency in the economy sense). Monitoring productivity is especially difficult for all health professionals who tend to work from a model of service in which all persons are entitled to the best professional service possible.

Assigning, staffing, and scheduling cannot be performed in isolation from the goals of the therapeutic recreation department. Moreover, because they interact on each other, they must be planned together.

# Therapeutic Recreation Process

A process is a series of planned actions or operations directed toward a particular result. The therapeutic recreation process is a systematic, rational method of planning and providing therapeutic recreation to the consumer (O'Morrow and Reynolds, 1989). To carry out the process at least two people must participate: the consumer and the therapeutic recreation practitioner. However, in some instances, a group or even a family may participate. A group is more likely to be seen in a community-based leisure service organization whereas a specific group would be involved in a leisure experience (e.g., wheelchair basketball).

The consumer or group participates as actively as possible in all phases of the therapeutic recreation process. The therapeutic recreation practitioner, by contrast, requires interpersonal, technical, and intellectual skills to put the process into action. Interpersonal skills include communicating; listening; conveying interest, compassion, knowledge, and information; developing trust; and obtaining data in a manner that enhances the individuality of the consumer. Within the group, interpersonal skills promote integrity both personally and collectively and contribute to the viability of the community. Technical skills are manifested in the use of specialized equipment and the performance of procedures. Intellectual skills required by a therapeutic recreation practitioner include problem solving, critical thinking, and making therapeutic recreation judgments. Decision making is involved in every component of the therapeutic recreation process (O'Morrow, 1986).

The therapeutic recreation process consists of a series of four components or steps. The four-step process includes assessing, planning, implementing, and evaluating. In some settings the process is assisted by protocols. An overview of the four-step process is given here:

1. **Assessing** is collecting, verifying, and organizing data about the consumer or group. Data is obtained from a variety of sources (e.g., formal or informal interviews, assessment instruments) and is the basis for decisions made in subsequent phases. Skills of observation, communication, and interviewing are essential to perform this phase of the therapeutic

recreation process. Once data are collected, problems or potential problems can be identified, and goals for the consumer can be developed.

2. **Planning** involves a series of steps in which the practitioner writes goals or expected outcomes, establishes therapeutic recreation interventions designed to solve or minimize the identified problems of the consumer, prepares a written plan, and informs others of the plan through announcements and meetings.

3. **Implementing** is putting the written plan into action. During this phase the practitioner continues to gather data and validates the therapeutic recreation plan. Continued data collection is essential not only to keep track of changes in the consumer's condition or group's reaction but also to obtain evidence for the evaluation of goal achievement in the next phase.

4. **Evaluating** is assessing the consumer's and group's response to therapeutic recreation interventions and then comparing the response to predetermined standards. The practitioner determines the extent to which goals or predetermined outcomes have been achieved, partially achieved, or not met. If the goals have not been met, reassessment of the plan is needed.

One must keep in mind that the various steps in the process are not discrete entities but an overlapping, continuing subprocess. As an example, assessing, the first step of the therapeutic recreation process, may also be carried out during implementing (i.e., intervention) and evaluating. Each step must be continually updated as the situation changes. Likewise, each step of the process affects the others; they are closely interrelated. For instance, if an inadequate database is used during assessment, the incompleteness will certainly be reflected in the next three steps. Incomplete assessment means unequivocal evaluations because the practitioner will have incomplete criteria against which to evaluate changes in the consumer and the effectiveness of the intervention. Table 20.1 provides a summary of the selected knowledge and abilities needed for the therapeutic recreation process.

## Accountability and Therapeutic Recreation Process

Accountability is the condition of being associable and responsible to someone for specific behaviors that are part of the therapeutic recreation manager's and practitioner's professional role. The therapeutic recreation process provides a framework for accountability and responsibility in therapeutic recreation and maximizes accountability and responsibility for standards of service (i.e., JCAHO, CARF, continuous quality improvement [CQI], NTRS, American Therapeutic Recreation Association [ATRA]). A brief re-

view of accountability and the therapeutic recreation process follows:

- **Assessing.** The therapeutic recreation practitioner is accountable for collecting information, encouraging consumer participation, and for judging the validity of the collected data. When assessing, the practitioner is accountable for gaps in data and conflicting data, inaccurate data, and biased data. In addition, the practitioner is accountable for the judgments made about the consumer problem. For example, is the problem recognized by the consumer? Did the practitioner consider the consumer's values, beliefs, and cultural practices when determining the problem? Especially in community-based service delivery the practitioner must consider a broad spectrum of consumer sociocultural backgrounds.

- **Planning.** Accountability at the planning stage involves determining priorities, establishing consumer goals, predicting outcomes, and planning activities. They are all incorporated into a written plan and shared with a team.

- **Implementing.** Therapeutic recreation practitioners are responsible for all their actions in delivering service. Although the manager has delegated or assigned practitioners to consumer activities, the practitioner is still accountable for the assigned action. Whatever action takes place, it should be noted after being carried out. In healthcare facilities it will be the chart which provides a written record. In other settings it may be in the consumer's file or if a group activity, it may be a daily or weekly activity report that is kept by the practitioner or manager.

- **Evaluating.** By establishing the degree to which the objectives have been attained, the practitioner is accountable for the success or failure of therapeutic recreation actions. The practitioner must be able to explain why a consumer goal was not met and what phase or phases of the process may require change and why.

Although the therapeutic recreation manager is ultimately responsible for practitioner activity relating to accountability and the therapeutic recreation process, the role of the manager relative to this process also incorporates the following: updates assessment tools; reviews treatment and program plans to ensure interventions match individual and group needs and objectives; audits evaluations to ensure achievement of individual, group, division, and department outcomes; facilitates documentation process via monitoring routine maintenance records; communicates to practitioner organization changes impacting division or department services and programming process; and last, ensures training on new interventions.

**Table 20.1   Selected Knowledge and Abilities Needed for the Therapeutic Recreation Process**

| Component | Knowledge | Abilities |
|---|---|---|
| **Assessing** | Biopsychosocial systems of humans<br>Developmental needs of humans<br>Health<br>Disability/illness<br>Etiologic factors of health problems<br>Pathophysiology<br>Family system<br>Culture and values of self and client<br>Normal measurement standards | Observe systematically<br>Communicate verbally and nonverbally<br>Listen attentively<br>Establish a helping relationship<br>Think critically<br>Develop trust<br>Conduct an interview<br>Understand consumers' attitude toward<br>   society<br>Identify patterns and relationships<br>Organize and group data<br>Make inferences<br>Reason inductively and deductively<br>Make decisions or judgments |
| **Planning** | Consumer's strengths and weaknesses<br>Values and beliefs of the consumer<br>Resources available to implement<br>   therapeutic recreation strategies<br>Roles of other healthcare personnel<br>Measurable outcome criteria that relate to<br>   the goals<br>Scope of therapeutic recreation<br>Organizational goals<br>Varied activities<br>Use of supplies and equipment | Problem solve<br>Make decisions<br>Write consumer goals that relate to<br>   therapeutic recreation process<br>Write measurable outcome criteria that<br>   relate to goals<br>Select and create therapeutic recreation<br>   strategies that are safe and appropriate<br>   to meet consumer goals<br>Sharing and eliciting the cooperation and<br>   participation of the consumer and other<br>   healthcare personnel<br>Adapting activities |
| **Implementing** | Leadership roles<br>Physical hazards and safety<br>Procedures<br>Use of supplies and equipment<br>Organization<br>Management<br>Change theory<br>Advocacy<br>Consumer rights<br>Consumer's developmental level | Observe systematically<br>Communicate effectively<br>Use self therapeutically<br>Perform psychomotor techniques<br>Act as a consumer advocate<br>Counsel consumers<br>Maintain confidence |
| **Evaluating** | Consumer's goals and outcome criteria<br>Consumer's responses to therapeutic<br>   recreation intervention | Obtain relevant data to compare with<br>   outcome criteria<br>Draw conclusions about goal attainment<br>Relate therapeutic recreation actions to<br>   outcome criteria<br>Reassess the therapeutic recreation plan |

# Protocols

In recent years therapeutic recreation practitioners and educators have given attention to the design, development, and implementation of protocols which provide for consistency and quality in therapeutic recreation practice (Ferguson, 1992; Olsson, 1992; Olsson, Groves, and Perkins, 1994). Knight and Johnson (1991, p. 137) note that "protocols distinguish therapeutic recreation's role in treatment and the uniqueness of our service."

A protocol is a series of actions required to manage a specific problem or issue. These problems are associated with the physical, psychological, social, and cognitive functioning of the individual. In addition, according to Smith-Marker (cited by Ferguson, 1992), a protocol may be collaborative, in association with other disciplines, may be independent wherein the problem is addressed specifically by the therapeutic recreation specialist, or may be interdependent from the perspective that the problem requires the skills of two disciplines and is so noted by the physician. While protocols have been developed for use in healthcare facilities, they are also found in community-based leisure service organizations.

The protocol provides instructions on "what to do" for a particular problem. A protocol may address a specific therapeutic recreation department program or service or a consumer's therapeutic recreation comprehensive treatment plan from admission to discharge including assessment, intervention, and outcome. Ferguson (1992) has added to these protocols teaching protocols (e.g., leisure education) and activity protocols (e.g., skill development).

While there is no specific standardized protocol found in use today, Figures 20.1 and 20.2 suggest an outline for the development of two types of protocols. Figure 20.1 shows the outline for a treatment protocol as developed by Lanny Knight and Dan Johnson as part of the 1989 Protocol Committee of ATRA and modified by Ferguson (1992). A program protocol outline is illustrated in Figure 20.2. This protocol outline was initially developed by Roy Olsson (1990) with modification by Ferguson (1992).

The development and application of protocols according to NTRS (1989, p. III):

Can (1) promote a better understanding of the therapeutic recreation service as it relates to the performance of others on the treatment team, (2) provide a process of systematic program and treatment planning, and (3) allow for program coverage by a replacement/secondary therapist without impacting the treatment plan.

In addition, according to Knight and Johnson (1991, p. 138), "protocols can be the basis for both the process and the evaluation of outcomes in quality assurance programs."

Figures 20.3 and 20.4 are sample protocols. Figure 20.3 reflects an aftercare services protocol at American Hospital, Los Angeles, California. Figure 20.4 (page 300) is a collaborative protocol involving rehabilitation staff at the Santa Clara Valley Medical Center, San Jose, California.

With the growing interest in protocols, the therapeutic recreation manager has three responsibilities associated with protocols: (1) overseeing the development and revision of protocols; (2) advocating the role of therapeutic recreation throughout the organization with protocols as an illustration of the contribution of therapeutic recreation to outcomes; and (3) supporting and conducting research and evaluation with protocol implementation and collection of data to verify outcomes of intervention application.

# Documentation

Professional responsibility and accountability in therapeutic recreation are among the most important reasons for documentation. Documentation is part of the practitioner's total responsibility in providing service, and it's the manager's responsibility to note its appropriateness and correctness through coaching, training, and auditing. With the development and initiation of the therapeutic recreation process as a framework for practice, documentation has evolved as an essential link between the provision of service and evaluation of service. The purpose of documentation is to facilitate service, to enhance continuity of service, to describe the service, and to evaluate not only the effectiveness of the service in achieving individual and/or group goals, but also the consumer's response to the

---

**Figure 20.1 Outline for Developing Treatment Protocols**

    I. Diagnostic Grouping
   II. Specific Diagnosis
  III. Identified Problem
  IV. Defining Characteristics
      A. Subjective Data
      B. Objective Data
   V. Related Factors or Etiologies
  VI. Process Criteria (Therapist will . . .)
 VII. Outcome Criteria (Client/Patient will . . .)

Used by permission of the Curators of University of Missouri, Columbia, MO.

**Figure 20.2 Outline for Developing Program Protocols**

I. Program Title
II. General Purpose
III. Description of the Program (very brief)
IV. Appropriate Presenting Problems Which *May* be Addressed
V. Referral Criteria
VI. Contraindicated Criteria
VII. Therapeutic Recreation Intervention Activities or Techniques to be Employed
VIII. Staff Training/Certification Requirements (Certified Therapeutic Recreation Specialist, Water Safety Instructor, etc.)
IX. Risk Management Consideration
X. Outcome Expected
XI. Program Evaluation (Frequency and Method)
XII. Approval Signature and Data

Used by permission of the Curators of University of Missouri, Columbia, MO.

service. Basically, evaluation of documentation ensures quality management.

While documentation is important regardless of setting, it is a requirement within healthcare facilities in response to meeting various regulatory standards. Probably the most notable regulatory agencies for healthcare and as related to therapeutic recreation are JCAHO and CARF.

As was mentioned earlier, without accreditation from JCAHO, hospitals are not eligible for any government funds such as Medicare or other healthcare insurance programs. Along with JCAHO's standards, healthcare facilities must comply with the documentation regulations issued by the state department of health in its state. In addition, NTRS (1994) and ATRA (1993) have established standards of

**Figure 20.3 Sample Protocol**

**American Hospital**
**Protocol Outline for Recreation Therapy Aftercare Services**

I. **PHILOSOPHY**
   A. **Statement of services**
      To provide opportunities for reorientation and adjustment to community environment for facilitating positive leisure time experiences and enhance activity in community lifestyle.

II. **PROGRAM CONTENT**
   A. **Special events—monthly**
      Organized group activity to encourage socialization and the development of peer relationships. To provide a support group by which an individual can trust and feel safe. Examples: Holiday events (i.e., Christmas dance, St. Patrick's Day party) or movies, field trips, guest speakers, etc.
   B. **Leisure education group**
      This group meets monthly and facilitates individual needs around group members' leisure time. Problems and barriers are processed. Peer support occurs and linkage of similar interests. Continuation of individual's awareness of the internal and external world and its relationship towards their sobriety and leisure time needs.

III. **LEISURE COUNSELING**
   A. **Individual**
      An individual can be referred to our staff for individual leisure counseling around specific issues needing to be worked on around his or her leisure time.

IV. **EVALUATION—ASSESSMENT**
   A. **Follow-up testing**
      Every six months an individual will be contacted to come back in for a follow-up assessment. This will give us data on how this individual is doing and our effectiveness within Recreation Therapy Services.

Source: National Therapeutic Recreation Society (NTRS). (1989). *Protocols in therapeutic recreation.* Arlington, VA: National Recreation and Park Association. Reproduced with permission.

## Figure 20.4 Sample Collaborative Protocol

**Santa Clara Valley Medical Center**
**Recreation Therapy Department**
**Protocol For Spinal Cord Injury Service**

### I. PURPOSE

To provide therapeutic recreation intervention to inpatients on the Spinal Cord Injury Service. Structured programs will be used to maximize an individual's potential as it relates to his or her leisure lifestyle.

### II. EVALUATION

An initial therapeutic recreation assessment will be completed within five (5) working days of a patient's admission. If a patient is unable to give input on his or her current and premorbid leisure interests the recreation therapist will seek input from the patient's family and/or friends. Based upon the patient's needs, interests, and functional skills the recreation therapist will develop goals and objectives for an appropriate treatment plan.

### III. PROGRAMMING LEVELS USED IN RECREATION THERAPY

**Level 1:** (New Patient—Total Care Unit [TCU])
**Goal:** Orient patient to recreation therapy program.

Recreation therapy intervention consists of monitoring patient's medical status as it relates to his or her future involvement in the recreation therapy programs. Patients at this level are confined to TCU and therefore activities will be done at the bedside. Modalities could include talking books, VCR movies, music for relaxation, and some table games. Evaluation will be ongoing.

**Level II:** (New Patient—Ward)
**Goal:** To orient patient to recreation therapy programs.

Recreation therapy intervention—individual and group. Patient to be seen at the bedside, and when medically stable the patient will be seen in the recreation therapy program areas. When the patient is up in wheelchair he or she should participate in all recreation therapy programs. Focus should be on socialization, increasing physical functioning and endurance. Modalities such as pet therapy, table games, special events, VCR movies, computer games and programs, leisure counseling, and leisure education. Evaluation is ongoing.

**Level III:** (Patient on Full Program)

    **Goal:** Community orientation.

    Recreation therapy intervention—individual and group. Patient should participate in all recreation programs. Patient should be given opportunities to make decisions and should be involved in the planning process. It is at this level that the patient begins to transition into the community. Community outings are designed to reinforce functional skills and activities learned in all therapies. Modalities such as swimming, special events, outside activities, and community outings are planned with the patient. Patient family involvement at this level is very important. Family members should be encouraged to participate with the patient in all programs, including community outings. Community resource and discharge planning should be completed with the patient at this level. Referrals to community programs should be made. Discharge note completed.

*Note:* Due to the uniqueness of spinal cord injury (SCI), it should be noted that a patient may go through each level or he or she may skip a level. Some levels may overlap. The patient's treatment plan is reviewed by the entire SCI treatment team. Goals and objectives are developed by the recreation therapist(s) in accordance with the rest of the team goals. Decisions involving recreation therapy intervention are the responsibility of the primary recreation therapist on the SCI service.

*Note:* Patient medical status may indicate that recreation therapy intervention may be inappropriate at a given time or level of cognitive functioning. The recreation therapist will note that the patient is "off program" and will reevaluate the patient's program potential every two weeks.

Source: National Therapeutic Recreation Society (NTRS). (1989). *Protocols in therapeutic recreation.* Arlington, VA: National Recreation and Park Association. Reproduced with permission.

therapeutic recreation practice which associate themselves with JCAHO and CARF regulatory standards. These standards of practice are based on the framework for providing service and the therapeutic recreation practice.

Documentation today has assumed new importance with the current emphasis placed on monitoring the quality of healthcare as evidenced by consumer outcomes. When financial resources were abundant and good service or care was assumed to be inherent, the evaluation of care was left to healthcare professionals, or no evaluation was done at all. Prospective payment systems and limited healthcare resources have made quality of healthcare a major issue. Consumers, insurers, and government agencies are seeking more information on clinical performance and related dimensions of good care. In response to these concerns, JCAHO adopted an *Agenda for Change* with the primary focus of evaluating organizational and clinical performance outcomes (JCAHO, 1987).

## Documentation Evaluation

While the therapeutic recreation practitioner will document the assessment, planning, and implementation phase of the therapeutic recreation process, documentation of the evaluation phase is an important and ongoing part of the process. Evaluation of the consumer's status, progress, or achievement of outcomes is provided through a progress note. Progress notes are not only vital for evaluation purposes, but they are also used for protection from liability and for reimbursement in healthcare facilities.

Progress notes document the consumer's status in relation to the desired outcomes. The consumer's responses are compared with the outcomes defined in the treatment or program plan. The frequency with which to document progress depends on organization policy. Within a community-based leisure service organization it may be on a weekly, monthly, or seasonal basis. In healthcare facilities the type of charting system used in the organization may define how often one should document an evaluation. Therapeutic recreation protocols may specify frequency. Last, the therapeutic recreation department, or its intervention procedures, may specify frequency.

In writing a progress note, the practitioner and manager need to be aware that such notes are used to document pertinent observations and responses to interventions. In addition, using specific, definitive words when describing a consumer's or group's status is very important. Such expressions as "appears" and "apparently" are not always appropriate. Objective observations should be included without qualifying phrases. Also, only specific pertinent comments should be included, and the use of stock phrases or basket terms which convey little or no meaning is to be avoided. Another common error is to project the future or potential outcome of participating in a specific activity.

Leisure education is an important activity in many settings. Unfortunately it is not always noted in progress notes, and the consumer's response to education is seldom noted. Merely providing information does not guarantee learning. That is why it is necessary to evaluate responses to any teaching or education effort. To determine whether learning is taking place the following methods may assist in deciding results of leisure education programs: demon-

strations, written tests, diaries, discussion, observation, questionnaires, problem solving, and simulation.

One last point on documentation evaluation specifically related to healthcare facilities is the transfer and discharge information. Transfer forms are used to communicate important information about the consumer's status when the consumer is moved within the healthcare facility, between two facilities, or between home and an agency. The consumer's most significant therapeutic recreation information should be discussed to provide a clear picture of the consumer's participation in therapeutic recreation service and the needs of the consumer for follow-up.

In some settings therapeutic recreation is incorporated in discharge summaries. Depending on the setting, therapeutic recreation discharge information would describe the consumer's involvement in the program (without going into extensive detail) and how well the consumer achieved the planned outcomes. In some agencies, the opportunity is provided for referral to a community-based leisure service agency if the consumer has been involved in a leisure education program.

## Legal Aspects of Documentation

Regardless of setting, legible, accurate documentation is imperative. Records communicate important information about the consumer to a variety of professionals. In the event of a lawsuit, the record may form the basis for the plaintiff's case or the therapeutic recreation practitioner's or manager's defense. This section briefly lists charting techniques and strategies to improve documentation:

1. **Write neatly and legibly.** Sloppy illegible handwriting creates confusion and wastes time. If the information is unclear misunderstandings can occur. In some settings computerized records have reduced difficulties associated with handwriting.
2. **Use proper spelling and grammar.** Progress notes filed with misspelled words and incorrect grammar create negative impressions. They imply that the practitioner has limited education or intellect, or he or she is careless and distracted when charting.
3. **Document in blue or black ink.** The use of either color has become a trend in healthcare settings.
4. **Use authorized abbreviations.** Most agencies have a list of approved abbreviations. This list needs to be available to all personnel who document.
5. **Use the consumer's name on every sheet.** Depending on the charting system, the consumer's name should be on every page.
6. **Chart promptly (if possible).** Chart as close as possible to the time of making an observation. When charting is left to the end of the morning or afternoon, details that are important are often forgotten.

7. **Chart after the delivery of service, not before.** Some practitioners get in the habit of charting before an activity since they believe they know how participants are going to behave. It is a dangerous practice if something happens to the consumer during the activity.

8. **Identify late entries correctly.** There are times when one cannot chart. Most healthcare facilities have a procedure for adding late entries.

9. **Correct mistaken entries properly.** Each healthcare agency has an approach for correcting mistakes. One of the more common ones is to draw a single line through the entry so that it is still readable and then to initial and date it.

10. **Do not tamper with the record.** This involves changing the date of entry, placing inaccurate information into the record, omitting significant facts, rewriting the record, and destroying the record.

11. **Chart only service provided.** Therapeutic recreation practitioners should sign only those notes describing service they provided or supervised. Cosigning others' notes is occasionally necessary. Student interns' notes are frequently cosigned by the practitioner, manager, or student intern coordinator.

12. **Avoid using charts to criticize others.** Finger pointing and accusations of incompetence do not belong in a chart.

13. **Document comments any consumer makes about a potential lawsuit against the agency or other drastic measures such as the consumer talking about suicide or harming others.** This type of information should be described in the progress notes and reported to the appropriate person in the facility. Other factors would include violent behavior and antisocial characteristics.

14. **Eliminate bias from written descriptions of the consumer.** Avoid using words that reveal negative attitudes toward the consumer such as abusive, drunk, lazy, spoiled, demanding, disagreeable.

15. **Document potentially contributing consumer acts.** There are situations when the practitioner needs to chart acts on the part of the consumer which may contribute to injury or failure to respond to a treatment or program procedure. These would include noncompliance with interventions, leaving an activity while on an off-grounds trip, without permission, or having on his or her person unauthorized items (e.g., alcoholic beverages, razors).

16. **Sign the progress note including one's position title, credential, and date of entry.**

## Charting Systems

Various methods of charting consumer healthcare plans in healthcare facilities have evolved over the years. Some of the more popular ones include narrative charting (i.e., describing the consumer's status, any interventions, treatment, and consumer response to the interventions), SOAP (i.e., subjective data, objective data, assessment, and plan), SOAPIE (i.e., same as SOAP but *I* for interventions and *E* for evaluation), PIE (i.e., problems, interventions, and evaluation), FOCUS (i.e., a method of identifying consumer concerns and organizing the narrative documentation to include data, action, and response for each identified concern), and CBE (i.e., charting by exception) (Iyer and Camp, 1991).

Today most healthcare facilities, especially hospitals, have shifted to computerized information systems. Hospital information systems (HIS) (as noted in Chapter 10), form a framework for electronically linking departments throughout the facility. In addition, personal computers (PC) can be found at the bedside. While computerized information systems, like other charting systems, have their advantages and disadvantages, it appears they are here to stay in this age of technology. Moreover, computerization provides the opportunity to integrate the best aspects of various documentation systems.

Data can be entered into the computer in a number of different ways. Depending on the type of terminal or PC that is used, the therapeutic recreation practitioner may use a light pen to touch the screen, a touch-sensitive screen that responds to a finger, a keyboard or keypad, a hand-held terminal, a bar code reader, or a mouse. Voice recognition is gaining more acceptance (Lansky, 1989).

Depending on the type of computer in use, the practitioner may enter data into the system by filling in blanks, entering words or phrases to construct sentences, using blank text or free-form data entry, or selecting from a menu to highlight critical pieces of data such as changes in consumer responses (Lansky, 1989).

Regardless of which documentation system is used, all incorporate assessment, planning, care plans, progress notes, and a discharge summary.

# Monitoring and Consulting Practitioner Performance

Monitoring and assessing new and experienced practitioner performance represents one of the more challenging responsibilities of a human service manager. The responsibility is a difficult one because of the complexity of making judgments about the very people managers rely on and the colleagues with whom they have developed close working relationships. Nevertheless, the manager is a supervisor whose task is to create and sustain within the department a work environment that supports and facilitates quality service delivery efforts of staff and encourages them to actualize their knowledge and skills in relation with consumers. As Schermerhorn (1987, p. 52) points out, "Even the most competent employee will not achieve *high* performance unless proper support for the required work activities is available." He goes on to say, "The effective manager, working in concert with upper management, helps to provide the requisite resources to achieve high performance from his or her employees" (p. 54). As research has noted, performance is one of the strongest predictors of an individual's general satisfaction with a job (Feldman, 1980).

It is important to recognize that policies and practices within the organization over which the manager has little control also constitute an important part of the work environment. Inadequate salaries, funding cutbacks, and unclear organizational directives are some of the many other factors that influence the attitudes and behavior of staff. While the manager can sometimes mediate the worst effects of these environmental influences, in the last analysis they will be part of the reality that impinges upon staff.

While these factors are important aspects of the work environment, the concern here initially is to consider the monitoring and informal assessment by the manager that takes place on a daily or weekly basis. In other words, the focus is on the work of practitioners including interns as related to the therapeutic recreation process and tasks that affect the recipients of service. Thereafter, the manager becomes a consultant who imparts knowledge and cultivates professional skills of the direct service practitioner. In some respects, the manager may serve as a kind of senior practitioner and role model; demonstrating valued behavior, attitudes, and/or skills that aid the practitioner in achieving competence, confidence, and a clear professional identity. To accomplish these specific functions, the manager must have:

1. knowledge of the delivery service deemed appropriate and used by therapeutic recreation professionals;
2. therapeutic recreation knowledge, techniques, and skills;
3. conceptualization of the social, cultural, and behavioral patterns of consumers (including individuals, groups, and organizations);
4. adequate interpersonal skills such as self-disclosure, conflict management, and giving and receiving feedback; and
5. knowledge and understanding of one's own interpersonal behavior including motives plus affective sensitivity to one's own feelings as they are experienced in interpersonal situations.

Before considering the functions in more detail, the amount of flexibility and autonomy allowed practitioners in the conduct of their work will be briefly addressed. It is well-known that practitioners who perceive their supervisors as directive, controlling, and restrictive of initiative and autonomy tend to be dissatisfied not only with the supervision they receive but with their jobs and other aspects of the organization as well.

At first glance, this might suggest that practitioners prefer a style of supervision that is detached and uninvolved, but this is clearly not the case in the authors' experience. It has been found that practitioners respond favorably to the opportunity to make practice-related decisions and to initiate ideas and activities that seem responsive to consumer needs and circumstances, but they prefer to do so in the context of a supervisory relationship marked by expert guidance, support, and corrective feedback. It was also found that, among the principle sources of job satisfaction, the opportunity to share responsibility and obtain support from management for difficult treatment and community-based plan decisions and receiving help from the manager in dealing with "problems with consumers in my work with consumers" are high on practitioners' list of positives. Conversely, the authors have heard practitioners cite lack of critical feedback and insufficient assistance in dealing with consumers as a major source of dissatisfaction with their managers.

These comments appear to suggest that a more intensive and individualized relationship between managers and practitioners will produce job satisfaction and professional growth in practitioners. Such a posture clearly places heavy interpersonal demands on the manager and practitioners alike. It requires frequent two-way communication, mutual problem solving, and the development of trust from both parties; however, the payoff is likely to make the investment worthwhile. In addition, the interpersonal skills acquired by the manager from experience in working with both consumers and colleagues provides a foundation for creating an effective working relationship which reflects a supportive, facilitating, growth enhancing climate. Feedback is essential to practitioner development. It not only helps practitioners correct mistakes before they become habits, but also it reinforces positive behaviors, encourages the development of desirable work habits, and helps practitioners achieve their goals. Lest one forget, the quality of a program's front-line practitioners—their knowledge, skill, and commitment—is a critical ingredient in successful program implementation. After years of schooling and some experience, practitioners, as noted in an earlier chapter, consider themselves capable of self-governance and believe they have the experience and knowledge to respond to the needs and demands of their consumers.

## *Monitoring Practitioner Performance*

Monitoring may be broadly defined as that managerial task concerned with checking and reviewing the day-to-day work activity of the practitioner. Monitoring is a means employed by managers to generate immediate ongoing feedback about work activities and accomplishments so as to determine whether corrective action is necessary. It may be an on-the-spot forum to collect and analyze information from the practitioner about work activity and outcomes while ascertaining whether steps should be taken to alter the activity of the practitioner or mode of operation. It may also be an individual conference as a result of reading case records or treatment plans. Previewing case records allows the manager to identify problem areas as practitioners pursue their responsibilities. Monitoring may or may not be associated with the annual performance evaluation or the formal appraisal interview. The rewards for this work consist usually of a bundle of intangibles including praise for a job well-done, dependence on practitioners as team players who "pull their own weight," or an unsolicited commendation letter from a consumer.

Close monitoring is most critical for inexperienced, new practitioners. At the same time, professional development continues throughout one's practice, and practitioners who have had experience also need assistance at times. However, the manager must be sensitive to possible defensiveness on the part of the experienced practitioner. Practitioners who have been monitored previously in their place of work may have positive or negative expectations about upcoming supervision. If the previous experience was negative, the present manager must overcome this mind-set.

What might be some reasons for daily or weekly monitoring? The following short list represents reasons for monitoring:

1. To assess practitioner's attitudes about the job, responsibilities, organization, and the supervision.
2. To further the manager's understanding of the practitioner.
3. To help the manager observe the practitioner more closely in order to improve the consulting or teacher relationship. The manager must keep in mind the timing and location of the coaching experience. Excellent coaching at the wrong time or wrong place may prove to be of more harm than help.
4. To obtain feedback on practitioner's work activity (e.g., complying with regulations, protocols, standards of practice and procedures, or achieving desired results).
5. To assist the manager in becoming more aware of differences among practitioners for better practitioner deployment.

6. To assist in clarifying activities associated with annual performance evaluations.
7. To assist the manager in analyzing practitioner strengths and weaknesses in order to enhance strengths and reduce weaknesses. Monitoring charting activities, for example, may demonstrate compliance with documentation as well as the staff's knowledge, strengths and deficits.
8. To assist the manager in making decisions about in-service training needs.
9. To assist the manager in verifying inadequate work performance demonstrated by a practitioner.
10. To assist the practitioner in his or her self-evaluation.
11. To enable the manager to represent the accomplishments of the program to the organization and to the larger community—a process that is crucial for building support, correcting misinformation, and defending against unwarranted criticism.

The manager must always keep in mind that the responsibility for monitoring is clearly shared by the manager and practitioner through the joint process of building a relationship which encourages free discussion of job-related responsibilities. It is assumed that practitioners will become more involved in their work when they utilize the freedom to discuss their work responsibilities. Monitoring is a productive, rather than reactive, management tool.

## *Consultant and Practitioner Performance*

Many managers view the term *consultant* as something reserved only for the expert or the outsider. While this view may be correct in some instances, its use here is viewed as a process whereby the manager, as a supervisor, provides assistance to others on the basis of a request for assistance or on the basis of developing an atmosphere for requesting assistance. From another perspective, consulting may be considered a method which gives service indirectly by assisting the practitioner in handling problems associated with the consumer. Regardless of the method, the ultimate goal of consulting is to increase the competence of the practitioner.

While the manager may be involved in consulting relative to giving colleagues insight into what is going on around them, within them, among them and other people, or in program consulting wherein the manager is invited by top management to assist in organizational planning and program development, the focus here is on therapeutic recreation process consulting. The consulting process begins with the recognition by the practitioner that his or her program responsibility could be enhanced by consulting with the manager. The manager assists practitioners in resolving particular problems which are related to a consumer or group for which the practitioner is responsible. The manager may engage in consulting related to helping the practitioner develop a more comprehensive diagnosis of the consumer's problems, expanding the practitioner's options regarding alternative methods of intervention and activities that might be used to bring about change, or assisting the practitioner in recognizing the relationship of the practitioner's personal feelings and anxieties to the consumer's problems. However, the manager should not confuse this consulting role with the previously mentioned process of monitoring and reviewing to assure effective service delivery to consumers which is an authority-accountability process.

The manager's method of intervention will vary according to his or her personality and professional background as an experienced practitioner, facilitator, and educator. These roles may be conceptualized along a continuum from most directive to least directive, most authoritative to least authoritative. As an experienced practitioner, the manager may be viewed as an expert and therefore authoritative and directive, one who imparts special knowledge or skill, and may be expected to have magical cures. A common occurrence is the desire of the practitioner to be as competent as his or her manager. While such aspirations of this type are a positive motivation for the practitioner to learn the knowledge and skills of the therapeutic recreation profession, it is wise for the manager to disclose his or her own errors, doubts, and disappointments. Good consulting requires that the manager not see himself or herself as an oracle but admits fallibility and devotes energy to furthering growth and building strength in the practitioner.

On the other hand, the manager as a consultant may assume a facilitator role. This involves the manager in a communication process which utilizes the collective resources of both the manager and the practitioner in problem solving. By skillfully using questions to help define and explore problems, the manager tries to generate alternative solutions from the worker and then discusses the pros and cons of each alternative. The manager might add alternatives not mentioned by the practitioner. Next, the manager helps the practitioner choose the approach that seems most likely to be successful and, equally important, one that is consistent with practice service delivery. By helping the practitioner to evaluate and choose an approach, the manager is not only assisting the practitioner with the development of professional competency, but also is communicating confidence in the practitioner's practice ability, thus encouraging the practitioner to take a major role in the learning process.

The role of the manager as consultant-educator to the practitioner is one of the most widely recognized roles. The educator role may involve anything from on-the-spot teaching (e.g., giving evaluative reactions to a specific service delivery approach to the consumer and offering sugges-

tions of what to do differently in order to be more effective) to citing specific articles or books relevant to the problem faced by the practitioner. The manager might also demonstrate a particular technique or approach by role playing with the practitioner. Then, too, the manager may offer strategies or techniques for the practitioner to implement.

Experience should suggest that educating and learning is a complex process and is affected by many variables in the subject, the context of learning, the educator, the learner, and the interaction among them. The practitioner as learner is not simply a passive object onto which the consultative can project already developed ideas. Rather, the practitioner is actively involved in the learning process. This view, elaborated by Dewey (1916, p. 46), maintains that "the organism is not simply receiving impressions and then answering them. The organism is doing something; it is actively seeking and selecting certain stimuli."

The practitioner is an active participant in the learning process. The consultant's job is to present ideas and to monitor the way in which the practitioner relates to the ideas. This may range from simply watching the practitioner's eyes to make sure he or she is understanding the directions for charting to having regard for the practitioner's feelings while trying to help him or her tackle a difficult total treatment plan. It can also mean being sensitive to the subtle interplay taking place between the consultant and the practitioner that has been described as the authority item. The effect resulting from this relationship can enhance the learning or can generate major obstacles to the integration of new ideas. Of course, some anxiety will be created by any supervisory technique or discussion, but most managers would agree that some techniques produce more anxiety than others. Also, some practitioners become anxious more quickly and to a greater extent than others. It is suggested that one should begin with a low-anxiety approach rather than a high-anxiety approach. However, the entire issue of supervisory intervention rests, to some extent, on the manager's belief about conflict. As noted in Chapter 11, conflict can have positive value as well as negative value. The authors view supervision here as the management of changes in the practitioner toward ideal professional behavior.

Much of what has been discussed in this section is associated with the term *coaching* which recently has appeared with some consistency in the literature. Coaching, according to Robbins (1995, p. 274), is a day-to-day, hands-on process of helping employees recognize opportunities to improve their work performance. There are three general coaching skills that managers should exhibit if they are to assist employees in their performance. They are (Robbins, 1995, pp. 281–82):

1. ability to analyze ways to improve an employee's performance and capabilities,

2. ability to create a supportive climate, and
3. ability to influence employees to change their behavior.

Effective coaching will develop strengths and potentials of practitioners and help them to overcome their weakness. It is a positive motivator when it is specific and behavioral. While coaching takes time, it will save time, money, and errors by practitioners, which in the long run will benefit all—the manager, the practitioners, the organization, and the consumers.

A criticism often heard about coaching is that it fosters a dependent relationship with the manager. Supposedly, the practitioner will become a skilled imitator of the manager and will not be able to integrate new or creative techniques into his or her service delivery. The counterargument may be that gaining such skills may very well assist the practitioner to become independent more quickly as his or her confidence increases.

The eventual goal of the consulting role is the engagement of the manager and practitioner in a mutually responsible collegial relationship that values the participation of the practitioner equally with that of the manager. The result of this engagement should assist the practitioner in being able to integrate and apply basic practice skills in the delivery of therapeutic recreation service with consistency. Competency gives a practitioner credibility so that others will tend to seek out and respond to his or her suggestions. As long as both the new and old practitioner and the manager communicate openly and recognize and respond to each other's needs and expectations mutual development will continue, and the satisfaction of all will be enhanced.

The challenges facing therapeutic recreation managers in delivering quality service are more numerous and complex than ever before. A prime example is the potential use of the computer to manage, supervise, and direct the work of practitioners at other sites resulting from changes in the delivery of services, downsizing, reengineering, and hospital mergers.

# Summary

Consideration was initially given to scheduling including the goals and problems associated with scheduling. Consideration must be given to many factors in developing a schedule such as consumer needs and staff skills. Thereafter the therapeutic recreation process and accountability for the process were reviewed. Associated with this review and accountability was protocols, actions which address specific programs or treatment plans. Outlines of a treatment and program protocol were provided. Documentation and its importance in evaluation was considered next. It was pointed out that while there are various charting systems in use in healthcare facilities, many hospitals have shifted to computerized information systems.

Last, attention was given to the monitoring process of practitioner performance and the role of the manager as a consultant to both the new and older experienced practitioner.

# Discussion Questions

1. How is scheduling related to other managerial functions and activities?
2. List and evaluate external factors affecting scheduling.
3. Develop guidelines to provide constructive criticism.
4. Ask yourself, "What do people have to do to get positive feedback from me?" Evaluate your expectations.
5. Develop program and personnel schedules using various computer packages.
6. Compare different progress note formats and charting systems in clinical and community-based leisure service organizations.
7. Review note taking and critique according to the 16 items presented in this chapter.
8. Visit a therapeutic recreation manager and "walk through" program development process reviewing the relationship between various types of schedules (e.g., individual-group, session-seasonal-annual).
9. Prepare either a program or treatment protocol based upon the outlines (Figure 20.1 and Figure 20.2) found in this chapter.

# References

American Therapeutic Recreation Society (ATRA). (1993). *Standards for the practice of therapeutic recreation, and self-assessment guide.* Hattiesburg, MS: Author.

Carter, M. J., Van Andel, G. E., and Robb, G. M. (1995). *Therapeutic recreation: A practical approach* (2nd ed.). Prospect Heights, IL: Waveland Press, Inc.

Carter, M. J., Van Andel, G. E., and Robb, G. M. (1985). *Therapeutic recreation: A practical approach.* St. Louis, MO: Times Mirror/Mosby.

Dewey, J. (1916). *Democracy and education: An introduction to the philosophy of education.* New York, NY: Macmillan Publishing Co.

Feldman, D. A. (1980). A socialization process that helps new recruits succeed. *Personnel, 57,* 163–174.

Ferguson, D. D. (1992). Problem identification and protocol usage in therapeutic recreation. In G. L. Hitzhusen, L. T. Jackson, and M. A. Birdsong (Eds.), *Global therapeutic recreation II.* Columbia, MO: Curators of University of Missouri.

Gunn, S. L., and Peterson, C. A. (1978). *Therapeutic recreation program design: Principles and procedures.* Englewood Cliffs, NJ: Prentice Hall.

Iyer, P. A., and Camp, N. H. (1991). *Nursing documentation.* St. Louis, MO: Mosby Year Book.

Joint Commission on Accreditation of Healthcare Organizations (JCAHO). (1987). *Agenda for change.* Chicago, IL: Author.

Knight, L., and Johnson, D. (1991). Therapeutic recreation protocols: Client problems centered approach. In B. Riley (Ed.), *Quality management: Applications for therapeutic recreation.* State College, PA: Venture Publishing, Inc.

Lansky, D. (1989). Hospital based outcomes management: Enhancing quality of care with coordinated data systems. In L. M. Kingland (Ed.), *Proceedings of the thirteenth annual symposium on computer applications in medical care.* Washington, DC: IEEE Computer Society Press.

National Therapeutic Recreation Society (NTRS). (1994). *Standards of practice for therapeutic recreation services.* Arlington, VA: National Recreation and Park Association.

National Therapeutic Recreation Society (NTRS). (1989). *Protocols in Therapeutic Recreation.* Arlington, VA: National Recreation and Park Association.

National Therapeutic Recreation Society (NTRS). (1982, May). *Philosophical position statement.*

Olsson, R. H., Jr. (1992). Assessment protocol in therapeutic recreation. In G. L. Hitzhusen, L. T. Jackson, and M. A. Birdsong (Eds.), *Global therapeutic recreation II.* Columbia, MO: Curators of University of Missouri.

Olsson, R. H., Jr. (1990). *Recreational therapy protocol design: A systems approach to treatment evaluation.* Toledo, OH: International Leisure Press.

Olsson, R. H., Jr., Groves, B., and Perkins, S. (1994). Recreation therapy programming: A protocol approach to treatment evaluation for quality assurance. In G. L. Hitzhusen, L. Thomas, and N. Frank (Eds.), *Global therapeutic recreation III.* Columbia, MO: Curators of University of Missouri.

O'Morrow, G. S. (1986). *Therapeutic recreation: A helping profession* (2nd ed.). Englewood Cliffs, NJ: Prentice Hall.

O'Morrow, G. S., and Reynolds, R. (1989). *Therapeutic recreation: A helping profession* (3rd ed.). Englewood Cliffs, NJ: Prentice Hall.

Robbins, S. P. (1995). *Supervision today.* Englewood Cliffs, NJ: Prentice Hall.

Schermerhorn, J. R., Jr. (1987). Improving healthcare productivity through high-performance managerial development. *Health Care Management Review, 12,* 49–55.

# Chapter 21

# Risk Management

## Introduction

During the past several decades there has been an increased emphasis on risk management which focuses on loss prevention and liability control as it relates to all activities or persons in a setting. Practiced by industry, governmental units, organizations such as hospitals, and individuals, the concept of risk management is not new; it goes back to ancient times. There are many reasons for the spreading of the practice of risk management. In the park and recreation arena it was not until after the mid-1970s that risk management programs became operational as a result of increased judgments against public entities and judgments for the plaintiffs who were injured in leisure activities (van der Smissen, 1990). Likewise, as a result of an increase in medical malpractice cases during the 1970s and 1980s, attention was given to loss prevention and risk management in healthcare facilities.

Therapeutic recreation managers need to participate actively in risk management programs as well as to practice those principles necessary to manage risk effectively. For example, one must be knowledgeable about therapeutic recreation practice and take appropriate action to ensure that one's staff and, in some situations, volunteers are competent in the performance of therapeutic recreation practices (e.g., proper lifting techniques regarding wheelchair transfers). Failure to do this indicates that one lacks an understanding of risk management. An active role in risk management contributes to health and human service organizations by identifying and decreasing po-

tential liability that will ultimately maintain or decrease the cost of services.

An interesting development in recent years, particularly in the healthcare industry, is the trend toward formalizing a relationship between risk management and quality management. Voelkl (1988) has suggested that risk management is a component of quality assurance in therapeutic recreation. She states: "Quality assurance and risk management appear to be natural partners in ensuring the highest level care for recipients" (Voelkl, 1988, p. 3). Because of similarities in the goals of these management activities, the trend is understandable. Both risk management and quality management must have ongoing monitoring and evaluating in order to improve financial and quality service continuously. In addition, risk management and quality management are concerned with patterns of noncompliance, either with safety practices or with goals, objectives, policies, procedures, and standards. The point of both management programs is to develop procedures that will provide feedback to the service providers so that services can be improved. As noted by Peters (1987, p. 79): "When quality goes up, costs go down. Quality improvement is the primary source of cost reduction."

This chapter introduces the reader to a variety of factors associated with risk management. The therapeutic recreation manager needs to understand the basic concepts of risk management, namely the risk management program and its elements, as well as the problems and concerns associated with risk management. This chapter does not attempt to provide answers to all risk management administrative matters; rather, it gives therapeutic recreation managers a better understanding of the importance of risk management in providing quality service.

# Risk Management Program

A risk management program consists of policies and tasks that must be in place and performed on a daily basis. A risk management program is a concern of top management as well as of every employee and should be an integral part of planning. It is an organization-wide program since it calls for a team approach involving all departments within the organization. Further, it incorporates input from staff and feedback to management to accomplish its objective. In large organizations and governmental units the program is formal; a risk management department and a full-time risk manager are in place. In smaller organizations the direction of the program is usually the responsibility of a manager who has other assigned duties. In some healthcare facilities the risk management manager and quality improvement manager may be the same.

Risk has been described as the probability or predictability that something will happen. A negative connotation is associated with risk. A consumer incident or a family's expression of dissatisfaction regarding service not only indicates some slippage in quality of service, but it also indicates potential liability. In this regard, Stein (1993, p. 37) notes that "too many recreation leaders—whether in regular or special programs—do not take all steps necessary and mandated to acquaint program participants with potential dangers in activities." A distraught, dissatisfied, complaining consumer is a high risk; a satisfied consumer is a low risk.

Risk management, on the other hand, usually refers to positive results achieved through some form of activity. Thus, a risk management program is a planned approach to risk problems or exposures to loss. Its purpose is to identify, analyze, and evaluate risks, followed by a plan for reducing the frequency and severity of accidents and injuries. Often, a risk management program focuses on general liability, general health and wellness within the environment, worker's compensation, and property or equipment loss due to vandalism, theft, fire, and fraud (Kaiser, 1986; Rios, 1992). According to Kaiser (1986, p. 229): "The objective of risk management is to effectively conserve the assets and financial resources of the organization and to achieve financial stability by reducing the potential for financial loss." West (1995, p. 180) points out:

> Agencies that have a well-developed risk management program will experience fewer lost work hours and cost associated with injuries and illnesses. When individual expectations are not met, liability

and the potential for litigation increase. A risk management plan provides a systematic approach for ensuring a safe environment and minimizing legal liability.

Last, Rios (1992, p. 163) comments that "risk management is simply a decision-making process to identify and control risk."

In brief, the development of risk management programs is the result of, but not limited to, the following:

- injury or death from environmental hazards found in parks, forests, and recreation areas;
- poorly maintained or dangerous equipment in parks and playgrounds;
- inadequately supervised recreation activities;
- user behaviors;
- changes in reimbursement and cuts in government health programs;
- consumer requirement for accountability in the health areas;
- increased cost of premiums for liability coverage;
- increased litigation;
- huge judgments or awards granted by courts;
- a demand for service when previously there was less demand; and
- expectations.

As a result of these factors and many others, management of these risks has gained significance in terms of priorities within community-based leisure service agencies and in healthcare organizations. In the final analysis, a risk management program serves as a deterrent to being sued and, if sued, as evidence of original intent to act responsibly.

The degree of involvement of therapeutic recreation managers in the development of risk management programs will vary from setting to setting. Some will be directly involved as a result of being a manager of a therapeutic recreation department within an organization. Managers of special recreation associations and community-based freestanding independent recreation centers for the disabled will certainly be responsible for the development of risk management programs in their specific settings. Others need both to be involved and aware of what composes exposure to loss and what are risk problems.

## *Elements of a Risk Management Program*

Elements of a risk management program include writing and disseminating policy statements; identifying, analyzing, and evaluating risks; and selecting, implementing, and monitoring the plan.

The key to an effective risk management program is the development of a philosophy regarding risk for the entire organization. Merely knowing about the program and what is involved will not do the job. There must be an emotional acceptance and positive attitude about a risk management program. The statements of policy:

> should set forth or delineate what risk management encompasses and its importance to the organization; the scope of authority and responsibilities of personnel and where risk management fits into the organization structure; and the extent and nature of the approaches to be used in managing risk. (van der Smissen, 1990, p. 4)

The organization board or policy-making body of the organization approves these statements.

The initial activity of the therapeutic recreation manager, like other managers, is to identify various risks within the department in terms of the potential loss to the organization and the likelihood of an accident. Kaiser (1986) notes four dimensions to risk identification: property loss, fidelity loss (e.g., employee dishonesty), contract liability (e.g., a specific therapeutic recreation service being provided by another), and tort liability (e.g., malpractice). Risks must be identified before they can be managed. Thus, the manager reviews policies, procedures, and activities in order to make recommendations regarding changes that will prevent or reduce potential loss.

According to Carter, Van Andel, and Robb (1995, p. 215) risk is associated with therapeutic recreation service in three ways: "(1) staffing, (2) program design, implementation and evaluation, and (3) participant intervention." In staffing, for example, consideration needs to be given to the practitioner's knowledge and experience including certification to successfully fulfill the responsibilities associated with the position. Managers, as noted by Stein (1993), are asking for legal problems if they assign a practitioner to conduct and supervise programs and activities without adequate training and education.

Program design, implementation, and evaluation uses American Therapeutic Recreation Association (ATRA, 1993) and National Therapeutic Recreation Society (NTRS, 1995) standards of practice as well as Joint Commission on Accreditation of Healthcare Organizations (JCAHO, 1993) and Commission on Accreditation of Rehabilitation Facilities (CARF, 1996) standards to ensure compliance with risk management. Other standards that need to be considered are those which have been legislated by law (e.g., statutes, ordinances, or regulations) and those set forth by organizations concerned with specific activities (e.g., American Camping Association, National Playground Safety Institute). "Ignorance of such standards is no ex-cuse for failing to comply" (van der Smissen, 1990, p. 45). A policy and procedure manual is another source which will provide insight into practices necessary to decrease losses and injuries (e.g., facility and equipment use and inspection, clinical privileges). It is extremely important in community-based leisure service agencies that sites, facilities, and programs conform with American with Disabilities Act (ADA) regulations. Consideration needs to be given to the procedures associated with handling emergencies, releases and waivers, injury precaution sheets, and agreements to participate. For example, contents of agreement to participate forms may need to be presented in large print or Braille. In other situations, sign language or visual supplements (e.g., videotape) will be necessary. Participant intervention focuses on such things as assessment guidelines and information including consumer chart updating and documentation of participation and degree of involvement. The broader the therapeutic recreation manager's knowledge of the department's operation, the more exhaustive and accurate will be the identification of loss exposures.

Other matters and concerns, not exhaustive, that need to be addressed by therapeutic recreation departments' are shown in Figure 21.1 (page 312).

After the identification of risks, the manager will probably be asked to analyze the frequency, severity, and causes of specific types of incidents which have caused injury to the consumer and staff in the past. Some managers will find that sufficient historical data are not available for reliable objective analysis. In such cases, intuitive analysis can be used, or the manager can compare data to that of a similar department within the same organization (e.g., occupational therapy) or to a like therapeutic recreation department in another organization. If the manager must forecast the future, consideration should be given to brainstorming, computer simulation, or asking "what if?"

Selecting is the first task of the last series of elements in the risk management program. Selecting focuses on the approaches to risk control: (1) elimination, (2) reduction, (3) retention, and (4) transference. Elimination is simply doing away with the service or activity because its risk is too great. Reduction considers minimizing the contingencies through planning, training, and better procedures. The keeping of risk is retention. There will always be risk, and the organization accepts a certain level of loss. Transference is having the responsibility of risk carried by an individual, contract, lease, bond, or harmless clauses.

The next step in the risk management process is implementation. This step incorporates implementation and inclusion of all aspects of the program and its administrative procedures within the organization's and department's policy and procedures manual including the various forms used to document incidents. Rios (1992, p. 172) suggests the following basics for inclusion:

---

### Figure 21.1 Therapeutic Recreation Department's Risk Management Concerns

1. Use of toxic materials.
2. Storage of flammable materials.
3. Kiln is periodically inspected and used by only experienced staff members.
4. Storage of equipment (to prevent people from using without proper supervision).
5. Proper space is available for program to be run safely.
6. Equipment is in good condition and regularly inspected.
7. Proper clothing is required for participation in certain activities (i.e., gym shoes for volleyball).
8. Staff-client ratio is an established policy.
9. Clients are informed of possible risks and means of preventing risks.
10. A first-aid kit is kept in the vehicle used for out trips. The kit is regularly checked to ensure it contains adequate supplies.
11. Out trip sites are inspected for accessibility, direct and safe entry ways, and services provided prior to taking clients.
12. Proper approval is obtained for clients to be involved in any activities.
13. Specific standards exist for the running of each program.
14. Assumptions are not made regarding clients' past experiences or skills.
15. Vehicles for out trips are regularly inspected.
16. Staff are involved in planning programs, policies, procedures, and standards.
17. Area is checked prior to activity.
18. Proper level and sequence of instruction is provided for each activity.
19. Proper supervision is provided for each activity.
20. All areas utilized in supervised or unsupervised activities are regularly inspected for safety.
21. Staff are always prepared to act in case of an emergency.
22. Clients are not allowed to participate in any general recreation or therapeutic recreation programs until staff have completed an assessment.

Source: Voelkl, J. E. (1988). *Risk management in therapeutic recreation.* State College, PA: Venture Publishing, Inc. Reproduced with permission.

---

1. a plan for supervision of all therapeutic recreation staff;
2. standards of practice referencing accreditation and professional standards;
3. ethical standards of conduct;
4. credentialing standards and clinical privileging;
5. process for reporting and investigating accidents and incidents;
6. process for safety inspections;
7. procedures for preventative maintenance;
8. procedures for routine maintenance;
9. emergency plans (e.g., search and rescue, fire evacuation, and power outage);
10. procedures for managing untoward behavior (e.g., unauthorized leave);
11. procedures for managing aggressive behavior;
12. safety guidelines for swimming;
13. specific program guidelines for any individual program of moderate frequency or severity of risk (moderate risk includes any injury such as minor fractures, strains, sprains, or infected lacerations versus inconsequential injuries such as minor lacerations, contusions, or abrasions);
14. job descriptions that include duties and responsibilities; reportability; minimum knowledge, skills and abilities to provide service; and level of supervision; and
15. internal peer review system.

Figure 21.2 illustrates the risk management process as developed by Kaiser (1986) and its modification to therapeutic recreation by Rios (1992) is illustrated in Figure 21.3 (page 236).

Once a risk management program has been developed, the therapeutic recreation manager will be involved in monitoring the program as it relates to the department recommending, if need be, preventive or corrective action. Certainly he or she will evaluate, on an ongoing basis, the effectiveness of the program and will provide reports to the administration or risk management manager for the agency or organization. The therapeutic recreation manager will gather information from staff and regularly inspect and observe current practices. The manager may find useful a checklist to adequately cover all aspects of risk exposure. Information gathered needs to be integrated into the department's computer risk management analysis program.

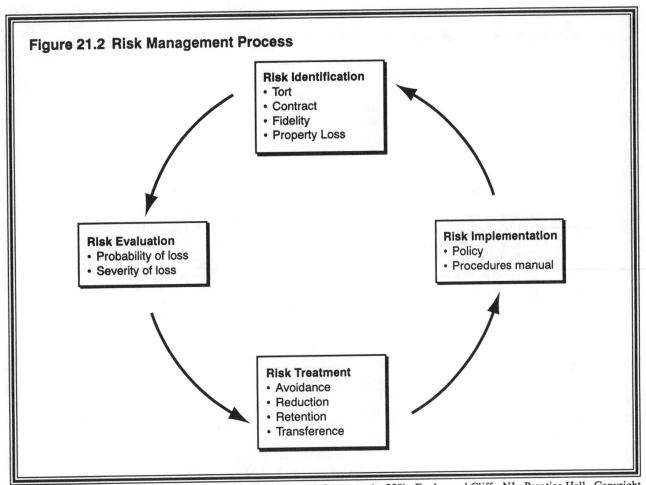

**Figure 21.2 Risk Management Process**

Risk Identification
- Tort
- Contract
- Fidelity
- Property Loss

Risk Evaluation
- Probability of loss
- Severity of loss

Risk Implementation
- Policy
- Procedures manual

Risk Treatment
- Avoidance
- Reduction
- Retention
- Transference

Source: Kaiser, R. A. (1986). *Liability and law in recreation, parks, sports* (p. 229). Englewood Cliffs, NJ: Prentice Hall. Copyright 1986 by Allyn & Bacon. Reprinted/adapted by permission.

In the review process of developing a risk management plan, volunteers and student interns need to be involved. Volunteers and interns are subject more and more to legal actions against them in a manner similar to regular paid employees although they are generally liable for their own acts of negligence. It is probably wise to include participants as a review resource especially in community-based agencies. It also may be wise to require students to have personal liability insurance prior to starting their internship; however, the organization undoubtedly has a policy on this matter which should be checked.

Education about risk is another major element. For a risk management program to be effective, every employee must be involved, including staff, volunteers, and interns. Staff and volunteers must understand the significance of hazards and associated liabilities. This means all those liabilities associated with negligence and/or malpractice. Merely knowing what to do and the liabilities associated with the risk is not acceptable. There must be an emotional acceptance, as has been noted, of risk management by the manager and practitioners of the department.

To close this section, the comments of Touchstone (1984, p. 25) are appropriate:

Although effective TR [therapeutic recreation] risk management will not guarantee complete protection from liability, the proper policies, procedures, programming and documentation should greatly reduce the chance of costly litigation and help to ensure reasonable healthcare.

## Incident Report

Regardless of safety rules and procedures as pertaining to consumer participation in program services and practitioners who deliver the services, incidents do occur. Incident reports are made for every accident, error, or anything unusual that could lead to legal liability. They are used to collect and analyze future data for the purpose of determining risk control strategies. The report needs to be completed with extreme care because it can be used as

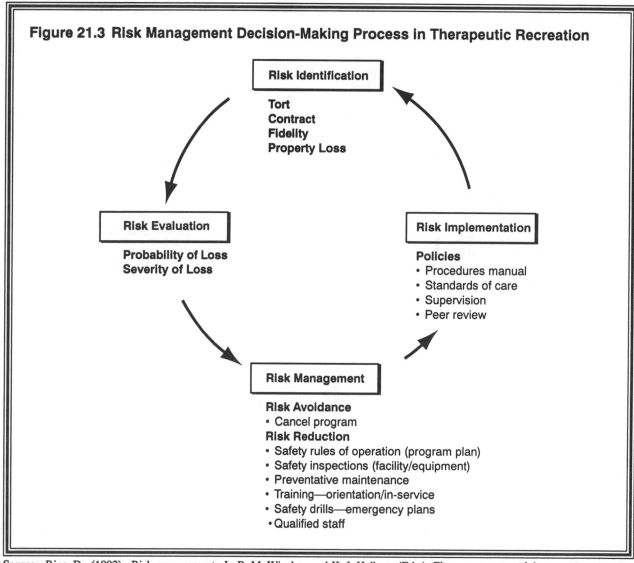

**Figure 21.3 Risk Management Decision-Making Process in Therapeutic Recreation**

Source: Rios, D. (1992). Risk management. In R. M. Winslow and K. J. Halberg (Eds.), *The management of therapeutic recreation services* (p. 168). Arlington, VA: National Recreation and Park Association. Used by permission of National Recreation and Park Association.

evidence if a lawsuit is brought against the organization or any person involved. Depending on the state, lawsuits can be filed until the statute of limitations runs out.

At times there is a reluctance on the part of practitioners to report incidents due to fear of the consequences. This can be alleviated by two techniques: (a) staff education programs that emphasize objective reporting; and (b) a clear understanding that the purpose of the incident reporting process is for documentation and follow-up and the report will not be used for disciplinary action. All incidents must be reported—even cases in which an unfavorable result follows the performance of a standard procedure. No segment of the department's staff is excluded from this responsibility.

According to Kaluzny, Warner, Warren, and Zelman (1982, p. 33), the principal purposes and functions of a prompt reporting system for all accidents and incidents are as follows:

• to provide a permanent record of the incident;
• to assist in refreshing the memory of the parties involved;
• to alert the risk manager of a possible claim situation for subsequent investigation;
• to allow for a timely investigation; and
• to provide a statistical base for incident patterns from which preventive recommendations can be made.

Although all organizations will develop their own incident report form and private instruction for completion, van der Smissen (1990, pp. 54–56) suggests the following items should be included on the form:

1. identification information;
2. location of accident;
3. action of injured;
4. sequence of activity;
5. preventive measures by injured (e.g., what could or should have been done to have prevented the accident?);
6. procedures followed in rendering aid; and
7. disposition.

Figure 21.4 (page 316) illustrates an incident report used by a community-based leisure service agency while Figure 21.5 (page 317) shows an example of a hospital incident report. This report would be used throughout the hospital.

## Risk Management Problems

Although there are many types of risk management problems, two categories will be considered here: negligence and malpractice. These two categories are associated with the term *liability*, which is used to describe a circumstance wherein an individual or organization has failed to carry out a responsibility required by law or through a contractual agreement. This responsibility may relate to the organization's judgment, professional practice, and/or negligence in conduct of activities and operations (van der Smissen, 1990).

*Negligence* is defined as:

> The failure to do something that a reasonable person guided by the consideration that ordinarily regulated the conduct of human affairs would do, or doing something that a prudent and reasonable person would not do. (Kaluzny, Warner, Warren, and Zelman, 1982, p. 324)

Negligence is not a fixed standard, according to Kaluzny, Warner, Warren, and Zelman, (1982), but must be determined in each case by reference to the situation and knowledge of the parties and the attendant circumstances.

Common acts of negligence associated with therapeutic recreation, regardless of setting, would include high-risk activities, falls, property loss, poor safety directions or measures, failure to communicate inappropriate activities, defects in equipment, and a variety of other activities or circumstances wherein the participant feels the agency or organization failed in its responsibility to prevent the incident or injury. In most of these examples, a number of principles must apply or be proven before a claim based on negligence can be won. In other words, there is an approved standard of behavior which protects the individual against risk. For a claim to be considered there must be a breach of this duty. While there are any number of breaches, the following are most common:

1. **Contributory negligence.** Conduct on the part of the injured party that helped to cause the accident.
2. **Comparative negligence.** The amount of contribution to the accident assessed each party, with damages assessed accordingly.
3. **Assumption of risk.** The injured party assumes part of the responsibility or participates in the activity knowing that harm may happen based on the activity and actions of others.
4. **Governmental immunity.** The government cannot be sued for its wrong action.
5. **Failure of proof.** The injured party is unable to demonstrate negligent action.
6. **Act of God.** The direct cause of the accident was the result of an unusual situation or circumstance (e.g., flood, tornado).

Damage or harm must have occurred, and the breach of duty must be proved as the proximate cause of the harm or damages (Kaluzny, Warner, Warren, and Zelman, 1982).

*Malpractice* refers to an unreasonable lack of skill in professional duties, illegal or immoral conduct, or professional misconduct. There are many forms of malpractice—educational, managerial. From a healthcare perspective, Kaluzny, Warner, Warren, and Zelman (1982, p. 324) defines it in these terms: "when a professional person, in treating or caring for a patient or client, does not conduct himself or herself with due care or reasonable skill." Malpractice also incorporates disregard of rules or principles, carelessness, and acts occurring as a result of a lack of knowledge that a professional should have (Richards and Rathburn, 1983). As with negligence, there must be a duty, a breach of duty, and an injury that resulted from the breach (Kaluzny, Warner, Warren, and Zelman, 1982). The major difference between malpractice and negligence appears to be the involvement of the professional. Any individual may be negligent, but the professional has a specific duty to perform in a way that requires some skill, knowledge, and behavior which meets a standard. Failure to meet the standard in performance of the duty by the professional constitutes malpractice (Richards and Rathburn, 1983).

While therapeutic recreation managers or practitioners, to the author's knowledge, have never been found guilty of negligence or malpractice, they have a responsibility to ensure that certain service expectations are met. Therapeutic recreation licensure laws, and to a lesser extent certification requirements, are designed to protect the public

## Figure 21.4 Leisure Service Agency Incident Report

**Alexandria, Virginia**
**Department of Recreation, Parks & Cultural Activities**
**1108 Jefferson Street 22314**

**Incident Report**

Date of Occurrence_____    Time of Occurrence_____

Location _____

TYPE OF INCIDENT:

❏  Vandalism             ❏  Trespassing        ❏  Assault
❏  Drug-Related Incident  ❏  Injury             ❏  Other
❏  Program Disturbance   ❏  Arson

— — — — — — — — — — — — — — — — — — — — — — — — — — — — — — — — —

Name of Injured _____

Address_____

Telephone No. (Daytime) _____    (Evening) _____

Parent's Name (If Applicable) _____

Telephone No. (Daytime) _____    (Evening) _____

Follow-Up Inquiry Date_____

**Narrative:  State in concise terms the details of the incident, include first aid administered and other action by staff.**

_____

_____

(Add attachment if additional space is needed.)

Name/Address/Phone No. of Witness(es) _____

_____

_____

**Equipment or Property Loss/Damage:**  Attach statement describing equipment loss to include manufacturer's name, serial number, quantity/value of each type item and total cost.  Include structural loss/damage if applicable: _____

_____

**Signature/Date:** _____

_____

(Type name, position and telephone number of reporter)

**Date Report Completed:**_____

Used by permission of the Department of Recreation, Parks, and Cultural Activities, Alexandria, VA.

# Figure 21.5 Hospital Incident Report

## CONFIDENTIAL OCCURRENCE REPORT
### Property of Hospital Attorney

**BRIEF DESCRIPTION OF OCCURRENCE:**

**ADMITTING DIAGNOSIS:**

**PREVIOUS OCCURRENCE REPORT THIS ADMISSION?**
❏ NO   ❏ YES   ❏ DON'T KNOW

**NAME & TITLE OF EMPLOYEE INVOLVED:**

**WITNESSES:**

**IDENTIFICATION—addresograph or handwrite**

OCCURRENCE DATE _____  TIME _____

❏ PATIENT   ❏ EMPLOYEE: _____
(Department & Job Title)

VISITOR: _____
(Address & Phone)

SEX: ❏ M  ❏ F   AGE: _____

**OCCURRENCE LOCATION**

❏ PATIENT ROOM NO.___ ❏ LABOR/DELIVERY   ❏ PHARMACY
❏ BATHROOM   ❏ AMBULATORY SERVICES ❏ CAFETERIA
❏ EMERGENCY SERVICES ❏ NURSES STATION   ❏ RADIOLOGY
❏ NURSERY   ❏ OPERATING ROOM   ❏ PATHOLOGY
❏ OTHER _____

**PATIENT STATUS BEFORE OCCURRENCE**

❏ ORIENTED   ❏ CONFUSED   ❏ SEDATED
PHYSICIAN ORDERS:
❏ OOB AD LIB   ❏ BRP   ❏ RESTRAIN
❏ BEDREST   ❏ OOB w/ASSISTANCE ❏ RESTRAIN PRN
RESTRAINTS IN PLACE: ❏ NO  ❏ YES
SIDE RAILS UP:   ❏ NO  ❏ YES
ADJUSTABLE BED:  ❏ UP  ❏ DOWN

**NATURE OF INJURY**

❏ NO INJURY OR ADVERSE EFFECT
❏ EMOTIONAL (fright, no physical damage) ❏ ALLERGIC REACTION
❏ ABRASION ❏ HEMATOMA ❏ IV INFILTRATION ❏ STRAIN/SPRAIN
❏ BURN ❏ FRACTURE ❏ LACERATION ❏ PUNCTURE
❏ OTHER _____

**IMMEDIATE FOLLOW-UP ACTION**

PHYSICIAN NOTIFIED?  ❏ NO  ❏ YES  TIME:____
PATIENT SEEN BY DR.? ❏ NO  ❏ YES  TIME:____
X-RAYS TAKEN? ❏ NO ❏ YES  RESULTS:____
RESTRAINTS APPLIED:  ❏ NO  ❏ YES

**HOSPITAL 24-HR. FOLLOW-UP**

**RELEASE FROM RESPONSIBILITY**

I certify that I do not wish to be examined or treated by a physician following circumstances described herein. I have been informed of the risk involved and hereby release the hospital from all responsibility for any ill effect which may result.

Signed: _____   Date _____

Witness _____

**OCCURRENCE TYPE**

❏ FALL
  ❏ FROM BED
  ❏ FROM CHAIR
  ❏ FAINTED/LOSS OF BALANCE
  ❏ FOUND ON FLOOR
  ❏ OBJECT ON FLOOR
  ❏ REACHING
  ❏ OTHER _____
❏ IV/INFUSION
❏ MEDICATION
❏ PROCEDURAL/PRACTICE
  ❏ PT. ID NOT CHECKED
  ❏ ORDER TRANSCRIBED INCORRECTLY
  ❏ PHYSICIAN'S ORDERS UNCLEAR
  ❏ PHYSICIAN'S ORDERS OVERLOOKED
  ❏ OTHER _____
❏ EQUIPMENT
❏ OTHER _____

**MEDICATION OCCURRENCE**

❏ DOSAGE
❏ DUPLICATION
❏ OMISSION
❏ LABELING
❏ ROUTE
❏ WRONG MED.
❏ TIME
❏ UNORDERED
❏ NOT CHARTED
❏ WRONG PATIENT
❏ TRANSCRIPTION
❏ IV INFILTRATE
❏ OTHER _____

❏ ADVERSE DRUG REACTION

❏ TRANSFUSION REACTION

**PHYSICIAN'S COMMENTS/Treatment Given:**
(including name of person receiving comments)

PHYSICIAN—DO NOT SIGN

FORM COMPLETED BY   DATE

SUPV./DEPARTMENT HEAD   DATE

ADMINISTRATION/RISK MANAGEMENT   DATE

and to ensure a safe environment. When consumer expectations are not met, liability and the potential for litigation are possible.

While it is not the intent to consider the legal process if litigation arises, since it would be extensive, it is important to define terms which are used in the process. Figure 21.6 provides a brief list of legal terms which will aid in better understanding the process.

Any professional person may be called upon to testify in court regarding standards of quality in his or her own agency or in some other agency or organization if there is a lawsuit. The expertise of a witness in a trial or hearing largely depends on education, experience, and recognition by colleagues in the field. Such testimony may have a profound influence on litigation involving therapeutic recreation services or the quality of service provided by an agency or organization.

Therapeutic recreation managers need to have a basic understanding of law or familiarity with types of law. There are a number of publications in the traditional parks, recreation, and leisure resource management field including several which focus specifically on legal aspects of parks and recreation (e.g., Grosse and Thompson, 1993; Kaiser, 1990; Peterson and Hronek, 1992; van der Smissen, 1990). *Parks & Recreation* also devotes a monthly column to this very issue. In addition, there are many health and human service publications which address all aspects of the law and legal process that affect health service organizations. An appreciation of the law and legal process and its applications is necessary for the successful manager.

Many healthcare facilities cover employees in the event of a lawsuit. On the other hand, some agencies require their employees to purchase professional liability insurance. Some agencies require students to show proof of personal liability before beginning an internship or fieldwork experience.

## *Other Risk Management Concerns*

This concluding risk management section highlights a number of additional concerns associated with risk management programs and the therapeutic recreation manager including patient rights, consumer charts, invasion of privacy, confidential communication, and research.

Some of the *rights of consumers* (i.e., patients) are spelled out in legal statutes or have been tested in court; others are not found in law books and might simply be considered the patient's human rights. Legal rights may vary from state to state, and therapeutic recreation managers should be aware of what their state laws require of them. Conversely, human rights are felt to exist by the very nature of the relationship between consumer and healthcare provider. As noted in the earlier chapter on ethics (Chapter 7), individuals have the human right to existence and, therefore, have the right to choose or make decisions concerning themselves as long as they are willing to accept any consequences. As also noted in Chapter 7, specifically defined sets of rights have developed in society by various agencies, organizations, and professional associations. Depending on the setting, therapeutic recreation managers need to be aware of these and adhere to them.

---

### Figure 21.6 Legal Terms

**Litigation:** Refers to a lawsuit.

**Complaint:** A document noting the complaint and asking for certain relief from the party against whom the plaintiff is complaining.

**Plaintiff:** The party who files the complaint.

**Defendant:** The party complained against, although the party may also be known as the respondent.

**Jurisdiction:** Refers to the rules governing where a case will be tried (i.e., federal, state, or local systems). May also include level of trial courts.

**Summons:** The complaint is filed together with a summons, and a U.S. marshal or the sheriff serves the summons and a copy of the complaint to all defendants.

**Answer:** A response to the various allegations in the complaint.

**Deposition:** The giving of testimony (by plaintiff or defendant) under oath, normally in an attorney's office based upon oral questioning.

**Interrogatories:** Questions in writing which must be answered by either the plaintiff or defendant in writing.

**Motion:** An application made to a court or judge for purpose of obtaining a rule or order directing some act to be done in favor of the applicant.

**Damages:** Parties to the litigation may be seeking either money or something other than money (i.e., "equitable relief").

**Appeal:** Once a judge makes a decision, either party may appeal to the appellate court. The appellate court does not retry the case but reviews the case and renders a decision. The decision may be to uphold the decision or reverse the decision and remand the case for further proceedings.

Source: Black, H. C. (1990). *Black's law dictionary* (6th ed.). Eagan, MN: West Publishing Co.

Malpractice claims are won or lost in many instances on the basis of *consumer charts* (i.e., patient charts); they are a legal document. Documentation has been identified as the most important nonmedical issue leading to liability for a hospital (Scott, 1990). Consumer's goals, objectives, and prognoses relative to their involvement in the program are key items to be charted. The court assumes that if one did not write something down, it did not happen. One should never wait, for instance, until the end of the day to chart if it can be helped. The quality service given will be compromised by charting the little that can be remembered.

As noted in Chapter 20, charting is to be as thorough as possible. It is important for the therapeutic recreation manager to instill in therapeutic recreation staff the habit of accurate and concise documentation. Sloppy, illegible handwriting creates confusion and wastes time. Likewise, misspelled words and incorrect grammar creates negative impressions. Improper or too many abbreviations creates unnecessary confusion when others try to decipher the charting. And one should chart as close as possible to the time an observation is made or service is provided. Last, one should *never* backdate or tamper with records. If this is detected the organization and anyone involved are in for problems.

Therapeutic recreation managers and their staff may become liable for *invasion of privacy* if they divulge information from a consumer's medical record to improper sources or if they commit unwarranted intrusions into the consumer's personal affairs. However, there are occasions when one has a legal obligation or duty to disclose information as required by law. While therapeutic recreation practitioners enjoy taking pictures of their programs with consumer involvement, pictures should not be taken without the consumer's consent. To be completely on the safe side, the consent of the agency's or organization's administrator should also be sought.

*Confidential communication* is also a concern as related to treatment, observation, or conversation. It is associated with invasion of privacy. One has a professional obligation to keep secret information relating to a consumer's illness or treatment which is learned during the course of professional duties. It is a tenet of the therapeutic recreation code of ethics. There are state statutes which address this matter and healthcare organizations have their own regulations.

Last, *research on humans* requires consent to be obtained in writing from consumers or their representatives. In all healthcare organizations there is a committee responsible for reviewing human research proposals. As thera-

peutic recreation research becomes more prevalent outside university centers, therapeutic recreation managers will find more requests for access to consumers. While research provides the opportunity to validate the theoretical or conceptual basis for practice, it must be proposed and conducted in a professional manner.

In conclusion, risk management is aimed at eliminating harm and reducing cost associated with harm. Cooperation between the risk management manager and the therapeutic recreation manager is essential in accomplishing these objectives.

# Summary

Initial consideration was given to the importance of a risk management program in reducing cost while at the same time improving quality service. Thereafter it was noted that the elements of a risk management program included a policy statement; identification, analysis and evaluation of risks; and selecting, implementing, and monitoring the plan. Examples of what should be included in a policy and procedures manual relative to risk management were provided. The importance of an incident report was discussed followed by identifying two major risk management problems: negligence and malpractice. In addition, a brief list of the legal terms that surround litigation was provided. The section concluded with a discussion of other concerns associated with risk management including consumer rights, consumer charts, invasion of privacy, confidential communication, and research.

# Discussion Questions

1. Collect and compare contents of incident forms.
2. Review policy and procedure manuals to identify risk management statements.
3. Visit with risk management and quality assurance personnel to consider their roles and responsibilities.
4. Ask a therapeutic recreation manager, regardless of setting, what advice would you give to your practitioners concerning avoidance of liability suits?
5. How have federal and state legislative enactments as well as professional standards of practice and organizational standards affected therapeutic recreation service?
6. How does planning, as a function of management, affect the development of a risk management program?
7. Visit a therapeutic recreation division or department, regardless of setting, and identify loss exposures.

# References

American Therapeutic Recreation Association (ATRA). (1993). *Standards for the practice for therapeutic recreation, and self-assessment guide.* Hattiesburg, MS: Author.

Black, H. C. (1990). *Black's law dictionary* (6th ed.). Eagan, MN: West Publishing Co.

CARF . . . The Rehabilitation Accreditation Commission. (1996). *1996 standards manual and interpretative guidelines for behavioral health, . . . for employment and community support services, and . . . for medical rehabilitation.* Tucson, AZ: Author.

Carter, M. J., Van Andel, G. E., and Robb, G. M. (1995). *Therapeutic recreation: A practical approach* (2nd ed.). Prospect Heights, IL: Waveland Press, Inc.

Grosse, S. J., and Thompson, D. (Eds.). (1993). *Leisure opportunities for individuals with disabilities: Legal issues.* Reston, VA: American Alliance for Health, Physical Education, Recreation and Dance.

Joint Commission on Accreditation of Healthcare Organizations (JCAHO). (1993). *1994 accreditation for hospitals* (Vol. 1). Oakbrook Terrace, IL: Author.

Kaiser, R. A. (1990). *Liability and law in recreation, parks, and sports.* Englewood Cliffs, NJ: Prentice Hall.

Kaluzny, A. D., Warner, M. D., Warren, D. C., and Zelman, W. N. (1982). *Management of health services.* Englewood Cliffs, NJ: Prentice Hall.

National Therapeutic Recreation Society (NTRS). (1995). *Standards of practice for therapeutic recreation society and annotated bibliography.* Arlington, VA: National Recreation and Park Association.

Peters, T. (1987). *Thriving on chaos.* New York, NY: Alfred A. Knopf.

Peterson, J. A., and Hronek, B. B. (1992). *Risk management.* Champaign, IL: Sagamore Publishing, Inc.

Richards, E. P., and Rathbun, K. C. (1982). *Medical risk management: Preventive legal strategies for healthcare providers.* Rockville, MD: Aspen Systems Corporation.

Rios, D. (1992). Risk management. In R. M. Winslow and K. J. Halberg (Eds.), *Management of therapeutic recreation services* (pp. 163–176). Arlington, VA: National Recreation and Park Association.

Scott, R. W. (1990). *Healthcare malpractice: A primer on legal issues for professionals.* Thorofare, NJ: SLACK Incorporated.

Stein, J. U. (1993). Critical issues: Risk management, informed consent, and participant safety. In S. C. Grosse and D. Thompson (Eds.), *Leisure opportunities for individuals with disabilities: Legal issues* (pp. 37–52). Reston, VA: American Alliance for Health, Physical Education, Recreation and Dance.

Touchstone, W. A. (1984). Fiscal accountability through effective risk management. *Therapeutic Recreation Journal, 28:4,* 20–26.

van der Smissen, B. (1990). *Legal liability and risk management for public and private entities* (Vol. 2). Cincinnati, OH: Anderson Publishing Co.

Voelkl, J. E. (1988). *Risk management in therapeutic recreation: A component of quality assurance.* State College, PA: Venture Publishing, Inc.

West, R. (1995). Management of therapeutic recreation in clinical settings. In M. J. Carter, G. E. Van Andel, and G. M. Robb (Eds.), *Therapeutic recreation: A practical approach* (2nd ed., pp. 157–188). Prospect Heights, IL: Waveland Press, Inc.

# Chapter 22

# Quality Service Management

## Introduction

Quality is a major concern of health and human service organizations and health and human service providers. The task of the therapeutic recreation manager focuses on ensuring high quality service to the consumer.

In the early 1960s health and human service organizations were viewed by society as providing low-quality and ineffective services. Over time these organizations were forced to raise the cost of providing services as a result of real budget problems or deficits coupled with the determination on the part of society to hold professionals, agencies, and organizations responsible for providing quality service and care.

One approach society used to assure higher quality was to take individuals, agencies, and organizations to court when services were inadequate, or outcomes in a healthcare facility were less than satisfying. Another was to lobby for stricter legal regulations. A third approach was simply to go elsewhere to participate in leisure experiences or, if it was health related, to seek a better service of care. In fact, all three of these approaches are very much alive today.

Each successive decade since the 1960s has seen the appearance of at least one concept or managerial method that was supposed to be the solution to improving health and human services. Many of these concepts and methods of management were borrowed from business and industry.

The 1960s saw the advent of program planning and budgeting (PPBS). Management by objectives (MBO) appeared on the scene in the early 1970s, followed in the latter part of the decade by zero-based budgeting (ZBB) and quality circles (QC). The decade of the 1980s has been called a period of consciousness raising regarding quality (Albrecht, 1992). It was during the early 1980s that quality assurance (QA) came into being. This concept gave way in the late 1980s to the application of total quality management (TQM) and continuous quality management (CQM). In the mid-1990s the Joint Commission on Accreditation of Healthcare Organizations (JCAHO) initiated a process in the healthcare field called "Improving Organizational Performance" (IOP) also referred to as performance improvement (PI). This process incorporated core concepts of TQM and CQI (Cunninghis and Best-Martini, 1996).

Historically, quality referred to the achievement of some preestablished standard of service. Today, quality has taken on a larger meaning. Health and human service organizations' focus and direction are provided by the quality preferences of the consumer (in healthcare TQM the consumer is referred to as a customer) and ongoing attempts to satisfy those preferences.

This chapter initially focuses on TQM and CQI and its unique characteristics. Thereafter, attention is given to TQM and CQI and therapeutic recreation service including its implementation into CQI. The topics are considered primarily from a healthcare facility perspective. While TQM was introduced into county and municipal governments nationwide during the late 1980s, according to Carr and Littman (1990), the extent of its application to community-based leisure service agencies is not known. However, a well-developed and stable quality movement in community-based therapeutic recreation divisions within public parks and recreation departments has been noted through a concept of QA since the 1980s. This concept which is also found in TQM and CQI will be discussed.

# TQM as a Philosophy of Management

TQM as a philosophy of management differs from previous managerial waves. Past managerial waves, like PPBS, MBO, and ZBB, were essentially tool-based systems. These tools could be adopted by a health and human service organization without any significant changes being made in its basic approach to management. TQM is different. TQM is a proactive, innovative management philosophy that is applied to all individuals, departments, and units within an organization. TQM or a variation of it is found in nearly all general medical hospitals as well as in other types of healthcare facilities. Its goal is to integrate the managerial process of quality planning, quality control, and quality improvement to provide focus for quality activities to measure existing performance while improving performance to desired levels (McCabe, 1992). McLaughlin and Kaluzny (1994) stress that TQM and CQI:

> is a structured organizational process for involving personnel in planning and executing a continuous stream of improvements in systems in order to provide quality healthcare that meets or exceeds customer expectations. (p. 3)

Thus, TQM is both process driven and consumer oriented. TQM recognizes that consumer requirements are the key to consumer quality, and that these requirements change over a period of time for various reasons (e.g., age, education, economics). As a result, these changes require continuous improvements in administrative and clinical methods to ensure quality service and care (McLaughlin and Kaluzny, 1994).

The success of TQM requires top management support and implementation over a period of time. As *Business Week* (1991) pointed out, many TQM efforts demonstrate some initial success and then fizzle out because top management support wanes. According to Kaluzny, McLaughlin, and Jaeger (1994), this is usually the result of internal political turmoil and cost.

A review of the literature notes the identification of six key elements of TQM as a philosophy of management (Carr and Littman, 1990; Milakovich, 1990). These six key elements are noted in Figure 22.1.

# CQI and Its Characteristics

A basic tenet of TQM as a philosophy of management is CQI. Other tenets or terms recognized and used are continuous improvement (CI) and total quality (TQ) (JCAHO, 1993a). CQI describes the conceptual framework for improvement of services. It blends or overlaps with earlier efforts initiated in the mid-1980s to improve quality through programs called quality assurance and risk management. CQI involves a systematic monitoring, evaluation, and improvement of the effectiveness and efficiency of work procedures through teamwork. A key characteristic of CQI is that it empowers staff to bring about improvements. As noted in an earlier chapter, there are three types of teams. One of these teams provides advice (i.e., improves quality). Problem-solving teams are the most frequently formed teams within TQM and CQI. They are empowered to discuss quality problems, investigate the causes of problems, recommend solutions, and, in some instances, take corrective action. According to La Vallee and McLaughlin (1994), teams are at the core of CQI.

Historically, hospital organizations have promoted the idea of discrete and separate departments with each department's functions and processes viewed as independent from each other. This type of organizational culture promoted departmental conflicts in a "turf-oriented" environment. The CQI process attempts to break down these departmental barriers and requires all hospital staff to work as teams (Smith and Hakill, 1994).

A basic assumption of CQI is that problems or quality deficiencies are neither the result of a single person, nor are they limited to a single department. Therefore, the development of multidisciplinary teams is used to realize improvements. A team approach requires cooperation and reduces or replaces competition as the interpersonal value to be maximized. At the same time it provides for a greater understanding of the function of each discipline in the process as well as a greater understanding of the roles and responsibilities of the various levels of management (Rosen, 1994).

The CQI program may include a hospital-wide committee with any number of subcommittees, work groups, or teams responsible for various aspects of CQI (e.g., problem awareness and evaluation, measurement, education). Another approach is to have teams associated with various services or units (e.g., psychiatry, physical medicine and rehabilitation, pediatrics, one-day surgery).

Last, CQI recognizes two groups of consumers as customers, internal and external. Internal customers are the professionals and employees of the organization as well as departments or units that provide services of various kinds to each other and to the consumer. External customers comprise the patients or clients (consumers), friends

---

**Figure 22.1 Elements of TQM as a Philosophy of Management**

1. **Quality** is a primary organizational goal.
2. **Customers** determine what quality is.
3. **Customer satisfaction** drives the organization.
4. **Variation** in processes must be understood and reduced.
5. **Change** is continuous and is accomplished by teams and teamwork.
6. **Top management commitment** to promoting a culture of quality, employee improvement, and a long-term perspective.

---

Source: Martin, L. L. (1993). *Total quality management in health services organization* (p. 24). Newbury Park, CA: Sage Publications, Inc. Reproduced with permission.

---

and family members of the consumer, and third-party payers. The community is also considered an external consumer since some of its needs are met by the healthcare facility (e.g., suppliers of equipment) (Macintyre and Kleman, 1994).

## Deming Cycle and CQI

CQI incorporates what has come to be known as the Deming cycle—"Plan-Do-Check-Act" (PDCA) cycle although it was adapted by W. Edwards Deming from Walter Shewhart (Deming, 1986). In short, this approach is similar in nature to active problem solving. Figure 22.2 illustrates the Deming cycle.

In brief, the Deming cycle begins with the plan stage. At the plan stage, a proposal is made to implement a change that hopefully will result in correcting a quality problem.

The proposed improvement has not been arrived at by "seat of the pants" guesswork, but rather by the analysis of data to determine the most probable cause of the quality problem and the most likely solution. One of the CQI tools used to generate as many ideas as possible about the causes of a quality problem is *brainstorming*. The do stage is the actual implementation of the proposed change while holding constant all other aspects of the system or process. At the check stage, the results of the change are evaluated. Did quality improve? At the act stage, the change, if successful in improving quality is made a standard operating procedure. If the change does not improve quality, then it is abandoned, and other probable causes of the quality problem are studied. In either case, the Deming cycle is never completed; there is no end state to the pursuit of quality improvement. It focuses on continuous improvement to increase consumer satisfaction, enhance productivity, and lower cost (Deming, 1986; Tindell and Stewart, 1993).

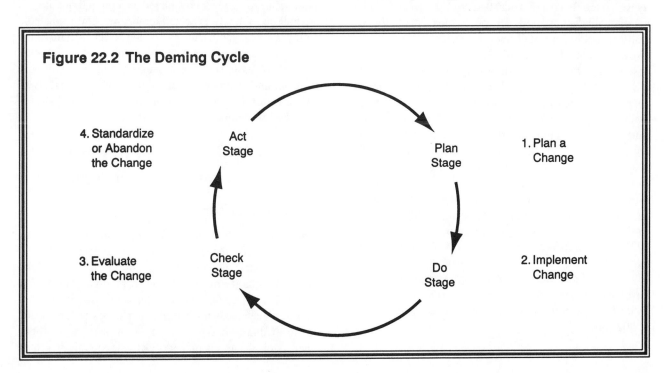

**Figure 22.2 The Deming Cycle**

4. Standardize or Abandon the Change — Act Stage

Plan Stage — 1. Plan a Change

3. Evaluate the Change — Check Stage

Do Stage — 2. Implement Change

# What is Quality?

In beginning this section it is interesting to note that the first recorded instance of quality of care in hospitals was instituted in France in 1793 by the National Convention of the French Revolution. The measure decreed that there should be only one patient in a bed, as opposed to the usual two to eight, and that beds should be at least three feet apart (Rosenberg, 1987). In the United States, the oldest recognized quality control is that of hospital accreditation which began in 1918 when the American College of Surgeons (1946) drew up a one-page list of basic criteria and standards for hospital facilities. In 1951 the Joint Commission on Accreditation of Hospitals (JCAH) (now the JCAHO), which included the Canadian Medical Association, was formed. Standards developed by the American College of Surgeons over a period of some 35 years were adopted by JCAH. JCAH officially began to survey hospitals in 1952 using 11 standards (Scalenghe, 1994). In 1966, the Commission on Accreditation of Rehabilitation Facilities (CARF) was established and entered into an administration relationship with JCAH (changed from JCAH to JCAHO in 1987) for accreditation purposes. It became an independent organization in 1971 (Toppel, Beach, and Hutchinson-Troyer, 1991).

No universally accepted definition of the term "quality" exists although one is aware of it when it is lacking. Quality, like beauty, lies in the eye of the beholder. What the professional considers to be a substantial achievement, the consumer may consider to be less so. In a society where a major automobile company proclaims that "quality is job one" and a small-town doughnut shop advertises that "quality isn't our only goal, it's our standard," the precise meaning of quality is obscured. The problem is that quality actually possesses several distinct dimensions. When people disagree about what quality is, they are often simply demonstrating preferences for differing quality dimensions. As O'Leary (1993, p. 219) has observed: "Quality of care is a judgment shaped by the interests of the individual or group making the judgment." In the conduct of healthcare utilization review, "quality" refers to the treatment process being reviewed or managed. Both provider and reviewer maintain their own perspective: the provider wants to correct the quality of his or her work, and the reviewer wants to assess the quality of that work. However, the provider is also interested in the quality of the review being conducted by the reviewer. According to Peterson (cited by Rhodes, 1991, p. 84) "between 54 and 78 percent of consumers feel that they can tell which hospitals provide quality care."

In TQM and CQI the consumer as a customer determines the relative importance of quality (Crosby, 1986; Juran, 1989). As Kaluzny and McLaughlin (1994, p. 202) note:

[It] . . . is a shift from a technical definition of quality to a recognition that effective care requires a subjective as well as technical evaluation. Specifically, a definition of healthcare quality is inadequate if it does not include the customer.

In general, this is the way it should be since consumers in healthcare facilities tend to judge quality of care by the interpersonal aspects of the clinical process because these aspects are the most obvious to them. Consumer-defined quality, regardless of setting, represents a way of achieving the health and human service goal of putting the needs of consumers first.

The consumer is not the only one concerned with quality. Each department within a healthcare facility is concerned with quality as determined by various organizational standards. Organizations such as JCAHO, CARF, Medicare, and community-based leisure services agencies have set expectations about quality that must be met. Quality is inherent in the American Therapeutic Recreation Association (ATRA) and National Therapeutic Recreation Society (NTRS) standards of practice. Third-party payers have specific perceptions of quality—ones that can be described by cost per case, length of stay, and other measurable criteria. Quality is also found in statutes which have been enacted over the years at all levels of government to protect the public. Other quality dimensions associated with health and human services would include accessibility, consistency, humaneness, outcomes, and licensure and certification.

Quality is a moving target. Because expectations constantly change, what is considered exceptional quality today will be routinely expected tomorrow. Unfortunately, quality is the most difficult, expensive (at times), and time-consuming factor to evaluate. Regardless of the quality views of professions and professionals, and the quality dimensions and standards specified in regulations and laws, the end result is quite clear: *Quality is determined, or defined, by consumers* (Martin, 1993).

# QA and CQI Comparison and Therapeutic Recreation

## *Quality Assurance*

Around the mid-1980s therapeutic recreation managers and practitioners became involved with the concept of QA, a process directed toward ongoing monitoring and evaluation of the quality of therapeutic recreation service provided in healthcare facilities through standards, and implementing mechanisms for ensuring that these standards were met to evaluate therapeutic recreation service. Others added to this the giving of feedback to individual and group providers of the service so that service could be improved. Over the intervening years, therapeutic recreation managers and practitioners working in community-based leisure service agencies and organizations integrated QA into their programs and services.

While several conceptual frameworks exist regarding quality service within health and human service organizations, Avedis Donabedian's (1969) approach to improving the efficiency and effectiveness of the services rendered had the widest application and is associated with QA. Donabedian's framework has the advantage of being simple yet comprehensive.

Comprehensive QA includes the *structure* in which service is given, the *process* of service, and the *outcome* of that service (Donabedian, 1969). The ATRA *Standards for the Practice of Therapeutic Recreation, and Self-Assessment Guide* (1993) are presented in the format of structure, process and outcome. Moreover, the standards are relative in two areas: (1) direct practice in therapeutic recreation and (2) management of the practice in therapeutic recreation. The latter area is concerned with monitoring and evaluating practice to improve services. These standards, according to ATRA, apply in a variety of settings. The NTRS *Standards of Practice for Therapeutic Recreation Service and Annotated Bibliography* (1995) note standards relative to treatment, leisure education, and recreation services respectively in clinical, residential, and community settings. Criteria are outlined within each standard but not in the structure, process, and outcome format. Consideration of the different measures of quality as applied to a therapeutic recreation department follows.

## Structure

Structure not only refers to the setting or location where services are provided but includes the resources. While the setting is perhaps the easiest of the three aspects to measure, it is many times overlooked in some evaluation procedures. The following offers examples of some of the structural aspects:

1. **facilities:** accessibility, adequate space to conduct programs, convenience of areas, safety;
2. **equipment:** adequate supplies and equipment, staff ability to use it;
3. **staff:** credentials (state licensure or certification), continuing education and professional development, performance evaluation, absenteeism;
4. **finances:** adequate budget, adequate salaries;
5. **management:** written statements of purpose, philosophy, and objectives, ethical statement of practice, scope of practice;
6. **organizational arrangement:** management structure, organization of practice, styles of supervision;

7. **legal authority:** accreditation, licensure; and
8. **program or treatment plan:** procedures associated with assessment, planning, implementation, evaluation, and documentation of treatment plan appropriateness.

None of these structural factors alone can guarantee that good service will be given, but they are factors that make good service more likely to occur. As Riley (1991, p. 57) notes: ". . . structure variables measure the probability or propensity for quality care." Without adequate policies and facilities, for example, the process of delivering service is impeded, and outcomes are adversely affected.

## Process

Process refers to the nature and sequence of activities carried out by therapeutic recreation management and practitioners. It usually involves two aspects—the technical and the interpersonal. Process standards assess the performance of specified and, at times, prescribed therapeutic recreation activities. It includes psychosocial interventions such as teaching a skill or leisure counseling, program leadership, formulating an individual treatment plan, assisting in discharge planning and referral, evaluating (e.g., formative and summative) and documenting intervention results as well as contributing to the advancement of therapeutic recreation as a profession through participating in research projects. It also encompasses what is and what is not done, and what should or should not be done. A critical difference between structural and process standards is that process standards require a professional judgment to determine whether a criterion has been met.

There are several ways to collect process data; the most direct is by observation of practitioner activities. Another is self-reporting done by the practitioner. A third source is a review of the chart or records that are kept, and last, various kinds of assessment tools can be used.

Whatever source of data collection is used, some set of objectives is needed as a standard against which to compare the activities. This set of objectives should be specific and measurable such as listing the steps in the development of a treatment plan. The objective is not only to collect valid, appropriate and comprehensive data, but also to collect these data in an efficient, standardized, and error-free manner.

## Outcome

An outcome is the end result of a process and is the product of actions. It refers to the results of the activities in which the practitioners have been involved. The result of a process must be consumer oriented; adequate quality leaves the consumer in a state or condition that is considered desirable. Outcome measures evaluate the efficiency and effectiveness of these activities by answering such questions as:

- Did the service to the consumer improve?
- Is the consumer more independent?
- Were there unexpected or unanticipated consequences to activity participation?

Other consumer outcomes might include rehabilitation potential, functional status, and quality of life including leisure-related knowledge, skills, and awareness. Although outcomes are the end result, they must be analyzed as part of the total picture (i.e., consumers and their environment) (Jennings, 1991).

Whether the questions are general or specific, a major problem in using outcome measures in evaluation is that they are influenced by many factors, not by just one factor or by just one person (e.g., medication, diagnosis, assessments by various staff disciplines, treatment plans, documentation, age of the consumer). Outcomes are particularly sensitive to subjective value judgments. Thus, it is extremely important to determine criteria that indicate if standards are being met and to what degree they are met.

Identifying and measuring all of the direct and indirect factors and their outcomes borders on the impossible. Nevertheless, direct and indirect measures do exist. Three forms of outcome measures are goals and objectives, standards and criteria, and instruments.

*Goals and objectives* are an important measurement device in any organization. Therapeutic recreation departments use goal and objective statements to provide direction and to identify whatever success has been achieved. Therapeutic recreation practitioners traditionally incorporate goals and objectives into the therapeutic recreation process.

The basic principles of outcome measurement rely on well-defined *standards*. Standards are a criterion for judging the work of a practitioner, team, or organization and they vary in their specificity. They supply a basis for comparison. Within an organization they form a consensus of professional thinking. In addition, standards are established and derived from a variety of sources. Managers must determine what standards will be used to measure the quality of therapeutic recreation service, then develop and implement a quality assurance program that can measure end results against the developed standards. Thereafter, managers have the responsibility to monitor the quality of the care or service to the consumer.

The major reason for setting standards is to increase objectivity by defining as clearly as possible what is acceptable and what is not acceptable. In addition, they must be achievable, practical, and flexible. Realistic standards that are achievable lessen the likelihood of frustration, increase the motivation to perform well, and are more ac-

ceptable to staff. Without this approach, the judgments that take place in the evaluation process can be variable, subjective, and susceptible to the biases of the evaluator. The ATRA *Standards for the Practice of Therapeutic Recreation, and Self-Assessment Guide* (1993) and the NTRS *Standards of Practice for Therapeutic Recreation Service and Annotated Bibliography* (1995) are the standards for quality in therapeutic recreation service. They also define the scope and dimensions of professional therapeutic recreation. ATRA (1993) has published a self-assessment guide with its standards. The guide incorporates a rating scale for use by the manager or practitioner in evaluating the various standards. The final score provides information about how well there is compliance with the standards. In addition to the guide, ATRA has developed a "documentation audit" form which focuses on whether or not standards of therapeutic recreation practice are being met. The audit provides the manager or practitioner with a means to determine the quality of services rendered.

The JCAHO has standards that relate directly to therapeutic recreation. A review of the *1996 Comprehensive Accreditation Manual for Hospitals* notes that in the section concerned with Initial Assessment (pp. 106–109), the initial standard refers to the assessment of each patient regarding his or her physical, psychological, and social status. Within this same section reference is made to a functional assessment of recreation therapy needs and social needs for patients referred for rehabilitation services. In another section specifically related to this text, Directing Departments (p. 298), a standard speaks to each department defining in writing the scope of services provided and its approval by the hospital administration. In addition, therapeutic recreation application is also found in the following sections: Reassessment, Care Decisions, Structures Supporting the Assessment of Patients, Planning and Providing Care, Rehabilitation Care and Services, and Additional Requirements for Specific Patient Populations (e.g., those with special needs due to age, disability, and specific characteristics of various patients). Last, the *1996 Standards Manual and Interpretive Guidelines for Medical Rehabilitation and . . . Behavioral Health* (CARF, 1996) makes reference to Therapeutic Recreation, Recreation, Leisure Skills, and Recreational Activities (see also Appendix E).

A second function of standards is to communicate clearly to everyone involved (staff, administrators, consumers, accreditors, and regulators) what level of service is expected in the department. This can be done only if the standards are available to everyone.

The implementation of standards and their measurements for evaluating performance may vary from organization to organization, the purpose of the evaluation, and the evaluator.

There are a variety of *instruments* that can be used to measure outcomes in therapeutic recreation practice. Some of these include Comprehensive Evaluation in Recreational Therapy (CERT)—Psych/Behavioral, Community Integration Program (CIP), and Leisure Step Up[4]. The therapeutic recreation practitioner in a medical rehabilitation setting will undoubtedly use the Uniform Data System for Medical Rehabilitation's Functional Independence Measure (FIM[SM]) (1993) which measures functional competence of the consumer in several areas that are important in rehabilitation and return to the community (see Figure 22.3). The findings can be applied to a treatment plan in association with leisure skills, leisure education and resources, and community reintegration. There are also instruments which are program oriented which involve a

[4]These instruments can be obtained from Idyll Arbor, P. O. Box 720, Ravensdale, WA 98051.

number of disciplines providing service as opposed to a single discipline-oriented instrument.

Further consideration of QA from a therapeutic recreation perspective is found in *Quality Management* edited by Bob Riley (1991) and in *Quality Assurance* by Richelle N. Cunninghis and Elizabeth Best-Martini (1996) as related to activity programs in long-term care facilities.

## Continuous Quality Improvement

With the advent of CQI in healthcare facilities in the early 1990s, QA became integrated into CQI. The major problem with QA was that it looked at the past or what had been delivered, identified areas for improvement, and made changes. In summary, it was retrospective in its approach,

---

### Figure 22.3 Functional Independence Measure (FIM[SM])

**Description of the Levels of Function and their Scores**

**Independent**     Another person is not required for the activity (NO HELPER).

7     **Complete Independence**—All of the tasks described as making up the activity are typically performed safely, without modification, assistive devices, or aids, and within reasonable time.

6     **Modified Independence**—One or more of the following may be true: the activity requires an assistive device; the activity takes more than reasonable time, or there are safety (risk) considerations.

**Dependent**     Subject requires another person for either supervision or physical assistance in order for the activity to be performed, or it is not performed (REQUIRES HELPER).

**Modified Dependence**—The subject expends half (50%) or more of the effort. The levels of assistance required are:

5     **Supervision or Setup**—Subject requires no more help than standby, cueing or coaxing, without physical contact. Or, helper sets up needed items or applies orthoses.

4     **Minimal Contact Assistance**—Subject requires no more help than touching, and expends 75% or more of the effort.

3     **Moderate Assistance**—Subject requires more help than touching, or expends half (50%) or more (up to 75%) of the effort.

**Complete Dependence**—The subject expends less than half (less than 50%) of the effort. Maximal or total assistance is required, or the activity is not performed. The levels of assistance required are:

2     **Maximal Assistance**—Subject expends less than 50% of the effort, but at least 25%.

1     **Total Assistance**—Subject expends less than 25% of the effort.

---

Reprinted with permission of Uniform Data System for Medical Rehabilitation. (1993). *Guide for the uniform data set for medical rehabilitation (Adult FIM[SM]) version 4.0.* Buffalo, NY: State University of New York at Buffalo. Copyright 1993 Uniform Data System for Medical Rehabilitation, a Division of U. B. Foundation Activities, Inc.

placed responsibility for quality on the person, and standards were either met or not met (Kaluzny, McLaughlin, and Simpson, 1944).

However, the implementation of CQI, according to Green (1991), does not preclude the use of QA which may serve as a foundation for the more comprehensive CQI transformation. According to Mayfield (1992), CQI complements and broadens the scope of QA. In many respects, QA can be considered the baseline of service delivery while CQI considers and implements improved service delivery. The integration of QA and CQI provides an opportunity to build upon the best of these two approaches in order to reach the goal of continual improvement in quality (Tindall and Stewart, 1993). There is a fine line that differentiates QA from CQI. The focus for CQI is not on assuring quality but rather on continuously improving the quality of consumer services. The concept is that there is always room for improvement (Peters, 1993). In reality, CQI is concerned with excellence.

CQI, as has been noted, is a movement from the standard definition of quality which looked back at the work already done, to a method of improvement. CQI involves defining and meeting consumer needs that eventually lead to exemplary services (Berwick, 1990). It requires the healthcare facility or any health and human service organization that adopts CQI to demonstrate a consistent endeavor to deliver consumer care and service that is optimal within available resources and consistent with achievable goals. Peters (1993) notes that CQI is concerned with improving QA. She further comments that quality monitoring and evaluation is an ongoing process, ". . . not retroactive and is based on reality, what is actually being done, not what was supposed to be done " (p. 82). In addition, according to Berwick (1990), QA is a specialized staff function while CQI is the primary job of every manager since it involves an organization-wide commitment to excellence. CQI is concerned not only with doing what is good now, but also improving or making it better than what it is. To modify an old adage, "If it ain't broke, it can be improved."

To assist an organization, department, or service, in monitoring and evaluating the quality and appropriateness of care and service, the JCAHO (1993b) developed the following ten-step process:

1. assign responsibility;
2. delineate scope of care;
3. identify important aspects of care;
4. identify indicators related to these aspects of care;
5. establish thresholds for evaluation related to the indicators;
6. collect and organize data;
7. evaluate care when thresholds are reached;
8. take actions to improve care;
9. assess the effectiveness of the actions and document improvement; and
10. communicate relevant information to the organization-wide quality assurance program.

Application of CQI to therapeutic recreation requires a different way of thinking about how to provide services to the consumer. The focus of attention is on the *consumer,* but the *structure, process,* and *outcome* are similar in nature to QA:

- **Consumer.** The term *consumer* (or *customer*) is used to signify the role that a person or unit plays when receiving the service. Consumers, as noted earlier, can be external: meaning the consumer, family, and the general community. Consumers can also be internal; internal consumers are all departments or units that exchange input or output to ensure continuous quality improvement. The therapeutic recreation department is a consumer in the hospital, but it is not the only one. Physicians are consumers for whom the therapeutic recreation department provides input. The therapeutic recreation department is a consumer of the medical records department if the department is requesting information about a patient.
- **Structure.** Structure incorporates all of those resources under which it is likely that good therapeutic recreation service will take place and that good consumer outcomes will occur. However, it does not ensure that consumer goals will be achieved; process and outcome are involved.
- **Process.** Process is the combination of activities, actions, or steps that repeatedly come together to transform input into output or have impact on the consumer. Typically applied to therapeutic recreation service, process tells what the practitioner will do and how—actual interaction between practitioner and consumer or consumer group. While outcomes are the ultimate measure, how one achieves the results or outcomes is extremely important. Process is analogous to a football game. One doesn't score any points looking at the scoreboard. The game is won and lost on the field. The scoreboard only records the outcome. Process focuses on setting standards, determining criteria to meet those standards, data collection, evaluating how well the criteria have been met, making changes based on the evaluation, and following up on change implementation.
- **Outcome.** Outcomes represent the ultimate goal of therapeutic recreation service measurement, for if the consumer outcome is unsatisfactory, it matters little what therapeutic recreation processes were used or what resources (structure) supported the treatment plan. Outcome focuses on the benefit to

the consumer. Benefit refers to a judgment that is made in relation to the values and expectations of the customer relative to the service. Managers have a responsibility to assess and promote consumer satisfaction whenever possible. One must keep in mind that outcome is in the eyes of the beholder. Thus, any study of benefits requires an understanding of and knowledge about the needs and expectations of the consumer. Only when the consumer is involved in the process can therapeutic recreation managers or practitioners truly understand the consumer's point of view. While there are obvious direct care outcomes, there are also behavioral, physiological, and psychosocial outcomes (Batalden, 1993).

To assist in determining better outcomes in association with CQI as well as fiscal responsibility, a tool called *critical paths* was implemented in many healthcare facilities in the late 1980s. Critical paths are a compilation of multidisciplinary input driven by a specific time oriented outcome. According to Heacock and Brobst (1994) critical paths provide an excellent opportunity for recognition, management, and resolution of structure, process, and outcome issues. Petryshen and Petryshen (1993/1994, pp. 111–112) describe the implications of critical paths as follows:

> Identification of critical steps in the management of patient care facilitates consistent treatment leading to discharge within the recommended length of stay. A consistent method of performing care activities is established, and caregivers are provided with advance knowledge of the outcomes toward which they are working, how these outcomes will be attained, and the time frame within which they should be achieved. Furthermore, because an entire course of care is outlined on a single care map, caregivers from all disciplines follow the same plan. A true interdisciplinary approach to care is created and, from an economic perspective, inappropriate, redundant, and excessive use of resources is minimized. As well, standard care plans for case types promote increased productivity through more efficient use of staff since the time required for caregivers to develop individualized plans for patients with similar needs is significantly reduced.

Petryshen and Petryshen (1993/1994) also note that critical paths have therapeutic recreation implications in providing opportunities for program evaluation and research. Specifically, managers and practitioners "will be in a position to make credible decisions, discontinue ineffective routines, and refine practice patterns to the benefit of the patient and the healthcare system" (p. 112).

## Indicators

Associated with QA and CQI are indicators. An indicator is a predetermined (i.e., written) and measurable, well-defined component of an aspect of care or service. Indicators may evaluate the structure, process, or outcome of service although they are more associated with outcome. Currently, JCAHO (1993b) expects every clinical specialty and clinical support service—both inpatient and outpatient—to develop indicators of the quality and appropriateness of care that it provides and to demonstrate that ongoing monitoring of these indicators is taking place. Structural indicators may include staffing, correct use of equipment, and adherence to policies. Processes consist of appropriate assessment of the consumer on admission and documentation of therapeutic recreation service given. The actual results of consumer service are the outcomes which show or reflect achievement or nonachievement of goals.

In developing indicators a few guidelines need to be kept in mind. The guidelines are as follows:

1. Decide whether the indicators should evaluate compliance, appropriateness, or outcome. Compliance refers to procedures found within policies while appropriateness is concerned with the adequacy of service, and outcome is the result of the performance (or nonperformance) of a process.
2. Indicators should be limited to a few important or critical indicators based on standards.
3. Indicators should be stated in positive terms.
4. Indicators should ask for one piece of information. Each point to be addressed should be the subject of a separate indicator.
5. Indicators should be reliable, valid, and tested. Indicators are usually selected from practice standards, policies, protocols, and guidelines. After they are developed, they should be reviewed by others for clarity. The reliability and validity of the indicators should be evaluated.
6. Determine the exceptions, if any, to the indicators. While there should be no exceptions, there may be situations that do develop.
7. Establish the threshold for evaluation. The threshold for evaluation of an indicator is established before the monitoring process begins. When the results are less than hoped for, some type of problem solving is indicated. The projected threshold is the number or percentage established when the monitoring activity is developed or planned. Thresholds are usually expressed by number or

percentage. It is unrealistic to set thresholds for evaluation at 100 percent although the percentage may change after testing.

Figure 22.4 illustrates an example of therapeutic recreation indicators which may form a therapeutic recreation section within a hospital or rehabilitation patient survey or be a separate form distributed to patients by the therapeutic recreation department at the time of discharge. The survey form can be either an open or closed questionnaire. The department would determine the threshold of acceptance. For example, 95 percent of the time consumers would rate each item as good or better.

Examples of other types of indicators might include:

- assessment: complete a leisure assessment of patient leisure abilities within 72 hours after admission to the unit 95 percent of the time;
- program: patient is seen by the therapeutic recreation specialist a minimum of once weekly during hospitalization 95 percent of the time; and
- discharge plan: complete a discharge plan with patient involvement no later than one week prior to discharge 90 percent of the time.

# CQI and Therapeutic Recreation Implementation

Once the hospital has committed to the concept of CQI, the therapeutic recreation department, like other departments in the hospital, must determine what values are important in providing services. Covey (1990) states that these values serve as maps and enable one to know where one is going. Every person and every organization has values that mark their way in life. People see the world through their values. Moreover, values are the motivation of their beliefs and actions and are the energy source of accomplishments. Managing by values is rendering services with personal and organizational values clearly defined. Decisions about future directions to take or about what to do in a given situation can then be based on those values. Thus the therapeutic recreation manager manages by facts (values) and not by intuition.

The values that are important to the therapeutic recreation department are set forth in the mission statement. Quality is determined by the degree to which the department adheres to its mission and those values or how well the department is doing what it set out to do as defined in its mission or purpose.

The next step is quality planning. In quality planning one looks to professional standards which are internal or external quality mechanisms set in place for the purpose of maintaining and/or improving certain aspects of quality. It is also important to note the relevance of identifying customer requirements since professional standards and accreditation standards do not necessarily respond at all times to customer needs. The identification of these needs or requirements can be determined through a variety of qualitative and quantitative approaches (Al-Assaf, 1993).

After the completion of quality planning, organizing quality becomes the next major task. This phase incorporates four parts:

## Figure 22.4 Therapeutic Recreation Survey Form

|  | Circle the number that best represents your feelings | | | | |
|---|---|---|---|---|---|
|  | very poor | poor | fair | good | very good |
| Courtesy of your therapeutic recreation therapist | 1 | 2 | 3 | 4 | 5 |
| Degree to which you were able to participate in setting your therapeutic recreation goals | 1 | 2 | 3 | 4 | 5 |
| How well did the therapeutic recreation specialist explain your treatment and progress | 1 | 2 | 3 | 4 | 5 |
| Adequacy of your therapeutic recreation program | 1 | 2 | 3 | 4 | 5 |
| Availability of recreational activities (e.g., crafts, games, entertainment) | 1 | 2 | 3 | 4 | 5 |
| Helpfulness of the instruction/information given about your postdischarge recreational activities | 1 | 2 | 3 | 4 | 5 |

1. translating the requirements of customers and/or professional standards into operational specifications,
2. selecting process performance measures or key indicators,
3. weighing process performance measures or key indicators, and
4. planning and implementing the proposed solutions.

This approach provides a scientific basis for making decisions.

The last step is evaluating quality using a systems approach with a feedback loop. The quality improvement process itself deals with structure and process while the ultimate improvement hopefully will be reflected in the outcome. Evaluating quality requires evaluating outcome of the implemented therapeutic recreation treatment plan. It is essential to monitor both process and outcome indicators to determine whether the plan is successful or unsuccessful. If the latter, a different plan with reevaluation and additional follow-up becomes necessary. On the other hand, the difference between successful and unsuccessful outcomes may just be a matter of how CQI is approached since the approach may vary from organization to organization. In evaluating quality it is also important that the therapeutic recreation manager and his or her staff evaluate their effectiveness—both their success and areas that need further improvement. Motivating the staff to participate in the total quality evaluating process may be the toughest part of the manager's job, but if staff are able to get motivated, the benefits will certainly make the effort worthwhile.

An example of a therapeutic recreation department quality assurance plan within a medical rehabilitation center is shown in Figure 22.5 (page 332). It was developed by the authors in association with Angie Anderson, Director, Recreation Therapy, Younker Rehabilitation, Iowa Methodist Medical Center, Des Moines, Iowa. The reader is reminded that such a plan will vary from setting to setting and even among like units depending upon the diagnostic groups being served.

Figure 22.6 (page 334) provides an example of a quality assurance program evaluation tool used in a therapeutic recreation unit within a community-based leisure service agency. The tool collects data for objective evaluation relative to improving services in various areas associated with quality management in the unit. Once standards have been developed, as noted earlier, consideration is given to setting up a system to evaluate whether standards are being met. It is important that the measurement form be used in a systematic way. Further, one needs to determine who will evaluate what at what times. Answers to these questions must be based on the organization's needs.

To summarize, CQI consists of four basic elements. The first of these elements is *teamwork*. A team approach

is essential to effective CQI, especially the ability to function as part of an interdisciplinary team in which each discipline is accorded recognition for its contribution to consumer care and service. *Consumer participation* is the next element. In the past, the consumer's point of view was often omitted. Today, both consumer outcomes and consumer satisfaction are considered. The third and perhaps most essential element of measurement is that of *work processes*. This includes both baseline measures and measures after changes have been instituted. The data collection and evaluation are as objective as possible. The final element is the adequacy of the resources available to support improvement. This ranges from administrative support for any changes indicated to adequate staff, adequate equipment, and so forth.

In conclusion, TQM is concerned with preventing problems in the healthcare delivery by creating the attitudes and controls that make prevention possible. TQM is a systematic way of guaranteeing that organized activities happen the way they are planned, or "doing the right thing right the first time" (Roster, 1990, p. 18). TQM is a prospective, proactive approach that involves each employee and reaches into every corner of a healthcare facility. At the same time, according to Richard C. Craven, administrator of Sheltering Arms Physical Rehabilitation Hospital in Richmond, Virginia, "in the race for quality there is no finish line" (Craven, 1995, p. 4).

Those interested in learning and understanding more about TQM may want to read the works of Dr. Joseph M. Juran (1989), Dr. W. Edwards Deming (1986), Philip B. Crosby (1986), and Armand Feigenbaum (1983). These individuals are considered "gurus" of TQM with Deming and Juran the patriarchs. In addition, McLaughlin and Kaluzny's (1994) *Continuous Quality Improvement in Healthcare* presents an interdisciplinary perspective on TQM and CQI in healthcare, taking into account a number of disciplines as well as operations management, organizational behavior, health services research, and information systems and CQI.

# Summary

This chapter focused initially on understanding TQM and CQI and its characteristics including the Deming cycle in health and human service organizations particularly healthcare facilities. Since the early 1990s, TQM has been used to identify an innovative management philosophy which focuses on quality service and is applied throughout many health and human service organizations today. TQM is *process* driven and consumer *outcome* oriented. With the advent of TQM came CQI which replaced QA. CQI is concerned with continuous service improvement to increase customer satisfaction while QA is retrospective in its approach to service improvement. However, QA can serve

## Figure 22.5 Therapeutic Recreation Department Quality Assurance Plan

I. **Purpose and Intent**
   The Therapeutic Recreation Department of Sullivan Medical Center (SMC) will monitor and evaluate the therapeutic recreation provided to patients to assure the patients, medical staff, and community that the services are of high quality, are appropriate to patient needs, are provided in a timely manner, are rendered in accordance with professional standards of practice, and are provided in a safe manner and appropriate setting to minimize patient risk.

II. **Objectives**
   The objectives of the therapeutic recreation review function include the following:
   A. To establish, maintain, and document an ongoing, systematic monitoring and evaluating process for the services provided to patients.
   B. To identify patterns of practice and utilization that need further investigation and review to improve the scope of service.
   C. To develop and approve policies and procedures for providing therapeutic recreation.
   D. To ensure patient safety and minimize medical center liability through protection of patient rights and in an environment that assures adequate safety to minimize patient risk.
   E. To establish an objective, timely, criteria-based peer review process.
   F. To assess the timeliness and appropriateness of the treatment plan.

III. **Plan Elements**
   The therapeutic recreation review will be performed in accordance with the following activities and functions:
   A. Authority and Responsibility for the Therapeutic Recreation Service Components.
      The Therapeutic Recreation Director at SMC is responsible for conducting the review of care provided by members of the Therapeutic Recreation Department. This authority is delegated to the Department by the Hospital Administrator of SMC. The patient services provided by the individual employee are specified in the employee job description and are compatible with the employee's required certification.
   B. Scope of Recreation Therapy Service.
      The Therapeutic Recreation Department's scope of care at SMC includes the following elements:
      1. Level of care:
         a. inpatient, outpatient, outreach;
         b. adults, pediatrics; and
         c. special units: interdisciplinary small group approaches treatment.
      2. Providers of patient services are certified therapeutic recreation specialists (CTRS) and trained volunteers.
      3. Approval of policies and procedures for assessment and treatment.
      4. Review of appropriateness of care provided.
      5. Review of process for care provided (includes timeliness and protocol compliance).
      6. Review of patient outcomes.
      7. Review of high risk situations.
      8. Review of high volume diagnoses and procedures.
   C. Aspects of Care.

| High Volume Services: | 1. Assessment of patient abilities. |
| | 2. Individualized and group activities for patients (enhance leisure life style). |
| High Risk Services | 1. Out trips for head trauma patients. |
| | 2. CVA. |
| | 3. Pet Therapy. |
| | 4. Cooking activities. |
| Low Volume Services Which Are High Risk: | 1. None. |
| Incidents Reported to Risk Management Department: | 1. Patient falls. |
| New Procedures and/or Equipment: | 1. One-on-one, one-half-hour sessions in therapeutic recreation during stay. |
| | 2. Interdisciplinary team modalities with two or more departments (speech, social group, patient recreational, functional outings). |
| | 3. Small group cognitive training. |
| | 4. Interdisciplinary team in-service—new approaches. |

## Figure 22.5 Continued

Infection Control Problems:   1. None.

Department Problems to
Be Monitored:
1. Patients not available to participate.
2. Scheduling patient for initial assessment around all other programs and departments.

High Volume Patients:
1. CVA.
2. Spinal cord.
3. Head injury.
4. Powell-3 substance abuse.

D. Criteria and Threshold

The Therapeutic Recreation Department will develop and approve criteria for each aspect of care that is monitored. The criteria are measurable, objective, valid, and relevant to current standards of care. Criteria are selected from three types:

1. Structure—assess resources, equipment, and staffing compared with needs.
2. Process—assess compliance to protocols, standards of care, and indications for treatment.
3. Outcomes—assess complications, adverse drug effects, patient recovery/client satisfaction.

Each criteria is accompanied by a threshold of acceptable compliance. This is a preestablished level of performance. The threshold can be a percentage, a ratio, or a number of occurrences.

## IV. MONITORING PROCESS

Rehabilitation review will be performed on a monthly basis and reported to the Therapeutic Recreation Department and the Continuous Quality Improvement (CQI) Committee quarterly. Initial screening will be performed on a concurrent and retrospective basis by the Therapeutic Recreation Director using the approved criteria. The screening will include a representative sample of the population. The number of cases is dependent on the volume of patients or treatments for the topics being monitored. If occurrence screening is used, each variance from the standard will be reviewed. Those cases not meeting screening criteria will be examined to determine if a problem or an opportunity exists to improve patient care. Variances are also examined to determine if a pattern exists.

If a problem is identified, it is referred to the staff therapists and administrative staff for corrective action. Corrective actions include the following:

A. Staff education.
B. Development of policies and procedures.
C. Counseling of staff.
D. Repair/replacement of equipment.
E. Request additional staff, equipment.
F. Changes in services provided.
G. Disciplinary action.
H. Monitoring for improved employee performance.
I. Communication of results to other departments and medical staff.
J. Other appropriate corrective action(s).

A follow up monitor is planned for any topic in which a problem is identified.

## V. Reporting and Integration

The results of quality assessment monitoring will be reported to the CQI office for review by the CQI Committee. The report will include the purpose, sample size, criteria, threshold of compliance, actual compliance, narrative findings, conclusions, actions, and effectiveness of actions taken.

If a multidisciplinary monitor is conducted, the results will be shared with each department involved. Results of department monitors will be shared with the appropriate members of the Therapeutic Recreation Department, and appropriate Medical Staff Sections, if applicable. The information will be distributed by the Therapeutic Recreation Director.

## VI. Annual Review

As part of the Therapeutic Recreation Department CQI program, the department's CQI plan, aspects of care, policies, and procedures will be examined and evaluated annually. Necessary revisions will be recommended, approved, and implemented.

**Plan Created:**    **March 1993**
**Plan Reviewed:**   **April 1996**

**e 22.6  Quality Assurance Evaluation**

### City of Los Angeles Department of Recreation and Parks
### Quality Assurance Program Analysis Evaluation
### (Valley Adaptive Unit)

Evaluator's Name _____

Evaluator's Name _____          Date of Annual Review _____

#### PROGRAM

___ Yes ___ No ___ Incomplete  1.  There is a current written program description.

___ Yes ___ No ___ Incomplete  2.  Program content is determined by program management and staff on a basis of program philosophy and the needs of the client.

___ Yes ___ No ___ Incomplete  3.  Particular program content offered by the program is specified in writing.

___ Yes ___ No ___ Incomplete  4.  Program content area includes one or more of the following skill areas: self-advocacy, employment, community integration, and self-care.

___ Yes ___ No ___ Incomplete  5.  Client to staff ratios are met, as well as state, local and federal qualifications.

___ Yes ___ No ___ Incomplete  6.  Program has written entrance and exit criteria definitions characteristic of clients served.

___ Yes ___ No ___ Incomplete  7.  The entrance and exit criteria are measurable.

___ Yes ___ No ___ Incomplete  8.  Program activities that occur in natural environments allow for maximum independence and productivity for clients.

Comments: _____
_____
_____
_____
_____

Items checked No or Incomplete in this section are to be completed by_____

#### SOCIAL INTEGRATION

___ Yes ___ No ___ Incomplete  1.  The program design includes a sequence and timing of activities that reflect, as much as possible, a "normal" day of adults without disabilities.

___ Yes ___ No ___ Incomplete  2.  Buildings and other facilities utilized by the program are similar in appearance and location to educational and business entities commonly patronized by the general public.

___ Yes ___ No ___ Incomplete  3.  Participation in community activities and resources for training and integration purposes take place in small groups (two or four persons per staff).

___ Yes ___ No ___ Incomplete  4.  Clients are taught basic skills and given opportunities to practice these skills as much as possible in natural environments.

___ Yes ___ No ___ Incomplete  5.  Clients have opportunities to engage in planned formal and informal interaction with nonhandicapped peers.

Comments: _____
_____
_____
_____

Items checked No or Incomplete in this section are to be completed by_____

#### INDIVIDUAL SERVICE PLAN

___ Yes ___ No ___ Incomplete  1.  The individual service plan (ISP) specifies functional and appropriate goals and objectives as agreed upon by the client, guardian, parent, conservator or Regional Center Case Worker and program staff.

## Figure 22.6 Continued

___ Yes ___ No ___ Incomplete   2. The ISP is reviewed and revised as needed according to the vendoring regional center standards, at least annually and the date for review is specified.

___ Yes ___ No ___ Incomplete   3. The ISP clearly indicates the persons participating in its development and meeting.

___ Yes ___ No ___ Incomplete   4. Goals and objectives are stated in measurable terms and in language that can be readily understood by most readers.

Comments: _____
_____
_____
_____

Items checked No or Incomplete in this section are to be completed by _____

### STAFF TRAINING

___ Yes ___ No ___ Incomplete   1. The program has a written plan for all employees that meets licensing and regional center requirements.

___ Yes ___ No ___ Incomplete   2. There is an orientation for all new employees.

___ Yes ___ No ___ Incomplete   3. There is ongoing training for all levels of staff.

___ Yes ___ No ___ Incomplete   4. There is a written job description for all staff.

Comments: _____
_____
_____
_____

Items checked No or Incomplete in this section are to be completed by _____

### CLIENT RECORDS

___ Yes ___ No ___ Incomplete   1. Client records are centrally maintained, except for community records which are secured with training staff.

___ Yes ___ No ___ Incomplete   2. Client records contain pertinent information which include, but are not limited to the following:

   ___ Yes ___ No ___ Incomplete    a. Admission agreement

   ___ Yes ___ No ___ Incomplete    b. Current medical information

   ___ Yes ___ No ___ Incomplete    c. Proof of TB clearance

   ___ Yes ___ No ___ Incomplete    d. Psychological data

   ___ Yes ___ No ___ Incomplete    e. Consents for emergency medical treatment

   ___ Yes ___ No ___ Incomplete    f. Personal rights

   ___ Yes ___ No ___ Incomplete    g. ISP—Individual Service Plan

   ___ Yes ___ No ___ Incomplete    h. Up-to-date emergency and personal information

   ___ Yes ___ No ___ Incomplete    i. Funding authorization

   ___ Yes ___ No ___ Incomplete    j. ISP documentation

   ___ Yes ___ No ___ Incomplete    k. _____

Comments: _____
_____
_____
_____

Items Checked No or Incomplete in this section are to be completed by _____

*Figure continues on page 336*

## Figure 22.6 Continued

### ADMINISTRATION

___ Yes ___ No ___ Incomplete   1. Program maintains adequate liability insurance coverage.
___ Yes ___ No ___ Incomplete   2. Program maintains personnel policies, procedures and records.
___ Yes ___ No ___ Incomplete   3. Program provides access on announced or unannounced basis, to regional center or other monitors designated by regional center.

Comments: _____
_____
_____
_____

Items checked No or Incomplete in this section are to be completed by _____

### FACILITY

___ Yes ___ No ___ Incomplete   1. The program's physical surroundings are suitable and safe for the individuals being served.
___ Yes ___ No ___ Incomplete   2. There is a posted disaster plan.
___ Yes ___ No ___ Incomplete   3. Facility is clean and adequately maintained per licensing standards.
___ Yes ___ No ___ Incomplete   4. Complete first-aid kit is provided per basic licensing standards.
___ Yes ___ No ___ Incomplete   5. License is current and posted.
___ Yes ___ No ___ Incomplete   6. Clients' rights are posted.
___ Yes ___ No ___ Incomplete   7. Grievance procedure is posted.
___ Yes ___ No ___ Incomplete   8. Consent for the release of information about an individual is:
       a. Obtained prior to the release of information.
       b. Specific information to be released and person or agency to whom the information can be released is indicated and signed by the individual, guardian, parent or conservator.

Comments: _____
_____
_____
_____

Items checked No or Incomplete in this section are to be completed by _____

Overall Summary: _____
_____
_____
_____

Reviewed by Evaluators with the following staff:

       _____
       _____
       _____

Date: _____

OFFICE USE ONLY:
Items requiring attention were completed and signed off by

Date: _____

as a baseline for CQI. Consideration was also given to defining quality from various perspectives—consumer, standards, and organization. Thereafter, the concepts of QA and CQI were compared in relation to structure, process, and outcomes in association with therapeutic recreation service. The function of critical paths and indicators to improve quality service was noted. This chapter concluded by giving attention to the steps involved in the implementation of therapeutic recreation service as part of CQI.

# Discussion Questions

1. What do you think a therapeutic recreation manager can do to increase the likelihood that the department successfully satisfies its consumers?
2. How can a therapeutic recreation manager determine a program or its services' effectiveness? Its efficiency?
3. Interview therapeutic recreation managers in various settings regarding how they measure the quality of their services. Compare results and discuss.
4. Why do you think the newer approach to quality assurance is called continuous quality improvement? How does it differ from the more traditional approach?
5. Generate examples of structure, process, and outcome indicators.
6. Discuss the differences and interrelations among risk management, quality assurance, and TQM and CQI initiatives.
7. Describe the therapeutic recreation manager's role in total quality management within a healthcare facility or a community-based leisure service agency.

# References

Al-Assaf, A. F. (1993). Data management for total quality. In A. F. Al-Assaf and J. A. Schmele (Eds.), *The textbook of total quality in healthcare* (pp. 123–156). Delray Beach, FL: Saint Lucie Press.

Albrecht, K. (1992). *The only thing that matters.* New York, NY: Harper Business.

American College of Surgeons. (1946). *Bulletin, 21*(4).

American Therapeutic Recreation Association (ATRA). (1993). *Standards for the practice of therapeutic recreation, and self-assessment guide.* Hattiesburg, MS: Author.

Batalden, P. B. (1993). Organization-wide quality improvement in health. In A. F. Al-Assaf and J. A. Schmele (Eds.), *The textbook of total quality in healthcare* (pp. 60–74). Delray Beach, FL: Saint Lucie Press.

Berwick, D. M. (1990). Quality: How do QI and QA differ? Expert illustrates the answer. *Hospital Management Review, 9,* 2–13.

*Business Week.* (1991, October 25). The quality imperative. [Special Issue]

CARF . . . The Rehabilitation Accreditation Commission. (1996). *1996 standards manual and interpretative guidelines for behavioral health, . . . for employment and community support services, and . . . for medical rehabilitation.* Tucson, AZ: Author.

Carr, D., and Littman, I. (1990). *Excellence in government—Total quality management in the 1990s.* Arlington, VA: Coopers and Lybrand.

Covey, S. R. (1990). *The seven habits of highly effective people.* New York, NY: Simon & Schuster.

Craven, B. C. (1995, June). Quality efforts yield reward. *QM,* 1–4.

Crosby, P. B. (1986). *Quality is free: The art of making quality certain.* New York, NY: McGraw-Hill.

Cunninghis, R. N., and Best-Martini, E. (1996). *Quality assurance* (2nd ed.) Ravensdale, WA: Idyll Arbor, Inc.

Deming, W. D. (1986). *Out of the crisis.* Cambridge, MA: MIT Center for Advanced Engineering Study.

Donabedian, A. A. (1969). *A guide to medical care administration, II: Medical care appraisal—Quality & utilization.* New York, NY: American Public Health Association.

Feigenbaum, A. (1983). *Total quality control* (3rd ed.) New York, NY: McGraw-Hill.

Green, D. (1991). Quality improvement versus quality assurance. *Topics in Health Records Management, 11,* 58–70.

Heacock, D., and Brobst, R. A. (1994). A multidisciplinary approach to critical path development: A valuable CQI tool. *Journal of Nursing Care Quality, 8*(4), 38–41.

Jennings, B. M. (1991). Patient outcomes research: Seizing the opportunity. *Advances in Nursing Science, 14*(2), 59–72.

Joint Commission on Accreditation of Healthcare Organizations (JCAHO). (1995). *1996 comprehensive accreditation manual for hospitals.* Oakbrook Terrace, IL: Author.

Joint Commission on Accreditation of Healthcare Organizations (JCAHO). (1993a). *1994 accreditation for hospitals* (Vol. 1). Oakbrook Terrace, IL: Author.

Joint Commission on Accreditation of Healthcare Organizations (JCAHO). (1993b). *The measurement mandate.* Oakbrook Terrace, IL: Author.

Juran, J. (1989). *Juran on leadership for quality: An executive handbook.* New York, NY: The Free Press.

Kaluzny, A. D., and McLaughlin, C. P. (1994). Managing transitions: Assuring the adoption and impact of TQM. In C. P. McLaughlin and A. D. Kaluzny (Eds.), *Continuous quality improvement in healthcare* (pp. 198–206). Gaithersburg, MD: Aspen Publishers, Inc.

Kaluzny, A. D., McLaughlin, C. P., and Jaeger, B. J. (1994). TQM as a managerial innovation: Research issues and implication. In C. P. McLaughlin and A. D. Kaluzny (Eds.), *Continuous quality improvement in healthcare* (pp. 301–314). Gaithersburg, MD: Aspen Publishers, Inc.

La Vallee, R., and McLaughlin, C. P. (1994). Teams at the core. In C. P. McLaughlin and A. D. Kaluzny (Eds.), *Continuous quality improvement in healthcare* (pp. 127–147). Gaithersburg, MD: Aspen Publishers, Inc.

Macintyre, K., and Kleman, C. C. (1994). Measuring customer satisfaction. In C. P. McLaughlin and A. D. Kaluzny (Eds.), *Continuous quality improvement in healthcare* (pp. 102–126). Gaithersburg, MD: Aspen Publishers, Inc.

Martin, L. L. (1993). *Total quality management in health services organization.* Newbury Park, CA: Sage Publications, Inc.

Mayfield, S. (1992). Quality assurance and continuous quality improvement. In R. M. Winslow and K. J. Halberg (Eds.), *The management of therapeutic recreation service* (pp. 137–162.). Arlington, VA: National Recreation and Park Association

McCabe, W. J. (1993, April). Total quality management in a hospital. *Quality Review Bulletin, 8:4,* 134–140.

McLaughlin, C. P., and Kaluzny, A. D. (Eds.). (1994). *Continuous quality improvement in healthcare.* Gaithersburg, MD: Aspen Publishers, Inc.

McLaughlin, C. P., and Kaluzny, A. D. (1994). Defining total management/continuous quality improvement. In C. P. McLaughlin and A. D. Kaluzny (Eds.), *Continuous quality improvement in healthcare* (pp. 3–10). Gaithersburg, MD: Aspen Publishers, Inc.

Milakovich, M. (1990). Total quality management for public sector productivity improvement. *Public Productivity and Management Review, 14,* 19–32.

National Therapeutic Recreation Society (NTRS). (1995). *Standards of practice for therapeutic recreation society and annotated bibliography.* Arlington, VA: National Recreation and Park Association.

O'Leary, T. (1993). Defining performance of organizations. *Journal of Quality Improvement, 19:7,* 218–223.

Peters, D. A. (1993). A new look for quality in home care. In D. F. Al-Assaf and J. A. Schmele (Eds.), *The textbook of total quality in healthcare* (pp. 80–90). Delray Beach, FL: Saint Lucie Press.

Petryshen, P. M., and Petryshen, P. R. (1993/1994). Managed care: Shaping the delivery of healthcare and creating an expanded role for the caregiver. *Annual in Therapeutic Recreation,* 108–114.

Rhodes, M. (1991). The use of patient satisfaction data as an outcome monitor in therapeutic recreation quality assurance. In B. Riley (Ed.), *Quality management: Appreciation for therapeutic recreation* (pp. 83–106). State College, PA: Venture Publishing, Inc.

Riley, B. (Ed.). (1991). *Quality management: Applications for therapeutic recreation.* State College, PA: Venture Publishing, Inc.

Rosen, A. (1994, December). Continuous quality improvement: Principles and techniques. *The Journal of Practical Nursing, 44:4,* 24–36.

Rosenberg, C. E. (1987). *The care of strangers.* New York, NY: Basic Books, Inc.

Roster, S. L. (1990, September/October). Total quality improvement. *Journal of Quality Assurance, 12:4,* 217–223.

Scalenghe, R. (1994). *In introduction to the JCAHO.* Presentation at the National Therapeutic Recreation Institute. Minneapolis, MN, October 13.

Smith, G. B., and Hakill, E. (1994). Quality work improvement groups: From paper to reality. *Journal of Nursing Care Quality, 8:4,* 1–12.

Tindill, B. S., and Steward, D. W. (1993). Integration of total quality and quality assurance. In A. F. Al-Assaf and J. A. Schmele (Eds.), *The textbook of total quality in healthcare* (pp. 209–220). Delray Beach, FL: Saint Lucie Press.

Toppel, A. H., Beach, B. A., and Hutchinson-Troyer, L. (1991). Standards: A tool for accountability the CARF process. *Annual in Therapeutic Recreation, 2,* 96–98.

Uniform Data System for Medical Rehabilitation. (1993). *Guide for the uniform data set for medical rehabilitation (Adult FIM$^{SM}$) version 4.0.* Buffalo, NY: State University of New York at Buffalo.

# *Appendix A*

# National Therapeutic Recreation Society Code of Ethics

## (Revised, 1990)

## Preamble

Leisure, recreation, and play are inherent aspects of the human experience, and are essential to health and well-being. All people, therefore, have an inalienable right to leisure and the opportunities it affords for play and recreation. Some human beings have disabilities, illnesses, or social conditions which may limit their participation in the normative structure of society. These persons have the same need for and right to leisure, recreation, and play.

Accordingly, the purpose of therapeutic recreation is to facilitate leisure, recreation, and play for persons with physical, mental, emotional or social limitations in order to promote their health and well-being. This goal is accomplished through professional services delivered in clinical and community settings. Services are intended to develop skills and knowledge, to foster values and attitudes, and to maximize independence by decreasing barriers and by increasing ability and opportunity.

The National Therapeutic Recreation Society (NTRS) exists to promote the development of therapeutic recreation in order to ensure quality services and to protect and promote the rights of persons receiving services. NTRS and its members are morally obligated to contribute to the health and well-being of the people they serve. In order to meet this important social responsibility, NTRS and its members endorse and practice the following ethical principles.

## I. The Obligation of Professional Virtue

Professionals possess and practice the virtues of integrity, honesty, fairness, competence, diligence, and self-awareness.

A. **Integrity:** Professionals act in ways that protect, preserve and promote the soundness and completeness of their commitment to service. Professionals do not forsake nor arbitrarily compromise their principles. They strive for unity, firmness, and consistency of character. Professionals exhibit personal and professional qualities conducive to the highest ideals of human service.

B. **Honesty:** Professionals are truthful. They do not misrepresent themselves, their knowledge, their abilities, or their profession. Their communications are sufficiently complete, accurate, and clear in order for individuals to understand the intent and implications of services.

C. **Fairness:** Professionals are just. They do not place individuals at unwarranted advantage or disadvantage. They distribute resources and services according to principles of equity.

D. **Competence:** Professionals function to the best of their knowledge and skill. They only render services and employ techniques of which they are

Approved by the NTRS Board of Directors in 1990. The National Therapeutic Recreation Society is a branch of the National Recreation and Park Association, 2775 South Quincy Street, Suite 300 Arlington, Virginia 22206–2204, (703) 820-4940, fax (703) 671-6772.

qualified by training and experience. They recognize their limitations, and seek to reduce them by expanding their expertise. Professionals continuously enhance their knowledge and skills through education and by remaining informed of professional and social trends, issues and developments.

E. **Diligence:** Professionals are earnest and conscientious. Their time, energy, and professional resources are efficiently used to meet the needs of the persons they serve.

F. **Awareness:** Professionals are aware of how their personal needs, desires, values, and interests may influence their professional actions. They are especially cognizant of where their personal needs may interfere with the needs of the persons they serve.

## II. The Obligation of the Professional to the Individual

A. **Well-Being:** Professionals' foremost concern is the well-being of the people they serve. They do everything reasonable in their power and within the scope of professional practice to benefit them. Above all, professionals cause no harm.

B. **Loyalty:** Professionals' first loyalty is to the well-being of the individual they serve. In instances of multiple loyalties, professionals make the nature and the priority of their loyalties explicit to everyone concerned, especially where they may be in question or in conflict.

C. **Respect:** Professionals respect the people they serve. They show regard for their intrinsic worth and for their potential to grow and change. The following areas of respect merit special attention:

   1. **Freedom, Autonomy, and Self-Determination:** Professionals respect the ability of people to make, execute, and take responsibility for their own choices. Individuals are given adequate opportunity for self-determination in the least restrictive environment possible. Individuals have the right of informed consent. They may refuse participation in any program except where their welfare is clearly and immediately threatened and where they are unable to make rational decisions on their own due to temporary or permanent incapacity. Professionals promote independence and avoid fostering dependence. In particular, sexual relations and other manipulative behaviors intended to control individuals for the personal needs of the professional are expressly unethical.

   2. **Privacy:** Professionals respect the privacy of individuals. Communications are kept confidential except with the explicit consent of the individual or where the welfare of the individual or others is clearly imperiled. Individuals are informed of the nature and the scope of confidentiality.

D. **Professional Practices:** Professionals provide quality services based on the highest professional standards. Professionals abide by standards set by the profession, deviating only when justified by the needs of the individual. Care is used in administering tests and other measurement instruments. They are used only for their express purposes. Instruments should conform to accepted psychometric standards. The nature of all practices, including tests and measurements, are explained to individuals. Individuals are also debriefed on the results and the implications of professional practices. All professional practices are conducted with the safety and well-being of the individual in mind.

## III. The Obligation of the Professional to Other Individuals and to Society

A. **General Welfare:** Professionals make certain that their actions do not harm others. They also seek to promote the general welfare of society by advocating the importance of leisure, recreation, and play.

B. **Fairness:** Professionals are fair to other individuals and to the general public. They seek to balance the needs of the individuals they serve with the needs of other persons according to principles of equity.

## IV. The Obligation of the Professional to Colleagues

A. **Respect:** Professionals show respect for colleagues and their respective professions. They take no action that undermines the integrity of their colleagues.

B. **Cooperation and Support:** Professionals cooperate with and support their colleagues for the benefit of the persons they serve. Professionals demand the highest professional and moral conduct of each other. They approach and offer help to colleagues who require assistance with an ethical problem. Professionals take appropriate action toward colleagues who behave unethically.

# V. The Obligation of the Professional to the Profession

A. **Knowledge:** Professionals work to increase and improve the profession's body of knowledge by supporting and/or by conducting research. Research is practiced according to accepted canons and ethics of scientific inquiry. Where subjects are involved, their welfare is paramount. Prior permission is gained from subjects to participate in research. They are informed of the general nature of the research and any specific risks that may be involved. Subjects are debriefed at the conclusion of the research, and are provided with results of the study on request.

B. **Respect:** Professionals treat the profession with critical respect. They strive to protect, preserve, and promote the integrity of the profession and its commitment to public service.

C. **Reform:** Professionals are committed to regular and continuous evaluation of the profession. Changes are implemented that improve the profession's ability to serve society.

# VI. The Obligation of the Profession to Society

A. **Service:** The profession exists to serve society. All of its activities and resource are devoted to the principle of service.

B. **Equality:** The profession is committed to equality of opportunity. No person shall be refused service because of race, gender, religion, social status, ethnic background, sexual orientation, or inability to pay. The profession neither conducts nor condones discriminatory practices. It actively seeks to correct inequities that unjustly discriminate.

C. **Advocacy:** The profession advocates for the people it is entrusted to serve. It protects and promotes their health and well-being and their inalienable right to leisure, recreation, and play in clinical and community settings.

# American Therapeutic Recreation Association Code of Ethics

Therapeutic recreation is the provision of treatment services and the provision of recreation services to persons with illnesses or disabling conditions. The primary purposes of treatment services which are often referred to as recreational therapy are to restore, remediate or rehabilitate in order to improve functioning and independence, as well as reduce or eliminate the effects of illness or disability. The primary purposes of recreation services are to provide recreation resources and opportunities in order to improve health and well-being. Therapeutic recreation is provided by professionals who are trained and certified, registered and/or licensed to provide therapeutic recreation.

The American Therapeutic Recreation Association (ATRA) acts as an advocate for members of the therapeutic recreation profession and consumers. ATRA's objectives include:

- to promote and advance public awareness and understanding of therapeutic recreation;
- to develop and promote professional standards for therapeutic recreation services with education, habilitation, rehabilitation, and medical treatment of individuals in need of services;
- to support and conduct research and demonstration efforts to improve service; and
- to support and conduct educational opportunities for therapeutic recreation professionals.

ATRA's Code of Ethics is intended to be used as a guide for promoting and maintaining the highest standards of ethical behavior. The code applies to all therapeutic recreation personnel. The term therapeutic recreation personnel includes certified therapeutic recreation specialists (CTRS), certified therapeutic recreation assistants (CTRA) and therapeutic recreation students. Acceptance of membership in ATRA commits a member to adherence to these principles.

## Principle 1: Beneficence/ Nonmaleficence

Therapeutic recreation personnel shall treat persons in an ethical manner not only by respecting their decisions and protecting them from harm but also by actively making efforts to secure their well-being. Personnel strive to maximize possible benefits, and minimize possible harms. This serves as the guiding principle for the profession. The term *persons* includes not only persons served but colleagues, agencies and the profession.

## Principle 2: Autonomy

Therapeutic recreation personnel have a duty to preserve and protect the right of each individual to make his or her own choices. Each individual is to be given the opportunity to determine his or her own course of action in accordance with a plan freely chosen.

March 1990  (Special thanks to Dr. Mary Ann Keogh Hoss, CTRS, and Ms. Sharon Nichols, CTRS.)

# Principle 3: Justice

Therapeutic recreation personnel are responsible for ensuring that individuals are served fairly and that there is equity in the distribution of services. Individuals receive service without regard to race, color, creed, sex, age, disability, disease, and social and financial status.

# Principle 4: Fidelity

Therapeutic recreation personnel have an obligation to be truthful, faithful and meet commitments made to persons receiving services, colleagues, agencies and the profession.

# Principle 5: Veracity/ Informed Consent

Therapeutic recreation personnel are responsible for providing each individual receiving service with information regarding the service and the professional's training and credentials; benefits, outcomes, length of treatment, expected activities, risks, limitations. Each individual receiving service has the right to know what is likely to take place during and as a result of professional intervention. Informed consent is obtained when information is provided by the professional.

# Principle 6: Confidentiality and Privacy

Therapeutic recreation personnel are responsible for safeguarding information about individuals served. Individuals served have the right to control information about themselves. When a situation arises that requires disclosure of confidential information about an individual to protect the individual's welfare or the interest of others, the therapeutic recreation professional has the responsibility and obligation to inform the individual served of the circumstances in which confidentiality was broken.

# Principle 7: Competence

Therapeutic recreation personnel have the responsibility to continually seek to expand their knowledge base related to therapeutic recreation practice. The professional is responsible for keeping a record of participation in training activities. The professional has the responsibility for contributing to changes in the profession through activities such as research, dissemination of information through publications and professional presentations, and through active involvement in professional organizations.

# Principle 8: Compliance with Laws and Regulations

Therapeutic recreation personnel are responsible for complying with local, state and federal laws and ATRA policies governing the profession of therapeutic recreation.

# Appendix B

# National Council for Therapeutic Recreation Certification, Inc.: The Nationally Recognized Certification Program for Recreational Therapists and Therapeutic Recreation Personnel

The field of recreational therapy has had a national credentialing plan for 40 years. The National Council for Therapeutic Recreation Certification, Inc. (NCTRC) is currently the recognized national credentialing body for recreational therapists. NCTRC provides a quality program for therapeutic recreation professionals and has gained national recognition by attaining accreditation from the National Commission of Certifying Agencies, NCTRC's certification program provides a valid and reliable method for identifying qualified recreational therapists.

NCTRC was founded as a nonprofit organization in 1981. NCTRC's mission is to protect the consumer of therapeutic recreation services by promoting the provision of quality services offered by the NCTRC certificants. By 1995, it had credentialed over 13,600 active therapeutic recreation professionals.

The professional level of certification requires a baccalaureate degree or higher, passing a national standardized certification exam, and leads to the award of the Certified Therapeutic Recreation Specialist® (CTRS®) certificate. There are three sets of standards that govern certification as a professional with NCTRC: (a) entry-level or initial certification standards, (b) conduct standards, and (c) recertification standards. Together these three sets of standards govern the expectation of professional knowledge, skills, and conduct that are expected as minimum competence for a professional recreational therapist.

Entry-level or initial certification standards include education and experience requirements and the passing of a national certification exam to be awarded the certification. Conduct standards govern and monitor certain professional behaviors to assure the public health and safety of the consumer as recipient of therapeutic recreation services. Recertification standards must be met every five years by the CTRS to show continued professional competence. All NCTRC standards are defined based on the analysis of the role and function of the CTRS on the job or in practice from the National Job Analysis Study which was conducted by NCTRC and Educational Testing Service (ETS). The NCTRC certification program is therefore tied directly to research from the field on the knowledge and skills necessary for competent practice in recreational therapy.

## Entry-Level or Initial Certification as a CTRS

There are two paths to professional certification as a CTRS. The academic path is for individuals who have completed a baccalaureate degree or higher with a major in therapeutic recreation. The equivalency path is for individuals with a related baccalaureate degree.

For the *academic path* to CTRS certification, the exam eligibility requirements are a baccalaureate degree or higher

Source: D'Antonio-Nocéra, A., DeBolt, N., and Touhey, N. (1996). *The professional activity manager and consultant* (pp. 16–17). Ravensdale, WA: Idyll Arbor, Inc. Used by permission of Idyll Arbor, Inc., P. O. Box 720, Ravensdale, WA 98051.

from an accredited college or university with a major in therapeutic recreation which includes the following:

1. **A minimum of 18 semester or 24 quarter units of therapeutic recreation and general education content coursework with no less than a minimum of nine (9) semester or 12 quarter units in therapeutic recreation content; AND**

2. **A minimum of 18 semester or 27 quarter units of support coursework including three semester or quarter units in each of the following three content areas: (i) anatomy and physiology, (ii) abnormal psychology, and (iii) human growth and development. The remaining semester or quarter units of the support coursework requirement must be fulfilled in the content area of human services; AND**

3. **A minimum of a 360-hour, ten consecutive week field placement experience in a clinical, residential or community-based therapeutic recreation program under the supervision of an on-site field placement supervisor who is certified by NCTRC at the Therapeutic Recreation Specialist Professional level.**

The professional *equivalency path* requires a baccalaureate degree or higher from an accredited college or university and the following:

1. **A minimum of 18 semester or 24 quarter units of upper division or graduate-level therapeutic recreation and general recreation content coursework with no less than a minimum of nine (9) semester or 12 quarter units in upper division or graduate-level therapeutic recreation content; AND**

2. **Supportive courses to include a minimum of 24 semester units or 36 quarter units from three (3) of the following six (6) areas: adaptive physical education, related biological/physical sciences, human services, psychology, sociology or special education; AND**

3. **A minimum of five (5) years of full-time, paid experience in a clinical, residential or community-based therapeutic recreation program.**

Initial professional eligibility is awarded for a period of five years to allow new applicants sufficient and fair opportunity to sit for and pass the national certification exam. Once an individual with professional eligibility passes the national exam, that individual is awarded the CTRS credential.

# Conduct Standards

NCTRC has established 14 statements regarding professional conduct. All NCTRC certificants must agree to abide by these conduct rules and to report truthfully information regarding any violation of a conduct matter. NCTRC may deny professional eligibility, revoke eligibility or certification, or take other appropriate action if a candidate for certification or a CTRS violates any of the 14 conduct statements.

# Continuing Professional Competence

During the five-year certification period, the CTRS must choose two of three potential recertification components. Each CTRS must earn a total of 100 points to renew certification at the end of the five-year cycle. The three components by which a CTRS can demonstrate continued professional competence are: professional practice or experience in therapeutic recreation, continuing education in therapeutic recreation, or passing the national exam at the end of the five-year period. The CTRS must complete at least two of the three components in order to recertify and retain the CTRS credential.

Each year of the five-year active certification period, the CTRS must submit an annual maintenance application and fee to retain certification. At the end of the five-year cycle, certificants must submit a recertification application documenting the completed continuing professional competence requirements.

During any period of time that an individual's certification is inactive, that individual is prohibited from (i) representing that he or she is a "Certified Therapeutic Recreation Specialist" or "CTRS"; and (ii) accepting the role of supervisor for a proposed internship requiring a supervisor that is certified by NCTRC as a CTRS. If an individual is not recertified for failure to meet the recertification requirements, that individual must return the NCTRC CTRS certificate and refrain from using the title "Certified Therapeutic Recreation Specialist" or "CTRS." Any individual who uses CTRS, or represents himself or herself as being NCTRC certified without having fulfilled the requirements of the NCTRC certification process is deemed in violation of the credentialing procedure and may be denied the right to future certification or may be subject to legal action.

For more information on professional certification with NCTRC or to request a *Candidate Bulletin* for application, please contact the national office by writing to NCTRC, P. O. Box 479, Thiells, New York 10984, or calling (914) 947-4346.

# Appendix C

# A Volunteer Manual for the Division of Therapeutic Recreation

## Cincinnati Recreation Commission

## Volunteer Placement Procedures

1. A volunteer brochure will be sent out to all prospective volunteers. This year, the division is varying the ages of volunteers for different programs. All individuals who work teen or adult programs must be 18 or over. For programs that include younger children, the minimum volunteer age will be 16. For programs that go on field trips, volunteers will be expected to provide their own transportation.

2. Specific volunteer job descriptions are written for the various program formats (i.e., aquatics, trimnastics, bowling) to give the volunteers a more specific idea of what their specific program responsibilities will consist.

3. All program directors must have a volunteer application on each and every volunteer before the volunteer will be permitted to work the program, (even if he or she is only going to come one time). Emergency numbers and release signatures (for individuals under 18) are *important* and must be readily available.

4. Since the program directors are the direct supervisors of the volunteers, they are responsible for their training, supervision and evaluation. The volunteer coordinator will assist in all areas. All new volunteers must attend a training and orientation session with their program director before they will be permitted to work the program. Each volunteer should set up a time to go over this information with the program director (can be before or after program or at another time to be decided by the director and volunteer). A volunteer orientation checklist will outline the information to be included in this training session. At this time volunteer manuals will be handed out, volunteer contracts signed and "volunteer skill bank" forms filled out.

5. All volunteer information (name, address, phone number, emergency number), should be reported to the volunteer coordinator to be put on a master volunteer list at the office. As soon as the names are turned in, a volunteer name tag will be issued.

6. Volunteer hours need to be recorded daily on the volunteer time sheet in/out log. These hours need to be turned into the coordinators on a monthly basis. All individuals who help out at a program need to be included on this log (even if they only come once). Be sure and put first and last names and total the hours. An ongoing month-by-month tab of volunteer hours is included in the program director's notebook so that each director can total the number of volunteer hours completed in a particular season. Each director can appoint an assistant director to handle this recordkeeping, but the program director is responsible for its accuracy.

7. Volunteer evaluations need to be done on the volunteers after each season. Mid-season evaluations should be done verbally by the program director so the volunteers know how they are doing and what areas need improvement. The written evaluation (which is due at the end of the ten-week session) should also be completed by the program director. These evaluations only need to be filled out for volunteers who come to at least eight out of ten weeks of the ten-week program session.

8. Volunteer recognition—volunteer hours are compiled from season to season with recognition as follows:

   - 25 hours—T-shirt,
   - 75 hours—letter to school or employer,
   - 100 hours—framed certificate, movie pass, and
   - 150 hours—plaque.

9. Volunteer dismissal—no volunteer can be dismissed without approval from the program coordinator following appropriate evaluations.

# Volunteer Application

Name:_____     Male:_____     Female:_____

Address:_____     Zip:_____     Phone:_____

Age:_____     Date of Birth:_____

Representative of: _____
                    (company or school)

## Program Choices

Program:   Mentally Handicapped____     Physically Handicapped ____     Learning Disability ____

Location:_____

Time Available:_____     Days:_____

## Education

Elementary/Junior High School: _____

High School:_____     Years Completed:_____

College/University: _____     Years Completed:_____

Degree: _____     Year:_____     Major:_____

Classes relating to recreation, physical education, or special education:

_____

_____

_____

Work experience with mentally retarded and/or physically handicapped or other special populations.  Please list length of time, place of work, age group, and disability:

_____

_____

_____

Other work experiences relating to recreation:

_____

_____

_____

Do you hold a current Lifesaving Certification? _____     Water Safety Certificate? _____

Adapted Aquatics Certification? _____     CPR (cardiopulmonary resuscitation)? _____

First-Aid Certificate? _____

Please list the activities in which you have interest and knowledge such as nature, gardening, drama, dancing, music, crafts, sports or other activities:

_____

_____

_____

Have you volunteered with the Cincinnati Recreation Commission before? _____

If yes, with what program? _____

How did you find out about our therapeutic recreation programs?

_____

     (Newspaper, friends, radio, television, etc.)

**RELEASE** (MUST BE SIGNED)
I hereby assume complete responsibility for any injury or damage sustained by the applicant and release the Cincinnati Recreation Commission of any and all liability for such injury or damage occurring during volunteer work for the Cincinnati Recreation Commission.

Signature: _____
If under 18, signature of a parent or guardian is required.

Person to call in case of emergency:

Name: _____

Address: _____     Phone: _____

# Volunteer Orientation Checklist

_____ 1. Discuss the division of therapeutic recreation—who we serve and how programs are set up on a seasonal basis (use program brochure, volunteer brochure).

_____ 2. How the division of therapeutic recreation is set up (use organization chart).

_____ 3. Policies and procedures of the division by which volunteers must abide (dress code, notification of absence, no smoking, no leaving the program site for lunch, no physical punishment, confidentiality).

_____ 4. Discuss your individual program (program goals, participants, disabilities involved, skill levels) show volunteer program goals and skill level descriptions.

_____ 5. Discuss volunteer job description for your individual program.

_____ 6. Discuss importance of safety of participants at all times (go over dealing with seizures and specialized equipment such as wheelchairs where applicable). This information is found in volunteer manual.

_____ 7. Discuss recordkeeping of volunteer hours (sign in/out sheet), recognition of volunteers, and volunteer evaluation—give volunteer copy of volunteer evaluation (point out that volunteer must attend eight out of ten seasonal programs to be evaluated).

_____ 8. Go over volunteer contract and sign. This contract should be kept with volunteer application in notebook. Need two copies (one for notebook and one for volunteer).

_____ 9. Be sure volunteer has submitted an application to be kept in program director's notebook. If volunteer is under 18, release must be signed by parent.

_____ 10. Be sure volunteer has numbers to call to notify program director of absence (staff and office number).

_____ 11. Give volunteer manual to volunteer.

_____ 12. Fill out following volunteer information to be put on master office list:

Name:_____     Phone number:_____

Who to contact in case of emergency:_____     Phone number:_____

As soon as this sheet is completed, and turned into program coordinator, volunteer will be issued a name tag which should be worn at all times.

This volunteer orientation was held on_____from_____to_____.
                                       date        time      time

_____     _____
Signature of Program Director                  Signature of Volunteer

# Volunteer Responsibilities

Under the supervision of the program director and/or assistant directors, volunteers in a therapeutic recreation program are responsible for assisting with or leading a variety of activities and supervision of participants.

The volunteer is responsible for:

1. Assisting in monitoring the safety of program participants, visitors, supplies and equipment.
2. Assisting in planning diversified leisure activities based on the needs and interests of the participants according to the continuum method.
3. Notifying the program director (at home or work) in case of absence. (Call one day or evening ahead, if possible.)
4. Attending at least one day of program each week for the entire program session.
5. Leading and/or assisting in conducting assigned activities.
6. Reporting progress and problems with participants and program to director and assistant directors.
7. Assisting with the evaluation of program and participants.
8. Dressing appropriately by wearing clothes that will allow volunteer to be actively involved in activities (i.e., wear gym shoes and loose fitting, comfortable clothes).
9. Being enthusiastic!
10. Being dependable and adaptable to various situations.

# Volunteer Contract

The Cincinnati Recreation Commission, Division of Therapeutic Recreation agrees:

a. To train volunteers to a level that will enable them to begin their work confidently.
b. To continue their training to whatever extent is necessary to maintain continuing competence.
c. To provide volunteers with working conditions equal to those of paid employees.
d. To make written evaluations of each volunteer's job performance at regular and suitable intervals and to provide references on request.
e. To offer volunteers promotion to more responsible jobs within the volunteer program.
f. To include volunteers in staff planning and evaluating when possible and generally promote their understanding of Division workings and decisions.

The volunteer agrees:

a. To work a certain number of hours a week according to a schedule acceptable to the program director.
b. To become thoroughly familiar with the policies and procedures (written and verbal) set forth by the Division for volunteers.
c. To be prompt and reliable in reporting for work and to provide the Division with an accurate record of hours worked by signing in and out.
d. To attend orientation and training sessions and undertake continuing education as necessary to maintain competence.
e. To respect the function of the program director and staff and to contribute fully to a smooth working relationship between staff and volunteers.
f. To accept the Division's right to dismiss any professional volunteer for poor performance, including poor attendance.
g. To notify the Division at least one week in advance of resignation or requested leave of absence.
h. To exercise caution when acting on the Division's behalf and to protect the confidentiality of all information relating to the Division and its participants.

_____     _____     _____     _____
Program Director                Date           Volunteer                           Date

# Volunteer Evaluation Form

*Directions:* This evaluation form is to be completed one week prior to the end of the program for all volunteers working 20 program hours or more. The evaluation is to be completed by all program directors supervising the volunteer or the director supervising the volunteer for the majority of service hours. This evaluation form must be filled out in duplicate (volunteer copy and office copy).

Name:_____  Address:_____  Zip:_____

Phone:_____  Birth date:_____

| Programs | Directors | Days | Times |
|----------|-----------|------|-------|
| _____ | _____ | _____ | _____ |
| _____ | _____ | _____ | _____ |
| _____ | _____ | _____ | _____ |

Rating Scale:

| (4) Always (exceeds requirements) | (3) Usually (meets requirements) | (2) Sometimes (needs improvement) | (1) Never (unsatisfactory) |
|---|---|---|---|

I.   Volunteer Responsibilities

| Program | Responsibilities | Rating |
|---------|------------------|--------|
| 1._____ | A._____ | _____ |
|  | B._____ | _____ |
|  | C._____ | _____ |
| 2._____ | A._____ | _____ |
|  | B._____ | _____ |
|  | C._____ | _____ |
| 3._____ | A._____ | _____ |
|  | B._____ | _____ |
|  | C._____ | _____ |

II.  Attendance

| Program | Number of Days Attended | Total Hours |
|---------|-------------------------|-------------|
| 1._____ | _____ | _____ |
| 2._____ | _____ | _____ |
| 3._____ | _____ | _____ |

a. Total number of hours served_____

b. Number of excused absences_____

c. Number of unexcused absences_____

d. Reports to program at scheduled time      4 3 2 1

e. Stays through scheduled time      4 3 2 1

Comments: _____

III. **Work Habits**

a. Contributes in the planning of program      4 3 2 1

b. Contributes in evaluating the program      4 3 2 1

c. Demonstrates ability to conduct group activity      4 3 2 1

d. Demonstrates ability to relate to participants on a one-to-one basis      4 3 2 1

Comments: _____

IV. **Learning Ability**

a. Knows when to ask for help and is able to follow through      4 3 2 1

b. Understands and retains training without continued supervision      4 3 2 1

c. Displays a grasp of knowledge of disabilities      4 3 2 1

d. Demonstrates an understanding of the goals of the program and participants      4 3 2 1

e. Suggests appropriate activities for the needs, abilities, and objectives of the participants      4 3 2 1

Comments: _____

V. **Personal Fitness**

a. Dresses appropriately for program activities      4 3 2 1

b. Demonstrates physical capacity to do the job      4 3 2 1

Comments: _____

VI. **Attitude and Initiative**

a. Accepts suggestions graciously      4 3 2 1

b. Displays interest and enthusiasm in work      4 3 2 1

c. Offers suggestions and introduces new ideas      4 3 2 1

d. Anticipates needs and performs without being told      4 3 2 1

Comments: _____

VII. **Interpersonal Relationships**

a. Exhibits a personable, outgoing attitude      4 3 2 1

b. Interacts well with staff, supervisors, and other volunteers      4 3 2 1

c. Recognizes individual behavioral differences and can adjust interactions accordingly      4 3 2 1

d. Supports discipline and behavior modifications employed by program staff      4 3 2 1

Comments: _____

VIII.   Overall Performance—Please use this space for any additional information regarding job performance of volunteer.

_____

_____

_____

_____

IX.   Volunteer Comments

_____

_____

_____

_____

Signature of Volunteer: _____   Date: _____

Signature of Evaluators: _____   Date: _____

_____   Date: _____

_____   Date: _____

For Office Use Only:

# *Appendix D*

## The Rocky Mountain Multiple Sclerosis Center
### Adult Day Enrichment Program
### 2851 West 52nd Avenue
### Denver, CO 80221-1259

# Therapeutic Recreation Internship Application

Date _____

Name _____
           Last                  First              Middle

Current Address _____
                              Street

_____
City                          State         Zip

Birth Date_____   Social Security # _____

Name of College/University_____

Title _____

Address_____
                            Street

_____
City                          State         Zip

Major_____  When do you expect to graduate? _____

1.  Will you have access to a vehicle (car, truck, motorcycle)?

    Yes_____   No_____   If yes, give type _____

2. Are you licensed to operate a vehicle other than a passenger car?

   Yes _____ No _____     If yes, give type _____     Licensed in what state? _____

3. Length of internship required by the college/university

   Available start date _____     Preferred ending date _____

4. Please summarize briefly your work/volunteer experience with individuals with a disability.

   _____

   _____

   _____

**EMPLOYMENT HISTORY SECTION (include any volunteer work)**
Complete this section unless resume is included with your application.

1. Name and address of employer _____

   _____

   Phone _____     Date of Employment: From _____ To _____

   Brief Description of Duties: _____

   _____

2. Name and address of employer _____

   _____

   Phone _____     Date of Employment: From _____ To _____

   Brief Description of Duties: _____

   _____

3. Name and address of employer _____

   _____

   Phone _____     Date of Employment: From _____ To _____

   Brief Description of Duties: _____

   _____

What do you expect from an intern experience?

_____

_____

_____

Provide a statement of your career objective:

_____

_____

_____

Include any other information you feel we should have; attach on separate page if necessary.

_____

_____

_____


_____          _____

Student's Signature                                                    Date

Please ask your college/university advisor to make comments that will help us plan your internship:

_____

_____

_____

# Recreational Therapy Student Intern Job Summary

The recreational therapy student intern will gain experience and expertise in the clinical setting through observation and work with professional staff in carrying out the recreational therapy program.

**Performance Requirements:**

Responsible for:

- Observation of therapeutic procedure with patients.
- Participation in treatment sessions with recreational therapists.
- Participation in in-services scheduled during the internship period.
- Preparation and teaching of sessions agreed upon by supervisor.
- Carrying out therapy objectives independently as assigned.
- Communication with supervisor and/or appropriate staff of any pertinent information concerning patients.
- Participation in interdisciplinary meetings as assigned.
- Preparation of materials for use in carrying out program.
- Familiarity with policies and procedures of the department and adherence to them.

**Physical Demands:** Moderate: Transferring patients, pushing patients in wheelchairs, handling of light equipment, directing exercise class and other physical activities: walking, cross-country skiing, swimming, moderate sports such as bowling, horse shoes, shuffleboard, volleyball, or others as they become available.

Able to tolerate complex learning environment and psychological stress.

**Special Demands:** The student intern is expected to work a 40-hour week for a minimum of 15 weeks. The student intern will be scheduled weekends and some evenings.

**Qualifications:**

*Knowledge:* Intern must have completed the classroom prerequisites of the referring educational institution in order to be considered for fieldwork placement.

Educational background should include courses which will provide the following:

- Psychology—introduction to psychology, abnormal psychology, some knowledge of instruments used in testing and evaluation.
- Basic knowledge of physical disabilities.
- Basic understanding of types of mental disorders.
- Knowledge of team approach.
- Knowledge of small and large muscle activities.
- Knowledge of crafts and a variety of related activities.
- Programming for physically, mentally, emotionally impaired.
- Some knowledge of written records, e.g., assessments, individual treatment plans, progress notes.

*Skills:*

- Good interpersonal skills—must be able to get along with staff in close work setting. Must be able to relate to patients.
- Must have good coping skills.
- Must be able to grasp new techniques and concepts and integrate them into treatment.
- Good written and oral communication skills—ability to take accurate notes.
- Ability to follow directions.
- Leadership and instructional skills—one-to-one, small group.
- Wide variety of recreation skills which can be applied in a therapeutic setting.

**Working Environment:** Chelsea Community Hospital (indoors and outdoors) and surrounding community. Working in large and small group settings or individually in recreational therapy room or in patient's room. May take patients to community functions occasionally.

**Job Relationships:** Unit Supervisor, Student Coordinator, Director of Therapy Services or Psych Nurse Manager.

**Dress Code:** Students are expected to serve as positive role models for patients. Dress will be geared to varying activities of the department.

**Standards of Grooming:** Appropriate and professional attire. Good personal hygiene.

---

Used by permission of Chelsea Community Hospital, Chelsea, MI.

# *(University Seal)*

# School of Education and Related Professions

# Exchange of Services Agreement

# Recreation/Recreation Therapy

This is an agreement between_____
and Ashland University to provide field-based experiences related to recreation and recreation therapy at the above named agency.

The University shall be represented in matters related to internships and off-campus field experiences associated with supervision by the recreation/recreation therapy faculty and the clinical supervisor employed by the University. The designated representative(s) of the agency shall be:

_____

_____.

The agency agrees to the following:

The Agency shall provide appropriate field-based experiences related to professional preparation in recreation/recreation therapy for students of Ashland University. The field-based experiences shall include field and other related experiences in the student's laboratory certification field(s). The recreation/recreation therapy faculty and clinical supervisor shall administer programs involving field-based experiences in recreation and recreation therapy.

Much responsibility for guiding the University student through the field-based experience rests with the cooperating supervisor. Accordingly, the work of the cooperating supervisor is vital to the success of field-based experiences related to recreation/recreation therapy. Cooperating supervisors shall be given all possible support and assistance in their work with university students by both the agency and the University.

Cooperating supervisors shall be selected by the designated agency and approved by the recreation/recreation therapy faculty and clinical supervisor. All professionals selected as cooperating supervisors shall have given their consent. To qualify as a cooperating supervisor, the supervisor shall hold an appropriate bachelor's degree, appropriate professional credential(s) (CLP/CTRS preferred) and have a minimum of three years of successful professional experience with at least one year in the current setting. (These are desired experience qualifications; consideration will be given to supervisors with comparable credentials and experience.)

Cooperating supervisor agrees to develop an individual contract with each student specifying placement objectives, student responsibilities and placement schedule. Additionally, the supervisor will meet weekly with the student and will review and sign weekly student reports/assignments. Cooperating supervisors will coordinate with clinical university supervisors to plan on-site observations and major student research/evaluation project(s).

Cooperating supervisors will be expected to attend Ashland University cooperating supervisor orientations and in-service sessions. Cooperating supervisors will evaluate the recreation/recreation therapy students' field-based experiences in writing on the basis of guidelines supplied by the University and agreed to by the agency.

Ashland University agrees to the following:

1. The student will assist the cooperating supervisor and will be given ample opportunity to demonstrate independently a variety of professional skills related to his or her certification field(s). The student will

---

Used by permission of Ashland University, Ashland, OH.

be expected to gradually assume as much responsibility for a series of regular programs and services as the cooperating supervisor and University clinical supervisor deem appropriate.

2. Students placed in field-based experiences will assist the cooperating supervisor with routine duties related to programs and services in their certification field(s). These duties reflect the job responsibilities identified in the job analysis of the Certified Leisure Professional and Certified Therapeutic Recreation Specialist.

3. The student will be expected to comply with agency and university policies. The field-experiences will be terminated immediately with violation of these policies and a grade of F will be issued for the experience. Permission to repeat the experience will be at the discretion of recreation/recreation therapy faculty and clinical supervisor considering agency input.

Before the placement of a recreation/recreation therapy student in a field-based experience is complete, the cooperating supervisor shall be supplied with a profile of essential information about the student. The cooperating supervisor, in consultation with the agency representative, may have the option of accepting or rejecting the student.

Guidelines for cooperating supervisors working with University students in field experiences are available and will be supplied to cooperating supervisors. All students placed in field-based experiences will be supervised by a University clinical supervisor, who will carefully assist and advise on matters related to the field-based experience. The University clinical supervisor shall be responsible for recording grades for field-based experiences.

## Provisions for Coordinating Ongoing Activities and Solving Problems

The Ashland University recreation/recreation therapy faculty and clinical supervisor in cooperation with the agency supervisor are responsible for coordinating the ongoing activities. Problems and concerns may be brought to the attention of the recreation/recreation therapy faculty and clinical supervisor by agency personnel, University clinical supervisors and/or recreation/recreation therapy students. The recreation/recreation therapy faculty and clinical supervisor will assist in the resolution of problems which may arise among participants in the field experience. The recreation/recreation therapy faculty will provide agency personnel, University clinical supervisors and recreation/recreation therapy students with handbooks, guidelines, calendars, and appropriate forms for each field-based experience.

## Means for Revisions to Meet Changing Needs and Conditions

The Ashland University recreation/recreation therapy faculty and the clinical supervisor are responsible for coordinating revisions that are necessary to meet changing needs and conditions. Agency personnel, University clinical supervisors and recreation/recreation therapy students are given the opportunity to make suggestions for needed revisions on the evaluation form(s) provided at the end of each field-based experience.

## Professional Development Programs for Persons Involved in the Preparation of Individuals for Recreation and Therapeutic Recreation Certification

To ensure the professional development of individuals involved in the field-based experiences, Ashland University, will provide orientation programs and in-service education for cooperating supervisors at no cost to the supervisor or the agency. The orientation session may be held on campus or off campus at the agency site. The University clinical supervisor is responsible for continuing the orientation process at the agency site.

In addition to the services provided by the students without cost to the agency, the University will assist the agency in the professional development of agency personnel.

We accept the conditions of this agreement and authorize the placement of Ashland University recreation/recreation therapy students for field-based experiences at:

_____.

This agreement is subject to annual review in April of each year by both the cooperating agency and Ashland University.

Entered into this _____ day of _____, 199___.

_____
University Representative

_____
Agency

_____
Recreation/Recreation Therapy Clinical Supervisor

_____
Recreation/Recreation Therapy Faculty

# Appendix E

# 1995 Standards Manual and Interpretive Guidelines for Medical Rehabilitation

## Commission of Accreditation of Rehabilitation Facilities

The following are references to therapeutic recreation, recreation, leisure skills, and recreational activity from the Commission on Accreditation of Rehabilitation Facilities' *1995 Standards Manual and Interpretive Guidelines for Medical Rehabilitation* which is effective on site surveys from July 1, 1995 through June 30, 1996.

### SECTION 4: PROGRAM STANDARDS

#### A. MEDICAL REHABILITATION PROGRAMS

21. For each person served, there should be a written plan of follow-up that includes:

   a. Referral and forwarding of clinical information to a designated physician and/or service program.

   b. As appropriate, specific recommendations for medical, physical, cognitive, behavioral, communication, vocational, recreational, educational, psychological, and family support.

#### B. OCCUPATIONAL REHABILITATION PROGRAMS

25. For each person served, there should be a written plan of follow-up which includes, as appropriate:

   a. Referral and forwarding of clinical information to the referral source, employer, and others.

   b. Specific recommendations for medical, physical, cognitive, behavioral, communication, vocational, recreational, educational, psychological, and family support.

### SECTION 5: SPECIFIC PROGRAM STANDARDS

#### A. COMPREHENSIVE INPATIENT CATEGORIES ONE, TWO, and THREE

**Program Description**

**CATEGORY ONE:** Hospital

4. Based on their individual needs, receive a daily minimum of three hours of services a minimum of five hours per week from the interdisciplinary team, which includes an occupational therapist, a physical therapist, a psychologist, a social worker, a speech-language pathologist, and a therapeutic recreation specialist.

**CATEGORY TWO:** Hospital

   **Hospital-Based Skilled Nursing Facility**

   **Skilled Nursing Facility**

4. Based on their individual needs, receive a daily minimum of one hour of services a minimum of

five days per week from the interdisciplinary team, which includes an occupational therapist, a physical therapist, a psychologist, a social worker, a speech-language pathologist, and a therapeutic recreation specialist.

**CATEGORY THREE:** **Hospital-Based Skilled Nursing Facility**

**Skilled Nursing Facility**

4. Based on their individual needs, receive a daily minimum of one to three hours of services a minimum of five days per week from the interdisciplinary team, which includes an occupational therapist, a physical therapist, a psychologist, a social worker, a speech-language pathologist, and a therapeutic recreation specialist.

3. The members of the interdisciplinary team in Comprehensive Inpatient Categories One, Two, and Three, should include, but not be limited to the following, though each may not serve every person:

 a. An occupational therapist.

 b. A physical therapist.

 c. A physician.

 d. A psychologist.

 e. A rehabilitation nurse.

 f. A social worker.

 g. A speech-language pathologist.

 h. A therapeutic recreation specialist.

**B.** **SPINAL CORD INJURY PROGRAMS**

6. Suitable staffing should be provided, including:

 a. Physician coverage seven days per week.

 b. Management of the care of the person under the direction of a single physician.

 c. In addition to the primary physician, availability of the basic medical consultation specialties including:

 (1) General surgery.

 (2) Gynecology.

 (3) Internal medicine.

 (4) Neurology.

 (5) Neurosurgery.

 (6) Orthopedics.

 (7) Pediatrics.

 (8) Physical medicine and rehabilitation.

 (9) Plastic surgery.

 (10) Psychiatry.

 (11) Pulmonary medicine.

 (12) Urology.

 d. Limitation of admitting and treating privileges on the spinal injury unit to those physicians with special interest and competence in spinal cord injury.

 e. Training and expertise of allied health specialists in the uniqueness of persons with spinal cord injuries.

 f. Availability of the following services seven days per week, 24 hours per day:

 (1) Rehabilitation nursing.

 (2) Respiratory therapy.

 (3) Intermittent catheterization.

 g. Provisions for the following services on a full-time basis:

 (1) Counseling for the persons served/family members provided by a social worker, psychologist, or vocational counselor.

 (2) Occupational therapy.

 (3) Physical therapy.

 (4) Social work.

 h. Provisions for the delivery of the following services:

 (1) Audiology.

 (2) Chaplaincy.

 (3) Driver education.

 (4) Nutrition.

 (5) Orthotics.

 (6) Psychology/neuropsychology.

 (7) Rehabilitation engineering.

 (8) Special education.

 (9) Speech-language pathology.

 (10) Therapeutic recreation.

 (11) Vocational rehabilitation.

7. In addition to the services previously identified, the following services should be provided:

 a. Community integration services, including supervised community excursions and provisions for overnight therapeutic leaves. There should be referral to appropriate available community services such as independent living, recreation, home health, education, vocational rehabilitation, and transportation services.

b. Recommendations regarding environmental modification—e.g., home, school, or work site modification.

c. Follow-up for health maintenance.

d. A formally organized and mandatory participation program for the persons served/family members in spinal cord injury education. The program should provide for, but not be limited to, education regarding:

(1) Bladder management.

(2) Bowel management.

(3) Equipment care and community resources for repair.

(4) Instructions in medications.

(5) The need for follow-up medical care and how to access it.

(6) The need for attendants and how to secure and manage them.

(7) Nutrition.

(8) Pulmonary care.

(9) Skin care.

(10) Substance abuse.

(11) Use of leisure time.

e. Provisions to facilitate the peer interaction and advocacy efforts of the persons served.

f. Sexual counseling and education, including information concerning fertility.

g. Urodynamic testing.

## C. COMPREHENSIVE PAIN MANAGEMENT PROGRAMS

21. The Chronic Comprehensive Pain Management team should be comprised of:

a. The person served.

b. Pain team physician.

c. Pain team psychologist.

d. At least three practitioners from the following list. Each program should identify the practitioners (other than physicians) who should be employed by or have a formal arrangement with the program (i.e., con-

tract or affiliation). The organization should also provide or assist each person, dependent upon his or her needs, to obtain services from those practitioners on this list who are not identified as needing to be employed by or have formal arrangements with the program.

(1) Biofeedback therapist.

(2) Case manager.

(3) Exercise physiologist.

(4) Nurse practitioner.

(5) Occupational therapist.

(6) Pharmacist.

(7) Physical therapist.

(8) Physician assistant.

(9) Psychiatrist.

(10) Registered nurse.

(11) Social worker.

(12) Therapeutic recreation specialist.

(13) Vocational specialist.

## D. BRAIN INJURY PROGRAMS

15. Initial or ongoing assessment should address:

a. Activities of daily living, including self-care, home skills, and community skills.

b. Adjustment to disability.

c. Affect and mood.

d. Alcohol and other drug dependency.

e. Behavior.

f. Cognition.

g. Communication.

h. Community reintegration, including appropriate postdischarge services.

i. Community resources.

j. Educational and/or vocational capacities.

k. Environmental modification.

l. Family systems and resources.

m. Financial resources.

n. Health and nutrition.

o. Interpersonal and social skills.

p. Issues related to human sexuality.

q. Legal competency.

r. Medical and neurological issues.

s. Perceptual ability.

t. Recreation and leisure skills.

u. Sensorimotor capacity, including gross and fine motor strength and control, sensation, balance, joint range of motion, mobility, and function.

22. There should be a written plan of follow-up which includes:

a. Designation of an individual within the program who is responsible for case management after discharge so that there is continuity and coordination of postdischarge services.

b. Identification of an individual within the receiving community who will be responsible for case management after discharge so that there is continuity and coordination of postdischarge services.

c. Referral and forwarding of clinical information to a designated physician and/or service program.

d. Specific recommendations for medical, physical, cognitive, behavioral, communication, vocational, recreational, educational, psychological/neuropsychological, and family support.

51. In addition to the disciplines listed for the core team in Section 5A, Comprehensive Inpatient Categories One, Two, and Three, the core team should also include:

a. A neuropsychologist.

b. A therapeutic recreation specialist.

60. The program should acquire sufficient information to assist it in determining the likelihood that the person can participate in and benefit from the program. A documented request for any missing information should be made within one week after entrance/admission. The program should obtain preentrance/admission information, both historical and current, including the person's:

a. Medical history.

b. Clinical status.

c. Alcohol and other drug dependency history.

d. Information on emotional and behavioral functioning, which should include, but not be limited to:

(1) The person's current and historical emotional and behavioral functioning.

(2) When indicated, the results of intellectual, projective, and personality tests.

(3) When indicated, language, self-care, and visual-motor functioning.

(4) Personality.

e. Social history, which should include:

(1) A statement of the presenting problem.

(2) The current and historical life situation, including, but not limited to:

(a) Domestic and household relationships.

(b) Emotional and health factors of family members.

(c) Alcohol and other drug dependencies of family members and attitudes towards such dependencies.

(3) Educational, financial, legal, military, occupational, and recreational status.

71. Assessment, coordinated planning, and direct services should be provided on a regular and ongoing basis by a core team of individuals with special interest, training, experience, and expertise in brain injury rehabilitation. Depending on the needs of the persons served and their stated goals, the core team should be comprised of at least four different professionals, including:

a. A clinical psychologist/neuropsychologist.

b. An educational specialist.

c. An occupational therapist.

d. A physical therapist.

e. A physician.

f. A rehabilitation nurse.

g. A social worker.

h. A specialist in behavior analysis—e.g., a behavioral psychologist or behavior analyst.

i. A speech-language pathologist.

j. A therapeutic recreation specialist.

k. A vocational specialist.

72. Dependent upon the needs of the persons served and their stated goals, the program should provide or make formal arrangements for:

a. Advocacy.

b. Alcohol and other drug abuse treatment.

c. Audiology.

d. Behavioral analysis.

e. Chaplaincy.

f. Creative arts therapies.

g. Dentistry.

h. Dietetics/nutrition.

i. Disability.

j. Driver education.

k. Education.

l. Health maintenance.

m. Occupational therapy.

n. Orthotics/prosthetics.

o. Pharmacy services.

p. Physiatry.

q. Physical conditioning.

r. Physical therapy.

s. Physician services.

t. Psychology/neuropsychology.

u. Rehabilitation engineering.

v. Rehabilitation nursing.

w. Respiratory therapy.

x. Sex education.

y. Social services.

z. Speech-language pathology.

aa. Therapeutic recreation.

bb. Vision care.

cc. Vocational rehabilitation.

E. **OUTPATIENT MEDICAL REHABILITATION PROGRAMS**

5. The team for an Outpatient Medical Rehabilitation Program is comprised of:

a. The person served.

b. The physician.

c. At least two practitioners from the following list. Each program should identify the practitioners (other than physicians) who should be employed by or have a formal arrangement with the program (e.g., contract or affiliation). Each organization should also provide or assist each person, dependent upon his or her needs, to obtain services from those practitioners on this list who are not identified as needing to be employed by or have formal arrangements with the program.

   (1) Case manager, either internal or external.

   (2) Occupational therapist.

   (3) Physical therapist.

   (4) Psychologist.

   (5) Rehabilitation nurse.

   (6) Respiratory therapist.

   (7) Social worker.

   (8) Speech-language pathologist.

   (9) Therapeutic recreation specialist.

   (10) Vocational specialist.

# 1995 Standards Manual and Interpretive Guidelines for Behavioral Health

## Commission on Accreditation of Rehabilitation Facilities

The following are references to therapeutic recreation, recreation, leisure skills, and recreational activity from the Commission on Accreditation of Rehabilitation Facilities *1995 Standards Manual and Interpretive Guidelines for Behavioral Health* which is effective on site surveys from July 1, 1995 through June 30, 1996.

### SECTION 3: SPECIFIC PROGRAM STANDARDS

**A.    ALCOHOL and OTHER DRUG PROGRAMS**

9.    Program personnel should acquire sufficient and current information to assist them in identifying the needs of the persons served by assessing their:

a.  Strengths, abilities, and preferences.

b.  Current physical and health history.

c.  Alcohol and other drug use history.

d.  Emotional and behavioral functioning, which should include, but not be limited to:

   (1)  Current cognitive, emotional, and behavioral functioning.

   (2)  A history of previous cognitive, emotional, behavioral, and alcohol and other drug dependency problems and treatment.

   (3)  When indicated, psychological assessments.

   (4)  When indicated, other functional evaluations of language, self-care, and visual-motor functioning.

   (5)  Thoughts and/or physically aggressive and/or self-injurious behaviors.

e.  Social history, which should include information relating to:

   (1)  A statement of the presenting problem.

   (2)  A description of the person's current and historical life situation including, but not limited to:

      (a)  Domestic and household relationships.

      (b)  Cultural, ethnic, and spiritual factors and experience.

      (c)  Emotional and health factors of the family.

      (d)  Alcohol and other drug use of the family and attitudes toward such use.

      (e)  Leisure skills.

      (f)  Abuse and neglect issues.

      (g)  Peer group functioning.

      (h)  HIV risk assessment.

      (i)  Sexual history.

f. Occupational and educational status.

g. Financial status.

h. Legal status.

i. Family members' roles within the developmental process as well as their potential for caregiving and supporting recovery.

## OUTPATIENT SERVICES

76. The program should also address the following, based on the needs of the persons served:

a. Family involvement.

b. Personal hygiene.

c. Recreation.

d. Social activities.

e. Culturally relevant activities.

## B.  MENTAL HEALTH PROGRAMS

2. The program personnel should acquire sufficient information and maintain the information on an updated basis to assist them in identifying the needs of each person served through addressing the person's:

a. Abilities.

b. Presenting problems.

c. History of previous mental health services, including psychiatric contact, pharmacotherapy, hospitalizations, use of community programs.

d. Medical history and status.

e. Diagnosis(es).

f. Mental status.

g. Emotional and behavioral functioning, which should include:

   (1) Current emotional and behavioral functioning.

   (2) History of previous emotional, behavioral, and alcoholism and other drug dependency problems and treatment.

   (3) When indicated, psychological assessments.

   (4) When indicated, other functional evaluations of communication, self-care, and visual-motor functioning.

h. Social history, including the current and historical life situation of the person served including:

   (1) Abuse and neglect issues.

   (2) Alcohol and other drug use of family members and attitudes toward such use.

   (3) Cultural, ethnic, and spiritual factors and expectations.

   (4) Domestic and household relationships.

   (5) Emotional and health factors of the family members.

   (6) HIV risk assessment.

   (7) Leisure skills.

   (8) Occupational, educational, vocational, financial, military, and legal status.

   (9) Peer group functioning.

   (10) Human sexuality.

i. Developmental history, including adult development.

j. Drug use profile, including:

   (1) Prescription and nonprescription drugs being taken at the time of entrance/admission and for the previous six months.

   (2) Drug allergies and/or adverse drug reactions.

   (3) History of ineffective chemotherapy.

k. The role of the family within the developmental process as well as the family's potential for caregiving activities.

l. Adjustment to disability.

5. Based on advance planning and the needs of the persons served, the program should provide or make arrangements for:

a. Alcoholism and other drug dependency treatment.

b. Case management.

c. Community housing programs.

d. Domestic violence services.

e. Emergency/crisis intervention.

f. Inpatient programs.

g. Medical services, including psychiatric, pharmacological, health maintenance, and dental services.

h. Medication management.

i. Outpatient therapy services.

j. Partial hospitalization programs.

k. Psychological services.

l. Psychiatric services.

m. Recreation/leisure services.

n. Residential treatment programs.

o. Social/protective services.

p. Vocational rehabilitation.

57. There should be common areas with adequate space for meals, group interactions, recreation, and therapeutic activities.

69. The program should be able to provide the following therapeutic activities based on the needs of the persons served:

a. Activities designed to incorporate family involvement.

b. Budgeting.

c. Cooking.

d. Personal hygiene.

e. Recreation.

f. Social activities.

79. Dependent on the needs of those served and their stated goals, the program should provide or make formal arrangements for the following services:

a. Alcohol and other drug dependency counseling.

b. Dietary services.

c. Occupational therapy.

d. Psychology.

e. Speech-language pathology.

f. Therapeutic recreation.

g. Vocational rehabilitation.

80. Based on the needs of the persons served as identified in their individual plans, the program should provide:

a. Activities of daily living.

b. Group therapy.

c. Individual therapy.

d. Recreational activity.

107. A daily activity schedule should be established that is consistent with the pattern of life of individuals without disabilities and that reflects the personal choices, age, and service needs of the person served. Based on the level of independence achieved by the person served, a daily activity schedule may not be appropriate.

a. The activity schedule should provide for reasonable amounts of personal free time.

b. Sufficient scheduled meaningful activity should be made available outside the person's home consistent with his or her choice and needs.

c. The activity schedule should reflect opportunities for integrated community, cultural, recreational, and spiritual activities.

d. There should be evidence that the choices of the person served have been respected whenever appropriate.

# Index

GERALD S. O'MORROW, CTRS, has over 35 years of professional park, recreation, and leisure services experience primarily in therapeutic recreation at the national and international level. He has served as a therapist, administrator and consultant within healthcare facilities and as an administrator and educator in academic settings. Dr. O'Morrow's scholarly activity in research and in books and journal article publications have added significantly to the philosophy, theory, and standards of therapeutic recreation practice. In addition, he is a frequent presenter at conferences, workshops, and institutes. Recently he was invited by the National Recreation Association of Japan to make several presentations about therapeutic recreation in Japan. He has been a visiting lecturer at colleges and universities in the United States and a visiting scholar at the University de Deusto, Bilbao, Spain. He has also served for many years as a consultant to public and private agencies including the World Health Organization and colleges and universities. Dr. O'Morrow has received the NRPA Distinguished Professional Service Award and National Literary Award respectively and the NTRS Distinguished Service Award. He has also been recognized by *Palestra* for his significant contributions to therapeutic recreation throughout his career. He holds a B.S. from Sacramento State College, M.Ed. from the University of Minnesota, and an Ed.D. from Teachers College, Columbia University.

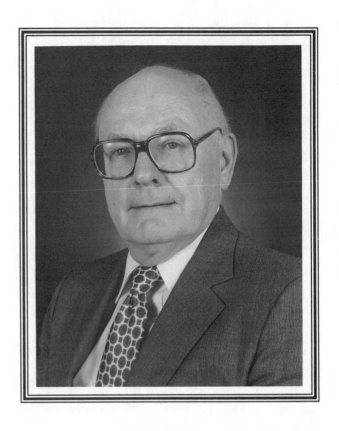

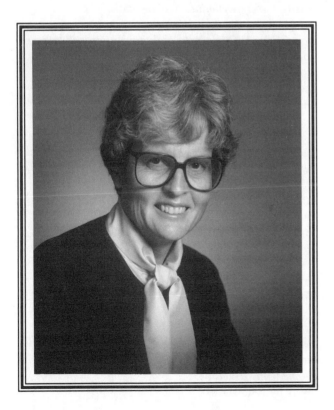

MARCIA JEAN CARTER, CTRS, received her Re.D. from Indiana University. She initiated the processes to create NCTRC, Inc. and was its first president. As Chair and Vice Chair of the National Certification Board, she was also instrumental in the development of the certification examination process for leisure professionals. Dr. Carter has been a member and Chair of the Council on Accreditation for Leisure and Recreation and the National Therapeutic Recreation Society. Dr. Carter has been awarded the Honor Award, Outstanding Achievement Award, and the Merit Service Award from AALR and the Distinguished Professional Award and the Professional of the Year Award from NTRS. Dr. Carter has been employed in mid-management positions with private and public agencies providing therapeutic recreation services. She has supervised interns, part-time staff, therapeutic recreation specialists and volunteers. Dr. Carter has held positions as undergraduate and graduate recreation and therapeutic recreation program director in higher education. Her presentations and publications have been in the areas of credentialing, programming, community therapeutic recreation services, aging, professional development, and foundations of therapeutic recreation.

# Other Books from Venture Publishing

*The A•B•Cs of Behavior Change: Skills for Working with Behavior Problems in Nursing Homes*
    by Margaret D. Cohn, Michael A. Smyer and Ann L. Horgas

*Activity Experiences and Programming Within Long-Term Care*
    by Ted Tedrick and Elaine R. Green

*The Activity Gourmet*
    by Peggy Powers

*Advanced Concepts for Geriatric Nursing Assistants*
    by Carolyn A. McDonald

*Adventure Education*
    edited by John C. Miles and Simon Priest

*Aerobics of the Mind: Keeping the Mind Active in Aging—A New Perspective on Programming for Older Adults*
    by Marge Engelman

*Assessment: The Cornerstone of Activity Programs*
    by Ruth Perschbacher

*Behavior Modification in Therapeutic Recreation: An Introductory Learning Manual*
    by John Datillo and William D. Murphy

*Benefits of Leisure*
    edited by B. L. Driver, Perry J. Brown and George L. Peterson

*Benefits of Recreation Research Update*
    by Judy M. Sefton and W. Kerry Mummery

*Beyond Bingo: Innovative Programs for the New Senior*
    by Sal Arrigo, Jr., Ann Lewis and Hank Mattimore

*Both Gains and Gaps: Feminist Perspectives on Women's Leisure*
    by Karla Henderson, M. Deborah Bialeschki, Susan M. Shaw and Valeria J. Freysinger

*The Community Tourism Industry Imperative—The Necessity, the Opportunities, its Potential*
    by Uel Blank

*Dimensions of Choice: A Qualitative Approach to Recreation, Parks, and Leisure Research*
    by Karla A. Henderson

*Evaluating Leisure Services: Making Enlightened Decisions*
    by Karla A. Henderson with M. Deborah Bialeschki

*The Evolution of Leisure: Historical and Philosophical Perspectives (Second Printing)*
    by Thomas Goodale and Geoffrey Godbey

*File o' Fun: A Recreation Planner for Games & Activities—Third Edition*
    by Jane Harris Ericson and Diane Ruth Albright

*The Game Finder—A Leader's Guide to Great Activities*
    by Annette C. Moore

*Getting People Involved in Life and Activities: Effective Motivating Techniques*
    by Jeanne Adams

*Great Special Events and Activities*
    by Annie Morton, Angie Prosser and Sue Spangler

*Inclusive Leisure Services: Responding to the Rights of People with Disabilities*
    by John Dattilo

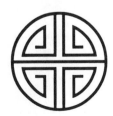

Venture Publishing, Inc.
1999 Cato Avenue
State College, PA 16801

Phone: (814) 234-4561; FAX: (814) 234-1651

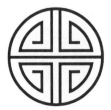